From Nursing Assistant
to Patient Care Technician

From Nursing Assistant to Patient Care Technician:

New Roles, New Knowledge, New Skills

Donna J. Brust, MS, RN,C
Staff Development Specialist
Educational Development and Resources
The Ohio State University Medical Center
Columbus, Ohio

Joyce A. Foster, MS, RN,C
Staff Development Specialist
Educational Development and Resources
The Ohio State University Medical Center
Columbus, Ohio

W.B. SAUNDERS COMPANY
A *Harcourt Health Sciences Company*
Philadelphia London New York St. Louis Sydney Toronto

W.B. SAUNDERS COMPANY
A *Harcourt Health Sciences Company*

The Curtis Center
Independence Square West
Philadelphia, Pennsylvania 19106

Library of Congress Cataloging–in–Publication Data

From nursing assistant to patient care technician : new roles, new knowledge, new skills / [edited by] Donna J. Brust, Joyce A. Foster.

p.   cm.

Includes index.

ISBN 0–7216–6046–0

1. Nurses' aides.   I. Brust, Donna J.   II. Foster, Joyce A.   [DNLM:
    1. Nurses' Aides.   2. Nursing Care.   WY 193 F931 1997]

RT84.F76   1997

610.73′069′8—dc20

DNLM/DLC   96–28910

FROM NURSING ASSISTANT TO PATIENT CARE TECHNICIAN:
NEW ROLES, NEW KNOWLEDGE, NEW SKILLS   ISBN 0–7216–6046–0

Printed in the United States of America.

Last digit is the print number: 9   8   7   6

Dedicated to:

Our families, who loved and encouraged us through the process.

Joyce's grandmother, Elsa Anderson, who knew she made a difference to her patients (retired as a Nursing Assistant at the age of 72).

The nurses, patient care associates, and other members of the health care team at The Ohio State University Medical Center, who struggle daily to find the way, to do it all, to do it right, and to provide "Intensive Caring" to patients and their families and to one another.

Joyce A. Becker, MS, RN,C

Instructor and Clinical Systems Consultant, Medica Logic, Inc., Beaverton, Oregon. Formerly Education Coordinator I, Mount Carmel Health System, Columbus, Ohio

Computerization of Health Care

Susan M. Bejciy-Spring, MS, RN,C

Clinical Associate, The Ohio State University College of Nursing; Clinical Associate, Division of Nursing, The Ohio State University Medical Center, Columbus, Ohio

The Endocrine System

Loretta Piombo Benton, MS, RN

Instructor, College of Nursing, Department of Maternal-Child Nursing, Rush University; Assistant to the Director, Nursing Professional Development, Rush-Presbyterian-St. Luke's Medical Center, Chicago, Illinois

Venipuncture and Point of Care Testing

Karen Boliek, MS, RN

Education Specialist, Suburban Hospital, Bethesda, Maryland

Assisting with Sterile Procedures

Donna J. Brust, MS, RN,C

Staff Development Specialist, Educational Development and Resources, The Ohio State University Medical Center, Columbus, Ohio

The Integumentary System

Michelle M. Budzinski-Braunscheidel, BSN, RN,C

Manager in Patient Access Services, The Cleveland Clinic Foundation, Cleveland, Ohio

The Renal Urinary System

Janice M. Crabill, MSN, RN

Professional Development Coordinator, Mercy Medical Center, Baltimore, Maryland

Organizing Your Work Assignment

Claire R. Esselman, EdD, RN,C

Instructor, Corporate Education, Tri Health— A Community Partnership of Bethesda Hospital and Good Samaritan Hospital, Cincinnati, Ohio

The Gastrointestinal System

Mara Ferris, MS, RN,C, CS, CRRN

Staff Development Instructor, Spaulding Rehabilitation Hospital, Boston, Massachusetts

The Nervous System

Anne Findeis, MS, RN

Clinical Instructor, University of Illinois at Chicago College of Nursing, Chicago, Illinois

Basic Concepts

Kathleen J. Fischer, MA, RN,C, CNA

Director of Educational Services for Nursing, University of Michigan Health System, Ann Arbor, Michigan

Leadership, Teamwork, and the Role of the Patient Care Technician

Joyce A. Foster, MS, RN,C

Staff Development Specialist, Educational Development and Resources, The Ohio State University Medical Center, Columbus, Ohio

Changing World—Changing Work: Thriving in the New World of Work

Susan Jenkins Galloway, BA, BS

LCDR, Nurse Corps, U.S. Navy, Graduate Student in Nursing Education, DePaul University, Chicago, Illinois

The Cardiovascular System

Linda Terry Godson, MA, BSN

Adjunct Faculty, University of Northern Iowa, Cedar Falls; Education Facilitator, Covenant Medical Center, Waterloo, Iowa

Self-Concept, Body Image, and Sexuality in Health Care

Esther E. Jones, MS, RN

Rush University College of Nursing, Chicago; Assistant to Director, Nursing Professional Development, Rush-Presbyterian-St. Luke's Medical Center, Chicago, Illinois

Venipuncture and Point of Care Testing

Jean A. Just, MSN, RN,C, CS

Staff Development Specialist, The Ohio State University Medical Center, Columbus, Ohio

Interpersonal Relationships and Communication

Shirley Fields McCoy, MS, RN,C

Adjunct Faculty Instructor, The Ohio State University College of Nursing; Staff Development Specialist, Department of Educational Development and Resources, The Ohio State University Medical Center, Columbus, Ohio

The Respiratory System

Juanita J. McDonough, MN, RN,C, CCRN

Clinical Nurse Educator, University Medical Center, Tucson, Arizona

Electrocardiogram

Laurie Miller, MS, RN, CS, CRRN, ANP

Rehabilitation Clinical Nurse Specialist, Massachusetts General Hospital, Boston, Massachusetts

The Nervous System

Dorothy H. Mundy, MN, RN, BSN

Professional Development Coordinator, Mercy Medical Center, Baltimore, Maryland

Organizing Your Work Assignment

Nancy R. Nelson, MS, BSN, RN,C

Nursing Instructor, Sierra College, Rocklin; Hospital Educator, Mercy Healthcare Sacramento, Sacramento, California

The Musculoskeletal System

Mildred Perlia, MSN, RN

Assistant Professor, Rush University, College of Nursing; Director, Nursing Professional Development, Rush-Presbyterian-St. Luke's Medical Center, Chicago, Illinois

Venipuncture and Point of Care Testing

Catherine Ricciuti, MS, RN, CCRN

Educational Nurse Specialist, University of Michigan Health System, Ann Arbor, Michigan

Leadership, Teamwork, and the Role of the Patient Care Technician

Ella Schulz, BSN, RN

Program Manager, The Ohio State University Medical Center, Columbus, Ohio

Emergency Care

Sherry Speer, BA, CHUC

Manager, Patient Management Services, Grant Medical Center, Columbus, Ohio

Clerical Skills

Shelley Uncapher, BSEd, BS, BA, CHUC

Staff Training and Development Coordinator, The Ohio State University Medical Center, Columbus, Ohio

Clerical Skills

Sandra L. Walden, MS, RN,C

Staff Development Specialist, The Ohio State University Medical Center, Columbus, Ohio

Emergency Care

Francie Wolgin, MSN, RN, CNA

Director, Operations Support and Practice Development, St. Joseph Mercy Hospital, Ann Arbor, Michigan

Challenges of the Cancer Patient

Economic forces are driving organizations to cut costs, improve quality, and increase customer satisfaction in order to survive in health care businesses. One strategy seen across the nation is to increase use of ancillary caregivers to assist registered nurses. This assistance is most beneficial when the participant is well prepared with a strong knowledge base related to patient care and safe clinical skills that reduce the RN's workload. Nurses want to know that the person they delegate to is responsible, accountable, and knows the important aspects of care that need to be reported. While this kind of multiskilled partner is in demand, the education materials with which to train these persons in today's health care environment have not been available.

This text, *From Nursing Assistant to Patient Care Technician: New Roles, New Knowledge, New Skills*, includes information about a variety of new skills that are most frequently included in the Patient Care Technician role. The person who fills this position, when taught the responsibilities and limitations of the role, can be a true multiskilled partner to the registered nurse. This text will reinforce the value and the necessity of guidance, delegation, communication, teaching, and direction provided by RNs.

Being a multiskilled worker does not mean just being able to do new tasks that previously were performed by others. It has to do with a new mindset—a new way for people to look at themselves and how they work with others. Part of the change includes gaining new information about the rapidly changing world of work and new skills to work effectively in it (Chapter 1). Skills help people thrive, not just survive! They include being able to quickly respond to a changing work setting and being comfortable dealing with uncertainty. They involve personal empowerment and performing your job as though you were in business for yourself and caring for patients as though they were your own family. Skills involve focusing care on patient needs and developing an attitude of customer service. Personal accountability, teamwork, and leadership are crucial to success, and practical information to assist caregivers with this is presented in Chapter 2. Chapter 3 focuses on basic concepts such as the nursing process, stress response, dealing with infection, and supplying nourishment and hydration. It also presents basic care procedures for surgical patients, patients undergoing diagnostic examinations, and processes to decrease pain and provide comfort. Because the work setting usually involves interaction with others, communication skills and tips to working effectively with others are given in Chapter 4.

The emphasis also is on working with new technology, and performing technical skills safely and effectively. Background information about body systems will help the learner understand why particular skills are performed, as well as how to adjust care to meet individual client needs. Chapters 5 to 12 each cover a different body system.

Throughout this text, the importance of coordinating care with other staff and departments as well as documentation of all care performed is stressed. Background information for safe practice is presented for all areas.

We believe that one of the keys to the effectiveness of this text are the icons found throughout all of the chapters for emphasis. The icons represent key aspects of performance. These icons highlight important messages within the text and signal crucial areas needing follow-up. They are:

In recent surveys, nurses indicated that they value advanced assistants who alert them when something is wrong with the patient. Therefore, the Megaphone icon indicates crucial elements or observations that need to be reported to the RN.

The practice of nursing and delegation to unlicensed caregivers are being closely monitored by many governing bodies. It is important that advanced assistants stay within the appropriate scope of practice. The "Scale of Justice" signals legal issues or awareness for boundaries of practice.

This icon alerts the reader to issues of safety for patients and staff that relate to the topic being addressed. Generally it signals unsafe intervention.

This icon indicates situations that need closer observation, more observation, or additional consultation. This additional information helps the PCT and ultimately the RN to assess progress and determine treatment.

This icon alerts PCTs when additional information and consultation can be obtained to help them deliver quality care. Resources such as clinical nurse specialists, educators, managers, and other members of the interdisciplinary team are often cited.

Suggested documentation appropriate for each skill or topic is signaled by this icon.

Individuals presently employed in health care settings may find the book very helpful in gaining new knowledge and preparing themselves to take on an expanded role where they work. Primarily, the text is suggested for use by those in hospitals and acute care facilities, community colleges, community vocational and technical school programs, as well as proprietary schools. Officials of Licensed Practical Nurse programs, nursing schools that also teach assistive caregivers, and other community agencies may find the book very valuable in their educational programs. Each chapter can stand alone and be taught separately, in a way that meets a variety of organizational needs. Chapters can also be used as part of an organized orientation/training program or individually, as inservice education. The Instructor's Guide, prepared by the authors and available from the publisher, contains a content outline, teaching strategies, worksheets, and review questions suitable for tests or quizzes. Registered nurses should always be providing the instruction.

We set a high priority on staying within the boundaries of Nursing State Board approved practice for unlicensed caregivers. We have provided basic practice guidelines. These guidelines support the Tri-Council for Nursing, *Statement on Assistive Personnel to the Registered Nurse*, Appendix 1, which states, "It is further incumbent on the nursing profession to define the appropriate educational preparation and role of any group providing services within the scope of nursing practice. The State Board of Nursing is responsible for the regulation of any other category of personnel who assist in the provision of direct nursing care. Professional and statutory provisions require that when the RN delegates and assigns direct nursing care activities to LPNs and assistive personnel, appropriate reporting relations are established and the RN supervises all personnel to whom these activities have been delegated." Practice guidelines identified in this text are general guidelines and readers are reminded to follow Nursing State Board practice guidelines determined in your own state.

Donna J. Brust
Joyce A. Foster

ACKNOWLEDGMENTS

We would like to thank Mary Simpson and Natalie Wittman, our supervisors, who knew we could do it and supported the process. Our co-workers, who supported us all the way, and especially, Jean Just, Shirley McCoy, Shelley Uncapher, Sandy Walden, Ella Schultz, and Susan Bejciy-Spring, who agreed to participate and be contributing authors in spite of the timing, just as we were beginning reengineering at the Medical Center. We also thank Shirley Alltop, Linda Biller, Cecilia Casey Boyer, Susan Evans, Nancy Franke, Betsy Heximer, Barb Montgomery, Theresa Slybe, Donna Smolen, and Lisa Troesch, all nursing specialists who provided valuable advice and assistance. Jim Brown, photographer for The Ohio State University Medical Center, was most helpful in adjusting to changing schedules and needs. His professionalism and suggestions are certainly appreciated.

We would especially like to thank all our contributing authors from around the country who were excited by the idea and anxious to be a part of the process. They provided creative ideas regarding the entire book, as well as their efforts in developing chapters that are interesting, complete, and relevant to current practice. Their enthusiasm kept us going when pressures mounted.

Lisa Biello, Vice President and Editor-in-Chief for Health-Related Professions, was our initial contact with W. B. Saunders Company. What a joy! We really believed that this project was possible after talking with her. She provided vision, excitement, and concrete ideas to get us started. Scott Weaver, our Developmental Editor at Saunders, was our rock throughout the entire process, taking us step by step and at the same time setting deadlines and keeping us to them. We thank them both very much.

CONTENTS

UNIT 3

PATIENT CARE TECHNICIAN ROLE IN BODY SYSTEM DISORDERS

UNIT 4

SPECIAL HEALTH CARE SITUATIONS

UNIT 5

CROSS-TRAINING OPTIONS FOR THE MULTISKILLED PARTNER

Mildred Perlia, MSN, RN, Esther E. Jones, MS, RN,
and Loretta Piombo Benton, MS, RN

Working Effectively with Other Staff

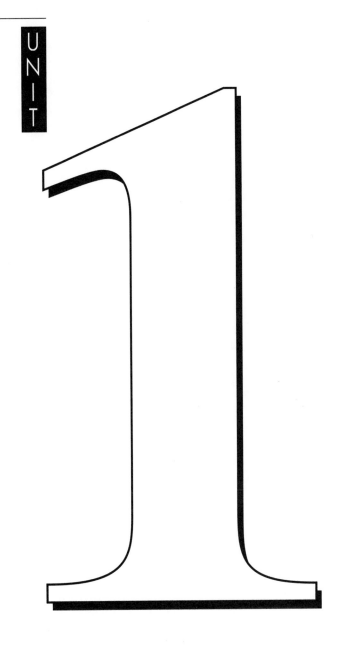

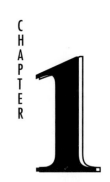

Changing World— Changing Work: Thriving in the New World of Work

JOYCE A. FOSTER, MS, RN,C

OUTLINE

PREREQUISITE KNOWLEDGE AND SKILLS

- Prior experience as a direct caregiver in a health care setting

OBJECTIVES

After you complete this chapter, you will be able to:

- Identify three historically significant technological changes that have affected the present work environment.

- Discuss how social and technological changes have affected consumers' expectations about their health care.

- Describe the impact of government health care programs and insurance companies on health care services.

- Identify at least three changes health care organizations have made in response to consumer pressures and changing payment for services.

- Discuss career and interpersonal skills required to thrive in a rapidly changing world of work.

- List specific strategies to provide customer service.

KEY TERMS

Customer Service Making all efforts to know your customers and being able to predict what they might need. In addition, it includes having the desire, and making all possible efforts, to meet your customers' needs promptly, accurately, and with a smile.

Patient Care Technician   This is an unlicensed patient care role. The role builds on the basic skills of a nursing assistant. It is often referred to as an advanced nursing assistant role. The role involves providing basic personal care to patients. Additional skills that also are included frequently within the scope of practice include performing 12-lead ECGs, assisting nurses with sterile procedures, performing simple dressing changes, drawing blood for laboratory tests, bedside testing of specimens, and clerical skills to enable the patient care technician to take the place of the unit clerk at the desk as needed.

Patient-Focused Care   A process of patient care delivery that focuses on the needs of the patient rather than the needs of the hospital. It usually involves:

- Designing services to come to the patient instead of bringing the patient to the service
- More flexible scheduling options for tests or services
- Encouraging all levels of staff to make on-the-spot decisions when necessary to benefit the patient
- Streamlining services to the patient to decrease the number of different staff who provide care, ask questions, or request information from the patient

Reengineering   The process of reorganizing and redesigning how an organization operates. In recent use, it has come to mean decreasing layers of management; bringing decisions down closer to the people who do the work; having fewer specialized departments and more multiskilled workers; emphasis on teamwork; and meeting needs of customers.

Scope of the Practice   The skills, duties, and range of responsibilities that are included in each job description. State nurse practice acts (laws) usually identify which skills must be performed only by professionals. This is the guide that hospitals use when deciding the skills to include in each job description written for unlicensed personnel.

OVERVIEW

Impact of Technology on Work

In the 1920s and 1930s, the internal combustion engine, powered by gasoline, began to change the way we lived and worked. Suddenly people could travel longer distances for work and recreation. Goods could be transported faster and more economically. Manufacturing began to replace farming and agriculture as a major form of employment and strength of the economy. Businesses began to manufacture new goods to support the expanding economy. Large businesses developed, and for the first time more people were employed by others outside the home than were self-employed in farming or other activities.

In the 1950s, '60s, and '70s the advent of television dramatically changed the lives of most Americans. Large numbers of people were exposed to new ideas, new cultures, and new consumer goods. This produced a major period of growth. Manufacturing boomed; the auto industry and the travel industry grew. The economy was steadily growing, and people took jobs in companies and expected to "grow with the company." There was emphasis on retirement plans and health care benefits. Insurance companies grew as they marketed health care and life insurance plans to businesses for their employees. Most employees just expected that that was the way it would be. Often several members of one family or several generations of families worked for the same company. They looked to the company for their welfare and their future.

Payment for Health Care Services

During this period, the health care industry also ballooned. Physicians and hospitals were being paid on a "fee-for-service" basis. In other words, they were able to bill and be paid separately for each X-ray, breathing treatment, physician visit, or medication. Physicians were often reimbursed "usual and customary" rates for services, which also contributed to increasing fees. With more and more health care being paid by third-party payors (insurance companies and the government, through Medicare and Medicaid programs), payment was virtually assured.

It was a logical step for the health care industry to grow and increasingly specialize. A number of medical specialties developed as medical research produced new breakthroughs in knowledge. Specialists began consulting with each other on more and more cases, and their services were billed to and paid individually by insurance companies. Hospitals expanded and diversified their departments. Specialized diagnostic and treatment areas such as radiology, respiratory therapy, pharmacy, and laboratories grew. Several new layers of managers, as well as new allied medical specialties, developed. As hospitals grew, more service workers and managers were needed to keep them going.

Computers Change Our Lives

In the 1980s, computers, fueled by an increasingly sophisticated array of software, hit the economy, and since then life has not been the same. With computers, businesses and the government could gather, store, and manipulate information more quickly and more accurately than ever before. The speed, power, and capacity of computers rapidly increased. Not only health care but everything from accounting to personal banking, food service to grocery shopping, and cars to homes was affected by the computer revolution. Very few people escaped the effects of computers on the economy or in their personal lives. In fact, by the 1990s 32 million computers were in homes; businesses linked the majority of their personal computers into networks; and communications via electronic mail, personal pagers, and cellular phones skyrocketed. This massive infusion of computers into the personal and business world has changed how businesses operate, how work is performed, and what jobs are like.

Cost Containment in Health Care

In the mid 1980s, as computerization was changing the world of work, computers were also beginning to change the face of health care. An extensive, nationwide, computerized data collection on health care costs was compiled by the federal government. This data collection examined the costs billed to the Medicare insurance program for the elderly and the Medicaid insurance program for the poor. This computerized picture of health care costs was the beginning of the end in the growth of the inpatient health care industry. Costs were spiraling ever upward, and strong efforts had to be made to stop the upward swing.

The initial changes came in the form of a new means of reimbursement for health care services called diagnostic related groups, or DRGs. In an effort to cut health care costs, the government said it would no longer pay for each service performed; instead, insurance programs would reimburse hospitals a set amount of money based on an average cost for care required for each particular diagnosis. In other words, if a person was admitted to the hospital because of a heart attack, the hospital and the physician would each be paid only a set amount of money. This amount was based on research gathered on what the average costs had been and how long a person usually was hospitalized for the particular diagnosis. This payment system *reinforced fewer separate costs and services* and forced the health care industry to begin looking at its entire way of doing business. DRGs and other similar forms of restricted payment increasingly became the form of reimbursement by insurance companies. The move was to "managed care," and the emphasis was on continuing to cut costs.

Insurance groups found they could "manage care" and control costs by joining with particular hospitals and clinics to form health maintenance organizations (HMOs). These HMOs guaranteed health care services for people who joined, but restricted consumers' use to the services within the HMO. This allowed insurance companies to market their HMOs to large businesses at a lower rate per employee. Hospitals that were left out of the HMOs were forced to adapt to the situation of fewer people with insurance coverage to use their services. Therefore, hospitals had limited survival options, all of which required them to make major changes:

1. They could join with other hospitals and physicians to form large managed care organizations.

2. They could decrease inpatient beds and increase outpatient services such as ambulatory surgery and specialized clinics.

3. They could cut hospital costs in every possible way, while at the same time making the hospital environment pleasant and the services focused on keeping patients comfortable, safe, and well cared for. While doing this, they could build a reputation for excellence so that consumers would demand that the hospital be included in their health plan.

4. They could close their doors.

Many hospitals struggled significantly with the first three choices. Many others, with fewer options, had to close.

Consumerism

At the same time that HMOs were limiting consumer choice in health care, consumer choice in all other areas of their lives was exploding. Customers began demanding more attention to their needs. As a society, people are used to instant everything. There are instant meals: freezer to microwave, or drive-through restaurants where people often think that 2 minutes is too long to wait for their food order. There is instant access to money with money machines and access to banks or credit card loans worldwide. Prescription eyeglasses can be made in an hour. There continues to be an unending array of goods and services with many options for personal preference. Everywhere there are companies that cater to time-conscious people. Consequently people have begun to expect that same quickness in all services.

Consumers are continuously exposed to both accurate and inaccurate information on medical topics through the media, families, and friends. This colors their views and expectations regarding their own health care. That may result in unrealistic expectations or fears. It can also result in a well-informed consumer who holds the health care system and workers to a high standard of care. When all goes well with the hospital experience, consumers are happy with the outcome. However, if they have been treated poorly or something they see as negative has happened during their hospitalization, they are quick to judge the health care agency and talk to all their family and friends about how "bad" their care or treatment was. One bad experience with their care or with a staff person may influence their view of the entire hospitalization.

Many who believe that something went wrong with their treatment will use the legal system in an attempt to get monetary awards. Lawyers advertise that they are ready to back people in demanding that their "rights" be served. The cost of preparing for possible legal recourse with every person treated adds significantly to the health care system.

Survival Skills in the Rapidly Changing World of Work

With computerization, rapid electronic communication, pressures for cost containment, managed health care and the change to a consumer-oriented economy, hospitals and health care organizations are rapidly and continuously changing. They must change to survive as well as to respond to ever-changing societal and economic demands.

Mary O'Hara-Devereaux and Robert Johansen in their text *Global Work: Bridging Distance, Culture and Time*, identify the following statistics that shed some light on the direction that the changing work place is taking.

- In 1991, nearly 1 of 3 American workers had been with his or her employer for less than a year, and almost 2 of 3 for less than 3 years.

- In the United States the number of temporary workers, consisting of roughly 45,000,000 self-employed, part-time workers, or consultants, has grown 57% since 1980.

- Going, if not yet gone, are 9–5 workdays; lifetime jobs; predictable, hierarchical relationships; and the perception that "the company will take care of you."

- Constant training, retraining, job-hopping, and even career-hopping are becoming the norm.

The Move to Patient-Focused Care

The issue of consumerism, or focus on meeting customers' needs, led to the examination of all health care delivery systems. What happens to patients when they come to the hospital? What do patients want to happen? Surveys found that in large hospitals 50–60 different people had contact with a patient in an average 3–4-day hospitalization! No wonder patients were often frustrated. They had to tell their story over and over to many different people, which often made them believe that staff members did not talk to one another. Patients never knew who would be in next to care for them. There were separate staff to provide personal care, draw their blood for laboratory work, do an ECG, take them to tests, bring them their lunch, get them clean linen, empty waste baskets, and restock supplies in their room. Conversely, because each staff person was doing the same job over and over for lots of different people, they never really got to know patients or had the feeling of satisfaction that comes from seeing people get better and go home, and knowing they had something to do about making it happen.

Patient surveys have shown that patients want to feel safe, to feel secure that their problems will be taken care of, and that they will be treated like individuals and not a part on an assembly line. They want to know that there is a plan for their hospital stay and that the people taking care of them know what the plan is and will work together to bring it to a successful outcome. They want information about what will happen to them and what they can expect. If a portion of the plan is delayed, they want to know why and what it means for them.

Patients recognize staff who make extra efforts to relate to them as people or who provide some extra service that makes a real difference to how they feel. Patients recognize staff for the human touches they bring to a difficult environment as well as for their expertise in the tasks they perform. Think about the last time you were injured, ill, or in an uncomfortable situation: What "extra efforts" made you feel better about your situation? How did you feel about the person who made the extra effort?

Patient-Focused Care

Providing patient-centered or patient-focused care has been the health care industries' response to the expanding impact of consumer interest, involvement, and demand for hospital care and health care services that meet their needs. The main goal of patient-focused care is to have only a few key staff coming in contact with patients, and to have them feel more ownership of patients' welfare and recovery than occurs in the more fragmented care delivery systems.

It involves bringing more services to patients than bringing patients to services. For example, in patient-focused care, patients often are admitted directly to the unit, and the entire admissions process occurs in their room. Patient-focused care encourages more flexibility in scheduling to meet patient/family needs. Instead of all processes and care provided for the convenience of hospital operations and staff scheduling, more attention is paid to meet the lifestyle and scheduling needs of patients. Patient-focused care also empowers all levels of staff to make decisions and choices on the spot to benefit the patient.

To implement this new care delivery system, hospitals have had to turn their systems upside down. The process has been referred to as reengineering and has swept the United States from coast to coast. Most hospitals are accomplishing this reengineering process by:

- Removing several layers of middle management to bring decisions closer to the patient.

- Closing or cutting back sharply on specialized departments or caregivers such as transportation, housekeeping, dietary, supplies delivery, ECG technicians, IV and transfusion teams, and phlebotomists (laboratory staff who go to patients and draw blood for tests). Physicians and RNs are also being expected to be less specialized and to function more as generalists in their practice.

- Organizing all care delivery into a team, with fewer job classifications: the RN, LPN, Patient Care Technicians and often a Patient Service Associate.

- Redefining roles and relationships.
  a. An RN who plans, coordinates, and evaluates all patient care and delivers professional aspects of care. The RN does the initial assessment of the patient and the patient's family situation and identifies a plan of care to meet needs. The RN coordinates care with the physician and other health care team members and delegates aspects of care to other team members based on their job description. The RN continuously evaluates patient progress and changes the care plan to meet changing needs. The RN also provides guidance to other team members about special needs for patients receiving particular medications, surgical interventions, treatments, diagnostic testing, or special emotional support or needs.
  b. The second staff member who is usually part of the team is an advanced caregiver. This text refers to that role as a Patient Care Technician (PCT). In practice the role may be referred to as a Patient Care Associate, Patient Care Assistant, or other similar title. The role fits under the generic term *Unlicensed Assistive Caregiver*, as defined by the American Nurses Association. The PCT often provides most of the personal care to the patient, observing for patient behaviors or changes that need to be reported to the RN and helping with essential, accurate measurements and documentation that aid

in determining treatment as well as assisting in tracking patient progress. The PCT also provides a variety of other services, including drawing blood for laboratory testing, providing simple dressing changes and assisting the RN with more complicated dressings, and performing limited bedside specimen testing. In addition, PCTs often perform 12-lead ECGs. They work closely with the service worker in setting up, delivering, and monitoring diet trays and transporting patients to and from tests or procedures. The PCT also may handle duties at the patient care station, such as answering phones and coordinating paperwork and communication to and from the unit. This PCT role is very demanding, but it is a role that provides much personal satisfaction. Because of the increasing importance of the role of the multiskilled worker on the health care team, this text has been developed to assist staff build on their prior patient care training and to learn additional personal and patient care skills.
  c. The third member of the team is frequently a service worker, often referred to as a Patient Service Associate (PSA). This staff person focuses on all aspects of the surroundings to ensure that supplies are available to provide care, the environment is clean and pleasant for the patient, and that rooms are promptly cleaned and prepared for a new admission. This worker also helps the PCT with basic patient care, assists with dietary needs, and transports patients when they have to go to other areas of the hospital.

- Encouraging staff in hospital departments that have closed or decreased in number to apply for one of the new positions on the team and to commit to learning new skills and duties. It involves tremendous responsibilities for education, retraining, cross-training, and helping staff understand and practice teamwork and customer service.

- Emphasizing teamwork and deemphasizing maintenance of a hierarchy with the manager giving orders. In some cases, self-managed work teams have been implemented (see Chapter 2). The focus is doing what has to be done efficiently and quickly, no matter whose job it really is. The rule, "never pass off what you can do yourself if it is quicker and more efficient," goes for all levels of staff. If the RN is in the room and the patient needs to get up to the commode, the RN would help the patient up. Someone who saw a water spill on the floor should get a paper towel and wipe it up, not call a service worker. It is not acceptable to say, Wait until so-and-so gets back, that's his or her job. Patient-focused care works best when team members trust and respect one another and do not impose unnecessary hierarchical standards.

The reengineering process is not without its struggles, however. Problems that at any time may turn out to be barriers to success occur at all levels of the organization. Following are some typical examples.

ORGANIZATIONAL ISSUES

- Struggling to cut costs and positions and realign departments and roles while maintaining a caring environment for staff and patients.
- Balancing the speed of the change with the ability of the organization to cope.
- Investing the time, money, and staff to adequately train, retrain, and educate all staff about the changes.

RN ISSUES

- Having to give up performing some direct patient care activities that often gave them the most rewards in their jobs.
- Fear that the new worker may not do things right and that patients will not get the care they need.
- Feeling legally responsible as a licensed professional while delegating tasks to newly trained caregivers.

⚖ Tasks that can be delegated to unlicensed personnel must be clearly identified in organizational position descriptions. They must be consistent with guidelines set forth by state licensing laws.

PATIENT CARE TECHNICIANS/PATIENT SERVICE ASSOCIATES ISSUES

- Resentment about having to give up a job they know how to do for a new one they are not sure about.
- Concern about their ability to successfully complete the course work and clinical skills required in the new training program. Not wanting to feel "dumb" or to embarrass themselves in front of others.
- Having to practice newly learned skills on a unit at the same time as several others and not having adequate time or support to learn.

🎓 Staff having difficulty getting support to learn new skills on the unit should contact their nurse-manager, Clinical Nurse Specialist (CNS), unit educator, or Staff Development Specialist (SDS) for further ideas or assistance.

These are realistic problems and concerns, ones that most organizations make an effort to address. It takes time to truly adopt the new role. There is a lot of information to

learn in a short time, and much of it takes clinical experience to master. When starting out in the new role, PCTs will not be feeling their most confident and at the same time the RNs may resent having to delegate to them. Delegation, assigning someone to do a job that one might do oneself, takes trust, and trust takes time to develop. Open communication is key, and understanding the struggles that each person may be going through is very important. It all takes time, planning, patience, and a sense of humor!

There usually are classes to help all staff on a new unit understand the pressures and issues and learn how to best work together to build trusting relationships. A patient-focused care delivery system is structured and its goal is to provide strong customer service and support. Part of that support is to help staff work together effectively.

Survival Skills for the Patient Care Technician

Survival skills include having a strong knowledge base to do the job well: gain or maintain technical competence with up-to-date skills and equipment; develop and use interpersonal skills to work effectively with others. Workers must be able to quickly respond to a changing work setting and be comfortable dealing with uncertainty. Staff must take responsibility for their own morale and seek out ways to feel competent and empowered while performing their jobs as though they were in business for themselves. In health care settings, a key to job survival is working toward customer satisfaction by caring for patients as though they were your own family.

Rapidly changing organizations are seeking workers who can respond readily to change. Resistance to change and an attitude of "it's not my problem" are dead-end roads in the current world of work. Employees must be prepared to change their roles, learn new job skills, deal with flexible work hours and see any change as a new opportunity. In fact, invite change! If there are processes or procedures that are not working well, do not just blame others or complain; offer suggestions on how things could work differently and then help to make the change. Take personal responsibility for responding to change. Treat your present job just as you would if you had accepted a new job with a new employer. Be enthusiastic, open, work hard, and be part of the team. "If the organization decides to turn on a dime, follow it like a trailer!"*

Organizations also need people who are committed to what they do, who work from the heart, and who invest themselves in their jobs. Whatever job you are doing, invest yourself in it. Make it personal. Put your own stamp of pride on any job you have. Organizations are looking for people who identify ways to do their job better, to be more efficient or more responsive. There is no

*Price Pritchett, New Work Habits for a Radically Changing World. Dallas, Pritchett & Associates, Inc., p. 11.

longer room for people who only go through the motions of their job, people who confuse longevity of employment with value to the organization, or people who equate activity with accomplishment. Organizations understand that consumers will no longer tolerate inattention to their needs. From a personal standpoint, commitment makes a job more interesting and satisfying. It feels good to do a job to which you have committed, that brings out your best, and that helps you and your employer. "The bottom line: Commitment is a gift you should give to yourself."* Committed employees are valued employees.

Lifelong Learning

Continue to learn. Lifelong learning is the only option in the rapidly changing world of work. A basic hospital aide or patient care course might have been the first step in learning about health care. You may have taken others. Whether this book is being read for personal development, as part of a training program, as an assignment for a course, or as portions for an inservice course, the text is only another step in the learning process. Continue to read, attend other classes, learn from coworkers, and learn about new equipment and new procedures. Learn as much as possible about your job and the jobs of others. Be prepared to step in and assist in someone's absence. Prepare yourself for other opportunities with your present employer or with others. Keep your skills current and yourself marketable. Do not hold on to the false notion that your employer owes you a job or is responsible for your learning or for your future. The future is now, and it is up to you to create it. Knowing customers and their needs and continually learning to meet them more effectively are the keys to success in today's work place.

Know Your Customers

Who are the organization's customers? Are they patients and families who rely on staff for kind, personal, knowledgeable, and safe care? Are they coworkers who look to you for fast, friendly, focused, and flexible service and who rely on staff to do their job well so that they can do theirs? Job security depends on knowing who your customers are, knowing their needs, and knowing how you can help them be successful. What are patients' fears, expectations, goals? What do they want to be the end result of their experience with the organization? What outcomes are the medical and nursing staffs working toward? What goals or outcomes does the organization want to achieve? Help all your customers work toward their goals. Assume responsibility for helping them reach their goals. If your customers are successful, your organization will be successful. If your reputation is that of a team player, a helper, a supporter of success, you also

will be successful and valuable as an employee (see Chapter 2).

Making Customer Satisfaction a Priority

"Customers don't care what you know, until they know that you care."*

Customer service is everyone's job. The goal of customer service is meeting customers' expectations and satisfying their needs. Strategies to provide customer service are defined by the organization. It has a plan and expects staff to follow the plan. The goal of strong customer service programs is to have staff know what their customers need or want and to offer it without being asked. It is making people feel secure, safe, and comfortable with their choice to come to your hospital. It is letting customers know that if something happens, staff know how to take care of it. It means listening to what people say and thinking beyond the words to recognize what they might really want or need. Are they scared? Do they need more information? Do they want someone to care for them, but cannot really ask? Learning how to understand, to help, and to work with people and *wanting* to provide top-notch customer service will guarantee you success with your job. Actually making it work and having highly *satisfied customers* should be the outcome!

Have you ever heard a staff member say, "I did everything for that patient, and he is still complaining. Some people are never satisfied." That staff member may have provided excellent service, but it may not have been what the particular patient really needed or wanted; therefore he was not satisfied. This is an example that just providing good service is not enough. Finding out what the individual really needs or wants and providing it leads to customer satisfaction. Customer service is defined by the organization; customer satisfaction is defined by the customer.

Customers with whom you interact do not care how many other patients you have, or what other things you have to do, or that someone called in sick and you are working short, or that you did not get the raise you thought you deserved, or any other personal issues you are dealing with. To them, their needs are most important. They are paying money to be there, and they expect to have their needs met. To them, you are "the company." The company hired you, and therefore if you cannot, or do not, do your job well and attempt to meet customers' needs, it means the company does not care. After all, look whom they hired!

The health care market is very competitive, and if patients are not satisfied with their care or with the way they are treated, they will go to another physician or another hospital. The realities of the present health care environment are that all needs cannot be met at the same

*Price Pritchett, *New Work Habits for a Radically Changing World.* Dallas, Pritchett & Associates, Inc., p. 7.

Digital Equipment Corp., Customer Service Dept., Maynard, MA.

time. Most people know if you are trying, if you care about what you are doing and about them. Often it is the uncertainty about time that is most upsetting to people. Keeping people informed helps most people to be understanding.

 Give people a realistic estimate of time. Have a good reason for the time schedule. Keep to the schedule and let people know that you have not forgotten them. Involve other staff or get more information, if necessary, to meet realistic expectations.

Keep in mind that patients are the reason you are here. Patients are not the enemy, they are not a bother, they are not an interruption—they *are* the job. Looking at your job in this way helps you to focus on patients' needs and to keep the pressures of your job in perspective.

The patient's family and friends who come to visit and support their loved one also are customers. They are constantly alert to the manner and timeliness in which information and care are delivered. They want to see that the organization and staff are competent, concerned, and sensitive to their loved one's needs.

Physicians also are customers. Patients shop for physicians, and physicians choose hospitals that they trust will provide safe, courteous, efficient, economical care to their patients. If their patients are not treated well, or if adequate services are not available, they can choose to take their patients to another hospital.

A fourth group of customers consists of coworkers. They rely on you to fulfill your responsibilities, communicate effectively and promptly, respect their needs and expectations of their roles, and function as an effective team member. Working together improves care to all customers!

Leebov and Scott (Fig. 1–1) have identified 16 house rules that specify key behaviors and attitudes that support quality customer service in health care settings. We have identified a few specific examples under each house rule.

- **Break the ice.** Make eye contact, smile, say hello, introduce yourself, call people by name, and extend a few words of concern. When possible, generate conversation by asking about their family, pets, work or hobbies.

 Introduce yourself to each new patient or staff member. Welcome him or her.

- **Notice when someone looks confused.** Stop and lend a hand. Give information; take persons where they need to go; phone ahead for them. Serve as their advocate in the system. If you pass a person on to someone else who can meet that person's needs, get the staff member's name and assurance that he or she now will be responsible for the guest.

1. Break the ice.
2. Notice when someone looks confused.
3. Take time for courtesy and consideration.
4. Keep people informed.
5. Anticipate needs.
6. Respond quickly.
7. Maintain privacy and confidentiality.
8. Handle with care.
9. Maintain dignity.
10. Take initiative.
11. Treat patients as adults.
12. Listen and act.
13. Help each other.
14. Keep it quiet.
15. Apply telephone skills.
16. Look the part.

F I G U R E 1 – 1

Sixteen house rules that specify key behaviors and attitudes that support quality customer service in health care settings. (Developed by The Einstein Consulting Group, Jenkintown, PA, 1990.)

Assist people to the right location to meet their needs.

- **Take time for courtesy and consideration.** Kind words and polite gestures make people feel special.
  - Recognize family members who come to visit. Help them be comfortable.
  - Compliment a coworker on a job well done.
  - Offer to get a patient a paper or magazine if the patient is well enough to read.
  - Involve patients in any conversation you have in their presence. Continuing or initiating a personal or social conversation with another staff member while caring for a patient, without involving the patient, devalues the patient and is disrespectful.

 Use *please* and *thank you* with every encounter.

- **Keep people informed.** Explain what you are doing and what people can expect. Clarify unit schedules, expected test times, physician visits. People are less anxious when they know what is happening.

Information related to diagnosis, laboratory results, the reason for a particular diagnostic test or operation, and medications should be presented by the physician or nurse. You may reinforce some information they presented or report patient/family questions to them.

- **Anticipate needs.**
  1. Safety
     - Know the "red flags" for the patients you are caring for and patient conditions that must be reported immediately.
     - Review CPR, role in code, recognizing and dealing with shock, and recognition of allergic reactions.
     - Keep bed in low position when not providing care.
     - Keep side rails up as directed.
     - Ensure that the call light is readily available, the phone is easily reachable, emesis basin is available for postoperative patients or the patient with nausea or productive cough, and urinal is available if needed.
     - Anytime you leave a patient's room ask, "Is there anything I can do for you before I leave?"
     - Offer to get a wheelchair for a visitor who appears to be having difficulty walking or is short of breath.

Know signs and symptoms of distress in patients returning from the operating room, invasive procedures, or diagnostic tests.

  2. Pain and comfort
     - Keep linens clean, dry, and wrinkle free.
     - Have an extra blanket available for new postoperative patients.
     - Reposition bedfast patients minimally q 2h. Position limbs for comfort with pillows.
     - Provide a lap blanket for a patient up in the chair or wheelchair.
     - Provide refreshment for family members who have been at the bedside for a long time. Offer information available on possible overnight accommodations in the area if that is necessary.
  3. Hydration
     - Keep water pitchers filled with cold water and readily available at the bedside.
     - Offer fluids every hour to those unable to assist themselves.

- **Respond quickly.** Learn to prioritize patients' needs and get assistance quickly when you need it. Let patients, family, or coworkers know if there will be a delay and about how long the delay might be. Give a reason if feasible. Get back to them when you said you would. When someone is waiting for medications, information or service, a minute seems like an hour.

- **Maintain privacy and confidentiality.** Do not access or pass on information about a patient unless you or the other person needs it to provide care. Knock and announce yourself before entering the room. Ask permission.

Do *not* agree to keep a patient's "secret." A caregiver cannot keep a patient's secret if the information relates to the patient's illness, hospitalization, or care. Caregivers are obligated to report it to the team.

- **Handle with care.** People are often physically and mentally slowed down from medications, illness, and bedrest. Take time to handle them gently when repositioning or assisting them up to a chair. Plan activities to allow periods of rest during care. Recognize that not everyone is comfortable with touch or close contact. Respond to their requests and nonverbal reactions.

- **Maintain dignity.** Give choices when possible.
  - Address the patient as Mr., Mrs., Miss or Ms. unless given permission to use first name.
  - Offer explanations or requests in words the person understands.
  - Show respect for cultural, racial, religious, or other differences. Seek additional resources to consult, translate, or meet special patient needs.
  - Maintain composure and nonverbal reactions when performing tasks such as emptying a bedpan or colostomy bag, assisting with infected wounds, or aiding a vomiting patient.

- **Take initiative.** Do not say, "That's not my job." Rather say, "I'm not sure how to take care of that, but I'll get someone who can."
  - Do not walk past a spill; wipe it up.
  - Use common sense and show common courtesy.
  - If someone needs help, pitch in.
  - In difficult situations, take charge, identify problem-solving options, draw on your training to assist others. Show patients and staff that the organization works as a team!
  - At shift change, when the previous workers are not finished with work, do not criticize—help them.

- **Treat patients as adults.**
  - Patients are not "Honey," "Sweetie," "Dude," or "Kid." Avoid use of baby talk or addressing patients as you would a child.
  - Do not talk to patients through family members who may be present. Address patients directly, allow time for them to answer, and give them as much opportunity to make their own choices and decisions as possible.

- **Listen and act.**
  - *Listen* to what people want and try to give it to them or give a good reason why you cannot.
  - *Listen* to peoples' complaints. Do not be defensive or blame other shifts, staff, departments, or administration. Try to understand why it is a problem to them. Involve others as necessary to *solve* the problem.
  - Never argue with a customer—you may win—then the customer loses and you lose a customer!

- Listen to your RN and follow directions. During stressful times, don't question requests. Involve others as necessary to get the job done. If you have a problem with the request, discuss it with the nurse later.

- **Help each other.** Patient-focused care cannot happen when staff are territorial about their jobs or when they choose to give their assistance. Assist other shifts and other staff as needed. The job is much more fun when team members help each other. Working together builds trusting relationships that are very powerful when emergencies arise or lots of work needs to be done.

- **Keep it quiet.**
  - Avoid conversations outside patient rooms. Use equipment as quietly as possible.
  - Pull patients' doors almost closed. Keep personal and party talk confined to the break room, not to the patient care station. Remember that the sickest patients are usually nearest the central station.
  - Look at your shift routines—are they planned for your convenience or the convenience of your patients?

- **Apply telephone skills.** Follow the telephone skills identified later in Chapters 4 and 19. Be professional, clear, and pleasant. Follow through with requests and take a message if necessary.

Phone message should include date, time, caller, whom the message is for, clear message, follow-up required, phone number to call, and name of person taking the message.

- **Look the part.**
  - Whatever your uniform, make sure it is clean, neat, and well-fitting.
  - Wear your ID tag where it can be seen.

- Maintain personal grooming.
- Have your language and behavior reflect concern and caring.

Taking Care of Yourself!

Working in the often hectic pace of a health care setting can be very stressful. Focusing on meeting other people's needs sometimes can lead to frustration and the feeling, When is it my turn? When is someone going to take care of me? The answer is, *you* need to take care of *you!*

The factor that has the most impact on satisfaction at work or at home is a positive mental attitude. Think of it as having a positive mental view of the world. When a new situation comes up, some people see the problems it will cause, and others see new opportunities. Negative people often are angry at what others have done to them or to someone else. Positive people tend to notice other's accomplishments. In the work environment as in personal life, it is your attitude that makes a difference in building and maintaining positive relationships. Your attitude shows in the way you look, talk to others, stand, and walk into a room. Are you relaxed, open, smile easily, and greet others cheerfully? Are people glad to see you when you walk on the unit, or does nobody notice? Building positive relationships at work goes beyond individuals' personalities. You do not always have to like someone's personality for a good working relationship. Having a positive mental attitude, and separating the person from the work required, make it possible to work with anyone.

This chapter has shown how change has affected the health care delivery system and how people function within it. Is it affecting you? Do you need to change to meet changing expectations?

Do it now; enhance your skills; think success; set in motion positive forces; start today.

The future will be different if you make the present different.

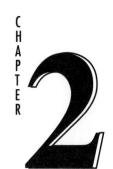

Leadership, Teamwork, and the Role of the Patient Care Technician

KATHLEEN J. FISCHER, MA, RN,C, CNA
CATHERINE RICCIUTI, MS, RN, CCRN

OUTLINE

Leadership

Model of Leadership

Understanding the Hierarchy

Concept of Team

Know Your Competencies/ Limitations: Know Yourself

Delegation Process
Steps of Delegation

Time and Stress Management
Participative Decision Making
Committee Member Questions
Meeting Management Skills

Conflict Management
Handling Conflicts

Living with Change

Opportunities for Personal Growth

PREREQUISITE KNOWLEDGE AND SKILLS

- Good communication skills
- Knowledge of other team member roles
- Knowledge of PCT scope of practice
- Willingness to resolve conflicts

OBJECTIVES

After you complete this chapter, you will be able to:

- Define leadership within your role.
- Describe the hierarchy system in the health care environment.
- Explain the importance of teamwork.
- Identify the importance of competency in delivering quality patient care.
- Explain your role in the delegation process.
- Identify ways to manage time and stressful situations.
- Review the role of the Patient Care Technician within the decision-making process.
- Examine your role in the change process.
- List potential opportunities for personal growth within the role of the patient care technician.

LEADERSHIP

In the past, leadership was considered the prerogative of managers or a very few people in superior positions. It assumed that people at the top of any organization were the leaders, having inherited unique, almost mystical skills. Leaders were viewed with awe by those within an organization and the position of leader as unobtainable. Many times the terms *manager* and *leader* were used interchangeably. Now we realize that leadership is not a position or place, but a process. It includes skills, abilities, and attitude that are useful in any position within an organization. The skills are both observable and learnable. Leadership is often defined in the eyes of the people with whom the leaders work. The myths or beliefs that leadership is for a selected few has been a major barrier to developing personal leadership skills.

Leadership can occur in any aspect of a person's professional or personal life. Patient care technicians (PCTs) can demonstrate leadership in caring for their patients, working with other team members, interacting with staff outside their unit, or assisting their agency in meeting its goals. Leadership can involve a simple or a complex project. For example, a PCT recommended a change in how a patient was ambulated that would better meet the patient's need to walk. Another PCT actively participated on a unit's committee and helped to institute changes in how the unit operates.

What is leadership? PCTs on an inpatient unit were asked to talk about what leadership means to them. They described leadership within their roles as follows:

Leadership is taking responsibility for what I do.
Leadership is knowing my areas of responsibility and fulfilling them to the very best of my abilities.
Leaders are open-minded and understanding, take into account other people's ideas, and treat everyone as equal.
Leadership is when responsibility is shared among all the team members.
Working together and communication help the unit to become cohesive. We help each other out because we all want the patients to get the best care. We want to do our best.
Leadership is being accountable to the patients and to the staff.

The word *guidance* can be used when describing leadership. Leadership is the ability to convince unit staff to work together toward the attainment of the organization, unit, and patient care objectives. It is through leadership that people are motivated to work together to improve patient care and work more efficiently as a team. It involves quality of work performance and service.

Research has shown that leaders demonstrate specific characteristics. The traits of honesty, competence, forward-looking, and inspiring have ranked among the most important characteristics of a leader. Other characteristics include being intelligent, fair-minded, supportive, dependable, caring, cooperative, mature, self-controlled, and loyal.

CHARACTERISTICS OF A LEADER

Honest
Competent
Forward-looking
Inspiring

Honesty has always ranked as the top characteristic. This is an absolutely essential characteristic. When you think of a person you want to follow, it is important that the person be trustworthy, ethical, and principled. If his or her trustworthiness is ever put in doubt, it is very difficult to regain trust. Honesty is measured by observing that persons do what they say they are going to do. It means that they keep their word, talk in an up-front manner, and follow through on promises. To trust people, you need to know where they stand on important issues and that they are willing to take a stand on those issues.

Competence is another important characteristic. Leaders must have the skills and abilities to do their job in an efficient manner. They must know what they are doing and that the people around them believe that they have these skills. What the specific skills are will vary with the activity. PCTs who recommend changes in a specific aspect of patient care must have credibility in their clinical skills. For an effective team, each member of the team needs to know the responsibilities and level of competence of all the other members. Then members can help each other when another member is unable to complete his or her work. For example, one team member who recognized that a patient was depressed and who was unable to sit with the patient asked the PCT, who had demonstrated good communication skills, to spend a little more time sitting with the patient.

Followers like to have a leader who is forward-looking. This is not the same as a visionary. As a leader it is important that the PCT plan for the future. A PCT can start being forward-looking by knowing what is going on in health care, understanding the direction of the organization and unit, and keeping in touch with new unit patient care activities. This can be done by reading the newspapers and other materials provided on the unit, talking with other team members, and attending educational activities.

Being a positive, energetic person adds the inspiration characteristic. People enjoy being around a positive person and are more willing to listen to the ideas of a positive individual. Positive attitudes inspire confidence in a person. Communication is part of inspiring. The clearer the ideas are articulated, the easier it is for other people to understand them.

These four characteristics—honesty, competence, planning for the future, and inspiration—address your credibility in the eyes of the people around you. Credibility means that other people believe you have the expertise or competence in what you are doing and you will do what you say you are going to do. Credibility is the basis for allowing a leader to make changes on the unit and for other members of the staff to believe and follow the leader's ideas.

MODEL OF LEADERSHIP

Kouzes and Posner* describe five aspects of leadership:

Challenging the process means that leaders look for opportunities to improve the surrounding area. They are willing to take risks, knowing that sometimes ideas work out and sometimes they do not, but they are willing to try. Along with looking for opportunities comes the responsibility of listening to ideas from other people. For example, a PCT recommended a different way of saving time in preparing a patient room for admittance and a system to efficiently communicate with staff when the room was available. In another example, a PCT recommended changing the place where clean and soiled supplies were kept, an idea that greatly enhanced the working environment for all the staff. Another PCT suggested a new system for protecting patient care belongings while the patient was in the operating room. There are many opportunities to improve the patient care areas in which PCTs work.

There is an old phrase, "If it ain't broke, don't fix it." Today the attitude is, "If it ain't broke, see if it can be improved." To do this the PCT needs to look at each new job assignment as an opportunity to make it better. Beware of the statement, "We have always done it this way." Think about whether it makes sense to do it the "old way," or if there is a "better way."

The second aspect of leadership is *inspiring a shared vision.* This includes having an idea that enhances the direction in which your unit is moving and getting others to support the idea. One PCT had the idea that her unit

Kouzes, J., and Posner, B.: The Leadership Challenge: How to Get Extraordinary Things Done in Organizations. San Francisco, Jossey-Bass Publishers, 1987.

FIVE ASPECTS OF LEADERSHIP

- Challenging the process
- Inspiring a shared vision
- Enabling others to act
- Modeling the way
- Encouraging the heart

---

could be the best working environment in the entire agency and that staff would want to work on that unit more than any other unit. The PCT talked and talked about what it meant to be the best. Surrounding staff supported the idea and came up with many ideas on how they could work together to become the number one unit. They looked not only at what would enhance their own satisfaction, but at the satisfaction of their patients, support staff, and physicians. One idea led to another. The unit staff became excited. Many changes occurred on the unit because one person had an idea and inspired others to work together.

Enabling others to act is important because one person cannot do or think of everything. Staff may have good ideas but are not comfortable or confident to share their ideas with others. A leader encourages other people to come up with ideas and supports the ideas that are realistic and promote the direction of the unit. One easy way to do this is to ask people their opinion. People enjoy sharing their thoughts when they believe that they are being heard. It makes them feel respected and important. Many creative ideas have been generated by asking other people about their ideas on a specific subject.

Leaders also share information and assist people to work together to get the job done. For example, a PCT can volunteer to work on a project with other staff members. By sharing different perspectives, the final outcome of the project is often more readily accepted and implemented on the unit.

Leaders are *role models*. Their behavior should be what they expect of others. Their words match their actions. They keep the promises they make. If the expectation on the unit is that everyone arrives on time, the leader is one of the first ones there. Not calling in sick when you are not sick is important. When a staff member takes advantage of the system by frequently calling in sick, other staff members have to pick up the extra work. This creates poor feelings and distrust on the unit. The PCTs can also be role models for positive behavior in how respect is shown to other team members. For example, the PCTs can show new orientees how to handle patient care assignments rather than tell them. They encourage ethical and honest behavior in themselves and in others. People depend on them and are not disappointed. Leaders have a strong belief in hard work and care for others around them. People depend on the leaders and try to model their behavior after them. In doing so, they win the respect of all the people around them.

The final aspect of leadership is *encouraging the heart.* Leaders enjoy working with the people they are with. They celebrate their accomplishments together, both the big and the small. Leaders recognize the work that others do and acknowledge it. This can be done at a staff meeting where the person or group is recognized with a thank-you or a small party. Some agencies have formal methods of recognizing staff achievements. Leaders can submit a person's or group's name so that the people and their accomplishments are recognized at higher levels within an organization. When leaders extend themselves to acknowledge others, the individual and the unit are recognized. Anyone on the unit can recognize the accomplishments of another. It has been found that the more that individuals and groups are recognized for their accomplishments, the more they are willing to participate in other activities. A PCT can be actively involved in recognizing other staff members' accomplishments.

Although the role of leader is an important one, being a follower is equally important. Most people change from being leaders to followers according to the situation. One PCT stated that sometimes the staff members as a group may come to consensus on an issue that the PCT does not agree with. At that time the PCT becomes the follower and supports the direction determined by the other staff members. A responsibility of the PCT is to understand why the group made the decision. Once the group decision is made, the PCT and other staff members need to support the decision in both their behavior and communications. Talking behind someone's back or negatively about the situation creates tension on the unit and reflects poorly on the individual. People lose respect for those who demonstrate destructive behavior.

UNDERSTANDING THE HIERARCHY

Almost anywhere you work there is a hierarchy. A hierarchy is the organization or unit structure that demonstrates who reports to whom. Understanding the hierarchy is important for getting the work done in an efficient manner. Who reports to whom varies within each organization and should be covered in the PCT's orientation. If it is not covered, it is the responsibility of the PCT to ask. Every organization has different titles for its staff. For example, in some organizations, PCTs may be called unlicensed assistive personnel, advanced nursing assistants, nurse aides, nursing techs, or other job titles. It is more important to learn how each member of the team functions and their relation to each other than being concerned about the titles.

In most organizations PCTs report to an RN (Fig. 2–1). PCTs receive their assignment and report their activities to the RN. How much direction the RN gives PCTs depends on the PCTs' experience and competence and the trust between them and the RN. RNs are responsible for the nursing care patients receive during their shift. RNs assess the status of the patients, determine the nursing diagnosis, set up the plan of care on the basis of nursing and medical orders, provide care, and monitor and document patients' progress. They are responsible for patient teaching and for working with both patients and patients' families and/or significant others. They also work with other RNs in helping patients take care of

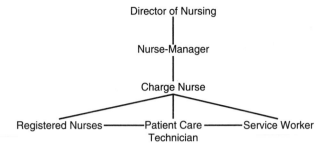

FIGURE 2–1
Patient care unit hierarchy.

themselves at home. The RN is the person who reports patient status to the physician and consults with him or her on the care of the patient.

In some agencies there are individuals who assist with the operations of the unit, but they do not directly care for the patients. They may be called service workers, unit workers, or a similar name. For example, these individuals may bring a tray of food to the patient, straighten up the patient's room, help with transporting a patient to an appointment, run errands for the nursing staff or the patient, or clean an unoccupied room. The service worker reports to the RN and works with the PCT.

Units practice nursing in different ways. If the unit practices primary nursing care, the RN is responsible for planning the nursing care for a selected group of patients. They are accountable for the patient care from the time the patient enters the unit until the patient is discharged. The primary RN may or may not actually be doing the hands-on care. The unit may practice team nursing, in which either RNs or RNs and assistive personnel work together to provide patient care. Other units may provide patient care by teaming one RN and one PCT. They work together the entire shift.

The charge nurse is responsible for the operation of the unit on a specific shift. For example, there may be a charge nurse on the day shift, another on the evening shift, and a third on nights. The charge nurse makes the patient care assignments to the RNs at the beginning of the shift. Charge nurses are also responsible for assigning new patients to an RN and changing patient care assignments if an emergency should occur. They also manage patient flow and check with nursing staff regarding work load issues. Many times, if there is a problem, patients and other support staff talk with the charge nurse. In some agencies, the PCT reports to the charge nurse.

RNs report to a nurse-manager; sometimes it may be the assistant nurse-manager. The nurse-manager is often responsible for the operations of the unit 24 hours per day, 7 days a week. The nurse-manager, along with the staff, sets the expectations and direction of the unit. Many times the nurse-manager is not on the unit because she or he must attend meetings to help make decisions or gain information that will impact on the unit. Nurse-managers often share what they have learned with their staff. They are responsible for evaluating their staff and working to continuously improve and develop them. Nurse-managers are often responsible for hiring, disciplining, and terminating nursing staff, including PCTs. They are also accountable for the unit's staffing and budgets.

Nurse-managers often report to the director of nursing or assistant director of nursing. The director of nursing may be called the vice president of nursing or the vice president of patient care services. Regardless of the title, this nurse is responsible for the entire nursing department and is a liaison with all the other departments. This role is very important. The director of nursing represents nursing in many of the important meetings across the agency. She or he also sets the direction of nursing services.

Physicians provide medical management of patients. They assess the status of the patient; determine the patient's diagnosis; write the medical orders, including the tests the patients will have; and monitor the patient's progress. They determine when a patient will be able to go home. Physicians are very dependent on quality patient care, provided by nursing staff, for their patients to get well. RNs are responsible for following the physicians' medical orders as well as the nursing orders. As a PCT, you are responsible for assisting the RN as he or she provides patient care.

CONCEPT OF TEAM

A *team* refers to a group of people who rely on each other to accomplish a goal. In the hospital, a common unit goal or mission of the team is to provide safe and effective patient care. Since PCTs are a vital part of the unit, it is important for you to understand how team members interrelate and rely on each other.

A team consists of a team leader and team members (Fig. 2–2). The team leader is the person who directs or assigns and oversees the work. On a nursing unit the team leader is the head RN or nurse-manager. In other cases the charge nurse is the team leader. The team members are the people who carry out the work. They are the ones responsible for completing tasks and providing appropriate feedback to the team leader. The RNs, LPNs, and PCTs act as team members. Some units may organize care delivery into smaller teams that include an RN, a PCT, and a service worker who jointly have responsibility for a group of patients. On some units, other personnel, such as physicians, social workers, and physical therapists, may be part of the team.

It is often helpful for team members to understand what makes an effective team. The box on the next page contains components of an effective team. Team members as well as the team leader have a responsibility to identify whether the team is working effectively and to resolve team issues. For example, if an individual is very busy and coworkers are not busy, it would be appropriate to ask either the other team members or the team leader for assistance. With the unit's mission in mind, it is easy to see that such requests are made so that the unit's mission is met.

Becoming a new member of an existing team is a challenging process. The new PCT will be faced with these challenges when joining a new unit. The PCT will be faced with learning not only the skills of his or her role but also the emotional components of the team.

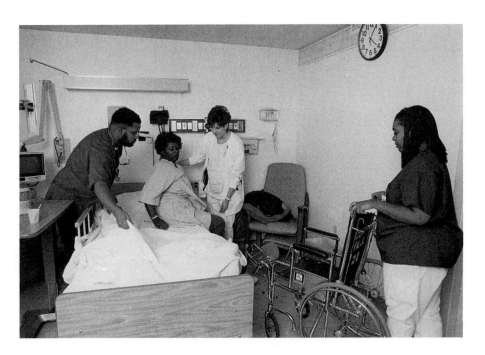

FIGURE 2–2
Team members working together.

CHARACTERISTICS OF WELL-FUNCTIONING TEAMS

- Members know why the team exists and are invested in accomplishing the unit's mission.

- Members know what needs to be done next, by whom, and by when to achieve goals.

- Members know their roles in getting tasks done and when to allow a more skillful member to do a certain task.

- Authority and decision-making lines are clearly understood.

- Conflict is dealt with openly and is considered important to decision making and personal growth.

- Members' diversity is valued.

- Members are able to share risky ideas and feel supported by the team rather than criticized.

- Members are competent.

- Members know clearly when the team has met with success and share this equally and proudly.

- Opportunities for feedback and updating skills are provided and taken advantage of by team members.

- Communications channels are clear and followed.

- Members receive honest and direct feedback.

- Members trust one another.

Finding out the team norms or operating procedures will be essential for the PCT's success on the unit. These team norms are not necessarily formal procedures. They can be unspoken ways of doing things that one observes and/or learns through trial and error. For instance, a team may have a team norm that everyone arrives for work on time. A team member arriving late for work may be reprimanded either with verbal statements or with nonverbal behavior, such as an undesirable work assignment. The team member soon learns that arriving late for work is unacceptable and results in undesirable consequences. Examples of other team norms the PCT will want to find out about are how breaks and lunches are handled and how birthdays are celebrated. The new PCT will also find that the team has a language of its own. An example of team-specific language is the term *clin spec* to indicate the clinical nurse specialist.

Following the team norms and using the team language are skills the PCT will develop over time. The new PCT's best plan for becoming a successful member of the team is to observe carefully the other team members during the first few weeks of employment. It is advisable to get to know members of the team gradually and identify team members that he or she feels comfortable with. These trusted team members can be relied on to share the team norms and share the team language.

Many times one of the first trusted team members that the PCT may identify is his or her preceptor. The preceptor is the individual who teaches the PCT about the unit during orientation, including the unit norms and actual work on the unit. The preceptor may be an RN or an experienced PCT. The PCT may choose to use the preceptor as a resource long after the orientation period.

KNOW YOUR COMPETENCIES/ LIMITATIONS: KNOW YOURSELF

Beginning in 1992, the Joint Commission on Accreditation of Healthcare Organizations (JCAHO) required that all nursing personnel demonstrate competency on specific topics. Demonstrating competency means that the individual has shown the capability to think about or do a certain task for another individual. It is a way to measure if one is capable to complete a task independently, with assistance, or not at all. Competence must be manifested before the PCT provides patient care.

While PCTs are in orientation they will be asked to demonstrate competency for a number of skills. This is so the RN who asks the PCT to complete a task can be assured that the PCT can complete the task in the expected way without direct monitoring. In most cases the competency check will require the PCT to demonstrate a skill for an RN. If the PCT is unfamiliar with the procedure, it is important that she or he review any relevant material and ask for someone (preferably the person who will be doing the competency check) to demonstrate the task. Next, the PCT may wish to demonstrate the task while being talked through it. The PCT is ready for the competency check once he or she thinks that the task can be comfortably completed without asking questions. In other cases the PCT may be asked to complete a short quiz to demonstrate knowledge or to talk-through a procedure. Regardless of the task it is important to be assured that the PCT is comfortable with it before being declared competent. Once considered competent, it is likely that the PCT will be expected to complete that task independently for the duration of employment in that agency.

Every year, new competencies will be developed based on certain criteria. Usually the tasks selected are high-

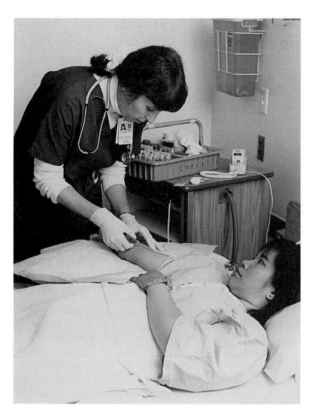

FIGURE 2 – 3
High-frequency task.

risk tasks or tasks that are likely to have life-threatening or legal implications, such as phlebotomy (Fig. 2–3). Low-frequency competencies involve tasks that are infrequently performed, such as use of a certain cooling blanket (Fig. 2–4). The PCT will be expected to demonstrate competency for these new tasks. The PCT also will need to demonstrate annually certain tasks that he or she

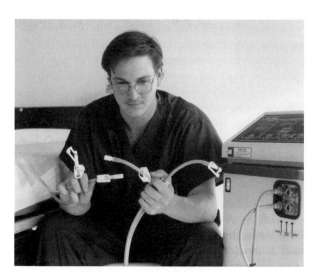

FIGURE 2 – 4
Low-frequency task.

presented in orientation. Typically these are the "mandatory" competencies, such as fire and safety, infection control, and bedside specimen testing. Some settings may require the PCT to demonstrate all of the orientation competencies annually plus any new competencies.

PCTs have an important role in the competency demonstration system. First, they must prepare themselves to complete the task at hand. This may require reading appropriate materials or requesting demonstrations. Second, PCTs should keep a record of the competencies they have demonstrated; the hospital will also keep a record. If PCTs should decide to seek a new place of employment, a competency list of skills is available to share with the new employer. Third, PCTs must take the responsibility to inform other staff members of the tasks for which they have not demonstrated competency.

When it comes to competency demonstration issues, PCTs' best defense is to know themselves, their limits, and their abilities. PCTs always have a responsibility to know what they can and cannot do and to share that information with others. Competency demonstration and record keeping are useful tools that will support the PCT on a daily basis.

DELEGATION PROCESS

Delegation is the act of transferring the responsibility for the performance of an activity from one person to another while retaining accountability for the outcome.* The RN determines what is delegated to Unlicensed Assistive Personnel (UAP), based on the protection of the public, and includes the needs of patients, the education and training of UAPs, the extent of supervision required, and the staff work load. Delegation is also based on the job description of the PCT. This means that at some point RNs on the unit in which the PCT is employed used the above criteria to determine what tasks the PCT will do on that unit (Fig. 2–5).

The types of tasks that are delegated to PCTs by RNs fall into two categories: (1) Direct patient care activities are those that assist the patient in meeting his or her basic needs, such as eating, bathing, or grooming. (2) Indirect patient care activities are those that assist in providing a clean, efficient, and safe patient care environ-

*American Nurses Association: Position Statement. Washington, DC, 1992.

DELEGATED TASKS
Direct
Indirect

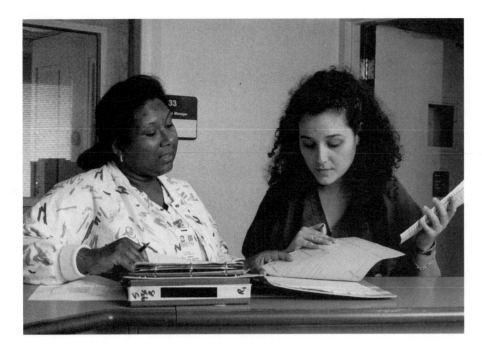

FIGURE 2 – 5

Nurse delegating to patient care technician.

ment. The PCT's role may include the above categories either alone or in combination.

Delegation is different from assignment. When a task is delegated, the responsibility for the performance of the task is transferred to the delegatee, but the accountability for the oversight of the task remains with the delegator. Delegation assumes that the delegator has greater knowledge than the delegatee and that the delegated task is only a subcomponent of a larger role. Assignment is the shift of the rights, responsibility, and accountability from one person to another. It assumes that the knowledge, skills, and judgment levels are transferable. Therefore, providing fresh water to all patients is an assignment, since the knowledge, skill, and judgment for completing such a task are the same for RNs, LPNs, and PCTs. On the other hand, feeding a patient is a delegated task because adequate patient nutrition is a component of the overall goal or outcome that the RN has set with or for the patient.

Regardless of the task that is delegated, it is important to realize that delegation is a process. It does not mean an RN tells a PCT what to do and he or she does it, but rather that the PCT follows specific steps to ensure safe and effective patient care or unit outcome. Both the delegator (RN) and the delegatee (PCT) should become familiar with the steps of delegation outlined below. If a problem does arise within the process, both parties are capable of analyzing the situation to improve the outcome.

Steps of Delegation

1. Determine if the task is appropriate to delegate. The responsibility for this task lies with both the RN and the PCT. The RN needs to determine if the task is one that can be delegated and within the PCT job description. The RN should also be assured that the PCT is competent in performing the task. The PCT also takes the responsibility for stating when she or he is not competent to perform a task.

 Do not accept an assignment outside your level of competency.

2. The appropriate delegatee is determined. The RN will determine if the PCT is an appropriate person to do the job. The PCT must provide feedback in this step to indicate whether there is adequate time to complete the task.

3. The desired outcome is stated. The RN must state what end result is expected upon completion of the task. For example, the RN may state, "Give Mr. B a bath."

4. The time frame for completion is stated. The RN must state in what time frame the task must be completed. It may be as broad as "today" or as specific as "at 1100 hours."

5. Authority is given. When PCTs accept authority for the task, they are given the responsibility to complete the task as determined most appropriate within defined parameters, which may be determined by the PCT's competency or the RN who is delegating. For example, a bath may be given while the patient is in bed or sitting in a chair or in the tub, provided the PCT is competent to complete the task in all of those ways.

6. Responsibility is assigned/accepted. Accepting responsibility indicates that the PCT will complete the task within the specified time frame.

7. Agreement is obtained. Once both parties agree to the delegation, work on the task may begin.

8. Progress is monitored. Both the RN and the PCT have a responsibility to keep each other updated on the task at hand. For example, if the patient has been emergently scheduled for a test or if the patient refuses to have a bath, the PCT would then notify the RN of inability to complete the task.

9. Provide feedback. Upon completion of the task, feedback should be provided. The mechanism of feedback may be agreed upon at the beginning of the delegation. This may mean that the PCT may be asked to record the completed task or that the RN may give feedback about the entire task such as what went well and what areas could be improved.

Communication is key to the delegation process. Asking questions for clarification as the process is delegated and providing feedback during or after the process is essential for an effective outcome. The box below identifies some important question-asking concepts that may help during the delegation process. The reader is referred to Chapter 4 for more information on maintaining an effective communication relationship with coworkers.

Given the complexity of the delegation process, it is easy to see that it may be challenging. These challenges may include reluctance on the part of the RN to delegate. For example, the RN may be concerned that it takes too much time to explain or may fear loss of control or that the job will not be done well. The PCT facilitates the delegation process by being willing and ready to accept being delegated, to assure that the steps are followed, and by providing feedback to the delegator.

Everyone benefits when the delegation process is followed. More work is accomplished. PCTs have the opportunity to demonstrate and learn new skills, and RNs can

concentrate on broader areas of responsibility requiring an RNs unique level of judgment and expertise. Finally, the sense of team provides for a positive and desirable work environment.

TIME AND STRESS MANAGEMENT

Stress is a normal part of life. It can be either positive or negative. When stress is positive it can help a person concentrate, focus, perform, and reach peak efficiency. When stress is negative, it can have long-term adverse effects on the body, leading to such problems as hypertension, migraines, and chronic back pain.

The body's initial response to positive and negative stress is the same—the heart races, the blood pressure increases, the hands become cold and clammy, and the stomach becomes tense—all because of the release of endorphins. The difference between the positive and negative stress response is the body's ability to relax after the stressor has occurred. When a negative stressor occurs, the body's initial response to stress persists long after the stressor is removed.

Individuals react differently to the same stressor. The presence of certain factors in an individual's life promote the perception of positive stress for the individual.* These factors include the ability to set priorities; help others; set achievable, realistic goals; and maintain a positive attitude. Other factors contribute to the ability to manage stress positively, including adequate sleep, periods of rest, meditation, muscle relaxation, well-balanced diet, exercise, and normal weight. The presence of supportive friends, family, and coworkers also contributes to an individual's ability to perceive stress in a positive light. Consequently it is in an individual's best interest that as many as possible of these factors are present in his or her life to improve the likelihood that the body will perceive a stressor as positive.

Deciding to manage the stress can be another appropriate way to make stress work to one's advantage. There are physical and mental skills that an individual can use when under stress to make it a positive experience.* Physical management may include such techniques as deep breathing, clearing the mind, progressive muscle relaxation, and stretching exercises. These techniques may be employed immediately after the stressful event to promote the essential relaxation phase of stress. Mental management may include such activities as positive self-talk, rehearsal, planning, using support systems, and making positive lifestyle changes that include exercise, adequate nutrition, and planned leisure time. These mental techniques require the individual to make stress man-

---

*Simon, S.: A self-instructional program on stress management. Journal of Post Anesthesia Nursing, Vol. 4, No. 4, 1989.

```
┌─────────────────────────────────────────┐
│           ASK THE RIGHT QUESTIONS         │
├─────────────────────────────────────────┤
```

Have a specific purpose to your questions. Know clearly what information you need so you can accomplish your goal. You may want to provoke thought, stress a major point, or make the listener more alert.

Your question must be understood. Use simple, concise language so the listener knows exactly what you mean.

Ask for a definite answer. Phrase your question for a specific answer and do not let up until you get it.

Don't guess. Inaccurate information is worse than no information at all.

agement a priority in his or her life. They need to occur before, during, and after the stressful event.

Managing time effectively may be another mechanism to support stress management. Effective time management means that one's efforts are focused on one's work and that work is accomplished within a reasonable period. Some individuals may find that time management comes naturally to them, and others may have to work at it.

There are certain methods that the PCT can employ to promote effective time management on the job. One important method is to prioritize work by setting realistic achievable goals. This can be done using the PCT's individual judgment in conjunction with input from the team leader and team members. It is crucial when prioritizing work that the PCT negotiate the priority level of all delegated tasks. If it becomes clear to the PCT that she or he will not be able to complete a delegated task, the appropriate individuals must be informed as soon as possible. This will minimize conflicts at the end of the day if work is not completed. Other team members will not appreciate the PCT who agrees to all tasks delegated to her but accomplishes only some of the tasks requested.

It is also helpful to write down a schedule for the day or use a unit worksheet such as the one presented in Chapter 15 and list the tasks to be accomplished every hour. The tasks then can be crossed out as they are accomplished. The schedule can also be a place to write notes for the day for future reference, note vital signs, record bedside specimen testing values for documentation on the chart, or place reminders to oneself. It can also be a ready reference for such questions as, "What did you accomplish today?"

Asking for help when it is needed is another time management technique. For example, it would take two people less than half the time to bathe a 300-pound new hemiplegic patient than it would one person. Be realistic about what can be accomplished as a team and as an individual.

Just as it is important to identify time management techniques, the PCT will also want to identify and avoid time wasters. Time wasters include getting caught up in "complaining sessions" that usually result in the participants' feeling worse than when they started the conversation and do not promote work completion. On

---

TIME MANAGEMENT TECHNIQUES

Prioritize work
Realistic goals
Written schedule
Communicate progress
Ask for help

---

the other hand, identifying problems and methods to improve them can be shared with the team leader and would be a good use of time. However, even this activity would be appropriate only if all other tasks for the day were completed or if it were an assigned task. Another time waster is attempting to complete a task for which the PCT has not demonstrated competency. This should never be done because it may cause harm to the patient. It will likely take the PCT longer to complete and may result in another individual having to do it over, therefore occupying two people's time.

Using effective time management for the PCT means completing the work assignment within the scheduled shift. Assertively writing and sharing the schedule for the day and setting realistic goals will assure that work gets completed, and the PCT feels a sense of accomplishment at the end of the shift.

PARTICIPATIVE DECISION MAKING

Participative decision making is becoming common practice in agency settings in which managers actively seek information from their staff prior to making a decision. This means that everyone in a group has the opportunity to share opinions about the issues. On a large unit, many of the staff will have the opportunity to share their ideas; however, not everyone may be involved in finding a workable solution. Nurse-managers may involve staff who are directly impacted by the issue, experts on the subject, and those who have strong opinions. Nurse-managers also may discuss the issues with people outside the unit. The nurse-manager wants to collect as much information as possible on the subject to make the best decision.

It is very important that staff, including PCTs, participate in sharing their ideas. Each person can respond from his or her area of responsibility and perception of the potential impact of the decision on patient care and the unit. It is important to listen to other staff members' points of view and to seek to understand their perspectives. Being open-minded is important. When staff members listen to each other and are willing to change their minds, the best ideas can come forward.

Once the decision is made, all of the staff need to support the decision. They need to make every attempt to make the solution work, even if it was not the solution they favored. If the decision does not produce the intended results, it is also the responsibility of each staff member to speak to the nurse-manager. Decisions can be changed if they do not work.

Being a member of a unit committee is an important responsibility (Fig. 2–6). A PCT asked to participate on a committee should consider the following important questions prior to agreeing to participate:

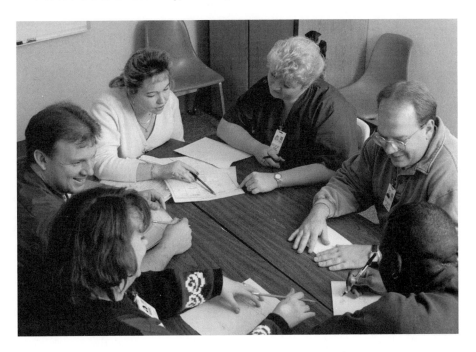

FIGURE 2-6
Participation on committees.

Committee Member Questions

- What is the purpose of the committee? Is the PCT interested in the topic? Does the PCT feel that he or she can contribute to and is interested in the committee work?

- What is the role of the PCT on the committee? It is important to be clear on the areas of expertise brought to the committee.

- Whom does the PCT represent—his or her own ideas or reflect the opinions of the PCTs on the unit or the perspectives of all staff on the unit?

- What level of decision making does the committee have? Does the committee make the decision or recommend to another group that makes the final decision?

- What is the time commitment involved in being a part of the committee? When will the committee meet, and what work is expected to be done outside the committee? What is the expected time of completion? Does the PCT have the time to participate? Will the nurse-manager support the attendance of the PCT on the committee? Will the nurse-manager authorize release time from patient care duties to complete committee assignments, if necessary?

- Who needs to be communicated to about the decisions of the group? Is the PCT responsible for keeping the unit staff informed about the progress of the committee or writing a report?

- Is the PCT interested in participating? It is very important to become an active participant once the PCT has agreed to become a member. A good participant will adhere to the following guidelines:

Meeting Management Skills

- Prepares for the meeting—doing an assigned reading, talking with other staff, and thinking about the upcoming agenda topics
- Arrives at the meeting on time
- Actively speaks up in the meeting to share ideas
- Asks questions
- Listens to the ideas of others and asks for clarification if not understood
- Thinks about the issues objectively
- Stays on the topic being discussed
- Gives feedback to the meeting leader and members as requested
- Follows up on any assigned tasks

Being a committee member is an important responsibility. It gives the PCT an opportunity to be involved in improving patient care and how the unit operates.

CONFLICT MANAGEMENT

Conflicts are a natural occurrence on every unit. They can occur wherever there is a group of people who come

---

CONFLICTS

Issues or events
Interpersonal relationships

together such as in the workplace. In the past, conflict was considered negative. Today, conflict is considered positive, an opportunity to work through issues. Usually conflict involves an issue or event that has occurred as well as interpersonal relationships. In working through conflicts, the interpersonal relationship is of more importance than the incident. For example, if staff members have a good working relationship and a disagreement occurs, usually the members can work it out. If they do not have a good working relationship, small conflicts often get bigger.

Conflicts can lead to disruptive behavior if they are not handled as they arise. For example, if a staff member thinks an issue is important and another staff member ignores it, the first person feels belittled and not important enough to have the issue resolved. Conflict, if suppressed over time, will continually recur between people, sometimes over very minor concerns. Some people also respond to conflict by becoming verbally or physically abusive.

Sometimes conflicts concern facts or opinions. For example, two people may attend the same meeting and understand something completely different. Two people may ambulate a patient differently. Conflicts can also be about values and beliefs. These are usually more difficult to resolve. One PCT might value working with patients, whereas another PCT may want to focus more on using technology and equipment or the social aspect of the unit. Another example might be a PCT who, because of religious beliefs, does not want to work with certain types of patients.

With conflicts inevitable, handling conflicts becomes very important. The following steps can help in handling conflicts.

Handling Conflicts

1. Provide a safe environment. Discussing issues needs to occur in a place where both people feel comfortable, such as an informal setting. When the staff feel more secure they are more comfortable in expressing their concerns. It is inappropriate to discuss conflicts in front of patients, their families, or visitors. It is also stressful and uncomfortable for many people to have conflicts discussed in a group. One-to-one conversations often offer the best chance of successful resolution.

2. Clearly identify the issue. What is the conflict? Is it an event or is it a relationship issue? Is it an issue of fact, opinion, values, or beliefs? Most importantly, do both people want to work through the conflict?

3. Determine the facts. What happened? Clarify generalizations. It is helpful to understand terms, for instance, who "they" are.

4. Clarify the perspective of both persons. Often conflicts are a result of miscommunication or misperceptions of a person's behavior. Honest communications by both

---

┌───┐
│ **CONFLICT MANAGEMENT SKILLS**   │
├───┤
│ Active listening   │
│ Assertive communication   │
│ Separating person from problem   │
└───┘

individuals will help each person understand the perspective of the other. Assertive communication and active listening are skills that help each person articulate and understand each other's concerns (see Chapter 4).

5. Look at acceptable alternatives to resolving the issue. Compromising may not be an acceptable resolution. Compromise implies giving up on important aspects of the issue. When compromise is completed, usually both parties are dissatisfied with the results. Identifying points of agreement and areas that both parties feel are important can lead to a resolution that both can support.

Active listening is a valuable tool in managing conflict. Many times we are so busy thinking about what we want to say next that we forget to listen. The first step in active listening is to stop talking and concentrate on what the other person is saying. At the same time, you can read the person's nonverbal language, such as eye contact and how the person uses his or her hands. When you listen, the other person feels that you consider her or him important and will take the time to hear what she or he has to say. You can also get an understanding of the other person's perception of the conflict. At the same time, listening builds relationships between people.

Assertive communication is also important. In being assertive, you speak from your own perspective and respect the other person. Using the pronoun *I* to share your concerns is important. *You* can be perceived as accusing the other person. Watch how you use your body. An aggressive stance or finger pointing can be perceived as an attack, while a calm manner has a quieting effect on everyone. Both people sitting down together creates an equal environment for communication.

Another skill is to separate the person from the problem. Ways to do this are to talk in specific rather than general terms and to ask concrete questions.

Finding a workable and agreeable alternative to the conflict is the desired outcome. Sometimes it is difficult for individuals to do it on their own. Using the nurse-manager or an RN that both staff members are comfortable with can help to resolve the issue. Some agencies have counselors or people trained in conflict management who can also be used as a resource.

LIVING WITH CHANGE

Years ago, rapid change was considered a rare event. The unit would implement a change and then stabilize.

One change would occur at a time. Today, change is the norm, and stabilization is the exception. Often many changes are occurring at the same time. Even before one change has been implemented another change is being planned. Although constant change can be stressful, it can also create a dynamic and exciting place to work.

Changes come from many sources. The health care environment and patients' expectations of care are changing. Agencies are needing to change to compete in health care. Regulatory agencies set expectations of agencies to protect the public. These expectations must be met; they change to be responsive to the needs of the health care consumer. Quality of care and lowering of costs are high priorities in every agency. Quality improvement is being integrated continuously into the daily activities of all agency employees. With both external and internal pressures to implement change, the unit constantly evaluates how patient care is delivered and how the unit team functions. Thus, change is the norm or constant part of any area within the health care field.

Identification of areas for improvement can come from any staff member. It is the responsibility of every staff member to look at the unit proactively to identify issues of concern. Once a concern is brought to the nurse's or nurse-manager's attention, he or she will bring people together to discuss the areas that need to be improved. Not all of the staff suggestions will be acted on. The nurse-manager and staff will prioritize the areas that need to be changed. Working through the change process takes staff time and unit resources. Therefore the areas that are selected to be evaluated must be important to the patients, unit operations, and staff satisfaction and have the most likelihood to succeed. For example, on one unit, the staff decided to change the visiting hours for patients. They believed that visitors and family members positively affected the healing process of the patient. The unit set up a committee to look at the visiting hours policy and to recommend changes. This was done, and the staff supported the committee's recommendation of more lenient visiting times. Communication with other units, physicians, and support staff on the change was completed. Unit visitation signs and patient information were changed. As a result of the change, patients, visitors, and family members were more satisfied, and the staff did not notice a difference in their being able to provide care.

Not everyone supports change. With any significant change, there will be a small percentage of staff who will actively support the change and a small percentage who will not. The majority of people are in the middle. Some of the middle-group members would like more information, whereas others may choose to wait and watch the results of the change. Either way, the active supporters and the middle group members can be engaged in clearly identifying the areas needing improvement, generating alternatives, selecting the best alternative, and evaluating the effectiveness of the change. The more people who are involved in planning the change, the more people will support the actual change.

People resist change for a variety of reasons. Change creates feelings of discomfort, insecurity, and anxiety. Staff feel more secure and comfortable in a working environment and in relationships that are known. Change can create less certainty in the future. Staff may see the change as a potential loss of their job, less money, or a different position. The fear of the unknown in and of itself provokes discomfort. People who are resistant to change will grieve over how things used to be. Allowing the grieving process to occur will help them accept changes.

Helping staff clearly understand what the problems are and involving them in seeking information on problem identification and alternative solutions will help staff feel that they are part of the change process. Giving staff support during the implementation phase is important. Lastly, it is important to monitor the results of the change and share this information with the staff. If the staff believe that the change will make a significant difference in the quality of care delivered or make their work loads more manageable, they are often more willing to support the change.

The PCT needs to become involved in the change process. This can be done by sharing ideas about the problem and offering alternatives for the group to discuss. Once the alternative has been selected, it is important that the PCT support the change and integrate it into practice.

OPPORTUNITIES FOR PERSONAL GROWTH

Goal setting is an important activity and should not be overlooked. Goals may be financial, social, or educational and may be job- or self-oriented. The important point is that realistic, measurable, and achievable goals are set for oneself. Job seekers may note that the PCTs who have set goals for themselves are the ones who are most likely to be hired. In general, people who do not set goals eventually feel helpless and dissatisfied with their job.

A sample goal may be to attend one inservice training session each month. This goal can be evaluated each month by asking oneself, Did I attend an inservice this month? If the answer is yes, then the goal has been achieved and a sense of accomplishment is felt. The PCT may choose to continue the goal or set another goal. If the goal is not achieved, the PCT needs to determine if the goal was realistic or if something in the environment prevented attaining it. The PCT may choose to continue the same goal, using an action plan to ensure that the goal is achieved. For instance, the PCT may share the goal with other team members and the team leader and ask for feedback and support in achieving the goal. The

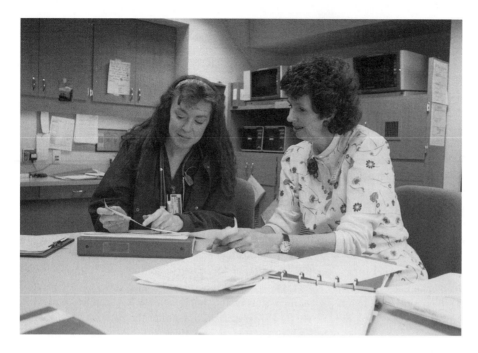

FIGURE 2–7

Assistant with mentor planning goals.

PCT may also decide to set a different goal or select a less difficult goal, such as reading the materials from an inservice each month.

One mechanism to help in goal setting is the identification of a mentor (Fig. 2–7). A mentor is a person who inspires others to achieve or realize their fullest potential. A mentor can be a teacher, a manager, or a coworker. The mentor will challenge the PCT to strive for the best and will provide insight into his or her character. Knowledge sharing is also part of the mentor relationship. In looking for a mentor, the PCT may identify someone she or he admires, respects, and feels comfortable talking with. The PCT–mentor relationship should include goal setting and ongoing feedback. The benefits for the PCT are a sense of direction and positive self-esteem.

Many PCTs select the PCT job as a stepping stone into another role in the health care field. It provides the opportunity to observe different roles firsthand and determine if a new role is worth striving for. The PCT may even select an individual in a different role as a mentor. Other PCTs select the career of PCT as their primary choice, with no intent of changing roles. Instead, becoming an expert PCT is the goal. Some of these individuals may ultimately decide to select another career path in the future. Regardless of the PCT's intent, education will undoubtedly be a large part in the job and personal endeavors.

When PCTs choose to be the best that they can be in their role, they are often asked to be a preceptor or resource for new PCTs. An excellent PCT may provide education for others in similar roles. Learning how to be a preceptor or educator to PCTs may require attending classes or learning from role models.

Educational and personal improvement opportunities are readily available in the hospital setting. Education from coworkers either with the same job classification or from other roles is easy to obtain. Many coworkers are ready and willing to share information. The PCT can take advantage of unit slow times by asking to learn new skills at those times. Other opportunities include unit-based inservices or hospital programs in the PCT's area of interest. Finding out about hospital-based programs may involve calling the nursing education or human resource department for information. The unit manager also will aid the PCT in finding information in an area of interest. Finally, formal education advancement is available. This may mean taking part in classes in the community, junior college, or university.

Financial support for career advancement may be available at several levels. The unit may provide funding for individuals to attend certain programs. The hospital may also offer tuition reimbursement for formal college classes. The unit manager can provide information about funding possibilities. Also the government may provide financial support for those striving for college degrees. The PCT can find out about this information at the college's financial aid office.

Goal setting and actively planning to contnue learning will ensure the PCT job happiness. It will make a valued employee, increase job satisfaction, and inspire other PCTs to look for opportunities for personal growth.

Advanced Care for Common Concerns

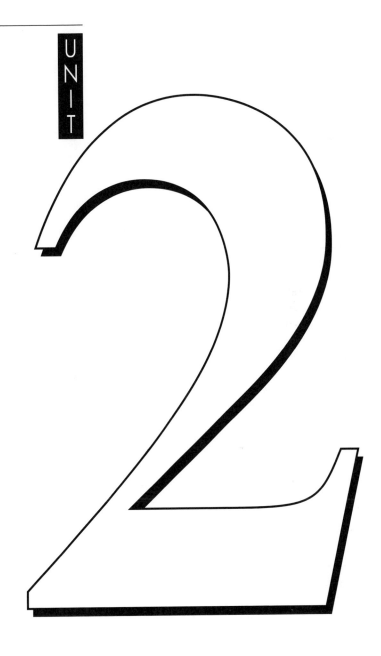

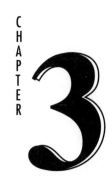

Basic Concepts

ANNE FINDEIS, MS, RN

OUTLINE

PREREQUISITE KNOWLEDGE AND SKILLS

- Handwashing
- Using gloves, masks, and isolation gowns
- Universal blood and body fluid precautions
- Sharps disposal
- Calculating fluid intake
- Feeding patients
- Basic nutrition concepts
- Basic preoperative and prediagnostic preparation procedures
- Repositioning patients

OBJECTIVES

After you complete this chapter, you will be able to:

- Describe how to use the nursing process to meet patient needs.
- Describe signs and symptoms of stress.
- Describe ways to help patients reduce stress.
- Discuss how various therapeutic diets contribute to health.
- Describe the importance of fluids to health.
- Calculate fluid restrictions.

- Describe the process of infection.
- Describe the body's defenses against infection.
- Describe ways to prevent the spread of communicable disease.
- List signs and symptoms of postsurgical complications.
- Describe ways to prevent postsurgical complications.

K E Y T E R M S

Antibodies   Proteins made by the body that help fight or prevent infection.

Cilia   Microscopic hairs that line the inside of the trachea; they sweep microscopic substances that have been inhaled up and out of the lungs.

CDC   Centers for Disease Control in Atlanta. Monitors the number and types of infectious diseases across the country. They write the national guidelines to help prevent the spread of infectious diseases.

Distal   A term that refers to the location (or distance) of a body part as it relates to the heart. For example, the fingertip is the most distal part of the arm; the ankle more distal than the knee.

Flora   A general term that refers to those microorganisms that normally live in or on the body. Under normal conditions they do not cause disease.

Hypothermia   Low body temperature.

Lesion   A general term for an abnormality. It usually refers to skin problems.

Microorganisms   A general term for microscopic forms of life, commonly used to refer to bacteria, viruses, fungi, or parasites.

MRSA   The abbreviation for *Methicillin Resistant Staphylococcus Aureus.* Pronounced *Mersah.* MRSA is a type of bacterial infection that is easily transmitted and does not respond well to antibiotic treatment.

Pathogens   Those microorganisms that cause disease.

Stoma   An opening in the body that has been created by surgery. A stoma may be temporary or permanent. If it is in the colon, it is known as a colostomy; in the trachea it is called a tracheostomy.

Stress   A physical or emotional condition that requires coping, change, or adjustment to try to achieve balance.

Stress Response   The ways in which the body attempts to adapt to stress.

Stressor   Anything that causes stress.

Tracheostomy   An opening made in the throat into the trachea to help breathing.

Vaccine   A specially designed chemical that will protect the body from a specific disease by causing antibodies to be produced against the disease.

This chapter covers many of the basic concepts needed to provide nursing care. Emphasis is placed on basic understanding of why we do what we do, rather than on specific technical skills. This chapter introduces the use of the nursing process—an organized system to assist with planning and carrying out nursing care to meet patient needs. In it we discuss patients experiencing stress, infection, surgery, and special nutritional needs. The relationship between stress, infection, and nutrition, especially in surgical patients, will be explored. Throughout the chapter the role of the patient care technician (PCT) is described as it relates to each aspect of patient care.

THE NURSING PROCESS

The PCT spends a great deal of time directly with patients. This advantage may lead the PCT to identify patient needs and problems before the RN does. This section describes the roles of the RN and PCT in using the nursing process to meet patient needs.

THE NURSE'S ROLE

The RN is ultimately responsible for developing a plan of care for each patient, for making sure the plan is carried out, and for evaluating whether the plan of care is successful in meeting patient needs. The RN uses the nursing process to accomplish this. When using the nursing process, the RN will do the following.

- Assess the patient's status to determine actual and potential health care needs or problems.

- Determine nursing diagnoses based on problems or needs.

- Plan the nursing care to meet patient needs and achieve the best possible outcome.

- Provide or delegate the nursing care that is planned.

- Evaluate how well the patient responds to the nursing care that has been provided, how well the expected outcomes have been met.

THE PCT'S ROLE

Although PCTs routinely assist the RN in carrying out nursing tasks, the PCT also assists the RN in planning the nursing care. By using a modified version of the nursing process, the PCT can help to plan and perform nursing care in an organized way that will assist all members of the nursing team. This will ensure consistency in the way nursing staff communicate, make decisions, and solve problems. It ensures efficiency in that each member of the team understands what others can and will do. The PCT can be guided by using the following approach:

- Collect information

- Determine the presence of a problem

- Identify problem-solving strategies with the RN

- Perform nursing care under the supervision of the RN

- Document the care provided.

Collect Information

Information can be collected about the patient in a variety of ways, all of which can be done as part of the PCT's routine work schedule. Valuable information is collected when you are taking vital signs, measuring intake and output, and observing eating, sleeping, mobility, and elimination patterns. Frequently medications and treatments are prescribed or withheld based on the PCT's measurements. Therefore, accuracy is critical when collecting information. Use the "Look, listen, touch, and smell" approach to collect information about the patient during daily care.

Look

Start by looking at the patient. It helps to start at the top (the head) and gradually move down to the bottom (feet) in an organized way. Do not forget the back, buttocks, and perineal areas. Bath time is the most obvious time to look at all these areas. However, any time you are working with the patient, e.g., changing a gown, repositioning the patient, or assisting the patient to use the bedpan or bathroom, there is much to be learned by looking. Chapters 5 through 13 review abnormalities to be recognized according to each body system.

Listen

Listening to the patient is one of the most important qualities of a PCT. Patients often confide in the PCT if they are the health care provider most often seen. Asking a patient to discuss feelings or problems in more detail often provides valuable information to be shared with the RN. Learning needs, emotional disturbances, or even side effects from medications can be discovered in this manner. Family members also have much to contribute about a patient's health problems, especially when the patient has limited communication. Be especially aware of statements such as, "I don't understand why I have to go through with this." If a patient or family member truly does not understand why a procedure is important, the doctor or RN must be notified so this can be explained. It is also important to listen to signs and symptoms of discomfort such as moaning, wheezing, shortness of breath, or crying during repositioning.

Touch

Touching the patient gives important information about the quality of the skin, presence of edema (swelling) or discoloration, tenderness, or other unusual characteristics. Abnormalities may indicate fluid, electrolyte, or nutritional irregularities; heart, kidney, or immune system disorders; infections or bleeding problems. Skin lesions may be (1) raised (pimples, bumps, tumors, swelling, or scars); (2) discolored (a bruise or rash); or (3) open (cuts, scrapes, wounds, or sores that are wet or glisten).

STOP Do not directly touch an open wound or drain site, even with clean gloves. Look only. Touching open wounds may spread infection.

Smell

Often a patient's breath or wound may produce an unusual or foul smell. If coming from a wound, it may indicate infection. If coming from the breath, it may indicate the presence of alcohol, gum disease, respiratory infections, lack of mouth care, or even diabetes.

STOP Be careful about smelling wound odors or breath. A mask is recommended when placing your face near or over an open wound or tracheostomy to prevent the spread of infection.

Developing the regular habit of observing the whole patient, listening, touching, and being aware of unusual odors is an organized part of collecting information that leads to the next step of recognizing problems that need nursing care. Figures 3–1 and 3–2 show situations requiring observation.

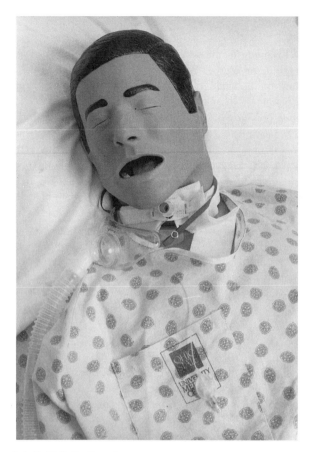

FIGURE 3-1

Notice the loose tracheostomy dressing and oxygen device.

Identify Problems or Patient Needs

The priority given to a patient situation is often directly related to the quality of the information collected. If your observations are complete and accurate, the value placed on them will be high. Also, information must be communicated clearly and in a timely manner.

Patient problems and needs may be actual or potential in nature. Actual problems may require immediate attention, for example, a patient with diarrhea. Potential problems require attention to prevent actual problems from occurring, for example, a patient who is confused may have many potential problems. This patient is at risk for falling, for skin breakdown, for nutritional deficits. The patient's need in this case is to prevent these from happening. The following questions may help to determine if a patient's need or problem exists.

- Is the patient's appearance changed or in some way unusual?

- Is the patient's behavior changed or in some way unusual?

- Are all dressings, drains, tubes, and other attached devices secure and functioning as expected?

- Is the patient able to manage basic self-care (e.g., eating, bathing, toileting, dressing)?

- Is the patient able to communicate easily?

If the answer suggests a problem, then more information needs to be collected to determine the patient's needs. This may require the RN to do additional assessment. Once the problems and needs have been identified, the next step in the process is to work with the nurse to identify strategies to deal with the actual or potential problems.

In addition to the staff RNs, RN specialists and therapists on your unit are also available as consultants if you are faced with a problem.

Identify Interventions

Identify interventions with the RN to prevent or solve a problem. Experiences from the past may lead to useful suggestions for solving problems now.

If you have an idea about trying something new to help solve a problem or meet a need, always consult with the RN first to ensure that the idea will be appropriate.

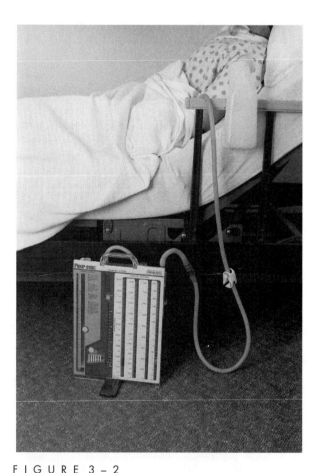

FIGURE 3-2

Note chest drainage system with tubing on floor and over side rail.

Examples of a few of the interventions that the PCT can carry out include:

- Comfort measures. Repositioning, skin care and back rubs, elevating an arm or leg, removing and reapplying support stockings or sequential compression devices, relaxation techniques, reinforcing a dressing, supporting the surgical area with pillows, assisting with deep breathing and coughing.

✔ Remember to consult with the RN about changing the position of any drainage device, tubing, traction weights, or splints when repositioning patients. Malplacement may injure the patient.

- Nourishment. Providing warm fluids, juices, snacks if allowed on diet.
- Activity. Helping the patient to move, ambulate, or perform range of motion (ROM) if not contraindicated.
- Recreation. Providing music, arranging for TV, books, magazines, puzzles, or games if available in your institution.
- Managing confusion. Using siderails, providing call light; reinforcing the date, time, and place to a confused patient; frequent monitoring and talking to the patient; safety straps when out of bed; and keeping commonly used items within reach.

Once the RN has approved specific interventions to be performed by the PCT, they are carried out promptly. When the PCT is providing care or performing procedures, it is important to monitor the patient for:

- Signs of intolerance or discomfort
- Signs that the care is ineffective

After completing the nursing care, the PCT completes the sequence by reporting back to the RN and by documenting what was done.

Documentation

This includes describing the problem, relevant observations, the intervention, and the result. For example: "1/1/95 9:15 PM. Patient complained of back pain. No redness seen on back. RN notified. Gave back rub, then turned to right side, supported with pillows, knees bent. Patient said he felt better." This documentation indicates that the PCT looked for abnormalities when the patient complained of discomfort, reported it, and provided care that helped. The RN would be responsible for any additional assessment performed or for documenting any medication given.

⚖ Each member of the nursing staff is responsible for documenting his or her own care.

The following example includes information that the RN asked the PCT to get. Although the PCT may take vital signs without a specific nursing order, when asked to do so at a nonscheduled time, results must still be documented. Because blood sugar monitoring is an invasive procedure, the RN must authorize a nonscheduled one before the PCT may perform it. "1/2/95 6 AM. Patient complained of nausea and dizziness; no emesis. RN notified. BP: 100/60, P: 110, R: 24, T: 97.6. Bedside testing of blood sugar reads 55. RN notified of reading and vital signs. Gave patient orange juice. Instructed patient to remain in bed until seen by RN."

⚖ Make sure you know the difference between tasks you can perform independently and those requiring an RN's order.

After documentation is complete, continue to monitor the patient's progress for changes. Using the nursing process will help improve the quality of your care as well as promote good working relationships with other health care workers on your team.

STRESS

Stress can be described as a demanding situation that taxes a person's ability to cope and adjust. Stress can be very threatening to a person's sense of well-being. Stress can have a negative effect on the way a person thinks about, reacts to, or even handles a situation. Physically, the body can also react in many unusual ways to stress. This can have unexpected and unwelcome effects on acute or chronically ill patients. This section discusses

- Physical and emotional causes of stress
- Physical and emotional effects of stress
- Strategies PCTs can use to help patients cope positively with stress

Causes of Stress

There are many emotional and physical causes of stress. In acute care settings, just being in the hospital is a major source of emotional stress. Uncertainty about their medical condition, lack of familiarity with procedures and the health care staff, and loss of control in managing their day-to-day lives are distressing to many people. In a long-term care facility, loss of home and lifestyle can lead to stress-related hopelessness and frustration. Children who are hospitalized experience special types of stress when surrounded by strange people and when they go through painful procedures they do not understand. Other sources of emotional stress include conflicts among family members and language or cultural differences.

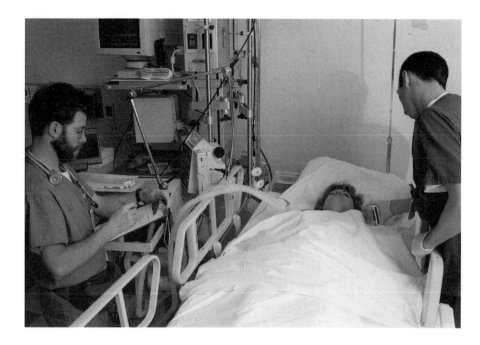

F I G U R E 3 - 3

Intensive care patients such as this with multiple IVs, and on respirators are at high risk of experiencing physical stress.

Physical causes of stress may include changes within our body or in our environment. Examples include injury after an accident, a tumor growing inside the body, an extremely hot or cold environment, pain, bleeding after surgery, an infection, or even lack of sleep. Among acutely ill patients, nearly any negative change in their condition may become a new source of stress. In such situations, stress may produce more complications and may make it difficult for a person to recover from illness or injury. One example is a person with diabetes who is hospitalized for an infection. The stress of having an infection will release chemicals in the body that cause blood sugar levels to rise. A person with diabetes whose blood sugar levels are not closely watched may develop severe complications from high blood sugar levels. Both emotional and physical causes of stress may lead to physical complications, and new and different signs and symptoms may appear. It is very important to note and report any such changes. Some of these are described below.

Effects of Stress

When stressed, the body tries to adapt to whatever is causing the stress. The cause of stress is called the *stressor*. The body's attempt to adapt is known as the *stress response*. The following effects of stress are important to consider. (1) The body uses up more energy when trying to adapt. This means more calories and nutrients are used and the person may need to eat more. (2) The body first tries to use positive ways to adapt to stress. A positive response may be an increase in motivation by the person to make decisions and solve the problem, if possible. For example, experiencing severe back pain when lifting heavy objects at work may motivate a person to seek

medical help, to take medication to ease the pain, to find a new way to lift the heavy objects without causing such pain, or to find a different job. (3) When stress is severe or lasts a long time or if positive responses do not help, then the body reacts in ways that may have a negative effect. Prolonged stress has been linked to many health problems, including heart disease, stomach ulcers, and even cancer.

Physical Effects of Stress

The body has specific ways to respond to stress. The longer or more severe the stress, the stronger and more severe the response. Examples of the physical effects of stress include the following. This is further demonstrated in Figures 3–3 and 3–4.

- Constriction of blood vessels
- Increase in blood pressure
- Increase in pulse
- Irregular pulse
- Faster or deeper breathing
- Decreased ability to fight infection
- Muscle tension
- Perspiration
- Cold hands or feet
- Headache
- Stomachache
- Nausea, vomiting, or diarrhea
- Change in appetite, weight
- Restlessness, inability to sleep

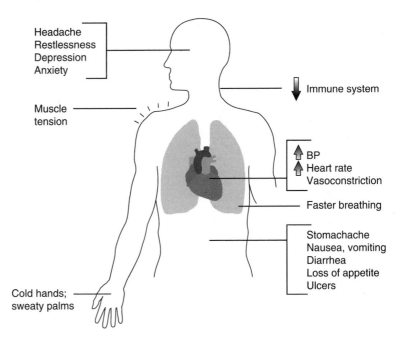

FIGURE 3-4

Stress and its impact on the body.

- Abnormal laboratory tests such as high levels of blood sugar and certain hormones

Figure 3–5 describes the relationship between stress and the effects of stress on the body.

Emotional Effects of Stress

Emotional effects include:
- Depression, withdrawal
- Anxiety, tension, nervousness

Stressed individuals may try to cope by smoking more, drinking more alcohol, taking drugs, overeating, or even denying the source of stress. Physical or verbal abuse of others is not an unusual way of trying to deal with stress. At its most extreme, stress may result in suicidal or homicidal behavior. Table 3–1 lists some of the signs and symptoms of stress that need to be reported.

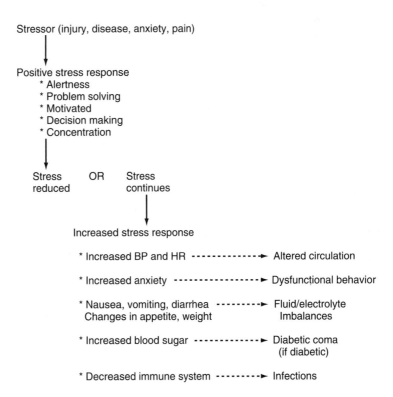

FIGURE 3-5

Relationship between stressors and stress response.

T A B L E 3 – 1
Signs of Emotional and Physical Stress

EMOTIONAL SIGNS OF STRESS
Suicidal thoughts
Noncompliance with nursing care
Anger, hostility, or violent behavior
Withdrawal, lack of communication with others
PHYSICAL SIGNS OF STRESS
Changes in vital signs
Changes in mental status, disorganized thinking
Changes in skin color or temperature
Changes in appetite
Nausea, vomiting, diarrhea

Coping Strategies

The PCT can be of great service to clients who experience stress: (1) Identify abnormal signs of stress. (2) Report abnormal signs and symptoms immediately to the RN in charge of the client. (3) Discuss interventions with the RN that will assist the patient to cope. Some ways to help clients cope with stress are described below.

Comfort

Basic comfort measures often provide relaxation for patients who are tense or uncomfortable or who cannot rest properly. Assist with repositioning as needed. Ensure that sheets are clean and dry and that the patient is warm enough. Providing a quiet, pleasing, relaxing, and comfortable environment often helps a patient feel better. If tubing, dressings, IVs, drains, or other devices are a source of discomfort, inform the RN.

Conversation

Talking with the client is another way to decrease acute or chronic emotional stress. In the acute care setting, anxiety is often highest among patients who do not know what to expect, especially those awaiting surgery. Although specific information can be given only by the RN or doctor, the PCT can provide reassurance that questions and information will be relayed and that staff will be looking out for them and be there to help. The PCT should avoid giving false reassurance and not tell patients that everything will be all right. This may not be true. If the client speaks of feeling depressed or wanting to die, report this to the RN.

Relaxation

This is useful for clients who have stress-related problems such as insomnia, headaches, muscle tension, or anxiety. Some hospitals and cancer centers offer relaxation therapy by experts as part of treatment. The PCTs should become familiar with relaxation therapy programs offered in their institution so they may assist and support patients through this valuable therapy.

Here is an example of a common method often taught that helps people relax. Start by providing quiet and privacy. Assist the patient to sit or lie in a comfortable position. Use a quiet, soothing tone of voice and have the patient close his or her eyes. Tell the patient to think of himself or herself as completely relaxed; then ask the patient to concentrate on the muscles, one part of the body at a time. Talk the patient through the relaxation training by focusing first on one part of the body and then another: for example, to feel the right arm becoming more relaxed, limp, and heavy, then the left arm, then each leg, head, eyes, and neck. Tell the patient that he or she is feeling restful, relaxed, and refreshed. The patient may need to continue this on his or her own for several minutes. It is not an exercise that can be done quickly, nor will it work if the PCT tries to hurry through.

Be sure to reinforce and assist patients in using relaxation therapies that worked successfully at home or have been taught in the hospital.

Imagery

Ask the patient to describe a pleasant, relaxing situation. Encourage the patient to fill in details. These scenes should not evoke strong emotion. Keep a quiet, relaxing tone of voice. Avoid adding your own thoughts or experiences or what you would enjoy. Once you know what the patient finds relaxing, you can refer to these scenes in the future when the person is feeling tense. For example, "Remember, Mr. Jones, how you told me about walking in the park, early in the morning, with your dog, hearing the birds singing? How peaceful that made you feel? How rested you felt? Think back to that now. Tell me more about it." And so on.

Gentle Massage

Massage can help to improve circulation, reduce tension, and promote relaxation. However, massage cannot be done on body parts that are injured, inflamed, or infected. This includes bony prominences that remain reddened from prolonged bedrest (stage I decubitus ulcers) or areas immediately around open bedsores. Massage is most effective when performed on a single body part at one time (e.g., arm, scalp, neck, back), by using circular motions, and gently kneading small muscle groups.

 The calves are not usually massaged because of the risk of dislodging blood clots, especially among bedridden patients.

Humor

The ability to laugh, when used appropriately, can be very effective in relieving short-term stress and anxiety.

Finding humor in an otherwise stressful situation can help a person cope with such a situation more effectively. Laughter has been shown to actually reverse some of the negative ways our bodies respond to stress. In some cases, laughter has been shown to decrease pain for a time, relax tense muscles, and even strengthen the immune system. Sharing humor in a natural and appropriate manner improves communication and relationships with patients.

INFECTION

Controlling the spread of infection is a major concern for all health care institutions. Both acute and chronically ill patients are at high risk for getting infections. Health care workers are at risk both for getting infections and for transmitting them to others. Therefore, it is crucial that PCTs understand the process of infection when protecting themselves and their patients from acquiring infections. This section discusses:

- The spread of infection
- The body's defenses against infection
- Precautions

The Spread of Infection

Microorganisms that survive on or in the body may be either pathogens or normal flora. *Pathogens* often come from sources outside the body (e.g., another person). Normal *flora* actually help maintain health by keeping pathogens away. However, normal flora may become disease producing under certain circumstances. This happens if normal flora travel to other parts of the body where it is not "normal." For example, if the normal intestinal bacterium *Escherichia coli* were transmitted to the bladder, it would cause an infection.

Several things must be present for an infection to occur:

1. A pathogen (source)
2. A place for the pathogen to grow (reservoir)
3. A way for the pathogen to leave the reservoir (exit port)
4. A way for the pathogen to spread (transmission)
5. A way for the pathogen to enter (entry port)

The ability of a pathogen to cause disease is related to several factors:

1. Susceptibility or resistance of the person. This is related to the immune system and the body's ability to resist infection. Stress and poor nutrition are two factors that may decrease resistance to infection. Many types of patients are at high risk, including postsurgical patients, patients with gastrointestinal disorders, cancer, AIDS,

emphysema, and diabetes. Chronic diseases put patients at risk because the body may be stressed for many years.

2. Strength or virulence of a pathogen. This is related to the pathogen's ability to survive, to reproduce, and to cause damage to the person's body tissues in spite of the body's defense mechanisms.

3. Number of pathogens that enter the person. The more pathogens present, the greater the chance of defeating the body's defense mechanisms and causing infection.

4. The environment. This may favor or interfere with the growth of the pathogen. Pathogens usually favor environments that are warm, dark, moist, and alkaline. A source of food is also necessary. Some pathogens thrive in an oxygen-rich environment like the lungs; others require total absence of oxygen.

The Body's Defenses

The body has many natural defense mechanisms designed to resist infection. These defense mechanisms are classified as primary or secondary. The role of the PCT is vital in maintaining the patient's defense mechanisms.

Primary Defense Barriers

The primary defense mechanisms consist of barriers to prevent pathogens from entering the body. Barriers to entry include the skin and mucous membranes. When the skin or mucous membranes are damaged, pathogens are more likely to enter into the body, where body tissues provide food for growth. Once inside the body, pathogens can create a reservoir directly under the skin or may travel to muscle, bone, blood vessels, and organs. Placements of IVs, drains, surgical wounds, and Foley catheters are examples of procedures that break down barriers, allowing microorganisms to enter the body and making the patient susceptible to infection at these sites. In the respiratory system, *cilia* in the trachea provide a barrier to respiratory infections. Cilia are destroyed by smoking, so smokers become less resistant to lung infections. Nasal hairs and the upper airway passages also help protect the lungs from the pathogens that are breathed in. Patients with a *tracheostomy* are at higher risk for lung infections because the *stoma* opens directly into the trachea, thereby bypassing the normal protection provided by the upper airway. See Figure 3–1 for placement of a tracheostomy.

Secondary Defense Barriers

Secondary defense mechanisms try to prevent pathogens from growing and spreading throughout the body if primary barriers have been unsuccessful. This mechanism involves the body's immune system. The immune system consists of the inflammatory response and the antibody response. When pathogens enter the body, the inflammatory response is activated. The inflammatory response is usually a local reaction that is limited to the site of the reservoir, where the pathogen first starts to grow. The body sends white blood cells to inactivate the pathogens and scavenger cells to remove them. In addition, the inflammatory response increases the blood supply to the area, which helps to promote healing of the area. Because of the inflammatory response, the site of inflammation may appear red, swollen, warm, and tender (painful). A low-grade fever (temperature 99°F) may be present.

When this initial inflammatory response is not successful in destroying the pathogens, infection develops and pathogens may spread to other areas. If pathogens enter the blood, the inflammatory response may spread throughout the body. In this case, a higher fever (temperature >101°F) is common. Weakness and loss of appetite are common. Blood vessels expand to try to meet the additional need for tissues to get blood, fluid, and nutrients. This is why with a fever the skin may appear flushed. The blood pressure may drop, and the pulse rate rise. This type of condition is very stressful for the body.

Severe inflammatory response could lead to shock and even death. Report temperatures greater than 99°F.

THE ANTIBODY RESPONSE. In addition to the inflammatory response, pathogens also trigger the antibody response. *Antibodies* are formed by the immune system to destroy specific pathogens whenever a person is exposed to them. This increases resistance to infection and may occur after exposure to the actual disease or to a *vaccine*. If antibody levels are high enough, immunity may occur. Examples of such immunity include immunity to measles, mumps, rubella, polio, and smallpox. Antibody-induced immunity may vary and last anywhere from a short time to lifelong, depending on the nature of the disease or the type of vaccine.

Be sure to report any signs of inflammation to the RN such as redness, swelling, pain, heat, tenderness, fever.

Primary and secondary defense mechanisms are affected when the immune system is weak or suppressed. This may occur when the diet is inadequate in protein, during times of severe stress when metabolism is high and nutrients are used up faster than they are replaced, or when drugs or disease weakens immune function. Patients with cancer or AIDS often have a weak immune system. Infections that develop in patients with a weak immune system are called opportunistic infections. The role of the PCT is to prevent transmission of pathogens to these patients and to report any new signs of infection.

Infection Control Practice

To effectively prevent transmission of communicable diseases, it is necessary to understand the types of pre-cautions that are taken. It is also important to understand *when* to use these precautions. The most important infection control practices are discussed below.

Category-Specific Isolation

Communicable diseases are a special class of infections noted by their ability to spread from person to person. Communicable diseases require special precautions to prevent the spread of infection; some require isolation. Precautions may be disease specific or category specific. Category-specific isolation protects patient confidentiality. Table 3–2 describes isolation categories.

Infection control nurses are responsible for infection control policies and procedures and continuing education for nursing staff. They collect information about the incidence and spread of infections, as well as pass on the latest Centers for Disease Control (CDC) and Prevention recommendations.

PCTs are responsible for ensuring that patients do not acquire infections during nursing care procedures that they perform.

Body Substance Isolation

Body substance isolation (BSI) is replacing the less restrictive universal precautions in some institutions. Body substance isolation requires the use of:

- Gloves whenever there is a possibility of hand contact with body fluids whether or not blood is present
- Gowns when frontal contamination is likely
- Mask and/or goggles when splashing or contact with sputum or other body fluid is possible

Gloves do not need to be worn when touching unbroken, intact skin or uncontaminated articles. Handwashing is still performed after removing gloves and between patients. Trash contaminated with blood is disposed of in *red* biohazard-labeled bags. Many institutions now treat all linen as potentially contaminated. Be sure to understand your institution's policy regarding disposal of linen, trash, and recyclable items.

Remember to place all needles or other sharp objects in the sharps container, *not* the garbage can. Needles are *not* to be recapped, since most needle sticks occur at that time. Assume that all used needles and sharps are contaminated.

Tuberculosis Precautions

Recently the incidence of tuberculosis (TB) has increased, especially in patients with AIDS. The *CDC* rec-

TABLE 3–2
Category-Specific Isolation Precautions

ISOLATION CATEGORY	PURPOSE	PROTECTION
Strict	To protect against highly contagious infections transmitted by both contact and air	Private room; closed door Gowns, gloves, masks for all who enter
Contact	To protect against direct physical or indirect contact with infected agents	Gloves and gown if contamination likely; masks if close to patient
Respiratory	To protect against inhaling infected air droplets	Mask at all times; keep door closed.
Enteric	To protect against contact with infected feces	Gloves and gown if contamination likely
Acid-fast bacillus (AFB)	To protect against tuberculosis (airborne)	Mask at all times
Drainage and secretion	To protect against contact with infected drainage	Gowns, gloves, and mask if contact with infected items or fluids likely
Blood and body fluid	To protect against contact with infected fluids	Gowns, gloves, and mask if contact with infected items or fluids likely
Immunosuppressed patient care	To protect patient from contact with potentially infectious organisms	Gowns, gloves, masks when coming in close contact with patient

ommends that all health care workers coming in contact with TB patients wear an approved TB respirator mask instead of traditional masks. A high-efficiency particulate air filtration (HEPA) mask (Fig. 3–6A and B) is one example of such a mask. These special TB masks offer much greater protection against the TB pathogen from entering the mask and being inhaled.

Methicillin-Resistant Staphylococcus Aureus (MRSA)

Another infection to be concerned about is MRSA. MRSA is a bacterial infection common in patients with reduced resistance to infection. It is very easily transmitted from patient to patient through the hands of health

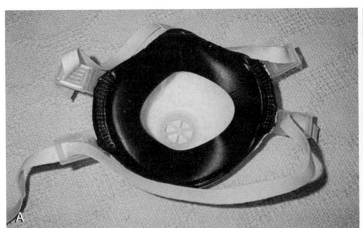

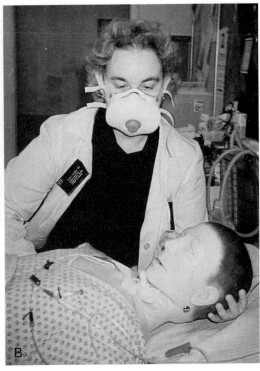

FIGURE 3–6
A, HEPA mask, inside. *B,* Nurse wearing mask when providing care.

workers. It can enter the body through the skin, nasal passages, mouth, lungs, and urethra as well as other body openings. Wounds, tracheostomies, and gastrostomy-tube–feeding sites are especially vulnerable to becoming colonized with these germs. Once transmitted, it is a difficult organism to treat. Therefore, scrupulous hand-washing is needed when the PCT is providing care to *any* patient who may be at risk. Because of the recent increase in infections that are resistant to antibiotics, appropriate isolation, BSI, and TB precautions are vital in preventing institutional epidemics of infections that cannot be treated.

NUTRITION

Proper nutrition has long been recognized as vital to maintenance of good health. Now it is also known that proper nutrition is vital for restoring health after injury or illness. To stay healthy, it is recommended that we eat a balance of foods from the different food groups. These include dairy products, meat and fish, fruits and vegetables, breads and cereals. To restore health after injury or illness, it is often necessary to change the proportion of foods in the diet. This section discusses:

- Nutrients needed by the body

- Diets used to help restore or maintain health

- Factors that affect the body's ability to use nutrients

- The importance of fluids in restoring health

- The role of the PCT in promoting health through nutrition and hydration

Nutrients

Nutrients are chemical substances found in food that provide the cells in the body with energy and enable them to function. At least 35 such nutrients are needed to live. These include vitamins, minerals, proteins, carbohydrates, fats, and water. Tables 3–3 and 3–4 list the major functions and sources of vitamins and minerals.

In particular, vitamin C is important for wound healing and vitamin K is important for normal blood clotting. These are especially important needs for patients after surgery. Vitamin K may also help prevent osteoporosis (loss of calcium from the bone). Vitamin C may also protect against heart disease and cancer. Potassium is a mineral needed to maintain muscle strength; the heart muscle in particular is sensitive to high or low levels of potassium. Life-threatening heart rhythms may occur if there is a deficiency. For this reason, attention should be paid to the pulse rate and rhythm when taking vital signs.

The fat-soluble vitamins A, D, E, and K do not need to be taken in daily; they can be stored in the fat cells in the body. They can, however, have toxic effects if taken in excessively large quantities. B-complex and C vitamins need to be taken in daily since they are not stored in the body. Excess amounts are removed through the urine.

T A B L E 3 – 3
Major Functions and Sources of Vitamins

VITAMINS	MAJOR SYSTEMS AFFECTED	PRIMARY FOOD SOURCES
Vitamin A	Vision, immune system, skin and hair	Liver, spinach, dairy products, eggs, yellow fruits and vegetables, green leafy vegetables
Vitamin B_1 (Thiamine)	Muscle and nerve function, metabolism	Pork, eggs, potatoes, whole grain foods, dried beans
Vitamin B_2 (Riboflavin)	Metabolism, growth	Milk products, whole grain products, liver, green leafy vegetables
Vitamin B_3 (Niacin)	Metabolism, nerve and intestinal function, skin	Meats, whole grain products, fish
Vitamin B_6 (Pyridoxine)	Nerve function, skin metabolism, blood cells	Whole grain products, meats, fish, potatoes
Folic acid	Red blood cells, metabolism	Liver, meats, green leafy vegetables
Vitamin B_{12}	Red blood cells, metabolism; bone, nerve and GI cell function	Meats, dairy products, eggs, fish
Vitamin C	Blood vessels, red blood cells, connective tissues, immune system	Citrus fruits, cabbage, tomatoes, potatoes, melons, strawberries, broccoli, green peppers
Vitamin D	Bones; helps body use calcium	Sunlight, fortified dairy products, fish liver oil
Vitamin E	Red blood cells; helps body use vitamins A and K	Green leafy vegetables, vegetable oils, milk products, whole grain products
Vitamin K	Blood clotting	Green leafy vegetables

TABLE 3 – 4
Mineral Chart of Functions and Food Sources

MINERALS	MAJOR SYSTEMS AFFECTED	PRIMARY FOOD SOURCES
Calcium	Bones, heart, muscle and nerve function, blood clotting	Milk products, green leafy vegetables, fish
Magnesium	Use of calcium, potassium, protein, and B vitamins; heart, nerve, and muscle function	Whole grain products, green vegetables, nuts
Phosphorus	Bones, muscle and nerve function, metabolism of nutrients	Meats, milk products, nuts
Zinc	Immune system, insulin formation, connective tissue	Meats, oysters, dried beans, nuts
Iron	Red blood cells, immune system, metabolism of vitamins	Liver, meats, whole grain products, green leafy vegetables
Iodine	Thyroid function, growth	Shellfish, iodized salt
Potassium	Nerve, muscle and heart function	Meats, fruits, vegetables
Sodium	Nerve and muscle function, fluid balance	Almost all foods, especially meats, processed and canned foods, condiments

Although fiber is not considered a nutrient, it is a valuable part of the food we eat. Fiber is not digested or absorbed; rather, it helps propel food matter through the bowel and is an important part of the diet to prevent constipation. It is also believed to help prevent gastrointestinal cancers. Fiber is found in many fruits and vegetables and in whole-grain food products. Some health problems may be helped by increasing the amount of fiber in the diet.

Therapeutic Diets

Special therapeutic diets may be ordered to increase or decrease the amounts of certain nutrients. The PCT plays an important role by monitoring food and fluid intake closely, restricting or encouraging intake of appropriate foods, and reinforcing the dietary education given by RNs or dieticians. Some important therapeutic diets are described below.

Low Sodium

Low sodium diets are salt restricted and are used primarily for those with heart or kidney disease. Low sodium diets may be mildly restricted, moderately restricted, or greatly restricted. Extra salt may not be added to foods, and salty foods are used sparingly or not at all. Although the body needs some salt to function well, too much salt in people with heart or kidney disease will cause fluid to be retained in the blood vessels. This puts a strain on the heart and makes it work harder. This can lead to problems such as swelling, high blood pressure, heart failure, and even death.

Diabetic Diets

Diabetic diets are specifically designed for persons with diabetes and are based on a person's weight and energy demands. Diabetic persons tend to experience high levels of blood sugar because of insufficient insulin. Whether diabetics are treated with oral medication, insulin shots, or neither, diet remains an important part of therapy. In general, diabetics are encouraged to maintain a balanced diet consisting of the four major food groups, with emphasis on natural fruits and vegetables rather than processed foods. Foods high in sugar or fat are limited.

Renal Diets

Renal diets are for patients who have some degree of kidney failure. Patients with kidney failure are unable to excrete some by-products of food breakdown. These build up in the body and become toxic. Nutrients that may need to be restricted include protein, potassium, sodium (salt), and phosphate. The amount of the restriction depends on the severity of the disease.

Hepatic Diets

Hepatic diets are for patients with liver disease. The liver assists in the breakdown of fats, proteins, and carbohydrates.

During acute liver problems (such as hepatitis), when patients are experiencing nausea, vomiting, and loss of appetite, they are likely to need a diet high in protein, carbohydrates, and liquids. They may have difficulty digesting fatty foods and are especially sensitive to strong odors. The PCT can help by offering the patient light meals in small portions several times a day. When liver disease is severe, patients may be placed on low salt and low protein diets. In this case, protein from vegetable and dairy sources (milk, beans) is better tolerated than protein from meats.

Cardiac Diets

Cardiac diets are for patients with some degree of heart failure. Restrictions may include sodium (salt), cholesterol, and fat. Cholesterol and fat tend to build up in the blood vessels and can lead to high blood pressure, heart attacks, and strokes.

High Metabolic Diet Needs

Some patients suffer from malnutrition and weight loss in spite of good eating habits. Increased metabolism is one cause. Increased metabolism means the body uses more energy, or calories, to function. Carbohydrates, fats, and proteins are used up at a faster rate. Patients with fever, infections, burns, cancer, or AIDS are examples of those with increased metabolism. To promote nutritional intake in these patients, the PCT can encourage patients to

- Take extra fluids and nutritional supplements *after* meals
- Eat regularly scheduled meals (do not snack intermittently)
- Take six small meals per day (if ordered)
- Add fat to foods (e.g., extra butter on vegetables)
- Add sugar to foods (e.g., in cereal, coffee)

Patients with AIDS and cancer may develop mouth sores. To encourage eating, offer foods that are cool, soft, bland, and nonacidic (i.e., no tomatoes or citrus fruits).

When patients with cancer or AIDS become nauseated:

- Avoid foods that are greasy, fatty, or spicy
- Minimize strong aromas

Calorie Counts

A calorie count may be ordered if the patient is not eating well. The nursing staff is responsible for recording *all* foods or fluids eaten that contain any calories. (Water, black coffee, black tea, or diet soda do not need to be included). The amounts ingested may be marked on the menu for convenience in cubic centimeters, ounces, teaspoons, or any other reference that can be used by the dietician to calculate calorie and nutritional intake. The physician changes diet orders on the basis of this information. An example of recording a calorie count might be as follows. "Mrs. Smith, Rm. 1123-A, Breakfast: ¼ cup orange juice, 2 tsp jello, 75 cc whole milk, ¼ slice rye toast with butter and jam, ½ slice bacon, ¼ pot coffee with 1 tsp sugar and 2 creams."

 The dietician is a good resource for information about calorie counts. She/he is responsible for calculating calories and nutrients taken by the patient.

Hydration

Fluids are vital in maintaining health. Just as every cell in the body requires nutrients, every cell also requires fluid. Usually the body's fluid needs are met by drinking when thirsty. Patients with increased metabolism, however, use up fluids very quickly. If fluid intake is inadequate, dehydration occurs. Dehydration can lead to health problems, such as poor wound healing, infection, kidney damage, dry broken skin, constipation, urinary stones, and abnormal heart rhythms. Blood pressure may drop, and a person may become weak or dizzy. The most important way to monitor for dehydration is by monitoring urine output. This is especially important to monitor in patients who have had recent surgery or who take medication to increase urine output (diuretics).

 The PCT observes if patients void regularly and reports urine outputs less than 250 cc per shift (or 30 cc per hour).

Fluid overload (or excess fluid intake) is a problem primarily for patients who already have heart or kidney failure. In these cases, too much fluid puts a strain on the heart. The heart loses the ability to pump, and death can result. The PCT works closely with the nurse to calculate, monitor, and regulate oral fluid intake. Many of these patients are on fluid restrictions.

Fluid Restrictions

Fluid restrictions may vary from 800 to 2000 cc per day. The more severe the heart or kidney failure, the more restricted the fluid intake. The PCT works with the RN and the patient to determine the amount allowed for the shift and for the meal. If the restriction does not include IVs, the PCT can calculate the amount allowed. There is no *one* right way to calculate how much fluid should be allowed at one time. Tables 3–5 and 3–6 offer one suggestion.

Post the fluid restriction at the bedside for other nursing staff as well as family members.

Other tips for managing fluid-restricted patients include:

- Do not fill the water pitchers for these patients.
- Use a glass to provide small amounts of ice chips throughout the shift for patients who are thirsty.
- Include ice chips when calculating intake. (1 glass ice chips equals ½ glass water)

TABLE 3 – 5
Calculating Fluid Restrictions

WHEN CALCULATING FLUID RESTRICTION

1. Allow for the following:
   ½ intake for 7–3 shift
   ⅓ intake for 3–11 shift
   ⅙ intake for 11–7 shift
2. Calculate about ½ to ⅓ of shift allowance for each meal.
3. Review totals to make sure patient receives at least 100 cc for night shift.
4. Make sure fluids are allotted reasonably and add up to the total fluid restriction.

- Check meal trays to make sure the right amount of fluid is present.

- If excess fluids are present on the meal tray, let the patient choose which should be removed.

- Document fluid intake immediately after ingestion.

SURGICAL PATIENT CARE

Patients requiring surgery have special needs both before and after surgery. Preoperatively, patients' most important needs include preparation for the surgical and postsurgical experience. Nursing staff must follow specific preoperative preparation instructions. Postoperatively, patients' most important needs include prevention of common postoperative complications and assistance in reaching the fullest recovery possible. This section discusses the role of the PCT in:

- Preparing patients during the preoperative phase

- Recognizing and preventing postoperative complications

TABLE 3 – 6
Sample Fluid Restriction

	800 CC/DAY	1000 CC/DAY	1200 CC/DAY	1500 CC/DAY
7–3 Shift	400	500	600	700
Breakfast	(150)	(200)	(250)	(250)
Lunch	(150)	(200)	(250)	(250)
Extra	(100)	(100)	(100)	(200)
3–11 Shift	300	350	400	500
Dinner	(200)	(200)	(250)	(300)
Extra	(100)	(150)	(150)	(200)
11–7 Shift	100	150	200	300

Preoperative Patient Preparation

Patient education is one of the most important aspects of preparing patients for surgery. Although RNs are responsible for preoperative patient teaching, the PCT is expected to reinforce patient teaching. Patients may not remember everything the first time they are told, especially if they are anxious. Patient teaching is especially important for patients who are going to have general anesthesia, since recovery can be more difficult than for those who have local or even spinal anesthesia. The better prepared a patient is *before* surgery, the greater the chance that the person will cope with the stress of surgery in a more positive way, improving the chances for a complication-free recovery.

The type of information (or reinforced teaching) PCTs need to give to patients consists of the following:

- Food/fluid restrictions: Patients may need to restrict their intake prior to surgery to prevent nausea, vomiting, and aspiration during or after the procedure. Instruct the patient whether or not to remain NPO, when, and for how long. Patients undergoing general anesthesia often must be NPO after midnight the night before surgery. In some cases, doctors will order for patients to be NPO after 4 AM or even after breakfast. Patients requiring local or spinal anesthetics might receive nourishment before the procedure or be NPO for only a few hours. This depends on the type of procedure as well as on the drugs that will be administered. Children and infants will be NPO for a specified period depending on their age or body weight.

Always check with the RN regarding diet or fluid restrictions for patients scheduled for any type of surgery or special procedure.

- Cleansing. If a special shampoo or shower is ordered the night before, instruct the patient to clean the area thoroughly. Cleaning the area thoroughly before surgery reduces the number of microorganisms present on the skin and reduces the chance of postoperative infection. Patients should avoid scrubbing too hard (this may cause irritation and inflammation).

- Enemas. If the order reads "Tap water enema (TWE) till clear" it will be necessary to look at the bowel contents after each enema to determine if more enemas are necessary. The goal is to give enemas until the return from the bowel is free from stool. Therefore, inform the patient that several enemas may be needed and not to flush the toilet. Emptying the colon of all stool helps the doctor see more clearly and also removes many of the bacteria present in the colon. If stool is still present after 3 TWEs, the RN is notified. After assessing the situation, the RN may require you to continue giving more enemas or may ask you to stop. This procedure is required before intestinal surgery or special diagnostic procedures.

• Bowel Evacuants. Go-Lytely is a drink that is commonly used to empty the bowel before bowel surgery or other special procedures. The PCT may be requested to assist the patient with this preparation. Instruct the patient to drink the whole quantity (4 to 5 liters) the evening before the procedure. Encourage patients to drink each liter over 30 to 45 minutes for it to be effective. If allowed, encourage the patient to walk around during this time to help the liquid pass through the stomach. Nausea may be a side effect, especially if the patient is drinking too fast. The patient may stop for a short time until the nausea subsides, then continue to drink. About 2 hours after drinking Go-Lytely, the patient will start to feel the urge to defecate. Bowel contents will become loose, and defecation will occur frequently.

Information related to preventing postoperative complications: If undergoing general anesthesia, patients should be prepared for the need to:

• Turn every 2 hours to prevent skin breakdown.

• Take deep breaths, cough hourly, and use an incentive spirometer (Fig. 3–7) to prevent pneumonia. To assist the patient to use the incentive spirometer, instruct the patient to place the mouthpiece securely in the mouth.

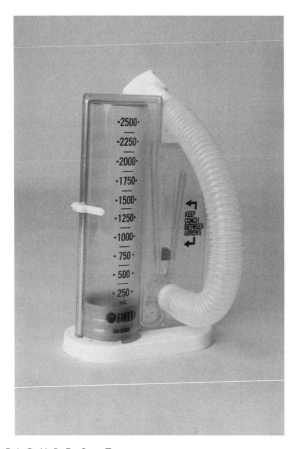

FIGURE 3–7

Incentive spirometer. Used to stimulate deep breathing and coughing after surgery.

Then holding the spirometer comfortably at eye level, exhale slowly and deeply to remove all the air in the lungs. Immediately inhale as deeply as possible. The white disk (or ball) will rise up to indicate the volume of air that the patient has breathed in. The RN or respiratory therapist will indicate the desired level to be achieved. Encourage patients to breathe in steadily and fully, keeping the blue float on the right in Figure 3–7 between the arrows. This allows for maximum lung inflation. Patients usually perform this 10 times each hour (while awake) during the first few days after surgery.

• Perform range of motion (ROM) exercises to stimulate circulation in the extremities.

• Wear thrombo-embolytic device (TED) hose or sequential compression devices (SCDs) to stimulate circulation and prevent blood clots from developing in the legs (Figs. 3–8 and 3–9). SCDs are sleeves that are wrapped around the patient's legs and attached to a machine that inflates and deflates the sleeves with a pre-set amount of air.

Pressure limits may be set on the machine and should be kept within the normal range of 35 to 55 mm Hg. If the pressure is too low, the sleeves are not adequately inflated and the SCD is ineffective. If the pressure is too high, overinflation may cause trauma to sensitive tissue. SCDs must also be the correct size. The correct size can be obtained by measuring the length of the leg and the width of the thigh 8 inches above the knee. Instructions for measuring and applying SCDs are located on the package. Some SCDs also have an optional sleeve cooling switch on the machine. This allows cool air to flow onto the skin periodically and helps prevent the skin from becoming too warm.

SCDs are kept on continuously while the patient is on bedrest. The PCT will be expected to remove the TED hose and SCDs to cleanse the legs. SCDs may also be removed temporarily to assist the patient to the bathroom or to the chair. Use of SCDs is usually discontinued once the patient is ambulatory.

ROM exercises, TED hose, and SCDs work by putting pressure on the muscles of the legs. This compresses the veins, pushing blood back up to the heart. Usually our muscles perform this activity when walking. Patients on bedrest or limited mobility need the additional help these supportive devices provide to prevent blood clots from developing in the veins.

Postoperative Care

Patients usually spend about 2 hours in the recovery room. Time spent in recovery allows the patient to waken from general anesthesia and for vital signs to stabilize. The RNs monitor the patient for signs of hemorrhage or

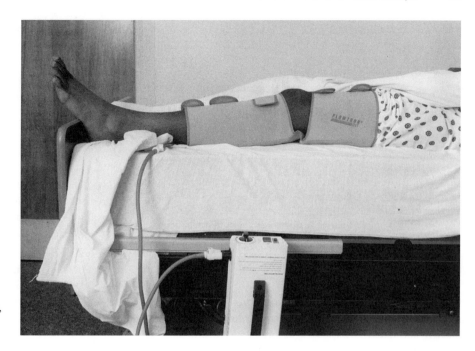

FIGURE 3–8

Sequential compression device sleeve, side view. Note opening over knee. This allows patient to bend leg.

other life-threatening complications. Once stabilized, the patient is transported back to the room. The PCT informs the RN that the patient has arrived. An RN should be present when the patient is transferred from the cart to the bed to complete an initial assessment. Special care must be taken during transfer because the patient is usually very weak and cannot offer much assistance. Also, the patient should be transferred gently to prevent incisional pain.

⚖ The RN is ultimately responsible for ensuring patient safety during the transfer and for performing a complete assessment.

The PCT provides a valuable service by:

- Organizing patient care supplies
- Noting relevant observations during the immediate postrecovery phase
- Assisting the patient to meet comfort and safety needs
- Providing care that will help the patient achieve the greatest possible recovery

Organizing Patient Care Supplies

Many items can be set up in advance. Once the recovery room nurse has given report to the RN on the unit, the room setup can be delegated to the PCT. This may include items such as:

- Suction setup

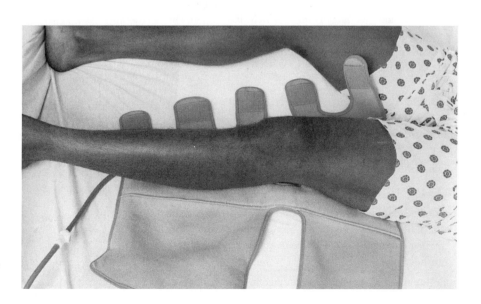

FIGURE 3–9

Sequential compression device sleeve, front view and open sleeve. Openings should fit over and behind knee.

- Monitoring equipment
- Emesis basin, bedpan
- Sequential compression pump
- Documentation records
- Disposable drainage pads
- IV poles
- Thermometer
- Extra blanket, towels, washcloth
- Incentive spirometer
- Oxygen flowmeter and setup

Observations During the Immediate Postrecovery Phase

When the patient is received from recovery, one of the first priorities after the patient is transferred to the bed is to take vital signs. This is of the utmost importance so the RN can determine changes and trends that indicate complications. Often patients are *hypothermic* and need to be rewarmed. Pulse and blood pressure may be lower than preoperatively as a result of the effects of anesthetics or other medications. Respirations may also be slow or irregular because of the effects of anesthesia or drugs.

✓ Although certain symptoms occur commonly after surgery, they are still considered abnormal and should be reported. It is the RN's responsibility to determine what, if any, action should be taken related to the symptom.

Often, vital sign determinations are ordered more frequently when patients return from recovery. It is not unusual to take them every 15 minutes for the first hour, every 30 minutes for the second hour, every hour for the next 2 hours, and then every 4 hours. This routine is also followed when a patient returns from a special diagnostic procedure, such as angiography, which may result in complications. By monitoring vital signs frequently, the PCT can quickly observe and report changes in the patient's condition.

🔔 Be alert to a drop in blood pressure with a rise in pulse rate at the same time. This is a classic sign of hemorrhage.

Other things to be watched for include:

- Comfort: Degree of pain or other discomfort
- Safety: Siderails and call lights are especially important if a patient is temporarily disoriented or receiving pain medication. Patients need more assistance until they are fully recovered.
- Equipment: Report if any equipment becomes loose,

disconnected, or otherwise appears to be malfunctioning.

- Changes in behavior. A patient who suddenly becomes confused, disoriented, or agitated could be experiencing physical abnormalities such as inadequate oxygen or electrolyte levels.
- Changes in skin color. Pallor or gray or blue-tinged skin may be a sign of poor circulation or inadequate oxygen.
- Nausea: Often patients are nauseated and vomit during the recovery phase because of general anesthesia and medication. Have an emesis basin, towel, and wash cloth readily available.
- Bowel activity: Peristaltic activity in the bowel is halted by the effects of anesthesia. The patient is not permitted to eat or drink anything until the RN notes that bowel sounds have returned. The RN guides gradual resumption of clear liquids, full liquids, and then food.

Hazards of Immobility

Postsurgical patients often have the same nursing care needs as those who have been on prolonged bedrest. Surgery sometimes lasts several hours. During that time the patient is confined to one position. Even in the recovery room patients are not usually repositioned, since positional changes could affect the stability of the heart. So by the time patients arrive on the unit they may already be experiencing some of the complications of immobility. In addition, anesthesia and other drugs may affect the body in various negative ways. See Table 3–7 for a description of common postoperative complications and nursing care.

Mobility is one of the most important aspects of nursing care after surgery that involves general anesthesia. Immobility can result in:

- Skin breakdown and ulcerations
- Muscle weakness and general debilitation
- Bone fragility due to loss of calcium (increases risk of fractures)
- Pneumonia
- Blood clots in the leg veins. These can break loose and travel to the heart and lungs, becoming life threatening.
- Urinary stasis, urinary tract infection, and urinary stones.
- Constipation
- Depression

In the immediate postoperative period, mobility is often limited. However, the nursing goal is always to increase activity as quickly as possible and as much as is safely possible. The PCT needs to understand each individual patient's activity level to include appropriate activity

TABLE 3-7
Surgical Complications and Nursing Care

BODY SYSTEM	POSSIBLE EFFECTS OR COMPLICATIONS AFTER SURGERY	NURSING CARE TO PREVENT COMPLICATIONS
Neurological	Sleepy, sluggish, confused, disoriented because of anesthesia or medication Patients at risk for falls	Monitor levels of consciousness; reorient patient to environment, date, and times Side rail up; assist with ambulation; put call light within reach; care with transfers
Respiratory	Shallow or slightly irregular respirations; accumulation of mucous secretions in lungs; pneumonia a common complication from immobility after surgery	To prevent pneumonia, turn q2h and have patient use incentive spirometer; coughing and deep breathing q1–2h; report dyspnea
Cardiac and vascular	Low blood pressure and/or higher pulse—in response to anesthesia, drugs, or blood loss High blood pressure if heart has to work harder than usual Blood clots in legs (deep vein thrombosis); if blood clots become loose, they can travel to the lungs (pulmonary emboli); if severe, can cause death	Monitor and report changes from normal or outside normal range Turn q2h to stimulate circulation Encourage drinking fluids if allowed, to help increase low blood pressure Apply antithrombotic stockings; apply sequential compression devices; perform ROM and leg exercises q4h
Skin	Pale, cool, blue tinged if circulation poor Decubiti over posterior bony prominences from prolonged positioning in surgery	Monitor and report changes from normal skin characteristics Turn q2h; avoid massaging any reddened areas
Gastrointestinal	Nausea and vomiting effect of anesthesia Constipation several days after surgery, due to anesthesia, lack of food, physical inactivity	Monitor and report any evidence of these symptoms Hold food/fluids if emesis occurs until consultation with RN If consistent with doctor's orders, offer fluids, and foods with fiber to prevent or treat constipation; also encourage ambulation
Urinary	Decreased urine output due to prolonged NPO status and possible dehydration Patients who are dehydrated and also on prolonged bedrest at risk for developing bladder stones and urinary tract infections	Monitor and report urine output less than 30 cc/h (if measuring hourly) or less than 250 cc/8-hr shift If allowed, encourage water and other liquids frequently Reposition q2h; ambulate often if allowed
Surgical wound	Bleeding the most important complication in the immediate postsurgical period Infection a complication that takes several days to appear	Monitor and report signs of bleeding through or around any dressing or drain Make sure tubes, drains, and dressings remain secure and do not become dislodged Avoid handling the surgical wound or drain sites directly—germs may be introduced that can cause infection. Do not reapply a loose dressing—report immediately to the RN
Fluid and nutrition	Dehydration, inadequate vitamin, mineral, and protein intake are most likely to occur in patients who are NPO or on liquid diets for several days Inadequate vitamin C and protein may interfere with wound healing Inadequate levels of vitamin K and vitamin C can interfere with blood clotting. This can lead to excess bleeding	If diet permits, encourage increased intake of protein—meats, fish, eggs, cheese, beans; vitamin C—citrus fruits, potatoes, cabbage, tomatoes; vitamin K—green leafy vegetables Encourage fluid intake

when providing care, thus preventing many of the hazards of immobility.

Care of Patients after Spinal Anesthesia

A patient who receives spinal anesthesia receives an injection in the spine that will cause numbness and immobility below that site, usually from the waist down. Spinal anesthesia has an advantage over general anesthesia because patients are awake during the procedure yet feel no pain. Also, spinal anesthesia does not have the many potential complications that general anesthesia does. However, because the anesthetic is placed into the person's spinal area, there is a risk of causing nerve damage. Sensation and movement must be checked frequently to determine that the condition is improving and that permanent nerve damage is not present. Awaiting the return of sensation and movement is often of great concern to the patient. Because it may take several hours for these effects to wear off, the patient is totally dependent on the nursing staff during this time to meet mobility and elimination needs. Feeling and movement gradually return to the patient from the toes first.

✓ Notify the RN if there is no apparent return of sensation or movement in the lower extremities.

Transferring Spinal Cord Patients

Special attention needs to be paid to transferring patients who have had spinal anesthesia. Do not assume that patients can move and transfer themselves easily just because they are alert, speaking, and cooperative. Because spinal anesthesia causes temporary paralysis, full support needs to be given to the back, hips, and lower extremities to avoid injury to the area where surgery was performed.

DIAGNOSTIC PROCEDURES

Occasionally the PCT will be required to care for patients who have special care needs after undergoing diagnostic tests. A few of these tests require nearly as much postprocedural attention as surgical procedures. The risk for complications is also high. Two of these, angiography and myelography, are discussed below.

Post-Angiography Care

Angiography is a special diagnostic procedure in which an IV injection catheter is inserted into an artery or vein, dye is injected, and X-rays are obtained to check the circulation in a particular part of the body. The femoral artery or vein is commonly chosen as an injection site. The IV injection catheter is removed after the procedure and the site covered with a Band-Aid if a vein is used or a small pressure dressing if an artery is used. The major potential complication after angiography is bleeding and subsequent loss of circulation. When receiving the patient back after an angiogram is obtained, it is important to check the following:

- Vital signs. A drop in blood pressure (about 10 mm Hg) should be reported immediately as a possible sign of bleeding.
- Injection site for bleeding, swelling, or bruising. Any new bleeding, swelling, or bruising should be reported immediately to the RN.
- Pulse at the injection site (unless a pressure dressing is applied). Check for pulse strength. It should be easily felt (Fig. 3–10).
- Distal pulses. For example, if the femoral site is used, also check the pedal pulse. If the brachial site is used, check the radial pulse at the wrist.

🔊RN A pulse that is weak or absence of a pulse is a sign of impaired circulation and should be reported immediately.

- Color, movement, and temperature of the distal part of

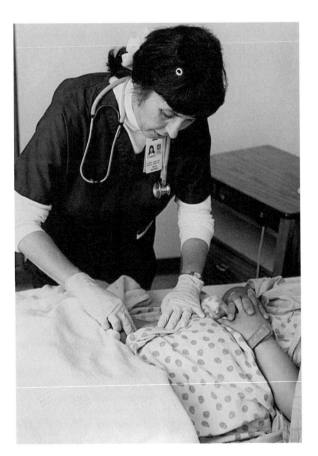

F I G U R E 3 – 1 0

Post-angiogram checks—locating femoral pulse and checking injection site.

the extremity. For example, check the toes if the femoral site is used or the fingers if a brachial site is used. Color and movement should be the same as before the procedure (or better). It should never appear worse. For example, the color might be described as pink, pale, or cyanotic. Among black or dark-skinned people, the term *pink* may still be used to describe healthy tissue. Usually the nail bed is checked, and this is normally pink among people of all races. A person who could "wiggle" the toes before the procedure should be able to do so afterward. Numbness, tingling, and burning should be reported immediately. Skin temperature should be the same as before the procedure. Cold skin implies poor circulation and should be reported if new. Compare both extremities to determine if abnormalities occur.

A patient should first be assessed by the RN after returning from this procedure. Thereafter, a PCT properly trained continues these measurements and observations and alerts the RN about any changes.

In some cases, sandbags or ice is applied to the injection site. Either may help prevent bleeding. However, the pulse and site must still be checked. Carefully remove the sandbag or ice bag, check the pulse and site, and replace the bag directly over the injection site so that it will not fall off.

Patients are also required to maintain bedrest for several hours afterward to immobilize the puncture, promote healing, and prevent bleeding. This means that the patient cannot bend the affected leg or use it to assist during transfer. Thus, this procedure may require up to 4 people to assist in a transfer. Once the patient is back in bed, the leg must remain flat for 8 hours. Use special precautions with meals or elimination. At no time should the head of the bed be elevated more than 45 degrees. To assist the patient with meals, either prop the head up

with a rolled towel or logroll the patient onto the side, keeping the affected leg straight. Logrolling is not recommended if sandbags or icebags are in use. Patients will likely need more assistance with meals at this time to avoid spilling or placing a strain on the injection site.

> Remember that an arterial puncture is more likely to hemorrhage than a venous puncture and therefore needs much closer monitoring.

Post-Myelography Care

Myelography is a special diagnostic procedure in which dye is injected into the lower spinal canal to detect spinal cord abnormalities. After the procedure, the patient remains on bedrest for several hours. Depending on the type of dye used, the orders may require the head of the bed to be elevated or to be flat.

> After a myelogram is obtained, the patient should be observed for fever, stiff neck, headache, seizures, or drainage. Any of these may indicate infection in the spinal canal.

Fluids are usually encouraged after both angiography and myelography, and voiding should be monitored. This is because the dye used in these procedures may contribute to dehydration. Therefore, intake and output should be strictly monitored for the first 24 hours after the procedure or until the RN changes the order.

The concepts discussed in this chapter are basic essentials to providing quality patient care. The PCT can apply the concepts of stress, nutrition, and infection control to the care of all patients, especially postoperative patients. The PCT now has the tools needed to work with the RN to plan and carry out nursing care in a coordinated and efficient manner.

4

Interpersonal Relationships and Communication

JEAN A. JUST, MSN, RN,C, CS

PREREQUISITE KNOWLEDGE AND SKILLS

- Patient-focused care
- Unit communication
- Teamwork
- Quality care and improvement
- Assisting family involvement
- Meeting needs and solving problems
- Stress: Body's response

O B J E C T I V E S
After you complete this chapter, you will be able to:

- Identify the building blocks of effective communication.
- Recognize barriers that commonly block the communication process.
- Define communication tools to strengthen work relationships.

- Cite communication strategies for relating to patients and families.
- Develop techniques to cope with challenging patient behaviors.

K E Y T E R M S

Anxiety Internal tension due to a general or specific fear

Communication Breakdown A block that stops the flow of information

Communication Process Methods to give and receive information

Conflict Disagreement between individuals

Defensiveness Protection from a perceived attack

Expectations What you want another person to do or say

Interpersonal Skills Ability to effectively deal with people

Verbal Abuse Personal attack that lowers self-esteem

With learning and practice, patient care technicians (PCTs) have no difficulty mastering those technical skills related to their advanced practice. What are difficult to master in most work situations are those skills known as interpersonal skills. Interpersonal skills refer to how we communicate, interact, and relate to other individuals, including coworkers, patients, and their families. Some of the most challenging work-related situations come from difficulties with interpersonal relationships and communication. However, interpersonal skills can be understood, practiced, and mastered just like technical skills.

BUILDING BLOCKS OF EFFECTIVE COMMUNICATION

Sender, Message, Receiver, Feedback

There are four main aspects to consider when communicating. They are the person giving the communication, the person receiving the communication, the message being communicated, and feedback. The person giving the communication is like a pitcher in a baseball game. The ball is the message to be communicated, and the catcher is the person who receives the communication. It is not possible to be successful in the game if you do not have a pitcher, catcher, and ball. A sender, message, and receiver are necessary for success in the communication process. The catcher lets the pitcher know she or he got the ball and signals if the pitcher needs to change the way the ball is being pitched. In the communication

process, when the receiver lets the sender know she or he got the message this is known as feedback (Fig. 4–1).

Verbal, Nonverbal Messages

There are two main ways to give a message and provide feedback. One way is by the spoken word or verbal communication. The other way is by use of body language or nonverbal communication. An example of nonverbal communication is looking at your watch or rolling your eyes when someone is trying to give you information. Often, nonverbal communication "speaks" louder than verbal communication and sends a very strong message to the receiver. Sometimes nonverbal communication is given without the sender's being aware it is happening. Remember, there is never a time we are not communicating. Even when sitting quietly in a chair, nonverbal communication is taking place (Fig. 4–2).

The following are examples of nonverbal communication:

- Foot tapping or jiggling
- Crossed arms
- Smile, smirk, or frown
- Heavy sighs
- Wringing hands
- Shrugging shoulders
- Squinting or glaring eyes

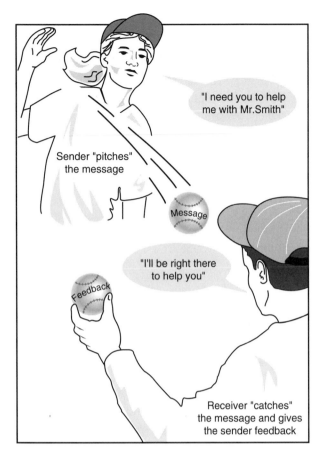

F I G U R E 4 – 1

The communication process.

BARRIERS TO THE COMMUNICATION PROCESS

Communication sounds like a simple process. As stated previously, it has four main parts—a giver, a message, a receiver, and feedback. The receiver lets the sender know he or she got the message by means of feedback. Although this should be easy to accomplish, the reality is there are many factors that can complicate the communication process (Fig. 4–3).

Background and Culture

Some of these factors are backgrounds and cultures of the two people involved in the communication. Each comes with individual past experiences, beliefs, and values. Often these are things learned while growing up in families. A person may have been raised in a culture in which it is disrespectful to look someone in the eye when speaking to him or her or has a belief that women do not question what is said by a man. These factors can get in the way of sending, receiving, and understanding the message, because both parties do not share common meanings. The message perceived by the receiver is not

the meaning intended by the sender, and miscommunication results.

Mixed Messages

Mixed messages can create barriers to communication. A mixed message occurs when verbal and nonverbal communications do not match. For example, a person may say he or she feels awful yet be smiling, or say everything is going great but be frowning and sighing. When a message is given and the verbal and nonverbals do not match, it is very confusing for the receiver to understand the true meaning of the message. Usually the receiver will associate the nonverbal communication with the true message. The adage "actions speak louder than words" tends to hold true.

Tone of Voice and Word Choice

Tone of voice and choice of words also can present a barrier to communication. Words spoken in a loud harsh tone take on an entirely different meaning than the same words spoken in a soft quiet tone. Thinking before speaking can help with choosing the "right" words to convey the message. Once communication with another person has occurred, it is impossible to take it back.

Poor Listening Skills

Poor listening skills are another barrier in the communication process. Often we are too busy thinking about our response and miss the intent or purpose of the mes-

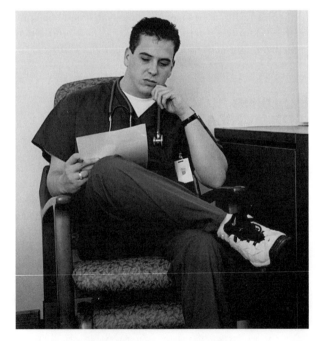

F I G U R E 4 – 2

This nonverbal communication sends a message of disgust and frustration.

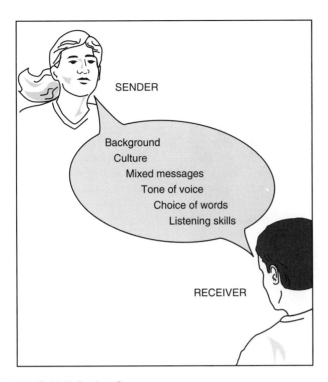

F I G U R E   4 – 3
Barriers to the communication process.

sage being sent. Listening takes work and is one of the most important parts of the communication process. Learning to be an "active" listener, someone who concentrates and focuses his or her full attention on listening, takes practice. Using the listening tips listed below will assist you in becoming a better listener:

- Maintain eye contact
- Give your full attention
- Avoid distractions
- Focus on the content of the message
- Hear out the other person
- Avoid jumping in with your reply

Tips to Avoid Communication Barriers

Although communication is a challenge, remembering these simple rules will help you communicate more effectively:

- Practice active listening skills
- Avoid sending mixed messages
- Respect and recognize the effect of individual differences
- Be aware of nonverbal communication
- Carefully choose your words and tone of voice
- Never forget that effective communication is hard work

COMMUNICATION TECHNIQUES TO STRENGTHEN WORK RELATIONSHIPS

There are specific communication techniques that can be used to support successful relationships with coworkers. The trend today in many work places is having individuals work together as a team. This is seen in health care with the emphasis on patient-focused care. Members of work teams need to have excellent communication skills to promote teamwork. Assertive communication is key for workers to function as an effective team and is an interpersonal skill valued by most employers.

Personality Styles

Individuals have different personality styles. A personality style or behavior style is the way a person presents himself or herself to others. The four main types of personality styles are passive, aggressive, passive-aggressive, and assertive.

Passive Behavior

When individuals exhibit a passive personality style their behaviors are generally labeled as meek or mild. They often are quiet and do not let others know what they think or feel. Passive individuals usually have difficulty making eye contact, have a slumped posture, and speak in a quiet voice. The tendency is for these individuals to hold everything inside because they do not want to risk hurting anyone's feelings or "stepping on toes." Their sense of self-esteem (feeling good about themselves) is not very high, so they do not feel comfortable communicating their needs to others.

Aggressive Behavior

Individuals with aggressive personality styles are easy to spot. They tend to be loud, pushy, and obnoxious. Their attitude is they are always right and the other person is wrong. A favorite blaming pose for aggressive persons is to stand with a hand on the hip and point a finger in another person's face. Since aggressive people do not feel too good about themselves they may try to intimidate or frighten others to get what they need (Fig. 4–4).

Passive-Aggressive Behavior

Passive-aggressive behavior tends to be sneaky and hidden. While the aggressive personality is downright nasty, passive-aggressive persons take out their anger in ways that are not always obvious. For example, someone who is passive-aggressive may "forget" to give an important message or not follow through on an assignment. You may walk away from an interaction with these individuals with a "gotcha again" feeling. The reason for passive-aggressive behavior stems from low self-esteem.

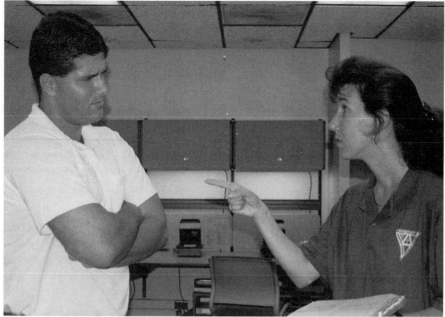

FIGURE 4 – 4

Finger pointing is a common pose for persons with an aggressive personality style.

These individuals have not learned how to directly ask for what they need, so they try to get needs met indirectly by manipulation.

Why are some people passive, aggressive, or passive-aggressive? Many times it is because these individuals have low self-esteem and are trying to provide a way to protect themselves. They use meekness, anger, and sneakiness as walls to hide behind and keep others away. These behaviors are usually learned in childhood and tend to be primary ways of relating to others. However, in specific situations, behavior may be altered. For instance, someone might risk being aggressive toward a spouse but resort to passive-aggressive behavior when relating to a superior.

Assertive Behavior

Assertive behavior is marked by direct, open, and honest communication. Assertive individuals have their needs met by asking for what they need. Because they have a high sense of self-esteem and do not need to build walls of protection, assertive individuals are respectful of the needs of others. They look you in the eye when speaking, have an erect posture, and speak in a clear firm voice.

Although it is impossible to be assertive 100% of the time, strive to be assertive as much as possible. How can you tell if you are being assertive? The following clues will help you determine if your behavior is assertive (Fig. 4–5).

- Respectful of self and others
- Increases feelings of self-esteem
- Decreases negative feelings

- Creates confidence
- Generates positive responses from others

Assertive Skills

There are specific skills that will help you be more assertive. These skills are knowing how to:

- Give an "I" message
- Make and refuse requests
- Clarify expectations
- Give and receive feedback

"I" Message

When an "I" message (messages that begin with *I*) is used, the giver of the message takes responsibility for what is communicated. The message "I feel frustrated when you don't help me" has a different meaning from the message "You make me frustrated when you don't help me." "You" messages (messages that begin with *you*) tend to place blame on the other person. When someone feels blamed, it becomes more difficult for that person to hear the message, and a breakdown in communication can occur.

I messages have three basic parts that are:

- I feel _____ (Describe your feeling.)
- When you _____ (Describe the other person's behavior.)
- I'd like you to do or say this instead _____ (How would you like the behavior to change?)

An example of an *I* message would be to say, "I feel angry when you return late from lunch and cut my lunch

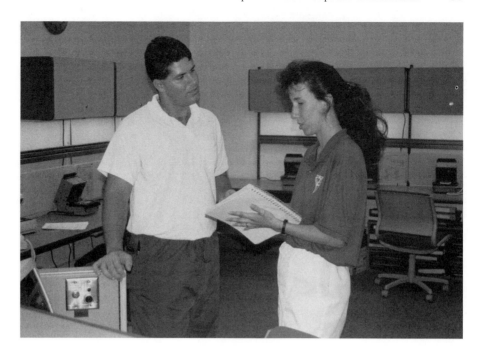

FIGURE 4-5
Assertive coworkers communicate respect and generate positive responses in others.

time short. I would like you to return from lunch on time so I am able to take my full break." It's important to add the part about what you would like the other person to do or say instead. Many people will not know how you would like their behavior to change unless you are direct in your communication. Giving an *I* message is not easy and does not come naturally, but it is an important assertive skill to learn. Using *I* messages will become easier with practice.

Make and Refuse Requests

Understanding how to make and refuse requests is another assertive skill that is important in the work place. To assertively make a request, directly state what you need or want from the other person. For example, "I need you to help me get Mr. Smith in a chair so I can make his bed" or "I want to be assigned to go to lunch first since Mrs. Martinez will be back from surgery early." Avoid the temptation to hint at what you want from the other person. Many times if you are indirect or vague, the other person will not understand your message.

Refusing a request can be tricky. Everyone has the right to refuse an unreasonable request, but the key is to learn the correct way. If a supervisor makes a request and you respond by saying, "Forget it, are you crazy?" or "No way am I taking care of Mr. Jones today!" you risk being viewed as an unhelpful member of the work team. Instead, refuse a request by saying "I'm not able to draw Mrs. Chen's blood because I have to do a stat ECG on Mr. Gomez" or "I'm not able to do 5 complete baths and all the blood draws and sterile dressings for the unit." Try to get the other person involved in a discussion of the situation by asking, "What other options or choices

do we have?" This type of question will help discover other solutions yet still convey your willingness to be a team player.

Clarify Expectations

Misunderstandings happen when clear expectations are not communicated between two people. An RN might say, "Take Mr. Smith's blood pressure." From this type of message the expectations are unclear and need to be clarified. To clarify expectations, ask questions such as "When would you like Mr. Smith's blood pressure taken?" and "After I take Mr. Smith's blood pressure, would you like me to tell you what it is or will you get the information from the documentation in the chart?"

Documentation, recording your observations of the patient in the patient's chart, is an important method of written communication among all members of the health care team (Fig. 4-6).

Sometimes people hesitate to ask questions because they are afraid the other person will think they are slow or do not know their job responsibilities. Asking questions that make assignments clear—who, what, when, and how—will help avoid misunderstandings and mistakes and strengthen teamwork.

Another method to clarify expectations is to repeat or paraphrase what you think you heard the other person say. If you have been asked by the RN to change a dressing, you would repeat back what you have been asked to do by saying, "You would like me to change the dry sterile dressing on Mrs. Green's abdomen, clean the suture line with hydrogen peroxide and saline, reapply

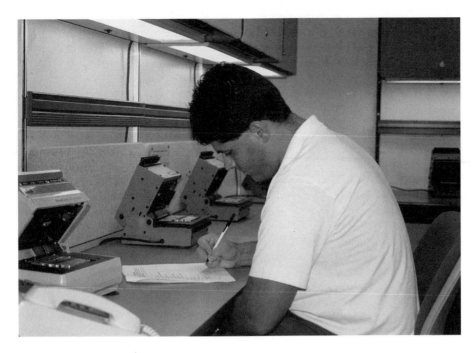

FIGURE 4 – 6
Documentation is an important method of written communication.

an occlusive dressing, and report my observations to you. Is that correct?" This gives the RN an opportunity to give additional information if needed to correctly complete the assignment.

It may seem as if it would take too much time to ask questions or paraphrase requests, but actually time is saved when everyone on the team has a clear understanding of each member's responsibilities. The team works more smoothly, and patients receive better care.

Give and Receive Feedback

Feedback involves giving another person information about behaviors you have observed. These behaviors could have had a positive or negative outcome. It is important to give both positive and negative feedback.

Positive Feedback

Positive feedback is usually easier to give than negative feedback. Everyone likes to be recognized for a job well done. Often we take the contributions of our team members for granted. Make an effort to give positive feedback by commenting, "Thanks for your help today with my assignment. I appreciate the way you always pitch in and help!" or "I noticed you talking to Mr. Winter. You really have the ability to communicate your concern to patients."

Positive feedback can be written. Think about starting a *brag book*. A brag book is a notebook that is kept on a unit and used as a place to write down positive comments about fellow team members. Comments can be read at staff meetings as a way to celebrate team accomplishments.

Receiving positive feedback can sometimes feel embar-

rassing. A common reaction is to feel that the positive feedback is something that is not deserved. Learning how to receive a compliment is as important as any assertive skill. Remember that everyone deserves recognition. Listen, hear, and take in what is being communicated instead of shutting it out because of feelings of low self-esteem.

Negative Feedback

Giving negative feedback can be a challenge. It helps to remember that coworkers cannot change or modify negative behavior unless they are made aware of the behavior. When observations and information on negative behaviors are not shared, the behavior(s) will continue and barriers are put up between coworkers.

When negative feedback is given it should be done in private. Describe the specific behavior, the effect the behavior is having on you, and how you would like the person to modify the behavior. The *I* message model is good to follow when giving negative feedback because it addresses those aspects and avoids putting blame on the other person. For example, you might tell a coworker:

- I feel uncomfortable . . . (Effect that the behavior is having on you.)

- When you ask me if I know what I am doing in front of a patient's family . . . (Describe the person's behavior.)

- If you have questions about how I complete an assignment, would you please ask me about it in a more private area? (How you would like the behavior to change.)

Use of labels and name calling are not an effective way to give feedback. Telling someone he or she is unprofessional, a bigot, or the worst nurse in the hospital will not get the results you want and will negatively affect the team. Feedback needs to be given in an honest yet respectful manner.

When receiving negative feedback, the biggest challenge is to focus on what is being said without interrupting. Listen for information that might be helpful in learning about yourself and improving work skills. If you think inaccurate feedback is being given, it is all right to ask for specific examples of the behavior. Try to remain open and understand the other person's point of view. When individuals on a team are comfortable giving and receiving honest feedback, the team improves and relationships are stronger.

Verbal Abuse

Verbal abuse should not be tolerated under any circumstance. Individuals use verbal abuse as a way to keep someone feeling put-down and "in their place." An example of verbal abuse would be telling someone he or she is stupid and no good. That type of remark usually takes an individual off guard and is a direct blow to his or her self-esteem. One way to handle such a remark is to call attention to the inappropriateness by saying, "Excuse me, what did you say?" or "What does that comment have to do with our discussion?" It's also all right to let the person know you will discuss the issue, but you will not allow yourself to be verbally abused.

Key Points

There are key points to remember when giving or receiving feedback

- Use *I* messages
- Use specific examples to describe behaviors
- Be open, honest, and direct
- Avoid personal attacks and name calling
- Give positive and negative feedback
- Learn to accept positive and negative feedback
- Make feedback an expectation for your team
- Have zero tolerance for verbal abuse

Resolving Conflict

Conflict and disagreement are a normal and unavoidable part of working with people. Resolving conflicts takes skill, practice, and time. Why is it important to learn how to resolve conflicts? When people do not understand how to work through or resolve a conflict, anger is not expressed or is expressed in a way that is not healthy for work relationships. Often anger turns into resentment, which can be like poison for a team. Examples of how resentment can affect a team are avoidance of certain coworkers, nasty remarks, and passive-aggressive behavior.

Identifying Defensiveness

The key to resolving conflicts is to learn to view them from your head—the thinking part of you—and not your heart—the emotional part. When people are in a situation in which they believe they are being threatened, the natural emotional reaction is to want to protect or defend themselves. This reaction happens during conflict, since conflicts involve people and their different values, beliefs, and self-concepts.

Many times the way we choose to defend ourselves causes the conflict to get bigger or escalate instead of getting resolved. It is important to know how you defend yourself when you feel threatened. Common ways in which people defend themselves on the basis of their emotional reaction is to:

- Fight back in an aggressive manner
- Leave the situation
- Shut down and not communicate
- Smile and pretend nothing happened

Setting the Stage

The problem with using these defenses is that nothing ever gets worked through, and the issues or problem that caused the conflict continues. If you can learn to respond to conflicts by thinking through your responses rather than reacting with emotions, you increase the chances of successfully resolving the problem. Some ways to accomplish this is to first determine how you defend yourself when threatened. Take a deep breath when feeling threatened, and identify what is happening (for example, your self-esteem is being threatened by a coworker's negative comment, and you want to defend yourself). Do not allow yourself to get caught up in defensiveness. Avoid becoming defensive by "shifting gears" from your heart (emotions) to your head (thinking). Once you are operating from your head it becomes easier to use the assertive communication skills you have learned.

Assertive Strategies

Ways to deal assertively with conflict include the following:

- Deal directly with the other person involved
- Avoid getting others caught up in the conflict
- Find a private place to talk
- Use an *I* message to describe the problem
- Allow enough time for discussion
- Listen to the other person's side
- Be prepared to look at different solutions
- Find a solution agreeable to both people

The following is an example of how to resolve conflict

in the workplace. Susan is a PCT who is upset because the RN she has been working with has been telling other members of the team that Susan is not doing a good job in completing her patient care assignment, yet has said nothing to Susan. Susan has been so angry lately about this situation it has been difficult for her to work with the RN. She thought about asking for another assignment but realized she must try to work through this problem. At the end of their shift, Susan asked the RN if she could speak to her in private before she went home. The RN agreed. Susan stated, "I have a concern I'd like to talk to you about. Janice told me you discussed my work performance with her. I feel angry that you talked to her instead of coming to me directly. In the future, if you have concerns about how I'm completing my assignments, please come and talk to me. How can I learn if you don't discuss things with me?" The RN apologized for not coming to Susan with her concerns and acknowledged that it was difficult for her to give negative feedback to someone. She agreed to speak to Susan about concerns she had related to the patient assignments. After this discussion, Susan and the RN felt that they had developed a closer working relationship because they were able to have an honest discussion.

Additional Considerations Related to Assertiveness

Acting assertively is not without some risks. You need to determine if it is safe for you to be assertive with another individual. How do you know if it is safe? If the person is a superior, does she seem receptive to feedback? How is her track record with individuals who have approached her in the past? Has she been able to react to the other person nondefensively or has her response been punitive.

You also need to determine what will happen if the problem is not dealt with assertively. Can you continue working in this job? What will you do with feelings of anger? How is not acting assertively affecting your self-esteem and feelings of self-worth?

These are not easy questions to answer. There are safe ways to deal with anger. One way is to use physical activity such as walking or hitting a pillow. Another way is to write your feelings in a journal or talk out your feelings with a friend you can trust or a mental health professional. Avoid letting your angry feelings build up inside. This can cause you to lash out at someone in anger or cause physical symptoms like stomach aches or headaches or emotional symptoms such as depression or anxiety.

A clinical nurse specialist with a background in psychiatric-mental health nursing is a mental health professional who can assist with assertive skills, conflict resolution, and strategies for improving interpersonal relationships.

COMMUNICATION STRATEGIES FOR RELATING TO PATIENTS AND FAMILIES

Understanding What Patients and Families Need

Changes in health care, such as the trend toward having the patient and family at the center of care, emphasize the importance of creating an environment that is concerned with the needs of health care customers. Hospitals are challenged to provide cost-effective quality care and maintain a high level of patient satisfaction. PCTs are key to maintaining customer satisfaction in the acute care setting and other settings where they are employed. To provide excellent customer service, it is helpful to understand the needs of patients and their families. Patients and families want the following:

- Information that is given in simple terms they can understand
- Trained staff who know how to provide for their needs
- Staff who truly care and are concerned about them as individuals
- Staff who will listen to their concerns

Information

Patients want to know what is going to happen to them while they are in the hospital. That is why it is important to clearly and simply explain the care you will be providing. Avoid using technical jargon or abbreviations that are familiar to you but make no sense to the patient. Repeat information that has been given by the RN. Patients often need to hear information more than once before they begin to understand. Encourage the patient and family to express their needs by using open-ended questions such as "Tell me what else you need" or "How may I help you today?"

If the patient or family member has questions you are uncomfortable with or unable to answer, notify the RN so the patient's need for information can be met.

Trained Staff

Patients want to feel safe and secure. Conveying your ability to provide competent care and working as an effective team contribute to the patient's sense of security. Move and turn the patient carefully and avoid rough, jerky movements. Never criticize or argue with another team member in front of a patient. Resolve conflicts and give feedback in private.

Care and Concern

Empathy is the term used to describe the communication of caring and concern for the patient. Ways to show empathy and establish a relationship with the patient are to:

- Sit down at eye level
- Make eye contact
- Touch the patient

✔ Some people are more comfortable with touch than others. If you do not feel comfortable touching the patient, do not use touch. Patients will be able to sense your discomfort. Ask permission before touching a patient. For example, "Mrs. Smith, is it all right if I hold your hand since you seem upset?"

- Address the patient by last name and preferred prefix
- Avoid calling the patient "Honey" or "Sweetie"
- Respect privacy and confidentiality
- Avoid giving advice or asking "why" questions

Sometimes, simply sitting with a patient in silence communicates caring and concern more than trying to find something to "do" for the patient (Fig. 4–7).

COPING WITH CHALLENGING PATIENT BEHAVIORS

Understanding Challenging Behavior

There are many factors that affect patients' behavior. In addition to concerns about their health, they may be worried about finances, family, or job. These multiple concerns can cause a patient to experience certain feelings. Common feelings experienced are anxiety, fear, powerlessness, and anger.

Anxiety and Fear

Anxiety causes internal tension and may be due to a general or specific fear. Patients can be afraid because they do not understand what to expect during their hospitalization or treatment. Fear of the unknown contributes to feeling anxious about a situation. Sometimes patients can feel anxious yet not know why they are having those feelings.

A way to tell if a patient is fearful or anxious is to listen. Anxious patients may describe feeling "stressed," "uptight," "nervous," or "all wound up." Outward signs of anxiety may include shaking, tapping or jiggling of the feet, wringing of the hands, or heavy sighing. Some patients may directly tell you that they are afraid of having a certain test or procedure performed. What may seem ordinary and routine to health care workers may seem frightening to a patient.

One way to help a fearful or anxious patient is to take time to listen to the concerns expressed. The patient may find it helpful if you are able to spend some time with him or her. If the patient is comfortable with touch, holding a hand or touching a shoulder may be reassuring. Answer questions or give information to increase understanding. When experiencing fear and anxiety, a patient may need to have information repeated several times before finally being able to understand. Notify the RN about the patient's concerns and any information or questions you were unable to answer.

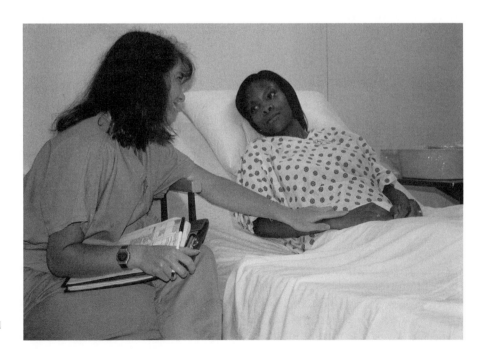

FIGURE 4–7
Sitting, making eye contact, and touching the patient show caring and concern.

Powerlessness

When patients come to get treatment at a health care facility they may be forced into routines that are sometimes more convenient for the staff. For example, hospital routines may be very different from the patient's routine at home. The patient may be so ill or injured that it is necessary to rely on staff to meet many needs he or she is used to doing independently. This loss of independence and control can cause a patient to have feelings of being powerless. To gain back a sense of control, a patient may become very demanding or refuse to participate in treatment.

It is important to allow patients to have as much control as possible in the hospital. Involve them in decision making and provide choices when possible. Allow as much independence as their condition permits. Inquire about routines at home, and determine if it is possible to follow those routines while they are hospitalized or receiving treatment. For example, many people prefer to bathe in the evening instead of the morning. Avoid ruling out an opportunity to be flexible in providing care because it is inconvenient for staff.

Anger

It is not unusual for patients to have angry feelings when ill or injured. Patients can be angry about the loss of control and feelings of powerlessness. They may perceive they are not getting answers to their questions or receiving enough information about their condition. When people experience any loss, angry feelings are a normal part of working through the grief process and accepting the loss.

Whatever the reason, patients can express anger in a variety of ways. Some patients are unable to state their feelings assertively. They may misdirect their anger at the first person they see, which may be you! Anger is expressed by some patients by yelling in a loud voice, being critical, and blaming staff for what they are experiencing. Staff may be unable to do anything correctly in the patients' eyes.

Strategies to Cope with Angry Behavior

It can be very challenging to deal with angry behavior. The following strategies will help you deal successfully with angry patients:

1. Do not take the angry feelings personally. The anger probably has no connection to you.

2. Remain calm. This will help you deal with the situation in an assertive manner.

3. Avoid raising your voice or arguing with the patient. This will keep the situation from escalating or getting worse. Ask a shouting patient to please lower his or her voice so you may help.

4. Help the patient identify what he is experiencing by saying, "Mr. Smith, you sound angry. Tell me what you are feeling."

5. Listen to the concerns of the patient without judging or jumping in.

6. If you are able, respond to the concerns without sounding defensive. "Mr. Smith, I can understand your frustration. I would be angry too if I had been told my discharge was going to be delayed."

7. If you are unable to help the patient or respond to his or her concerns, get assistance. Be yourself—you do not need all the answers. Many times patients only want someone to listen and show caring and concern.

STOP All staff need to be aware if the patient has a history of violent behavior. Steps should be taken to protect staff and other patients from harm. A psychiatric Clinical Nurse Specialist can consult with staff to develop a safety plan.

When to Get Assistance

Since you work as part of a team, there are certain situations in which you need to get assistance for a patient. The RN is the most available resource for assistance. It is essential that you communicate closely with the RN and provide feedback related to the patient's condition. Notify the nurse if:

- The patient is angry or appears sad and/or tearful.

- There is a change in the patient's emotional state, for example, the usually upbeat patient appears sad or the pleasant patient seems upset.

- The patient needs information or education you are unable to provide, such as understanding a disease process or procedure.

- The patient seems hopeless or helpless and is talking about harming himself or herself.

A patient who is talking about harming himself or herself and seems to have lost hope needs to receive immediate evaluation. Stay with the patient and notify the RN to come and assess the patient's condition. This psychological emergency can be just as serious as a physical emergency.

SUMMARY

Interpersonal relationship skills and effective communication are important for success as a PCT. Interpersonal skills strengthen work relationships and assist with development of relationships with patients and their families. People skills take practice to master just like task-related skills. Make a commitment to practice assertive communication on a daily basis.

Understanding what patients and their families want can help with meeting their needs. This will result in greater patient satisfaction. Patients are affected by certain feelings while in the hospital. PCTs will be more effective at providing patient-focused care if they attend to the patient's emotional as well as physical needs.

Patient Care Technician Role in Body System Disorders

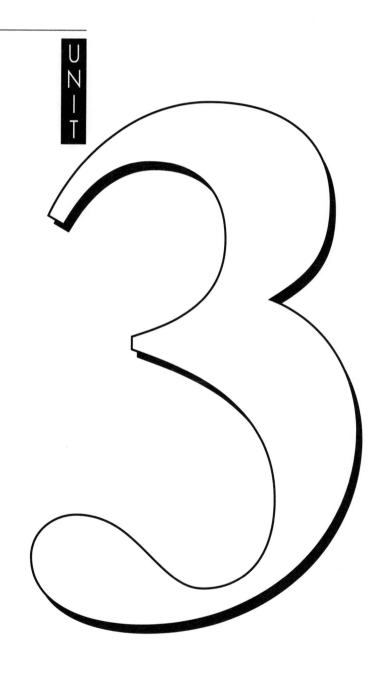

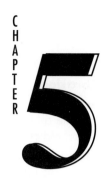

The Nervous System

MARA FERRIS, MS, RN,C, CS, CRRN
LAURIE MILLER, MS, RN, CS, CRRN, ANP

OUTLINE

The Central Nervous System (CNS)
Structures of the CNS
Protection for the CNS
Cells of the Nervous System

The Peripheral Nervous System
Structures of the Peripheral Nervous System

Common Neurological Disorders and Conditions
Head Injury
Cerebrovascular Accidents
Brain Tumors
Altered States of Consciousness
Seizures
Spinal Cord Injuries

Degenerative Diseases of the Nervous System
Delirium and Dementia
Sensory Losses

Care of the Patient with Neurological Disorders
Neurological Testing
Observations
Physical Care
Emotional Care
Equipment
Medications

Neurosurgical Care
Preoperative Care
Postoperative Care

Summary

PREREQUISITE KNOWLEDGE AND SKILLS

- AM and PM care
- Personal hygiene for complete care patient
- Maintaining the musculoskeletal system
- Obtaining vital signs
- Preoperative and postoperative care
- Documenting findings

OBJECTIVES

After you complete this chapter, you will be able to:

- List structures and functions of the nervous system.
- Describe behavior changes associated with head injury.
- Discuss common diseases of the nervous system.
- Describe physical care to be provided for patients with varying levels of cognition.
- Identify interventions for patients preparing for neurological testing.
- Recognize changes in vital signs or behaviors that need to be reported to an RN.
- Select and implement treatment interventions, together with the RN, for the neurologically impaired patient.
- Document observations and care given.

K E Y T E R M S

Abrasion Scrape of the skin or scalp

Activities of Daily Living (ADL) Tasks done by individuals to maintain hygiene and personal appearance, toileting, eating, and performing household chores

Alopecia Loss of hair on the scalp or body; may be partial or complete; the causes may be natural (for example, balding associated with aging) or caused by malnutrition, disease, medication, or radiation

Alzheimer's Disease A progressive and fatal disease that gradually destroys areas of the victim's brain, causing increasing memory losses, impaired thinking, changes of mobility, and speech

Amyotrophic Lateral Sclerosis (ALS) A rapidly progressing and fatal disease that destroys muscle cells along the spinal cord, causing loss of mobility, including the mobility needed for breathing

Analgesic Medication given to reduce or to stop pain

Anticoagulant Medication given to increase the time needed for blood to clot

Anticonvulsant Medication given to reduce or to stop seizure activity

Antihypertensive Medication given to reduce blood pressure

Arachnoid A membrane that lies between the dura mater and the pia mater

Aura Sensation or awareness that some patients may experience immediately before a seizure begins

Axon Thread-like extension of a nerve cell that carries impulses away from the cell body

Brain A large soft organ made up of nerve cells and protected by the cranium and meninges; the functions of this organ are to control the body and to interpret sensory information. *(The following are parts of the brain referred to in Chapter 5; each is listed in the glossary. See Brainstem, Cerebral Hemispheres, Cerebellum, Cerebrum, Frontal Lobe, Parietal Lobe, Occipital Lobe, Temporal Lobe.)*

Brain Tumor A tumor that occurs in the brain
  Primary brain tumor A tumor that begins in the brain
  Secondary brain tumor Cells from a tumor in another part of the body travel in the blood and begin to form a new tumor in the brain.

Catheter Any tube inserted into the body to carry fluid into or out of the body; often used to refer to urinary catheters

Cell Body The central part of the nerve cell that contains the cell nucleus

Cerebral Edema Condition characterized by too much cerebrospinal fluid (CSF) within the skull, which causes too much pressure on the brain and may cause temporary or permanent damage to the brain

Cerebrospinal Fluid (CSF) Clear fluid that surrounds and protects the brain and spinal cord within the skull and vertebra

Cerebrovascular Accident (CVA) Condition caused by interruption of blood flow to an area of the brain, which causes permanent damage; commonly referred to as a stroke
  Hemorrhagic stroke A stroke caused by a ruptured blood vessel
  Ischemic stroke A stroke caused by a blocked blood vessel

Chemotherapy Term for any "chemical" or medication used to treat a disease, but the term is generally used only for the drugs used to treat cancers

Clonic   Spastic muscle activity that causes rigidity and relaxation

Cognition   Process of recognizing, knowing, understanding, and interpreting

Coma   Condition of unconsciousness or of being unaware

Computed Tomography (CT); CAT scan   A diagnostic test that takes detailed pictures of the brain and spinal cord; used to show areas of injury, disease, or abnormalities

Concussion   Condition caused by the brain being shaken within the cranium or skull and characterized by a momentary change in brain function (for example, a brief loss of consciousness)

Consciousness   Condition of awareness

Contusion   A bruise that causes bleeding underneath the skin within the subcutaneous tissue

Cranial Nerves   Twelve pairs of nerves that provide motor and/or sensory function

Cranium   The bones of the skull or head that enclose the brain

Delirium   Temporary condition of confusion or excitement that may include hallucinations; a patient who is always confused because of a disease or an injury may have periods of delirium in which the confusion or hallucinations are worse

Dementia   Condition of progressive confusion; the progression may be slowed in some diseases but cannot be reversed or cured

Dendrites   Small finger-like projections of the nerve cells that receive information from the environment or from other neurons

Diuretic   Medication given to increase the production of urine

Dura Mater   Outermost of the meninges, lying immediately below the cranial bones

Edema   Condition in which too much fluid accumulates in the tissue

Electrocardiogram (ECG)   Diagnostic procedure that records the electrical activity of the heart

Electroencephalogram (EEG)   Diagnostic procedure that records the electrical activity of the brain

Epilepsy   Chronic condition caused by disturbances of electrical or neurological activity in the brain that causes various motor, sensory, emotional, and cognitive changes

Glial Cells   Specialized cells of the nervous system that function to support the neurons by providing nutrition, production of myelin, and protection

Grand Mal Seizure   Life-threatening type of seizure activity characterized by tonic/clonic movements of the limbs and trunk

Guillain-Barré Syndrome (GBS)   Neuromuscular disease that causes demyelination of the peripheral nerve pathways characterized by progressive muscle weakness

Halo Vest   Device secured to the skull and attached to a rigid vest used to stabilize the neck

Head Injury   General term used to describe any injury to the skull or brain that affects function

Hematoma   Swelling caused by bleeding into tissues or an organ
   Epidural Hematoma (EDH)   A hematoma between the skull and the dura mater
   Intracerebral Hematoma (ICH)   A hematoma into the cerebrum

Subdural Hematoma (SDH) A hematoma between the dura and the arachnoid

Hemiplegia Condition characterized by loss of motor and/or sensory function on one side of the body, usually caused by stroke or head injury

Hypothermia Unit Device used to lower very high body temperatures; also called cooling blankets

ICP Monitoring Process of assessing the progress of patients' conditions at risk for changes of intracranial pressure; includes monitoring the patient's level of consciousness, changes of motor function, complaints of headache or vision changes, changes in breathing and vital signs, vomiting

Insomnia Condition in which sleep is difficult or impossible and is characterized by inability to fall asleep or to stay asleep for adequate periods; may be due to emotional or physical conditions

Intracranial Pressure (ICP) Term to indicate the force (pressure) of the cerebrospinal fluid within the ventricles of the brain. (See also *ICP monitoring*)

Intravenous (IV) Term to describe being within or entering a vein; often used to refer to the administration of medications or fluids directly into a vein via a small catheter

Korsakoff's Syndrome A dementing and terminal illness often but not always associated with alcoholism; characterized by increasingly severe memory loss, difficulty in walking, and constant uncontrolled movements

Laceration A tear or cut of the skin

Lou Gehrig Disease (See *Amyotrophic Lateral Sclerosis*)

Lumbar Puncture Diagnostic procedure to obtain samples of cerebrospinal fluid (CSF); involves insertion of a needle into the subarachnoid space of the lumbar spine

Magnetic Resonance Imaging (MRI) Diagnostic test that takes detailed pictures of the brain and spinal cord; used to show areas of injury, disease, or abnormalities

Meninges The three membranes lying on the outside of the brain and spinal cord and beneath the bones of the skull and vertebral column. (See also *Dura Mater, Arachnoid,* and *Pia Mater*)

Multi-infarct Dementia (MID) Condition caused by many successive, small strokes that progress rapidly or slowly or may be stable for long periods, the severity of the impairments being determined by the location and size of the small strokes

Multiple Sclerosis (MS) Progressive and sometimes fatal disease characterized by destruction of myelin, which causes loss of motor and sensory function

Myasthenia Gravis (MG) Chronic progressive disease characterized by muscle weakness

Myelin Sheath Fatty substance that surrounds and protects neurons

Narcotic Medication or drug that slows the activity of the central nervous system (CNS) and that may be used to reduce or stop pain

Neoplasm (See *Tumor*)

Nervous System Intricate network of communication of the brain and body that receives, relays, and interprets information, controls the body's movement and organ functions

   Central Nervous System (CNS) Includes the brain and spinal cord
   Peripheral Nervous System (PNS) Includes the cranial nerves, spinal nerves, and autonomic nervous system

"Neuro Signs" Information used to assess the neurological status of patients; includes usual vital signs (BP, pulse, respirations, and temperature) and level of orientation and consciousness, behavior, and change of movement

Neurons Specialized nerve cells that receive and transmit impulses

Non-narcotic Medication used to reduce or stop pain that is not a narcotic

Orientation Condition of being able to recognize and to understand one's environment

> ***Orientated X 3*** Condition in which individuals know who they are, where they are, and the date or time
>
> ***Orientated X 2*** Condition in which individuals know who they are and where they are, but do not know the date or time
>
> ***Orientated X 1*** Condition in which individuals know who they are but do not know where they are and do not know the date or time

Paraplegia A condition characterized by the inability to feel or to move the legs or the lower portion of the trunk

Parkinson's Disease (PD) Progressive and ultimately fatal disease characterized by fine motor tremors, shuffling walk, little facial expression, and difficulty in swallowing; some victims of PD also develop dementia

Persistent Vegetative State (PVS) Condition of continuous deep coma without signs of improvement or awareness

Petit Mal Seizure A non-life threatening seizure characterized by altered consciousness

Postconcussive Syndrome (PCS) Period following a concussion, which may be brief or as long as a year, characterized by one or more of the following symptoms: nervousness, irritability, insomnia, extreme fatigue, changes in memory and ability to concentrate

Postictal The period following seizure activity that varies in length and may be characterized by one or more of the following symptoms: confusion, lethargy, weakness, headache, nausea or vomiting, and amnesia due to the seizure

Ptosis Drooping of the eyelids

Quadriplegia Condition characterized by inability to feel or to move the legs, trunk, and arms

Radiation Therapy Treatment involving exposure to radioactive substances or rays used to destroy or shrink malignant tumors or to slow their growth

Restraint Device used to restrict the movement of an individual for purpose of reducing the risk of injury to the patient or others by the patient when the patient is agitated or may become violent; restraints may also be used to prevent dislodging of equipment being used in patient care (for example, breathing tubes, urinary catheters, or intravenous therapy apparatus)

Reticular Activating System (RAS) An area of the brainstem responsible for the control of sleep and wakefulness

Sedation Condition in which the nervous system is slowed

Sedative/Hypnotic Medication used to calm or to slow the nervous system

Seizure Condition of uncontrolled and abnormal electrical activity in the brain that may be characterized by spasms or convulsions of muscles; abrupt changes in thinking or mood, or sudden changes in sensation. (See also *Aura, Clonic, Epilepsy, Grand Mal Seizure, Petit Mal Seizure, Postictal, Tonic*)

Sense The ability to perceive conditions; the five major senses: sight, hearing, touch, taste, and smell

Sensory Loss Inability to perceive or to recognize and understand one or more of the five senses

Skull The 14 bones of the head and all of the teeth, includes the bones of the cranium (those that cover the brain)

Skull Injury An injury to any of the bones in the head; therefore, may involve the bones of the cranium but also the facial bones and teeth

Spinal Cord A column of nerves from which nerves to the trunk and limbs originate; the cord is contained within the vertebral column

Spinal Cord Injury (SCI) Injury to any part of the spinal cord resulting in temporary or permanent loss of motor and/or sensory function; may be caused by concussion, contusion, laceration, or hemorrhage

Spinal Nerves Thirty-one pairs of nerves originating in the spinal cord and carrying sensory and motor impulses

Spinal Shock A complication of spinal cord injury characterized by low blood pressure, slowed heart rate, and low body temperature

Stroke (See *Cerebrovascular Accident [CVA]*)

Subarachnoid Space The space beneath the arachnoid (See *Arachnoid*)

Subdural Space The space beneath the dura mater (See *Dura Mater*)

Synapse A space between two neurons in which nerve impulses are transmitted or communicated

Tonic An uncontrolled muscle contracture or rigidity

Total Parenteral Nutrition (TPN) A solution containing all the nutrition the body needs in a formulation delivered directly into the circulatory system (blood); used for patients who are unable to eat and cannot receive food through a tube to the gastrointestinal system

Tube Feeding A method of providing nutrition to patients who are unable to eat or to eat enough; a solution containing necessary nutrients is administered through a tube into the digestive tract; these tubes are referred to as follows:
  Gastric Tube (GT) Inserted through a surgical opening on the abdomen; delivers food to the stomach
  Jejunostomy Tube (JT) Inserted through a surgical opening on the abdomen; delivers food to the jejunum (a section of the small intestine)
  Nasogastric Tube (NG) Inserted through the nose; delivers food to the stomach

Tumor Abnormal growth or mass of tissue
  Benign Tumor Tumor that does not spread as a cancer
  Malignant Tumor Tumor that may spread to involve more tissue or other organs

Unconsciousness A condition of no awareness of self or of the environment

The nervous system is an intricate network of communication. It is responsible for controlling all of the cells in the body and integrating their functions. The development of the nervous system begins in the embryonic stage of life and proceeds until birth. After birth, no new nerve cells will develop; however, further refinement of existing ones will continue through adolescence. The nervous system has two subdivisions: the central nervous system and the peripheral nervous system. Each subdivision is discussed separately; however, keep in mind that both work together to integrate function.

THE CENTRAL NERVOUS SYSTEM (CNS)

Structures of the CNS

The CNS includes the brain and the spinal cord and is the control center for integrating functions. The brain is capable of performing very high level activities and allows the ability to memorize, make complex decisions, think logically and creatively, and have emotions.

The brain is divided into three areas: the cerebrum, the brainstem, and the cerebellum.

CEREBRUM. The cerebrum is divided down the middle (from front to back) into two hemispheres, a right one and a left one. Many nerve fibers travel through the cerebral hemispheres and help control movement. Each hemisphere is further divided into lobes—frontal, temporal, parietal, and occipital (Fig. 5–1). It is important to have an understanding of the functions of each lobe, as damage to a certain lobe will cause specific symptoms.

FRONTAL LOBE. The left side of the frontal lobe receives sensory information, and the right side receives motor information. There is an area within the frontal lobe called *Broca's area* that allows the ability to produce language. Other functions of the frontal lobe are concentration, problem solving, and memorization. Although individual personalities are the result of life's experiences, characteristic moods and behaviors are also heavily influenced by activities in the frontal lobes. These include humor, anger, modesty, sorrow, and happiness.

PARIETAL LOBE. The parietal lobe is the primary area for analyzing sensory information, such as pain, temperature, and pressure. The parietal lobe also allows the body to know where it is positioned in space. For example, a person knows when he or she is lying down or standing up and is aware of where the body parts are in relation to one another.

OCCIPITAL LOBE. This is the primary area responsible for vision. The occipital lobe interprets visual images and allows the ability to see and read.

TEMPORAL LOBE. The temporal lobe receives and processes all information heard. An area within the temporal lobe is *Wernicke's area*, which interprets sounds as words. This area of the temporal lobe allows a person to know and understand what another person is saying. For example, a person with damage to Wernicke's area may hear a person say "What a nice day," when the person actually said "Aren't you going to eat your lunch?" This example is somewhat extreme; however, this is important to know when you are caring for patients who have damage to this area, since they will not always understand what you say to them.

THE BRAINSTEM. This is the second major subdivision of the brain and is composed of the midbrain, pons, and medulla (Fig. 5–2). The parts of the brainstem work together to integrate the higher functions such as thinking and feeling with the life-sustaining functions of the nervous system. The medulla, specifically, contains the centers for cardiac, vasomotor, and respiratory functions, so damage to the medulla may result in death.

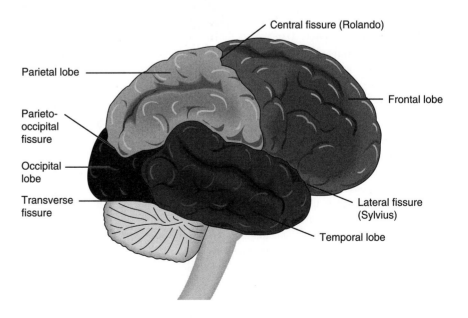

FIGURE 5–1

Lateral aspect of left cerebral hemisphere.

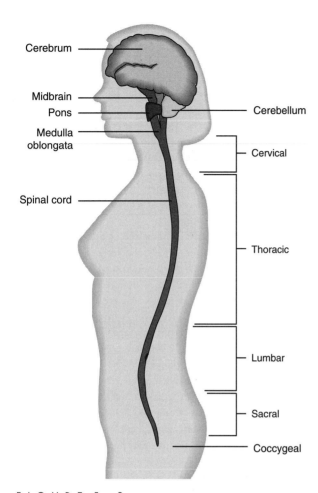

F I G U R E 5 – 2

Anatomical divisions of the central nervous system.

THE CEREBELLUM. The cerebellum attaches to the back of the brainstem, and its functions are related to motor activity and balance. It can either excite or inhibit muscle tone, coordinate muscle group activity to produce smooth movements, and coordinate fine motor movement and balance. Damage to the cerebellum can result in ataxia, poor balance, poor coordination, and the inability to judge distances between objects (dysmetria).

Protection for the CNS

The CNS structures are soft and fragile. They are protected by three mechanisms; the first is the **bony structures**. The bones of the cranium, which are named for the underlying cerebral lobes discussed earlier, enclose the brain and act as a protective vault. The spine has 33 vertebrae bound together by ligaments that also provide support and protection to the spinal cord.

The second protective mechanism is the **meninges**. These are tissue-like membranes covering the brain and spinal cord. The *dura mater* is the outermost layer, lying just beneath the cranial bones. Underneath the dura is a small space called the *subdural space*. This space is a

common site of bleeding in head injury. The middle layer of meninges is the *arachnoid layer*. It gets its name from the many blood vessels that resemble the legs of a spider. The space underneath the arachnoid layer is the *subarachnoid space*. This is the area where the *cerebrospinal fluid* (CSF) flows. The *pia mater* is the innermost layer and is very vascular. This layer is in direct contact with the cerebrum and provides blood and nutrients to the cerebral tissue.

The third protective mechanism is the *cerebrospinal fluid* (CSF). CSF is a clear, colorless, odorless fluid that functions as a shock absorber. It cushions against injury caused by motion. Any tearing or damage to the walls of the subarachnoid space where the CSF flows can cause CSF leakage. This is most commonly seen when CSF leaks from the nose or ears after trauma or surgery. The CSF circulates through the spinal cord and enclosed cavities in the brain called ventricles. *Intracranial pressure* (ICP) is the pressure exerted by the CSF within the ventricles of the brain. The ICP is affected by many factors such as blood pressure, oxygen, drugs, and body temperature. Because the CNS is completely enclosed in the skull and spinal cord, increased volume or pressure in an area will increase pressure throughout the system. With the rising pressure and no place for the brain to expand within the bones of the skull, the increased pressure destroys brain cells, and symptoms are noted. Any of these symptoms of increased ICP must be reported immediately.

Monitor patients for decreased level of consciousness, loss of motor function, complaints of a headache, changes in breathing, changes in vital signs, or vomiting and report these to the RN immediately.

Cells of the Nervous System

There are two types of cells in the nervous system: glial cells and neurons.

GLIAL CELLS. There are far more glial cells in the nervous system than there are neurons. There are many different kinds of glial cells, all of which support the activity of the neurons. Some functions of the glial cells are to provide structural support (similar to that of the foundation on a house), nourishment, and protection for the neurons. Other glial cells produce myelin for the nerves (myelin will be discussed later in this chapter), and still others are responsible for producing CSF.

NEURONS. Also called nerve cells, neurons are very specialized cells that receive and transmit impulses from one cell to another. Neurons can be either motor or sensory; the anatomy is similar, however. Each neuron (Fig. 5–3) has a *cell body*, which is the metabolic center. *Dendrites* are small finger-like projections that receive information from the environment (sensory) or from other

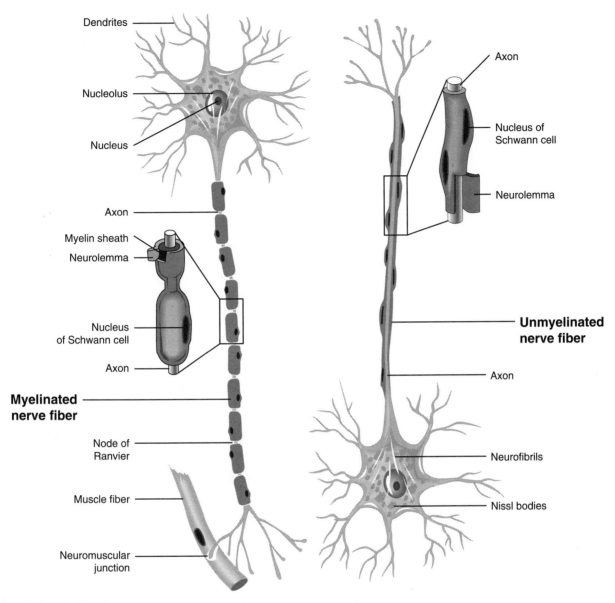

Dendrites

Nucleolus

Nucleus

Axon

Myelin sheath
Neurolemma

Nucleus
of Schwann cell

Axon

**Myelinated
nerve fiber**

Node of
Ranvier

Muscle fiber

Neuromuscular
junction

Axon

Nucleus of
Schwann cell

Neurolemma

**Unmyelinated
nerve fiber**

Axon

Neurofibrils

Nissl bodies

F I G U R E 5 – 3
Efferent neuron.

neurons (motor). One *axon* leaves the cell body and conducts electrical signals to the next cell. The axon is covered by a *myelin sheath* which acts as insulating material. Along the axon there are unmyelinated areas called the *nodes of Ranvier*. These allow the signal (impulse) to "jump" from one to the next. This allows the signal to travel faster, covering more distance in a shorter amount of time. Finally, the impulse reaches a *synapse*, the last part of the neuron. The synapse is the communication area between the axon of one neuron and the dendrite of the next.

THE PERIPHERAL NERVOUS SYSTEM

The peripheral nervous system consists of the cranial nerves, the spinal nerves, and the autonomic nervous system. The autonomic nervous system is further subdivided into the sympathetic nervous system and the parasympathetic nervous system.

Structures of the Peripheral Nervous System

THE CRANIAL NERVES. There are 12 pairs of cranial nerves. Each nerve has either a motor or sensory function or a combination of both. The cranial nerves originate at different areas in the brain between the cerebral hemispheres and the medulla. The cranial nerves play a role in functions such as seeing, moving the eyes, hearing, smelling, tasting, chewing, swallowing, speaking, and making facial expressions (Table 5–1).

THE SPINAL NERVES. There are 31 pairs of spinal nerves that emerge from between the vertebrae in the

T A B L E   5 – 1
Functions of Cranial Nerves

NUMBER	NAME	FUNCTIONS
I	Olfactory	Nerve of smell
II	Optic	Nerve of vision
III	Oculomotor	Adjustment of eye to distance Regulates light reaching retina Most important nerve in eye movements
IV	Trochlear	Responsible in eye movements
V	Trigeminal	Nerve of pain, touch, heat, and cold to skin Chewing movements
VI	Abducens	Movement of lateral rectus muscle Eye movements
VII	Facial	Taste to anterior tongue Motor and muscle sense to face
VIII	Acoustic	Nerve of hearing Balance in position
IX	Glosso-pharyngeal	Taste to posterior tongue Pain, touch, heat, and cold to pharynx Circulatory and respiratory reflexes
X	Vagus	Secretory to gastric glands and pancreas Inhibitory to heat Motor to muscles of larynx and pharynx Constrictor to coronary arteries Respiratory, cardiac, and circulatory reflexes
XI	Accessory	Motor and muscle sense to sternocleidomastoid, trapezius, and muscles of larynx
XII	Hypoglossal	Motor and muscle sense to tongue Important in speech and mastication

From Chaffee, E. E., and Lytle, J. M.: Basic Physiology and Anatomy. Philadelphia, J. B. Lippincott Co., 1980.

spinal column. Each nerve has a sensory and a motor fiber that carry impulses. The sensory portions of the nerve receive information related to pain, temperature, or pressure on the skin and carry the impulse to the brain. The brain interprets the information it receives from the sensory nerve and determines if the input hurts, feels good, and is cold or hot. The motor portion of the nerve carries a message from the brain to the skin related to movement. This automatic response, such as pulling the hand away from a hot stove, is called a *reflex*. Reflexes are subconscious responses to a stimulus. Reflexes are made up of sensory and motor nerves and act as protective agents.

THE AUTONOMIC NERVOUS SYSTEM. The autonomic nervous system is the last part of the peripheral nervous system. As stated previously, it is divided into the sympathetic and parasympathetic nervous systems. The autonomic nervous system is made up of only motor neurons and regulates the activity of smooth, involuntary muscles (heart, glands, and the gastrointestinal muscles).

The sympathetic nervous system is activated during stressful situations. This is called the fight-or-flight phenomenon or reaction. During these situations heart rate and blood pressure increase and blood vessels constrict. The parasympathetic nervous system acts to balance sympathetic activity and stimulates activities that will restore normal functioning. Blood pressure and heart rate return to normal when the parasympathetic nervous system is activated. The autonomic nervous system is stimulated by areas in the spinal cord, brainstem, and hypothalamus.

COMMON NEUROLOGICAL DISORDERS AND CONDITIONS

Head Injury

Head injury is an injury to the skull or brain, or both, that causes a loss of function and requires treatment. It is one of the leading causes of death and disability in trauma patients. The highest incidence is among males (two to three times higher than in females) ages 15–29 years. Half of all head injuries occur in motor vehicle accidents, most of which are associated with alcohol or drug abuse. Other causes of head injuries include falls, sporting injuries, gunshot wounds, assaults, and occupational injuries.

Types of Head Injuries

SCALP INJURIES. These injuries include abrasions, contusions, and lacerations. The extent of damage is related to the type of object, as well as the force of the object causing the injury. An *abrasion* is a minor injury that scrapes away the top layer of skin. There may be some slight bleeding, but essentially abrasions are not serious. A *contusion* is a bruise with possible leakage of blood into the subcutaneous layer. There is no break in the integrity of the skin. In treatment of a contusion, the application of ice over the site will prevent formation of a hematoma. A physician may order X-rays of the skull just to be certain there is no fracture of the bones. A *laceration* is a wound in the tissue of the scalp that usually causes profuse bleeding. Once the bleeding has been controlled, the surrounding scalp is shaved. All lacerations should be cleansed with normal saline to remove any debris, and a physician will usually explore the laceration with surgical tools to look for any foreign objects such as glass or bone fragments. Once the wound is cleansed and any foreign objects have been removed, the physician will suture the wound closed.

SKULL INJURIES. Skull injuries are injuries to the cranium (bones covering the brain) and/or the facial bones. The type of injury that occurs is called a deformation injury. This means that there is a distortion of the skull (usually an inward denting) disrupting the contour. Factors that influence the amount of deformation include the speed and force of the impact and the weight and type of the object. There are many different types of skull fractures; however, the most important to be familiar with is the *basal skull fracture.* Basilar skull fractures and their consequences are much more serious than other fractures to the cranium. Many basal skull fractures disrupt the integrity of the bones over the nasal air spaces. The underlying dura is then exposed, and CSF leaks out. Drainage of the CSF is serious because of the potential for infection to the brain. Visible leakage of CSF indicates an opening of the CNS to the outside environment. This opening provides a route for microorganisms or bacteria to enter the CNS. Anytime there is a CSF leak there should always be monitoring of the patient for signs and symptoms of infection, as well as changing neurological status.

BRAIN INJURIES. Brain injuries occur when there is bruising, tearing, or bleeding of the dura. There are many kinds of brain injuries, and this section will focus on the most common.

Concussion. Concussion is caused when a mechanical force hits the head, causing the brain to "shake" within the bones of the cranium. Concussion means to shake violently. The result is a momentary malfunction of the cells within the nervous system. This may result in loss of consciousness, lasting as little as a few seconds or as long as hours. The episode may also include temporary loss of reflexes and/or respirations and may involve possible amnesia for the events occurring just prior to and at the time of injury. The patient may also complain of headache, drowsiness, confusion, dizziness, visual disturbances ("seeing stars"), and difficulty walking.

Recovery takes minutes to hours; however, some patients may develop *postconcussive syndrome.* Postconcussive syndrome can last from several weeks up to 1 year (extreme cases) and includes such complaints as nervousness, irritability, insomnia, and extreme fatigue, as well as poor memory and inability to concentrate.

A *cerebral contusion* is bruising of the surface of the brain, whereas a *laceration* is actual tearing of the brain tissue. Although a cerebral contusion does not involve tearing of tissue, there is an area of hemorrhage. Both contusions and lacerations can cause swelling and increased intracranial pressure. Another potential complication of severe swelling is herniation. This occurs when the brain has swelled to such a tremendous extent that it pushes downward through the bones surrounding the base of the brain near the neck. Once this occurs the damage to the brainstem is irreversible, and the ability to perform life-sustaining functions is lost. Signs and symptoms are related to the area of the brain damaged. Diagnosis is by *computed tomography* (CT), and treatment is based on the symptoms.

Intracranial hemorrhage can occur into the epidural, subdural, or subarachnoid spaces. It may result from blunt trauma to the cranium or by tearing of tissue, which may rupture blood vessels. The neurological signs and symptoms appear when enough bleeding has occurred to occupy space within the brain and put pressure on other brain tissues.

An *epidural hematoma* occurs in the space between the skull and the dura. Diagnosis is made by CT. A *subdural hematoma* refers to bleeding between the dura and the arachnoid layer of the meninges. Bleeding from a subdural hematoma results in immediate pressure on the brain, since the arachnoid layer is so close to the brain. Bleeding directly into the cerebrum is called *intracerebral hematoma.*

Cerebrovascular Accidents

A cerebrovascular accident (CVA) is usually referred to by the public as a *stroke.* CVAs occur when the blood supply to part of the brain is interrupted by either a blocked blood vessel (ischemic stroke) or a ruptured blood vessel (hemorrhagic stroke). Because the brain is unable to store oxygen or glucose, it must receive a constant blood supply. When the supply is interrupted, the damaged area of the brain is referred to as *infarcted* and is permanently damaged within minutes.

When the blood supply is only briefly interrupted, the patient may experience brief sensory, cognitive (thinking), or motor losses, but these functions return within 24 hours and sometimes within minutes. These *transient ischemic attacks* (TIA) are important indicators of blood vessel changes that may lead to a CVA.

If the cause of the stroke occurred in a small blood vessel, the damage will be limited to a very small area of the brain. Some strokes occur without causing any noticeable changes in the individual's function. Patients admitted to a hospital for care following a CVA, however, will have significant functional losses. These patients have had damage to areas of their brains that govern important functions. The losses may range from minor changes of motor function to coma. The types of losses are determined by the area of the brain that has been damaged. For many patients, the interruption of blood flow occurs in a major artery supplying blood to an entire hemisphere. When this occurs, motor and sensory function on the opposite side of the body is lost. Total loss of function on one side of the body is referred to as *hemiplegia.*

Brain Tumors

Brain tumors (brain neoplasms) are classified in one of two categories, primary or secondary. A primary brain tumor develops from the cells and other structures within the brain, while a secondary brain tumor is usually the result of cancer beginning elsewhere in the body and spreading. Tumors may be present at birth, related to hereditary factors, or may develop on their own for some unknown reason. A tumor that arises from the neurons is called a *neuroma* and one that begins in the glial cells is termed a *glioma*.

Neoplasms occurring in the brain are categorized as benign or malignant. *Malignant* tumors indicate a poor prognosis; *benign* refers to a better prognosis. The term *benign tumor*, however, can be misleading. Although a tumor may be considered benign, it may exist in a location that makes surgery difficult. A surgeon may be able to remove only a small portion of the tumor, if any at all. In this circumstance, the tumor will continue to grow and eventually cause further neurological damage or death.

A tumor will continue to grow until it reaches a more rigid structure, such as bone. When this happens, the growth will continue in different directions. As the tumor enlarges, it compresses other structures and cells within the brain. *Cerebral edema* (swelling) and *increased intracranial pressure* (ICP) result, causing further neurological damage. Treatment involves the use of drugs to minimize symptoms, surgery to remove the mass, and radiation therapy or chemotherapy to reduce the size of the mass or remove it by killing all the tumor cells.

Signs and Symptoms

There are no classic signs of brain tumors, and the neurological symptoms identified relate to the location of the tumor, the size and degree of compression from the tumor, and the related cerebral edema. In general, most patients have alterations in their level of consciousness (ranging from alert to coma and agitated to sedated). Headache is an early symptom of the presence of a brain tumor, and it is related to the increased intracranial pressure. Close to half of the patients with a brain tumor develop seizures related to abnormal electrical impulses generated by the enlarging mass (see Seizures).

Care of the Patient

Patients with either malignant or benign tumors may be treated with radiation therapy, which is intended to reduce the size and spread of the tumor. These patients are at risk for a number of complications (see Chapter 13). Skin breakdown is common at the irradiated site, and proper care should be taken to prevent further breakdown. Many skin creams contain oils that are not compatible with radiation.

 Before applying anything to the skin, check with the nurse or radiation therapist.

The skin becomes reddened and the tissue may flake off (called *radiation dermatitis*). No tape, creams, cosmetics, powder, or alcohol-based products should be used on the skin receiving radiation. Do not wash off the skin markings; they are used to indicate the area receiving radiation.

 Nausea, vomiting, and diarrhea may result from radiation therapy.

The nurse can administer medications to relieve these side effects. Because of the nausea and vomiting, patients will not want to eat and may become anorexic (loss of appetite). To manage this, offer small portions of food that are liked by the patient and easily digestible (for example, toast, rice, crackers, tea, ginger ale). Fatigue is another common side effect of radiation. Allow the patient frequent, uninterrupted periods of rest. The side effects of chemotherapy and radiation therapy can be overwhelming. Reassure patients that after the therapy has ended, the side effects will resolve.

Along with the physical side effects of radiation therapy, it may also be a very sad and scary time for the patient and family. Emotional support should be provided to the patient and/or family. Encourage them to discuss their concerns and fears. Some people will have difficulty expressing their feelings. You may help them by asking general questions about their experiences and feelings.

Chemotherapy may be offered to a patient with a malignant brain tumor. The side effects of chemotherapy are similar to those of radiation (nausea, vomiting, fatigue) and also include alopecia (hair loss). Be sensitive to the patient's feelings about hair loss and reassure him or her that very often hair grows back after chemotherapy is complete. The care of the patient receiving chemotherapy is similar to that of the patient receiving radiation therapy.

Altered States of Consciousness

Consciousness is a person's awareness of himself or herself and the environment. A patient's level of consciousness is determined by orientation to time, place, or person, the level of understanding of the written and spoken word, and the ability to express ideas verbally and in writing. An area within the brainstem, called the *reticular activating system (RAS)*, is the section of the brain responsible for the ability to fall asleep and wake up. When this area is damaged by trauma or changes in ICP or is affected by medications or drugs of abuse, the awareness of surroundings and the ability to respond to the environment are lost. These are also noted in persons as they recover from the effects of anesthesia.

There are varying degrees of consciousness. A patient

who is oriented to person, time, and place and who is able to understand what is being said, is said to be fully conscious.

Coma

Prolonged and profound loss of consciousness is called coma. A patient in coma may show no reaction to painful stimuli or may react only by grimacing or withdrawing the limb to which stimuli were given. Sometimes the eyes will be open and sometimes closed, giving the appearance that the patient is falling asleep and waking up. It is uncertain if coma patients are able to hear, so it is best not to discuss private information at the bedside or information that may distress the patient. Encourage family members and other staff members to talk to the patient about familiar things and day-to-day activities. The patient's situation should be discussed outside of the room, especially if it is information one does not want the patient to hear. The opening of eyes is usually a reflex action and can sometimes be confused by the patient's family as a sign of recovery. Although it is important not to take away the family's hope of recovery, it is important to give them factual information. Let the family know things they can look for, such as asking the patient to squeeze and let go of a person's hand on command, or asking the patient to stick out his or her tongue on command. These are motions that cannot be confused as a reflex action.

⚖️ It is the responsibility of licensed personnel to provide the family with the education they need regarding neurological deficits and potential for recovery. The PCT can reinforce the information that has been provided to the family.

Patients can remain in a coma for as little as a day or for as long as years. This can be very frustrating for both the family and for the caregivers. The length of coma depends on the extent of damage caused to the brain. The patient will usually have a CT scan or an MRI of the head to determine how much damage has been done. Patients who remain in a coma for years without signs of improvement or recovery are said to be in a *persistent vegetative state*.

Seizures

Seizures are the result of abnormal firing of impulses from the neurons and cause a disturbance of motor and sensory functions as well as changes in behavior or level of consciousness. Seizures can occur because of swelling or cerebral damage from head injury, or the cause can be unknown. A chronic syndrome characterized by recurrent episodes of seizure activity is known as *epilepsy*. Seizure activity is diagnosed by an *electroencephalogram* (EEG),

which is a record of brain wave activity. Epilepsy is treated with *anticonvulsant* medications.

There are many types of seizures, all with different characteristic symptoms. Most dramatic to witness and traumatic to the patient is the *grand mal seizure*. This type of seizure causes tonic/clonic movements (muscle contractions that consist of a pattern of rigidity and relaxation) that cause a thrashing and flailing of the extremities. Many patients will experience an *aura* prior to the onset of a seizure. An aura is a particular sensation that immediately precedes the symptoms of a seizure. Individuals will have different characteristic auras, such as a peculiar taste or smell, ringing in the ears, dizziness, or others.

 Auras are a good clue to prepare for the onset of a seizure.

When you are with a patient in whom seizure activity begins note the exact time the symptoms began. Call for assistance from an RN by using the call light or yelling for help, as the patient should not be left alone. The thrashing that occurs during a seizure places the patient at risk of injury from banging the limbs on furniture or siderails. The PCT can minimize the risk of injury to the patient by padding the siderails of the bed with pillows or blankets. Seizure pads are long cushions that extend the length of the siderail. Check to see if your facility has them available.

🛑 Patients at risk for seizures should have the siderails padded at all times.

If the patient is not in bed at the onset of a seizure, assist him or her to the floor and move all furniture, chairs, and equipment out of the way.

🛑 Never attempt to hold a limb still during a seizure as you may get hurt or the patient may break a bone.

The patient's airway must also be kept open during a seizure. The teeth often clench shut during seizure activity, and the mouth fills with secretions.

🛑 Never make any attempt to unclench the teeth or put your fingers into the patient's mouth during the tonic/clonic phase of a grand mal seizure.

 The nurse is responsible for suctioning the airway, if needed, once seizure activity has stopped.

The PCT can have all of the suction equipment available to assist the RN with this procedure. Also be sure to obtain an oral airway in case it is needed after suctioning. Immediately after the seizure activity has ceased, raise the head of the bed for continued protection of the airway or turn the patient into the side-lying position in case of vomiting. A set of vital signs should be taken immediately after the seizure activity stops and then every few minutes until the RN or physician determines that the vital signs are stable. Also be sure to note the exact time the seizure activity stops.

The duration of seizure activity is very important for the physician to know. Be sure to document the time the seizure began and the time that it ended.

A postictal phase (postseizure) is common and may last a few minutes to hours. It can be characterized by symptoms of confusion, lethargy, weakness, nausea/vomiting, incontinence, amnesia of the seizure, headache, or any combination of symptoms. Unconsciousness is common during a seizure. As the patient begins to awaken, take time to provide emotional support and comfort. Patients can be very frightened by not remembering what just occurred and to waking up to numerous people watching over them.

If the PCT is present at the onset of the seizure, she or he should document the time the seizure started, the progression of symptoms, length of time of tonic/clonic phase, and vital signs postseizure.

A licensed person will explain to the patient what has happened, but a PCT can continue to reassure the patient that he or she is safe.

Spinal Cord Injuries

Spinal cord injury results when excessive force is exerted on the spinal column (Fig. 5–4), resulting in temporary or permanent loss of motor and/or sensory function. The injury can be similar to those occurring to the brain, such as concussion, contusion, laceration, or hemorrhage. A transection is the slicing of the spinal cord and may be complete (cord is severed) or incomplete. Depending on the type of injury and the location within the spinal cord, a patient may have no neurological deficits, total loss of motor and/or sensory function, or any range in between.* Quadriplegia is the loss of motor and/or sensory function to both the arms and the legs and can occur with an injury to any of the cervical vertebrae. Paraplegia

---

General rule of thumb: All spinal and motor tracts below the level of injury will be affected.

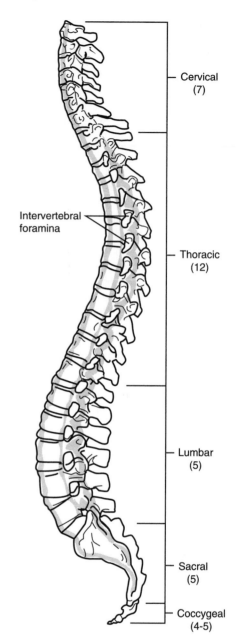

F I G U R E 5 – 4
The vertebral column.

is the loss of motor and/or sensory function to the lower extremities only and may occur with any injury below the level of the thoracic vertebrae. Paraplegic patients will have full use of the arms and will be able to participate in care; however, quadriplegic patients will require total assistance with performing activities of daily living.

Care of the Patient

HALO VEST. The halo vest (Fig. 5–5) is a device designed to stabilize the neck in a fixed position. It is used after injury to the cervical spine to achieve stabilization of the spinal cord. A halo ring is secured to the

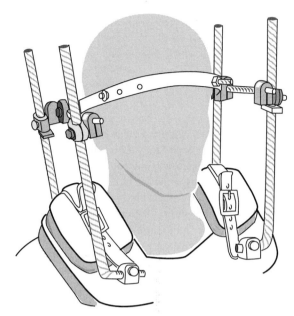

F I G U R E   5 – 5
Halo traction.

skull with titanium pins and is attached to the vest by metal bars.

Care of the Vest. The vest lining should be kept dry at all times. If the fleece should get wet, it can be dried with a hair dryer set on a cool setting. Moisture in the lining will predispose the skin to breakdown. When the patient changes position, areas under the vest (shoulders especially) may come in contact with the vest edges and be subjected to pressure. Extra pieces of fleece can be placed over bony areas to prevent the development of pressure sores. Each vest is supplied with a set of instructions regarding the procedure for removal of the vest for skin care.

Consult with licensed personnel, Clinical Nurse Specialists, or staff development to learn the proper procedure for removing the vest.

PIN CARE. Pin care is the cleaning of the titanium pins and the skin around the insertion site. There is no universal agreement on how pin care should be accomplished. It is strongly recommended that it be done once a day and that the cleaning substance be able to remove crusting. Usually hydrogen peroxide or alcohol on a cotton-tipped applicator is used to cleanse the pin site. Soapy water may be used if the hydrogen peroxide or alcohol burns. It is not recommended that bacteriostatic or other ointments be used on the pin sites as part of routine care.

HYGIENE AND GROOMING. A sponge bath will be necessary as showering will wet the vest liner. When the hair is washed, the shoulders and neck of the vest should be protected with plastic. A mobile patient can

kneel over a tub or lean over a sink for this procedure. If the patient is immobile the hair will be washed in bed or on a stretcher, using a basin to catch the water. Clothing will need to be altered to fit around the vest because the halo will remain in place for about 3 months.

OBSERVATIONS. In the acute phase of spinal cord injury, monitoring of the patient's status is very important. Vital signs and neurological signs should be checked at least every 4 hours, if not more often.

 The RN will complete the neurological examination, but as a PCT providing care, you may be the first to notice changes in the patient's condition.

Talk to the RN caring for the patient about what neurological changes to watch for.

Vital Signs. Spinal shock is a common complication after spinal cord injury and may last a few days to months. It results because the brain can no longer transmit impulses to the areas below the level of injury. Vital signs are important because the signs of spinal shock include hypotension (low blood pressure), bradycardia (slow heart rate), and decreased body temperature.

A change in vital signs reflective of these symptoms should be brought to the attention of the nurse.

Treatment of the blood pressure and the heart rate will rely on the physician and the RN; however, the PCT may apply blankets to a patient for comfort when the temperature is low. This will also prevent a further drop in temperature.

Respiratory Function. The nerves that innervate the muscles of the respiratory system arise from the cervical vertebrae. Therefore, a patient with a cervical spinal cord injury may have difficulty breathing or may be unable to breath on his or her own. In the latter instance, the patient will require intubation, tracheostomy, or mechanical ventilation. Depending on the type of injury and the damage that occurred, these interventions may be permanent (see Chapter 6).

Degenerative Diseases of the Nervous System

Myasthenia Gravis

Myasthenia gravis (MG) is a chronic progressive disease of muscular weakness caused by a defect in the area where a nerve and a muscle meet. The muscles do not always get the message from the nerves to perform their usual function. Patients with MG usually first notice weakness in the eyes. The eyelids droop (ptosis), and the patient is likely to have double vision. MG progresses and eventually causes weakness in the muscles responsible for chewing, swallowing, speaking, and breathing. Patients will often show improvement of muscle strength with rest. They are maintained on drug therapy to control symptoms and to slow the progression of the disease. Most myasthenic patients are managed at home and are hospitalized for medication adjustment or observation of symptoms when their condition worsens.

Guillain-Barré Syndrome

Guillain-Barré syndrome is a neuromuscular disease believed to result from an immune response to a viral infection. Destruction of the myelin sheath (demyelination) around the motor portion of a peripheral nerve pathway is the characteristic that causes the progressive weakness that follows. Along with the demyelination, there is swelling and inflammation around the nerve. Individual patients will have varying degrees of motor loss. Sensation is mildly affected and is usually characterized by numbness. Recovery from Guillain-Barré syndrome can take weeks to months, and as nerves remyelinate, the patient may experience heightened sensation characterized as pain. Patients spend long periods on bedrest.

There are many potential complications of immobility. These include pressure sores, depression, and constipation from loss of peristalsis; however, the most serious complication is loss of respiratory function. Any of these symptoms should be brought to the attention of a licensed person.

If Guillain-Barré syndrome affects the muscles of the chest, a dangerous decrease in respiratory function can occur. If the status of a patient with Guillain-Barré syndrome progresses to this point of weakness, intubation or tracheostomy will be required along with mechanical ventilation.

Multiple Sclerosis

The cause of multiple sclerosis (MS) is unknown; however, there is some thought that it may be related to a virus. Multiple sclerosis affects transmission of messages in the brain and spinal cord by causing scattered areas along the motor and sensory pathways to lose myelin.

Remember myelin is necessary for an impulse to travel along the pathway to reach its destination.

The destruction of the myelin causes the nerve pathway to degenerate. The result is the loss of motor and sensory function to the area where the nerve malfunctioned. The

disabilities that occur are permanent, unlike those seen in Guillain-Barré. Often the symptoms begin with weakness to the legs, which eventually spreads and then progresses to the inability to move. Sensory changes begin with numbness and tingling and eventually progress to loss of sensation. The course of multiple sclerosis is unpredictable, and the disease progresses differently in individual patients. Care provided to a patient with multiple sclerosis depends on how limited the patient's movement is. Some patients will require only minimal assistance with performing activities of daily living, especially if they are in the early stages of disease and have not yet developed limited mobility. Patients further along in the disease process may require total care with special attention to skin and passive range of motion.

Amyotrophic Lateral Sclerosis

Amyotrophic lateral sclerosis (ALS), also known as *Lou Gehrig's disease*, is a progressive, fatal degenerative disease. It is characterized by destruction of muscle cells along the spinal cord resulting in wasting of the muscles of the body. All muscles can be affected with the most serious being deterioration of the muscles of respiration. Death usually occurs from infection, aspiration, or respiratory failure. Depending on the stage of disease, patients may require minimal assistance with activities of daily living or may need total care. Either way, the muscles of respiration can become very weak with activity, and rest periods should be provided at frequent intervals.

Delirium and Dementia

Delirium is a temporary or correctable period of confusion. Delirium can be caused by emotional shock, depression, anesthesia, medications, infections, fluid or chemical changes in the body, or physical trauma, including surgery. Patients with dementia may experience periods of delirium during which their confusion is worse than usual.

Dementia is progressive loss of intellect, reasoning, and memory. Dementia is not a normal part of aging, although it is common. People with dementia gradually become more confused and disoriented and eventually lose motor function and coordination. Delirium or dementia cannot be distinguished by behavior alone. Medical tests and time are needed to determine which condition is present.

The PCT should know the baseline mental status of the patient and should observe and report changes in the patient's mental status. This will be presented later in this chapter.

Delirious and demented patients will both need close supervision by the skilled PCT to ensure their safety, since both are at risk of injury because of impaired judgment. There are many dementing diseases. Among the most common are Alzheimer's disease, Parkinson's disease, multi-infarct dementia, and Korsakoff's syndrome.

Alzheimer's Disease

Approximately 4 million people in the US currently have Alzheimer's disease. The disease usually begins in late life but may occur in adults in their 40s or even 30s. Nearly half of Americans 85 years and older have Alzheimer's disease. When the disease begins, the victims have difficulty remembering recent events and new information. As the disease progresses, more types of memory are lost. Speech becomes confused and is gradually lost. Coordination changes slowly, eventually making it difficult or impossible to walk, to perform ADLs, to maintain continence, and finally to chew and swallow. Alzheimer's disease is a terminal illness. Persons with advanced Alzheimer's disease need to be monitored constantly. Their forgetfulness and confusion allow them to get lost or put themselves or others at risk for injury.

Parkinson's Disease

Most of the 1.5 million elderly Americans who have Parkinson's disease began developing the early signs and symptoms of their illness when they were in their 50s or 60s. Movement is affected very early in Parkinson's but not in Alzheimer's disease. Parkinson's disease begins with fine motor tremors that stop during sleep and become worse when the affected limb is being used. When walking, Parkinson patients shuffle their feet and lean forward. Another characteristic of Parkinson's disease is that patients show little facial expression, making it difficult for family and caregivers to understand what the patient may be feeling. Not all Parkinson patients develop dementia. As the disease progresses, Parkinson's causes severe swallowing difficulty and risk of aspiration. Parkinson's disease is also a terminal illness in which symptoms may progress over a period of years.

Multi-infarct Dementia

Multi-infarct dementia (MID) is caused by many successive, small strokes or infarcts. People at risk for strokes are also at risk for MID. A patient with a major stroke or one of the other dementing illnesses may also have MID. MID may begin any time during adulthood, but its progression is variable. Some patients remain stable for long periods, but many become progressively more demented. MID is not a terminal disease, but these patients are very likely to die from a major cerebrovascular accident.

Korsakoff's Syndrome

Most but not all patient's with Korsakoff's syndrome have a history of significant alcohol abuse and the thia-

mine deficiency associated with alcoholism. Korsakoff's can occur at any age following long periods of malnutrition or alcoholism. The early signs of Korsakoff's are short-term memory losses, even when no alcohol has been used. As the syndrome progresses, there are more severe memory losses. Walking becomes a stagger, and dyskinesia (purposeless movements) of the limbs, mouth, and eyes develops. Korsakoff's syndrome is a terminal disease.

Sensory Losses

Sensory deficits include impairment of vision, hearing, touch, taste, or smell. These deficits are not limited to patients who have neurological disorders. Individuals may be born with deficits (congenital) or may develop the deficit later in life (acquired). The acquired deficits may develop with no other related disorders or may occur as the result of an injury or disease. Some neurological disorders and injuries are associated with sensory losses.

Just as with any other deficit a patient may have, it is important for the PCT to recognize the patient's limitations as well as his or her abilities. If the patient has had the deficit long enough, he or she may already be able to compensate effectively for the deficit. On the other hand, if the deficit is more recently acquired, the patient may feel frustrated, isolated, or overwhelmed by the loss. Other patients may be unaware of their sensory deficits and therefore find themselves in unsafe situations and will require close monitoring.

VISION. Many patients of all ages wear glasses. The PCT should know how the glasses are used and assist the patient to use the glasses appropriately. For example, some patients need their glasses all of the time, but many others need them only for reading or for watching television. Not all older people need glasses, but many do. They also tend to need more light, but have difficulty seeing when there is glare.

After a stroke or head injury, even though the eyes have not been injured, a patient may not "see" from one or the other eye. Although the eye functions normally, the message it sends goes to an injured part of the brain and so is not interpreted or recognized. Frequently these patients are not aware that they do not "see" things on one side. They are easily startled by objects or people approaching them from their blind side. For these patients, the PCT should try to approach the patient on the sighted side or to announce himself or herself if compelled to approach from the impaired side. These patients will also need cues and supervision to protect themselves from hazards on the impaired side.

HEARING. The number one cause of hearing impairments among all ages is too much wax in the ear canal. Because many people think hearing loss is a normal part of aging, older adults may accept their difficulties without consulting a health care professional. If the hearing loss is due to ear wax, the patient may have irrigations to the ear to loosen and remove the wax. Most older adults do lose some ability to hear high-pitched sounds.

TOUCH. Many neurological injuries and disorders change the sense of touch to one or more areas of the body. The sense of touch may be absent (numb) or overly sensitive, or the patient may have sensations of pain or pressure without touch occurring. Stroke and head-injured patients often lose sensation on one side of their body or in one limb. The PCT will need to help the patient protect the affected body parts, because the patients are at extreme risk to injure themselves. If the patient is not too confused or dependent, this may be done by reminding the patient to protect the part. Other patients will require protective positioning. Patients who have increased sensation of pressure or pain will need extra gentle care when the affected body part is touched. They may also be made more comfortable with padded positioning devices.

TASTE/SMELL. When an individual's sense of taste is altered, usually their sense of smell is also, and vice versa. Few neurological injuries cause changes of taste or smell, but it may happen. Neurological diseases are more frequently implicated in these changes. Cancers and the therapy used to treat cancers often alter patients' sense of taste and smell. Favorite foods often become revolting to patients. For these patients, bland foods with mild odors may be more appealing. Some cancers cause the individual to "smell" scents when none is present. Before a seizure, some individuals will briefly experience unusual smells or tastes. A person who has had a seizure disorder for some time may recognize the sensation as the preictal aura and may warn the PCT that a seizure is about to take place. If this occurs, stay with the patient, summon the RN, and ensure that seizure precautions are in place.

CARE OF THE PATIENT WITH NEUROLOGICAL DISORDERS

Neurological Testing

Computed Tomography

Diagnosis for each type of brain injury is made with a computed tomography (CT) scan. While the patient is hospitalized a repeat CT scan may be done to evaluate a worsening neurological status. During CT scan the patient lies on an X-ray table and the head is moved into the scanner. The head is scanned many times at different angles. The hair should be clean, with all hairpins removed, and all jewelry should be removed from the head and neck. There are no dietary restrictions before CT. If the patient does not have a Foley catheter, assist him or her to urinate prior to testing, as it is important to be comfortable and remain still during the test.

The patient will usually be sent by stretcher for a CT scan. A patient who needs to be restrained should be secured properly once he or she is on the stretcher. Be sure to let any transport person taking the patient for testing know that the patient is restrained and why. In some instances (i.e., severe agitation or confusion), it may be necessary for a PCT to accompany the patient for a CT scan. Report off to another RN or PCT and let him or her know where you will be. Completion of the test takes about 30 minutes.

⚖️ If the patient has a tracheostomy, needs suctioning, or possibly requires another skilled nursing procedure, an RN should accompany the patient.

When necessary to obtain further enhancement of brain tissue on the CT films, a small amount of radiopaque dye is administered intravenously by the physician or an X-ray technician. The patient may experience feelings of warmth, headache, nausea, and possible vomiting after receiving the injection. Warn the patient in advance that these symptoms may be experienced. A patient who is to receive contrast dye will not be allowed food or fluids for up to 8 hours before testing. Once the test is complete, there is no postprocedural care for patients who did not receive contrast dye. However, the patient who received an injection should be encouraged to drink fluids and should be monitored for signs of delayed allergic reaction.

📢 Notify a nurse if any of these allergic reaction symptoms should occur and stay with the patient. This may include hives, skin rash, itching, nausea, or headache.

📓 Documentation might include: "Patient returned from CT and assisted into bed; 30 minutes later red, raised bumps to arms below elbow and legs below knees. Patient complains of itchiness and headache. Nancy Jones, RN, notified. Mary White, PCT."

Magnetic Resonance Imaging (MRI)

Magnetic resonance imaging (MRI) differs from CT scan because no radiation is used. The images obtained are sharper and more detailed than CT images. Patient preparation for MRI is similar to that for a CT scan without contrast dye, and there is no postprocedural care.

Electroencephalogram

An electroencephalogram provides a recording of the electrical activity of the brain (brain waves) on graph paper. It is used to diagnose abnormal cerebral function that cannot be seen by CT or MRI, such as seizure activity. Testing is done with the patient comfortable in a reclining chair or stretcher. The patient's cooperation is essential to the quality of the test. Electrodes are placed on the scalp, and a baseline reading is established. The patient is then exposed to stimuli, such as nerve stimulation or flickering lights, which may provoke seizure activity. The brain waves are recorded throughout the test.

Prior to the procedure, the PCT assures the patient that the testing is painless. Caffeinated beverages are sometimes withheld for 24 hours before testing as they can stimulate the brain wave activity. Check with a licensed person to establish if the patient has any pretesting dietary restrictions. If a sleep deprivation study will be done, the patient will not be allowed to sleep the night before testing. This type of testing is done to determine the effect of sleep deprivation on the brain waves. The patient will, of course, be extremely tired after testing is complete and should be provided with rest periods to catch up on sleep. The patient's hair should be clean and no oils, sprays, or lotions should be used on the hair or scalp before the test. These interfere with adherence of the electrodes to the hair. Once testing is complete, the hair is shampooed to remove the paste used to affix the electrodes.

Lumbar Puncture

Lumbar puncture (LP) involves a physician placing a needle into the subarachnoid space of the lumbar spine. A sample of CSF can be obtained and analyzed in the laboratory for blood (indicating a hemorrhage) or white blood cells (indicating infection). An LP is performed at the patient's bedside. An RN or physician will prepare the LP kit for use. A PCT may be asked to help position the patient in bed. Prior to positioning, the patient should be assisted to empty the bladder for comfort during the procedure. The patient will be positioned in the lateral recumbent position with the back along the edge of the bed (Fig. 5–6). The knees should be flexed up to the chest with the chin touching the knees. The PCT can talk with the patient to help him or her relax. It may also be helpful for the PCT to place his or her hands on the patient's legs and back to remind the patient to lie very still.

When the LP is complete the patient remains lying flat in bed for 6–24 hours; this is determined by the physician, hospital policy, and the degree of the patient's headache. Neurological and vital signs are monitored frequently (check your institution's policy), and the patient is encouraged to drink fluids if able.

 Be sure to document all vital signs on the clinical data sheet as they are obtained.

Observations

A PCT with the proper training has the knowledge and skill to make basic observations of the comatose patient.

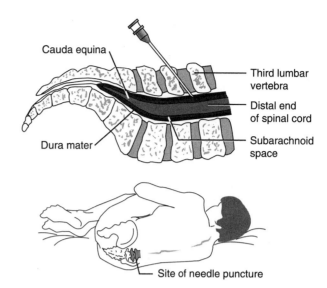

FIGURE 5-6
Positioning for lumbar puncture.

An RN is responsible for completing the full neurological examination of a comatose patient.

Because it is PCTs who will be providing the greatest amount of direct patient care, they are the ones who are most likely to determine subtle changes in the patient. Become familiar with the patients you care for, including how they behave and how they look. Use this as a baseline to recognize differences from day to day.

VITAL SIGNS. The center of the brain that controls vital signs is located within the brainstem. Stability of vital signs then may be affected by damage to the brainstem, swelling from surrounding tissues, or tumors that cause pressure. Measurement of vital signs should include blood pressure, temperature, pulse, and respiratory rate. Vital signs are crucial in a neurological patient because the first sign of further damage to the brain is often demonstrated by a change in vital signs. The frequency of assessing vital signs is determined by the stability of the patient. This is ordered by the physician, and if the RN does not inform you how frequently to check vital signs, you should ask.

NEUROLOGICAL SIGNS. A PCT relies on his or her own knowledge of the patient's previous condition and notes any changes. For example, yesterday during the patient's bed bath, the patient was calm and quiet. Today while providing care, you notice that the patient seems agitated (moving his or her extremities all over the bed, making a lot of grimaces). This would be considered a change in status and an RN should be notified.

A PCT can also provide this basic observation of a patient who is not comatose but may have a head injury. In this situation, an observation can be made regarding the patient's mental status. This observation is completed by asking the patient a few questions. First ask the patient his or her name. Next ask the patient the month and year. Most patients who have been hospitalized for longer than a couple of days are unable to know the exact date unless a calendar has been provided in the room. Finally, ask the patient where he or she is. If the patient is able to answer one question correctly, he or she is considered to be "Oriented times 1." Two correct responses is "Oriented times 2," and the correct response to all three questions is "Oriented times 3" or "Fully Oriented." For any neurologically injured patient it is also important to note any changes related to the following:

1. Ability to follow commands (e.g., lift your hand; turn on your side)
2. Behavior/mood
3. Ability to communicate
4. Ability to perform ADLs
5. Ability to move extremities

 Be sure to notify the RN of changes in any of these categories.

Physical Care

HYGIENE. The extent to which a PCT will need to provide care to the patient will depend on the severity of the neurological deficits. For example, a comatose patient will require total assistance with physical care or ADLs. This includes a total bed bath, mouth care, shaving, and hair shampoo. Monitoring bowel and bladder function is also very important. Patients may be incontinent, as the comatose patient does not have control of the bowel and bladder. It is also important to make sure that the patient is urinating or passing stool. These functions may be affected by the neurological disorder also. On the other hand, a patient with mild concussion may need assistance only in gathering supplies and be able to wash himself or herself with supervision. PCTs use their own judgment to determine what care needs to be provided and take into consideration the patient's status (motor deficits, judgment or safety issues, and level of consciousness). Remember to respect the patient's dignity and close doors and/or bedside curtains during care. Even though a patient may not appear to be aware, it is important to provide privacy.

Consult with licensed personnel, staff education personnel, and Clinical Nurse Specialists when there is uncertainty about the extent of care that needs to be provided to the patient.

SKIN CARE. Neurological injury predisposes the patient to multiple risk factors leading to skin breakdown. Loss of sensory and motor function from stroke or spinal cord injury prevents the patient from experiencing and reacting to pain or discomfort. Therefore, there is little,

if any, awareness that body parts have been in the same position for too long. The continued pressure may lead to the development of a pressure sore. Patients with head injury may be agitated and move around a lot in bed. This causes friction on the skin as it rubs against the sheets and is another risk factor for tissue damage. Friction may also result from the rubbing of wrists or ankles against restraints. Finally, immobility resulting from loss of motor function, as in a coma or a quadriplegic patient, also places the patient at risk for pressure sore formation.

Once pressure sores develop, healing is difficult because of decreased blood flow to the tissues. Skin care should be provided at least every 2 hours. Monitoring the skin for signs and symptoms of redness and breakdown is a crucial role of the PCT.

FEEDING. The cranial nerves responsible for the ability to chew and swallow may be temporarily damaged or permanently destroyed with a neurological injury. If the patient is unable to eat normally, a gastrostomy tube (a tube placed through the abdomen into the stomach) will be placed to provide nourishment. When the patient's condition is stable, and it has been determined that the ability to swallow is present, the enteral feedings will be stopped and oral feedings will resume. Still other patients, because of stomach ulcers, chronic diarrhea, or malabsorption, will receive total parenteral nutrition (TPN) through a central IV line.

Monitoring of the TPN is the responsibility of licensed personnel.

Speech therapists are specially trained professionals who make assessments of the patient's ability to chew and swallow and then determine the safest foods a patient may eat. The oral diet may initially consist of only thick liquids because they are easier to swallow. As the muscles of the throat continue to strengthen, the diet will progress to solid foods and eventually include regular liquids.

A PCT who is uncertain about a patient's ability to swallow should consult with speech therapists, licensed personnel, or Clinical Nurse Specialists prior to feeding the patient.

For those patients able to eat orally, modifications may be needed to achieve independence with eating. Occupational therapists will work with patients to find adaptive equipment that may assist patients with feeding themselves. Some patients may require total assistance with feeding (quadriplegia), while others need only supervision. Remember that most head-injured patients lack good judgment skills and are a safety risk when eating. They may burn themselves on hot coffee or choke because they have not swallowed between bites of food. Even if your patients are able to feed themselves, be sure to check on them frequently to be certain they do not need assistance.

MOBILITY. Any patient with loss of motor function from neurological injury or degenerative disease is at risk of muscle and joint deterioration from immobility. Range of motion exercises are provided to weak or inactive limbs to prevent contracture.

 The PCT should consult with physical therapists, licensed personnel, and Clinical Nurse Specialists to determine which range of motion (ROM) exercises are appropriate for individual patients.

When there is no further risk for increased ICP or further damage to the spinal cord after injury, the patient will be allowed to sit up out of bed. If the patient is unconscious, or has limited ability to assist with a transfer, obtain assistance from other caregivers. There are many pieces of equipment to assist with transfers such as mechanical lifting devices and slide boards. Check your facility for which equipment is available and consult with physical therapy to determine the most appropriate method and technique for transferring a patient to the chair.

The patient remains in the chair as tolerated and should be checked every 15–30 minutes for safety. For alert patients be sure the call light is within reach.

BOWELS AND BLADDER. The movement of food and waste products from the stomach to the rectum can slow down after neurological injury. The result is constipation; it is primarily caused by immobility or side effects of medications given for discomfort.

 Licensed personnel are responsible for performing a complete assessment of the bowel and bladder. A PCT evaluates any changes in the pattern of elimination, changes in color of urine or stool, and changes in consistency of stool and reports these to the nurse.

Diarrhea can also be a complication resulting from side effects of antibiotic therapy or a reaction to enteral feedings, or it could be a sign of infection.

The reflexes of the bladder and the control over urination may also be affected by damage to the nervous system. A Foley catheter is inserted initially to monitor urine output. It will be removed, however, as soon as possible, as it predisposes the patient to urinary tract infection. Once the catheter is removed, incontinence of urine may result from lack of sensation to the bladder or inability to get to the bathroom. Male patients may have a condom catheter placed to contain the urine; however, it should be removed every shift to provide skin care. Female patients should have pericare with each episode of incontinence to prevent skin breakdown.

Document episodes of incontinence by the number of times per shift.

SAFETY. If the patient exhibits confusion or lack of judgment, care will need to be taken to provide a safe environment. Restraints may need to be used to prevent an attempt at getting out of bed without assistance or to inhibit the ability to pull on tubes such as IV lines. Each state has different regulations governing the use of physical restraints on patients. Check your institution's policies regarding the application of physical restraints. There must always be a physician's order for a restraint.

The PCT may not decide to use a restraint without an order.

There are many types of restraints. One of the most common is the jacket type of restraint that is applied to the patient's trunk area and either zips or ties in the back. There are two long ties that come off the side of the vest jacket that should be tied to the back of the chair the patient is sitting in. If the patient is lying down, they should be tied to the frame of the bed near the middle of the bed. The ties should never be attached to the siderails. This type of restraint is useful in preventing a patient from getting out of bed or out of the chair without assistance. However, it can also be harmful, as the patient can slide down in bed and choke. Another type of restraint is the extremity restraint. This can be made of a soft cotton material. For the more agitated patient leather restraints can be used that can be locked with a key. These types of restraints are applied to the wrists and ankles either alone or in combination with a jacket restraint for further restriction of the patient's movement. Extremity restraints prevent patients from pulling at tubes, IVs, and other equipment, as well as inhibit the patient from striking out at the nursing staff. These types of restraints may also be used on patients who have been determined to be at high risk for suicide attempt.

When a patient is physically restrained, care must be taken to prevent the skin from breaking down. Restraints should be removed every 2 hours for skin care and range of motion exercises. If the patient is at high risk of injury when restraints are removed, then take only one extremity restraint off at a time. Once care to that extremity is complete, replace the restraint and move to the next limb. The other option is to have another PCT with you when restraints are going to be removed. The patient whose extremities are restrained will also require assistance with ADLs and feeding. For the patient with a jacket restraint, repositioning in the bed or the chair should occur every 2 hours to aid in the prevention of pressure sore formation.

 Documentation for the patient in restraints might include the following (include date and time): "Patient found attempting to climb out of bed on three occasions. Notified RN, who obtained order for vest restraint. Restraint applied without incident at 11:00 AM. Patient checked every 30 minutes for safety. Restraint removed at 1:00 PM and patient toileted. Skin care provided and restraint reapplied. Patient resting quietly in bed. J. Smith, PCT"

To prevent injury, sharp objects should be out of reach and moved out of the room if the patient is ambulatory. The call light should be within reach of the patient. All confused patients should be checked on frequently, and siderails should remain up at all times. A majority of head injuries or brain tumors cause uninhibited behavior. Patients may expose themselves, use profanity, or make sexually provocative and inappropriate remarks. Remember that this behavior is not intentional, and it is important not to take it personally. When it happens, protect the patient's dignity and remind the patient that the behavior is inappropriate, then continue with your care. If the patient has memory problems, you may have to deal with this situation on a continual basis. Try to maintain your patience.

Emotional Care

PCTs provide more than physical care for their patients. They also provide emotional support and comfort for patients and their families. By spending more time with the patient the PCT often knows the patient's emotional needs better than any other member of the health care team.

The feelings of loss, anger, denial, and grief are all normal reactions to serious illness or injury. For the patient with a neurological disorder, the feelings may be made more complicated to face, control, and resolve because of difficulty in speaking, moving, and even thinking. Some neurological disorders also cause uncontrollable moods and even rapid mood changes.

The PCT provides support and comfort to patients with neurological disorders and their families in many ways. This includes all of the same methods used by the PCT for all patients (Table 5–2). Patients with impaired judgment because of dementia, delirium, or neurological injuries require close supervision to minimize the risks of injury. Patients with uncontrolled moods or mood changes will need support to reduce the stimulation that triggers their moods, to contain their behaviors when they are unable to do so themselves, and to redirect their energies and attention from provocative situations.

Equipment

INTRACRANIAL PRESSURE MONITORING. Intracranial pressure (ICP) monitoring is instituted for brain-injured patients when there is increased ICP or a

TABLE 5–2
Some Causes of Acquired Sensory Losses

DISEASE	TYPE OF LOSS	INJURY
Glaucoma, retinopathy due to diabetes, stroke	Vision	Trauma to the eye, burns of the eye (often chemical), head injury
Accumulated ear wax, ear infections	Hearing	Trauma to the ear, medications that damage nerves, head injury
Diabetes, peripheral vascular disease, herpes zoster (shingles)	Touch	Trauma to the site, head injury
Cancer, seizure disorder (preictal)	Taste/Smell	Anticancer medicine

risk for it. In the operating room, a small thin catheter is placed in a ventricle of the brain where the CSF flows (Fig. 5–7). The catheter is connected to a monitoring device, and the pressure in the ventricle shows up as a waveform on a screen, much like that of an electrocardiogram (ECG). The physicians and nurses will interpret the waveform and determine the amount of pressure in the ventricle. A rise in pressure above normal is called increased ICP. ICP monitoring is done in the intensive care unit or on a specialized unit where there is skilled nursing staff to care for the patient.

When a patient has an ICP catheter in place, caution must be taken not to dislodge it when providing care. A sterile dressing covers the area where the catheter has been placed.

⚖️ The ICP monitor dressing should not be changed or removed except by a physician or other licensed personnel.

A PCT should be aware of the dressing when providing care and notify a licensed person immediately if it is falling off or is missing. The patient's position in bed can significantly alter ICP or the waveform on the screen. If the patient is moved in the bed from side to side let a licensed person know so he or she can make a note of how the ICP was affected. The head of the bed should remain at a 30–45-degree angle at all times.

 Never change the position of the bed without first asking an RN

Patients should be turned every 2 hours and provided

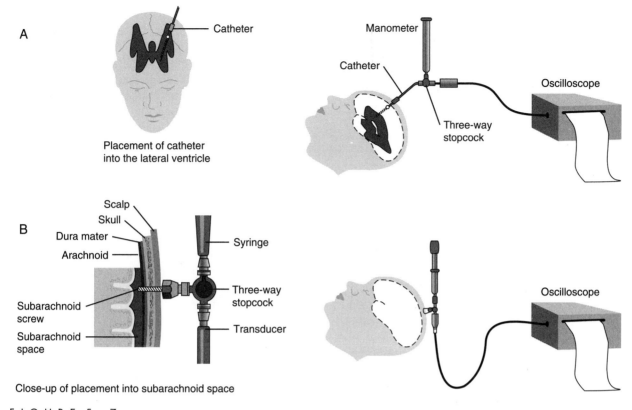

A

Catheter

Placement of catheter
into the lateral ventricle

Manometer

Catheter

Three-way
stopcock

Oscilloscope

B

Scalp
Skull
Dura mater
Arachnoid

Syringe

Three-way
stopcock

Transducer

Subarachnoid
screw

Subarachnoid
space

Oscilloscope

Close-up of placement into subarachnoid space

F I G U R E 5 – 7
ICP monitoring.

with skin care to prevent breakdown from pressure and moisture. Water retention can further increase ICP; therefore the patient may be on fluid restriction.

 The PCT must accurately document all oral fluid or tube feeding given to the patient.

 A licensed person is responsible for documenting any IV fluid given to the patient.

Urine output will be closely monitored by means of a Foley catheter. The PCT should check and document the amount of urine per order (usually every 1 hour).

HYPOTHERMIA UNITS. Hypothermia units, also called cooling blankets, are used to lower elevated body temperature in patients with neurological disorders. A unit is ordered by a physician when the body temperature rises to or above 102.5°F. The unit consists of a blanket, which lies flat under the patient and connects by hoses to a motorized temperature controller filled with water. When the unit is turned on, a licensed person will set the machine at a water temperature ordered by the physician. The machine will fill the blanket with water and will cool the water to the preset temperature. As the patient lies on the cooling blanket the body temperature will decrease.

Careful monitoring of the patient on a cooling blanket is necessary to prevent hypothermia or rapid lowering of body temperature. A PCT should obtain the rectal (unless otherwise indicated) temperature every 15 minutes and a full set of vital signs every half-hour. When skin is exposed to cold for an extended period it can be damaged. Lanolin cream or another oily emollient should be applied to the skin on the entire back of the body. Also place a sheet or thin blanket between the cooling blanket and the patient. This will prevent the cooling blanket from directly touching the patient's skin, further protecting it from breakdown.

 Report any signs of chills, shaking, goosebumps, and >2°F drop in temperature within one-half hour to a licensed person.

Also report and document any changes in the skin's integrity. Be sure to document all vital signs on the clinical data sheet.

✔ Notify the nurse when the temperature reaches 101°F.

The cooling blanket will usually be turned off then, as the patient's temperature will continue to drop 1–2°F even after the blanket is off.

Medications

When a physician orders a medicine for a patient, the drug chosen will be intended to reduce or stop the cause or consequence of a problem. Like all medicine, the drugs used to treat neurological disorders are powerful and may cause side effects. As a PCT you will not give patients medicines. Your familiarity, however, with the medicines used and possible side effects are important to protect patients from complications and identify problems early to allow for correction.

Anticonvulsants

Seizures may be caused by many conditions, including infection, rapid rise or fall of body temperature (especially in children), tumors, or increased pressure on the brain. If one of these is the cause, the physician will use antibiotics for the infection, control fluctuating temperatures, reduce or remove the tumor, or reduce the pressure inside the skull. No matter what the cause, all seizures involve disturbances of electric activity in the brain. So for all patients with a seizure disorder, one or more *anticonvulsant* medications will be ordered. These drugs interrupt or calm the electric activity in the brain. Because of this, they may also affect thinking and movement (like walking) and may cause drowsiness.

Anticoagulants

Most strokes (CVAs) are caused by ischemia and not hemorrhage. To reduce the risk of additional clot formation, *anticoagulants* are given. Lay people often call these drugs "blood thinners," but the blood is not thinned; instead, the clotting activity of the platelets (a component of blood) is slowed. The risk of too much anticoagulation is bleeding. The bleeding can be noted anywhere on the body as unusual bruising or petechiae (tiny spots of bruising noted on the skin or mucous membranes). Most common, however, is to find blood in the urine or feces, so the PCT will routinely check the urine and feces for blood.

Antihypertensives

Antihypertensives are the medicines used to treat high blood pressure (hypertension). They include vasodilators, calcium channel blockers, and diuretics. *Vasodilators* and *calcium channel blockers* relax the walls of the cardiovascular system, allowing blood to circulate with less pressure. *Diuretics* increase the amount of urine produced by pulling fluid from the body. With less circulating fluid, the pressure exerted on the vessel walls is decreased.

Analgesics

Pain medications are called *analgesics* and can be grouped into two very large categories: *narcotics* and *non-narcotics. Narcotic analgesics* are generally used for moderate to severe pain. The doctor may also select a narcotic for pain control if the side effects might be helpful for the patient. For example, many narcotic analgesics will calm and relax an anxious patient. If, however, a patient has a history of drug abuse the doctor may select non-narcotic medication or lower doses of narcotics. Whether or not there is a history of drug abuse, narcotics may cause confusion, drowsiness, changes in vital signs, constipation, and urinary retention. All of these can be identified early by the PCT.

Most *non-narcotic analgesics* are non-steroidal anti-inflammatory drugs (NSAIDs). All NSAIDs are likely to cause bleeding by disrupting the clotting function of platelets. The PCT will monitor the patient taking any NSAID the same way he or she would monitor patients receiving anticoagulation therapy (see above).

Sedatives/Hypnotics

Patients whose thinking is confused because of illness or injury often experience severe anxiety and may have unsafe or uncontrolled behaviors. To reduce both the feelings and the problem behaviors, *sedatives/hypnotics* may be ordered. These drugs act on the CNS. Unfortunately, these drugs affect the entire CNS and are not limited only to the problem feelings or behaviors. Patients may become more confused, more unsafe in their movements (including walking), and drowsy, or they may breathe too slowly. Monitoring levels of alertness and vital signs is essential.

NEUROSURGICAL CARE

Preoperative Care

The preoperative care of the patient undergoing a neurosurgical procedure is similar to the care given any person having surgery. The patient is restricted to nothing by mouth (NPO) after midnight; the usual morning care is delivered the day of surgery. For intracranial surgery, most patients will be ordered to have an antimicrobial shampoo to the hair. PhisoHex is used to decrease any microorganisms on the hair and scalp. Prior to intracranial surgery the hair is cut and the scalp is shaved. This is to prevent infection and to allow the incision to be cleaned postoperatively. Most patients will find this thought very distressing, and a PCT can provide emotional support.

A licensed person will complete a neurological assessment to establish baseline data. A PCT can help by obtaining the patient's weight and vital signs. The patient will be sent to the operating room wearing thigh-high elastic stockings to minimize the risk of clot formation during surgery. If a urinary catheter has not yet been placed, assist the patient to empty the bladder before surgery.

Postoperative Care

After surgery the patient is taken to the recovery room, then to the intensive care unit, where he or she will stay 2–3 days or until in a stable condition. Next the patient will be transferred to an acute care unit where RNs will continue to monitor the patient for postsurgical complications. A PCT should be aware that after surgery the patient may be restricted as to food and drink, and movement may be restricted. Before allowing the patient food or drink or moving the patient in the bed or the position of the bed, check with a licensed person.

Postsurgical equipment usually includes a urinary catheter, nasogastric or gastric tube, IV lines, and oxygen and may also include a tracheostomy or endotracheal tube, a ventilator, and an ICP monitor or ECG monitor. Recovery from neurosurgery depends on the procedure, the extent of the problems requiring surgery, postoperative complications, and the patient's determination to recover.

Patients may be hospitalized for as few as 3 days or as long as weeks or months.

SUMMARY

The PCT has an important role in the care of a neurologically impaired patient. Whether it is the astute observation of a change in vital signs or the task of providing skin care to prevent breakdown, the actions of the PCT can make a positive impact on the recovery of the patient. Caring for people with disorders of the nervous system challenges not only your mind but also your patience as a caregiver. Respond to inappropriate behavior in a professional but gentle way, as most often the patient is not able to control his or her behavior.

Finally, look at each neurologically impaired patient as a learning experience. With practice you will feel comfortable caring for these patients and will eventually anticipate their needs long before they are able to express them.

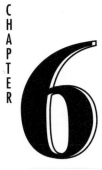

The Respiratory System

SHIRLEY FIELDS McCOY, MS, RN,C

OUTLINE

Tracheostomy Equipment
Closed-Chest Drainage System
  (CCDS)
**Caring for Patients on
Ventilators**

The PCT's Caregiver Role in Patient
  Education
Respiratory Isolation
Summary

PREREQUISITE KNOWLEDGE AND SKILLS

- Counting Respirations (Vital Signs)
- Cardiopulmonary Resuscitation (CPR)
- Choking Victim Rescue Techniques
- Mouth-to-Mouth Rescue Breathing
- Use of Mask with One-Way Valve
- Use of Manual Resuscitator
- Collecting Sputum Sample
- Fire Safety: RACE
- Respiratory Isolation Procedures

OBJECTIVES

After you complete this chapter, you will be able to:

- List the structure and functions of the respiratory system.
- Describe normal observations associated with the respiratory system.
- Identify and discuss common disorders of the respiratory system.
- Describe observations associated with respiratory distress.
- Identify interventions to respond to respiratory distress.
- Demonstrate use of equipment associated with respiratory system.
- Deliver basic care for patients who are dependent on oxygen and ventilator equipment.

KEY TERMS

Atelectasis   Collapse of the alveoli or air sacs of a portion or all of a lung. Reduces the amount of air exchange that can take place.

Breaking Point   The length of time a person can voluntarily hold the breath before sensors in the brain respond to low oxygen and high carbon dioxide and force the person to breathe.

Intercostal   Between the ribs. The intercostal muscles, located between the ribs and attached to them, help move the ribs in and out to breathe.

Metabolism   The work of the cells. The process that each cell of the body goes through to take in nutrition and oxygen, generate heat and energy, and eliminate carbon dioxide and waste products; often referred to as relating to the demands of the body as a whole. Adequate respiratory system functioning is required to support metabolic activity.

Orthopneic Position   An upright sitting position that allows full expansion of the lungs with the least physical effort. Position used for someone experiencing respiratory distress. The person may fold arms over several pillows placed on a table in front of him or her for support.

Ventilator   A machine that takes over the work of breathing for persons who are no longer able to breathe on their own due to injury or illness.

Weaning   The process of gradually allowing persons who have been on a ventilator to breathe on their own again, after their condition has been treated.

The chemistry of the body is constantly changing, and body systems work to maintain the right chemical balance for the body to function properly. As you will see throughout the book, a change in one system often causes changes in others. Sometimes this is noted by a change in the blood or urine chemistry; skin color, temperature, or moistness, or a change in vital signs. When these changes extend outside of the normal range due to illness or trauma, we refer to them as symptoms, because they indicate that something has changed in the body and may require intervention such as medications or treatments. Changes in the rate, depth, and regularity of respirations are often noted in many body system problems, as well as in primary respiratory illness.

No matter where the patient care technician (PCT) works, patients with respiratory conditions will be encountered. These conditions may be acute or chronic and require supportive care. PCTs need to be familiar with patient's physical and emotional needs, as well as the type of care they can provide to patients.

A basic understanding of the respiratory system structures and functions will be the foundation on which to build the PCT's ability to make and report observations. Appropriate communication, interventions, and documentation will be identified. Safe use of basic respiratory equipment will be explained. Teamwork, patient care, and family support will be emphasized.

STRUCTURES—BASIC ANATOMY AND FUNCTION OF THE RESPIRATORY SYSTEM

The structures of the respiratory system provide the mechanism to bring oxygen into the body and eliminate carbon dioxide by the act of breathing, or respiration. The respiratory system consists of the nose, pharynx, larynx, trachea, bronchi, and lungs. The diaphragm, along with the intercostal muscles of the rib cage and the abdominal muscles, provides the muscular action that actually moves the chest in and out (Fig. 6–1).

During respiration, air rich in oxygen is inhaled through the mouth or nose, passes through the back of the throat called the pharynx, through the larynx (called the voice box) into the trachea. The trachea branches into two bronchi that go to the right and left lung. In the lungs, the bronchi branch into smaller and smaller tubes and then into tiny air pockets called alveoli. The blood stream provides circulation of the blood to each alveolus. These blood vessels take in oxygen (O_2) and pass carbon dioxide (CO_2) out to the alveoli. With exhalation the carbon dioxide is breathed out from the alveoli through the bronchi, trachea, larynx, pharynx, nose, and mouth.

The respiratory system provides oxygen to support cel-

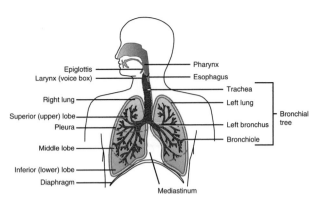

FIGURE 6–1
Respiratory tract.

lular activity and releases carbon dioxide, a waste product of the metabolism of body cells, to the outside. Respiration is very much a chemical process. The carbon dioxide dissolved in the blood acts as a chemical and reacts with other body chemicals. A portion of the brain called the medulla is responsible for regulating the respiratory rate. It responds to the level of carbon dioxide in the blood and increases or decreases respirations to maintain a normal chemical balance. This chemical balance is called acid-base balance and is measured by pH of arterial blood.

Certain drugs, such as narcotic pain medications, depress the respiratory center and prevent normal removal of carbon dioxide since respirations are shallow and slow. Some illnesses result in structural changes to respiratory tissues that decrease their effectiveness. Less oxygen is made available to body tissues and more carbon dioxide is retained. An increased level of carbon dioxide in the arterial blood is referred to as respiratory acidosis, low pH. Situations that result in increased respiratory rates may blow off more carbon dioxide and result in respiratory alkalosis (high pH). Table 6–1 describes common situations that result in these two states. Further discussion of the illnesses identified and care needs, will be found later in this chapter. The table serves as a reminder that changes in respirations have much more impact on body systems, and are much more important, than you might have thought in the past.

STRUCTURAL FUNCTIONS

Nose

As air is inhaled through the nose, it is warmed by the body temperature, moistened by body fluids, and filtered by the large hairs in the nasal cavities (nares). The nares are separated by a narrow wall called the nasal septum. The nasal sinuses are pockets in the cheekbone near the

T A B L E 6 – 1
Acid-Base Conditions

CONDITIONS	CAUSES	ACTIONS
Respiratory acidosis (Retention of carbon dioxide)	COPD (chronic obstructive pulmonary disease) such as: emphysema or chronic bronchitis Respiratory depression from narcotic medication	Monitor patient for level of consciousness, decreased respirations, headaches, restlessness, irritability, blurred vision, and depressed reflexes. Maintain head of bed at 45 degrees and low-flow supplemental O_2. Notify RN of changes by means of the call light and stay with patient.
Respiratory alkalosis (Decrease of carbon dioxide)	Hyperventilation due to hypoxia, anxiety, fever, exercise, or excessive mechanical assist to breathing	Monitor patient for numbness and tingling, c/o's, light-headedness, dry oral mucosa, inability to concentrate, mental confusion, and increased respirations. Try to decrease patient's level of anxiety. Notify RN of changes by the call light and stay with the patient.

nose that contain fluid. There are small openings between these sinus cavities (pockets) and the back of the nose that aid in draining the sinuses. With a cold or allergies the nasal tissues swell and block off sinus drainage. A sinus infection often develops in the blocked sinuses.

Pharynx (Throat)

The pharynx, the back of the mouth (throat), serves as the common passageway for air and food. The pharynx consists of 3 portions. The nasopharynx extends from the nose to the soft palate. The oropharynx, the middle portion that lies behind the mouth, is the common passageway for food. The laryngopharynx, the lower portion, leads to both the larynx, which extends downward to the lungs, and the esophagus, which leads to the stomach.

Larynx (Voice Box)

The larynx, or voice box, serves as a passageway for air between the pharynx (throat) and the trachea (windpipe). It lies in the middle of the neck. The larynx acts like a valve guarding the entrance of the trachea. It controls the air flow and prevents anything but air from entering the trachea.

When food is swallowed a flaplike structure called the epiglottis in the throat covers the larynx. This allows food to bypass the larynx and trachea as we swallow and not enter the lungs, but go to the stomach. Should food or any foreign matter enter the larynx, a cough reflex will occur to expel it. This is commonly said to be getting something caught in your windpipe or swallowing the

wrong way. This most commonly occurs when someone tries to talk and eat at the same time.

The larynx houses the vocal cords, which vibrate as expired air passes out, allowing people to speak. The opening between the vocal cords is called the glottis. Any obstruction of this area can easily lead to death by suffocating if not relieved promptly (see Chapter 16).

The PCT should know the international sign for choking (Fig. 6–2), signs of a choking victim (such as being unable to talk, turning blue, and making a high-pitched gasping sound), and how to rescue a conscious or unconscious choking victim of any age.

Trachea (Windpipe)

The trachea is a flexible, tubular structure that continues from the larynx into the thoracic cavity and divides into the right and left bronchi. It is open at all times to allow for air to pass to and from the lungs.

Bronchi

The right and left bronchi enter into the lungs. These bronchi then divide into smaller branches (smaller tubes) and continue still farther to form even smaller branches called terminal bronchioles. These are all located in the lobes of the lungs. When you look at Figure 6–1, you will see how this these branches form a respiratory network that resembles an upside-down tree. It is referred to as the bronchial tree.

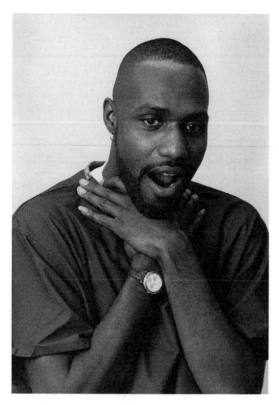

FIGURE 6-2
International sign for choking.

Alveoli

At the end of the terminal bronchioles are clusters of little air sacs called alveoli. In fact, the interior of the lungs looks like a sponge, with the alveoli as the holes. These clusters located deep within the lungs are the site where the gas exchange process occurs.

Gas is exchanged between the lungs and the blood by diffusion through thin walls of the alveoli and the capillaries of the circulatory system. Oxygen goes through a thin wall into a red blood cell, and the red blood cell sends back carbon dioxide into the alveoli to be exhaled (Figs. 6–3 and 6–5).

Lungs

The lungs are the essential organs of respiration. When air reaches the bronchi and alveoli in the lungs, this allows for the process of gas exchange. When oxygen reaches the alveolar sacs, the exchange of gases takes place.

The lungs are cone shaped. Their broad bases rest upon the diaphragm. The apex or the pointed top extends above the first rib. The lungs are enclosed by a transparent, serous membrane called the pleura.

Pleura

The pleura is a closed sac consisting of two layers that are attached to the chest wall and diaphragm. There is a small amount of fluid between the layers. This allows the layers to glide freely over each other during expansion and contraction of the chest.

Mediastinum

The mediastinum is the space between the right and left lungs. This space extends from the sternum to the spinal column. It contains the heart, large blood vessels connected with the heart, trachea, esophagus, various veins, lymph nodes, and nerves.

Diaphragm and Intercostal Muscles

The diaphragm is the primary muscle of respiration. It is a flat muscle attached to the back as well as to the rib cage in front and separates the thoracic and abdominal cavities. The diaphragm is located beneath the lungs and above the abdominal organs. During inspiration the upward-curving diaphragm contracts, pulling downward, and increasing the vertical length of the thoracic cage. At the same time the intercostal muscles, between the

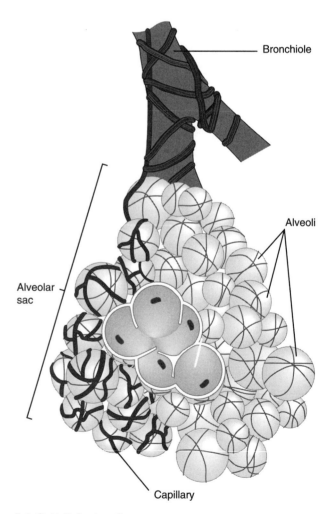

FIGURE 6-3
Lobule of lung showing alveoli.

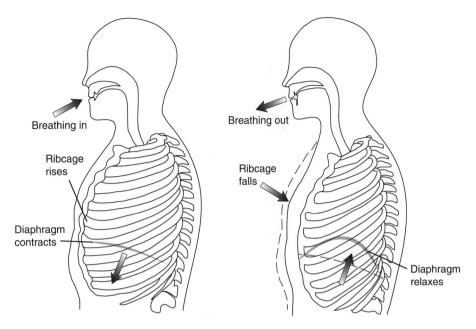

F I G U R E   6 – 4

Thoracic cage during inspiration/
expiration.

ribs, pull the ribs upward and outward. It is this activity, increasing the size of the thoracic cavity, that causes lung expansion and the pulling in of air (Fig. 6–4).

Expiration is passive and all the contracted respiratory muscles relax. The alveoli empty, and air high in carbon dioxide is pushed out of the lungs.

Voice Production

As exhaled air passes through the larynx, it may also be used to produce sound. Two folds of tissue, known as the vocal cords, extend across the inside of the larynx. Changes in the length of these folds and the opening (glottis) between them produce sounds we use to speak as air passes outward. These sounds are further changed by being bounced against the walls of the sinuses (cavities in the head) and being shaped by the tongue, teeth, and lips. When someone has a cold, the sinuses often become filled with mucus and may be blocked, and changes in the voice as air resonates against full sinus cavities are easy to detect.

HOW THE RESPIRATORY SYSTEM WORKS AND RELATES TO OTHER BODY SYSTEMS

Respiration is simply the act of breathing. Respiration involves the taking up of oxygen and giving off of carbon dioxide. "In with the good air and out with the bad." Each cell in the body must have a constant supply of oxygen. The oxygen is used to produce the energy for cellular activity.

Nutrients (food) + oxygen (air) → energy
+ water + CO_2 (toxins)

This reaction is known as cellular respiration. Blood transports nutrients and oxygen from the lungs to the cells where an energy exchange takes place. This produces water and carbon dioxide from the cells; the carbon dioxide travels back to the lungs.

The carbon dioxide is brought to the lungs by the pulmonary artery from the right side of the heart. It passes through tiny capillaries that surround the alveoli. The carbon dioxide escapes through the walls of the alveoli and is exhaled. The oxygen absorbed by the blood is carried back to the left side of the heart by the pulmonary vein. It is then pumped through the general circulation (Fig. 6–5).

The center of respiratory control is in an area of the brain called the medulla. The need for oxygen is sensed by the cells of this special area. The medulla then transmits this message through nerves to the diaphragm and the intercostal muscles to cause the movement of breathing.

Breathing is an involuntary action of the body. However, there are times when we can control or hold our breath, for example, when talking, singing, eating, and swimming. This voluntary control is limited. The respiratory center in the brain will override our voluntary control and make us breathe to meet the body's basic need for oxygen. The breaking point for this is usually around 23–27 seconds. If the lungs are aerated by forced breathing (deep breathing), the breaking point has been postponed in some people for as long as 8 minutes.

Respiration is the physical (breathing) and chemical processes by which an organism supplies its cells and tissues with the oxygen needed for metabolism and relieves them of the carbon dioxide formed in energy-producing reactions. The mechanics of the respiratory cycle (one respiration) consists of two phases: inspiration and expiration.

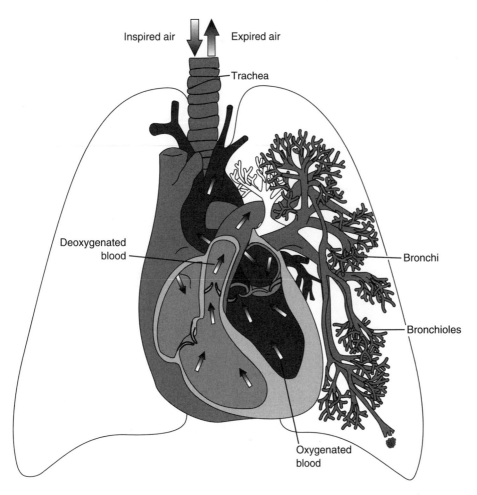

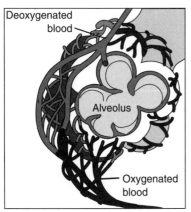

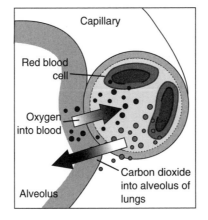

FIGURE 6-5
Oxygen diffusion into blood.

Factors Affecting Respiration

There are many factors that can affect our ability to breathe; some we can control, and some we cannot. They are:

- Conditions of acute or chronic illness
  Whether the illness is of a respiratory nature or not, illness affects how people breathe. For example, in patients with cardiac conditions or neuromuscular conditions, the respiratory system is often compromised.

- Elevated temperature
  When the body has an increase in temperature, as during fever or strenuous muscular exercise, there is an increase in the respiratory rate to blow off excess body heat. On the other hand, a subnormal temperature, as during hypothermia, results in a decrease in respiratory rate to maintain body heat.

- Exercise
  Spontaneous or infrequent exercise activity tends to increase the respirations of the patient, but patients

who do aerobic type of exercise regularly over time will tend to breathe easier with any type of activity.

- Drugs/Medications
  Medications that are narcotics, such as morphine, cause respiratory depression, slowing the respirations.

- Obesity
  Increased body weight requires increased oxygen demand and therefore increases respiratory effort. Extra weight around the abdomen or chest also interferes with the ability to breathe.

- Emotions/Pain
  The body's stress response increases the respiratory rate. Depression may decrease the respiratory rate. Patients in pain may have greatly altered respiratory rates.

- Position or Immobility
  When a patient is on prolonged bedrest, the inactivity, along with the decreased ability to expand the lungs, increases the opportunity for pneumonia, an infection in the lungs, to develop.

- Smoking
  Nicotine, tars, and other irritants in inhaled smoke damage lung tissue and decrease the amount of functional lung capacity. Cancerous tumors of the lung also are associated with smoking.

Respiratory Changes due to Aging

Because aging lungs over time have been exposed to environmental and internal stresses and irritants, lung disease is not uncommon in older age. It is often difficult to determine causation. Even in the absence of disease there are changes in the respiratory structures that lead to decreased elasticity and increased rigidity. Changes that are thought to occur as a result of normal aging are:

- Loss of elasticity in the lungs causing difficulty in inhaling and fully exhaling.

- Reduced musculoskeletal ability to tolerate stressful exercise, resulting in more "work" and increased respiratory demand.

STOP Close observation of older adults and their endurance for activity is needed. The PCT may need to adjust the pace of activities to reduce the potential for respiratory distress in the older adult.

Aging Changes in Older Adults

Think of the lungs as balloons that have been inflated for a long time. When the air is released, the balloon does not go back completely to its original shape. As aging occurs, it becomes more difficult to breathe deeply because the lungs have become less pliable or elastic. The enlarged alveoli may collapse and not open, and thus

there is diminished breathing capacity. Fibrotic muscular changes in the diaphragm and intercostal muscles cause rigidity, producing decreased functioning of the respiratory muscles.

In some older adults, changes in posture affect the thoracic cage. These changes, known as *kyphosis,* which refers to a posterior curvature of the spine, and *scoliosis,* which is a lateral curvature of the spine, cause a reduction in lung volumes. Along with the above structural changes related to aging, the older adult is more susceptible to frequent respiratory infections, partly because of the decreased ability to fully expand the lungs and keep secretions moving. Also, the older adult's voice tends to become higher pitched and weaker as fibrotic changes occur in the vocal cords.

DISORDERS OF THE RESPIRATORY SYSTEM

It is important to have a basic understanding of the respiratory disease processes affecting your patients, so that appropriate interventions can be made. The respiratory tract can be affected by a wide variety of disorders.

When respirations are inefficient, there is less oxygen in the blood available for use, carbon dioxide may be retained, maintenance of body temperature may be affected, and other systemic effects can result.

$$\text{Increase in } O_2 \text{ or } CO_2 = \text{Problem}$$
$$\text{Decrease in } O_2 \text{ or } CO_2 = \text{Problem}$$

STOP The PCT will need to learn the abnormal symptoms of each of the following disorders and alert the RN when they are observed.

The following are some categories and specific major respiratory disorders that you will encounter as PCT.

Inflammatory Disorders of the Upper Airway

Inflammatory disorders are most likely caused by viruses. These disorders are common and usually treated on an outpatient basis. The upper respiratory organs include the nose, sinuses, and throat. A common cold, which is caused by a virus, is an example of an upper respiratory infection (URI). It is one of the most common upper respiratory illnesses.

 Symptoms include elevated temperature, runny nose, and watery eyes.

A URI usually runs its course over a period of 10 days and can be treated with an antipyretic, like aspirin, to reduce the fever and relieve aches; rest; and increased fluid intake to liquefy secretions.

Sometimes a URI can move down into the chest and result in bronchitis or pneumonia. Since mucus tends to settle into the alveoli of the lung in a patient on bedrest, it is important for patients to change their positions frequently, ambulate if able, use incentive spirometer devices to assist in keeping the lungs open, and mobilize mucus as much as possible.

Influenza

Influenza is an acute disease accompanied by fever and systemic symptoms such as cough, sore throat, generalized muscle aches and pains, and sometimes gastrointestinal (GI) distress like vomiting or diarrhea. There are 3 types of flu (A, B, C); they usually occur in the winter and affect children first and spread to adults. Influenza is time limited, usually about 10 days, followed with a 1–2-week period of fatigue. Again, there can be further complications like pneumonia in adults with underlying heart or lung disease.

Sinusitis

Inflammation of the mucus lining of sinuses located throughout the facial bones may be acute or chronic and result in blockage of drainage with nasal congestion. Patients may complain of constant severe pain in the forehead, cheek, upper teeth, base of skull, or behind the eyes (locations of various sinus cavities). Symptoms are treated with medications and antibiotics if an infection develops.

Inflammatory and Other Restrictive Disorders of the Lower Airway

Acute Bronchitis

Acute bronchitis is an inflammation of the bronchi. Most episodes are caused by viral infection. A person with acute bronchitis usually has a cough and muscular-type chest pain. Production of sputum may occur along with fever and chills. Unless there is an underlying disease process, dyspnea (shortness of breath) does not usually accompany bronchitis. The bronchitis is usually time limited and can be treated with antibiotics.

Pneumonia

Pneumonia is a serious inflammation of the lungs. It can be caused by a variety of infectious organisms. Three common causes of pneumonia are: viruses, *Streptococcus pneumoniae* (a bacterium), and *Pneumocystis carinii* (a protozoan). It may involve only a portion of one lung or affect both lungs.

Today, most pneumonias, though serious and potentially life threatening, respond favorably to antibiotic therapy. For people on steroid therapy and those who have depressed immune systems, pneumonia can be very dangerous. *P. carinii* is most often noted in people who have poorly functioning immune systems.

Pneumonia is most typically seen as a sudden onset of shaking chills, high fever, pleuritic chest pain, cough, and production of greenish sputum. The pain is worse with inspiration and sometimes radiates to the shoulder or abdomen. To splint the pain the patient may lie on the affected side. Abdominal distention and nausea and vomiting may occur. The patient may also have tachycardia (increased heart rate) and shallow respirations.

Atypical pneumonia has a gradual onset that may seem to be generalized fatigue. This may be characterized by symptoms of headache, sore throat, earache, rash, or dry nonproductive cough. Later the cough may become productive, and there will be accompanying chest soreness from coughing. In the older adult, the symptoms may appear as agitation or lethargy, with or without fever.

Aspiration pneumonia is pneumonia that develops after food or fluid gets into the respiratory tract, due to the failure of the epiglottis to close over the larynx. This often shows as a localized bacterial infection with a gradual onset of low-grade fever and cough over several days to weeks. Later, copious foul-smelling sputum is coughed up.

Tuberculosis (TB)

Tuberculosis is an inflammation of the lungs caused by a bacterium *(Mycobacterium tuberculosis)*. In response to the bacteria, which destroy parts of the lung tissue, the body develops fibrous connective tissue around the infection sites in an attempt to isolate them. These fibrous structures are called tubercles. Because the tubercles are inelastic, they interfere with the full recoiling of the lung during expiration. In addition, the thick fibrous tissues increase the difficulty of gas passing through the alveoli.

Pulmonary tuberculosis is treated with special drugs and by giving the infected lung as much rest as possible. In mild cases this may be accomplished by keeping the patient in bed. In advanced cases, the lung may be temporarily or permanently collapsed by various surgical procedures.

TB is one of the oldest known diseases. It still ranks high as a cause of death. It is caused by microorganisms that are transmitted to others by droplets from sneezing and coughing. The organisms usually attack the lungs, but other parts of the body may be invaded. The person with TB usually does not have clinical symptoms. Diagnosis is made with chest X-rays or positive bacterial cultures. The presence of the disease is detected through a positive reaction to a tuberculin skin test and Gram stain and culture of sputum.

STOP When caring for patients with active TB, the PCT must protect himself or herself from exposure by wearing a HEPA-filtered mask for special respiratory isolation (see Fig. 3–6).

✔ Report to the RN when caring for TB patients: fatigue, fever, weight loss, spitting up blood, night sweats, and excessive coughing.

Sleep Apnea

Sleep apnea is a disorder of breathing during sleep. Apnea is characterized by the presence of a 10-second or longer pause in breathing. Sleep apnea is diagnosed when 30 or more of these periods occur per 7 hours of sleep or more than 5 such episodes during 1 hour of sleep. Sleep apnea syndrome is a potentially lethal condition associated with episodes of unusually loud snoring and excessive daytime sleepiness. It is diagnosed after overnight observation in a sleep laboratory.

Obstructive Respiratory Disorders

Chronic Obstructive Pulmonary Disease (COPD)

COPD refers to any chronic lung disease that results in the blocking of the bronchial airways. Chronic pulmonary inflammation results in narrowing and irreversible damage to the bronchioles and alveoli and the pulmonary blood vessels. There is increasing loss of lung elasticity, so the lungs do not fully inflate on inhalation or deflate on exhalation. Carbon dioxide is trapped in the lung, and levels increase in the blood stream.

Normally, increased levels of carbon dioxide in the blood stream stimulate respirations. People with COPD, however, adjust to high levels of carbon dioxide. Eventually they depend on special receptors that are sensitive to low levels of oxygen for respiratory stimulus (hypoxic drive).

If too much oxygen is given to the patient (flow rates are too high), the stimulus to breathe is lost. For this reason, patients with COPD are usually given oxygen at 1–2 liters/min with a low-flow oxygen delivery device like a nasal cannula.

Several conditions may develop into COPD. They include asthma, bronchitis, and emphysema.

ASTHMA. Asthma is characterized by attacks of difficult breathing, coughing, wheezing, raising of mucoid sputum, and a sensation of tightening of the chest. It is the result of bronchial muscle spasms and swelling of the mucous membrane tissue. This narrows the airways. It is usually a result of inhalation or ingestion of substances to which a patient is sensitive and is part of the allergic response.

The body responds by:

- Increasing mucus production in the air passageways
- Producing spasms in the bronchial musculature
- Causing the mucous membrane lining the respiratory tract to swell

The flow of air is obstructed on expiration. The patient experiences dyspnea (shortness of breath) and wheezing. Chronic asthma leads to COPD.

BRONCHITIS: RESTRICTIVE AND OBSTRUCTIVE. Chronic bronchitis develops from frequent infections or chronic irritations of the respiratory tract such as occurs with smokers.

Chronic bronchitis is a severe obstruction of airflow characterized by:

- Excessive mucous secretions in the bronchi
- Variable levels of dyspnea
- Tendency to be overweight
- Severe hypoxemia (low oxygen levels)
- Enlarged heart, leading to right-sided failure
- Peripheral edema
- Thickened, reddened bronchial walls
- Chronic, recurrent, productive cough

EMPHYSEMA. An increasing number of Americans die from emphysema every year. This condition develops gradually, usually over a period of years.

Characteristics of Emphysema
- Tiny alveoli lose some of their elasticity.
- The alveoli cannot become smaller as they should during expiration.
- A portion of carbon dioxide stays trapped in the alveoli.
- There is less possibility of good gas exchange.

Results of Emphysema
- Interference with gas exchange in the lungs puts additional strain on the blood vessels and heart.
- These patients are susceptible to infections.
- Expiration is difficult so that patients with emphysema characteristically lean forward with their shoulders raised as they try to force the carbon dioxide out of their lungs by pursing their lips to exhale. Known as "pink puffers."
- Patients show great efforts to breathe.
- Patients usually have to sleep with the head of bed raised or sleep on several pillows.

🛑 The following interventions should be initiated by the RN. The PCT can assist and reinforce these actions.

Interventions and general care of emphysema and bronchitis patients include all of the care provided to a COPD patient:

- Assisting with proper breathing techniques such as pursed-lip breathing
- Encouraging breathing exercises
- Positioning to improve ventilation by raising the head of bed or use of several pillows

- Assisting with postural drainage
- Providing care during low-flow oxygen therapy
- Monitoring patients receiving antibiotic therapy for overgrowth with a vaginal or oral infection
- Encouraging patients to avoid crowds, especially during flu season
- Encouraging patients not to go outside when the temperature is 35–40°F or lower, since the cold can trigger spasms.
- Encouraging patients not to smoke
- Maintaining humidity with a room humidifier if ordered

Bronchiectasis

Bronchiectasis is the chronic dilatation of the bronchi associated with airflow obstruction. This is usually caused by viral infection such as measles and flu; bacterial infection such as tuberculosis; or fungal infection such as histoplasmosis.

Cystic Fibrosis

Cystic fibrosis is usually thought of as a childhood disease, and indeed many persons with this disease process do not survive into adulthood. With better medical treatment the survival rate into young adulthood is increased, and you will see these patients on medical units with increasing frequency.

Cystic fibrosis is a multisystem genetic disease. Abnormalities of the exocrine glands and formation of thick mucus are characteristic symptoms. The most important organs involved are the lungs, pancreas, bowel, and sweat glands. The thick mucus blocks the bowel, destroys the pancreas, and fills the bronchi. Respiratory symptoms noted are similar to those of COPD, particularly chronic bronchitis. The primary symptom is thick copious mucus with a productive cough, and with progression of the disease there is increasing shortness of breath and decreasing exercise tolerance. Bowel problems cause dietary deficiencies, and nutritional intake has to be monitored closely.

Cancer of the Larynx

The incidence of laryngeal cancer is low, but it primarily affects the male population. Chronic irritation of the larynx from cigarette smoke is believed to lead to cell changes that develop into cancer. Any person who complains of hoarseness for 2 weeks should be checked for cancer. The first symptom may be painful swallowing or difficulty in swallowing due to obstruction by a tumor.

If the glottic area (vocal cords) is involved, the choice of treatment is usually surgery with adjunctive radiation therapy. *Laryngectomy* is the excision of the larynx. The patient is unable to speak and may use an external voice box to simulate the vocal cords and allow limited speech.

Though this surgery is disfiguring, the prognosis is generally good.

Lung Cancer

The incidence of lung cancer is increasing; it is the second most common type of cancer in the United States. Some cases of lung cancer are due to metastasis—the transfer of abnormal cells from one organ (the primary site) to another not directly connected with it. For example, cancerous cells from a kidney tumor may break free and be carried to the lungs by way of the blood or the lymphatic system. This is called metastatic cancer of the lung.

Primary pulmonary cancer, which begins in the lungs, is the most common form of cancer in males today, and it is becoming increasingly common in females. This great increase in the incidence of lung cancer appears to be directly related to years of heavy cigarette smoking.

The general clinical symptoms of lung cancer may be difficult to recognize because they are nonspecific and may not be pulmonary in nature.

Treatment may include chemotherapy, radiation therapy, surgery, or a combination, depending on the type of cancer. Patient care interventions should be centered around the control of pain and discomfort from coughing or dyspnea. The use of narcotics can cause side effects that result in respiratory depression, constipation, and decreased levels of consciousness. The PCT's observations of the above should be reported immediately to the RN, so corrective interventions can be implemented. Also, emotional support of the patient's grieving process is essential during this time. (See Chapter 13 for further discussion of care of cancer patients.)

TRAUMATIC CONDITIONS AFFECTING RESPIRATORY FUNCTION

Trauma to the respiratory system can involve structures of either the upper or lower respiratory tract.

PULMONARY SYMPTOMS
Dyspnea Productive cough or change in cough Hemoptysis (blood-tinged sputum)
NONPULMONARY SYMPTOMS
Anorexia Loss of appetite Weight loss Nausea and vomiting (N/V) Weakness

Epistaxis (Nosebleed)

Epistaxis is frightening but is usually not dangerous when it results from a trauma. The bleeding occurs because there is a layer of small blood vessels in the nose covered by a thin mucosa. Trauma to the nose causes the vessels to tear open. Epistaxis can also occur from an underlying disease process that interferes with the blood's ability to clot, such as hemophilia, or in patients receiving anticoagulant therapy like Coumadin.

Bleeding from the nose may be obvious, but the PCT should be aware that the patient may also be swallowing blood. In fact, major blood loss could occur down the back of the throat if that went undetected. Look in the back of the throat for any signs of bleeding. The patient should be placed in a Fowler's position and assisted to lean forward to expectorate blood. Pressure can be placed on the vessels by squeezing the bridge of the nose. A cold pack may also be placed on the nose. Patients need close observation and support.

Nasal and Maxillofacial Fractures

Fractures may be isolated or associated with other facial injuries. Characteristics to observe for are epistaxis, pain, swelling, and bruising of the face. Potential airway obstruction may be related to the swelling. The patient may have an altered appetite related to the facial immobilization. A special diet may be ordered, and the patient may require assistance to eat. Attention to comfort management is needed. The patient may need assistance in many self-care measures, depending on the extent of injury.

Chest Wall Injuries

Approximately 25% of all traumatic deaths in the United States are due to chest trauma. Chest trauma is classified into two categories: blunt and penetrating. Blunt trauma is usually the result of deceleration or compression due to a motor vehicle accident or fall. Penetrating injuries occur most commonly as the result of gunshots and stabbings, although other projectiles may occasionally cause penetrating wounds. Each type of injury results in different care issues.

Acute Respiratory Failure (ARF)

ARF is a sudden impairment in the respiratory system that results in failure to take in sufficient oxygen and/or failure of sufficient carbon dioxide elimination to meet the metabolic requirement of the body. This failure can be monitored by arterial blood gas values. Chronic respiratory failure occurs slowly over time, usually in patients with COPD.

Adult Respiratory Distress Syndrome (ARDS)

ARDS is a serious respiratory complication of trauma to the lungs or to other body systems. It is the breakdown of the lung's structural integrity that results in ineffective gas exchange. ARDS is characterized by severe hypoxemia and dyspnea.

The patient is vulnerable to fluid overload and is usually on mechanical ventilation to control the forced inspiratory oxygen flow. Sepsis, a systemic infection, can either cause or complicate ARDS. Strict handwashing and other infection control measures must be followed with these patients. Fever and other signs of infection must be reported.

Thoracic Surgery

Thoracic surgery usually involves the organs located within the thoracic cage, of which the heart and lungs are the primary organs. Any surgical procedure in which a patient receives general anesthesia will slow down the respiratory function. The patient may or may not be on a ventilator to provide for respiratory function. Patients recovering from surgery will be weaned from the ventilator and encouraged to take deep breaths to help expand the lungs and decrease the incidence of any respiratory complications. The patient often will have chest tubes in place to provide for drainage of fluids and the escape of air from the intrapleural space. This helps the lungs to reinflate. Intravenous fluids are monitored closely to reduce the risk of fluid overload and pulmonary edema.

OTHER PULMONARY COMPLICATIONS ASSOCIATED WITH MEDICAL/ SURGICAL CONDITIONS

Pulmonary Edema

In pulmonary edema, fluid fills the bronchioles and alveoli, decreasing oxygenation and increasing dyspnea, and is often accompanied by a protective cough. The respirations may sound wet. This usually is the result of fluid overload and congestive heart failure.

Pulmonary Embolism/Pulmonary Infarction

Often called PE, this refers to the obstruction of one or more pulmonary arteries. An embolism is obstruction of the arterial system of the lungs by a foreign substance. This substance can be air, fat, blood clot, or amniotic fluid, or it can be parasitic in nature. The substance causes a blockage that results in damage to the surrounding tissue. Historically this has occurred with long-term bedrest when antiembolism measures, such as use of leg compression devices and leg exercises, are not carried out. Cardiac arrhythmias also may produce clots that result in PE.

 Pulmonary embolism is like a heart attack to the lungs! Sudden onset, decreased blood pressure, increased heart rate, and severe shortness of breath are symptoms. Report as an emergency to the RN.

RESPIRATORY DIAGNOSTIC PROCEDURES/COMMON TESTS

Apart from the general physical examinations of the patient, further diagnostic studies may be needed to confirm a diagnosis. The PCT should be familiar with the commonly ordered tests to answer patients' questions and prepare them properly for tests.

Radiographic Examinations

The most common type of radiographic examination is a chest X-ray (CXR). CXRs are used as screening tests, for diagnosis, for measuring progress of therapy and extent of disease process, and for determining placement of various types of tubes and catheters. X-rays are produced from an X-ray tube that is directed so that the rays pass through the chest and are recorded on photographic film.

To avoid shadowing on the X-ray film, the patient should remove any clothes with buttons or metal clips and all jewelry or other metal objects above the chest. The CXR is taken after the patient has had a deep breath, so the lungs are fully expanded. The PCT should make sure the patient is clothed appropriately before going for the test.

Other diagnostic techniques are computed tomography (CT) and magnetic resonance imaging (MRI). These examinations provide more specific diagnostic capabilities, defining anatomical changes. They usually require no preparation, except removal of all metal and jewelry.

Arterial Blood Gases (ABGs)

Arterial blood gas (ABG) measurements are taken to assess gas exchange. Serial measurements help to determine the effectiveness of both nursing and medical interventions to improve oxygenation and gas exchange.

Blood samples are drawn from an arterial line or aspirated directly from the radial, brachial, or femoral artery. The PCT may be asked to apply pressure to the site after the stick for at least 5 minutes to assure that bleeding has stopped. Observations for hematomas and infections at the site should be ongoing. ABGs need to be put on ice and taken to the laboratory immediately.

Pulmonary Function Tests

Pulmonary function tests are used to evaluate dyspnea, to evaluate lung disease preoperatively, to detect early-stage pulmonary disease, to evaluate the effects of medication, and to follow the progression of pulmonary disease. They are also helpful in determining the degrees of

disability in patients with chronic lung disease. A lung volume study measures the amount of air entering or leaving the lungs during different respiratory movements.

These tests can be done at the bedside for simple screening and in a pulmonary function laboratory for more definitive testing. A type of spirometer is used to measure and provide a graphic readout of inspiratory and expiratory volume. The patient is asked to breathe as deeply as possible and to blow out hard and fast as long as possible into a mouthpiece attached to the machine (Fig. 6–6). Respiratory therapists conduct these tests.

Bronchoscopy

Bronchoscopy is the direct visualization procedure in which a rigid or flexible fiberoptic lighted bronchoscope is passed through the mouth and respiratory tract for inspection of the pharynx, larynx, trachea, and bronchi. The procedure can be performed at the patient's bedside, in an operating room, or in a procedure room. The patient is medicated so that he or she is in a form of twilight sleep that blocks the gag reflex. The purpose can be diagnostic, to determine a pathological problem, or therapeutic, to remove a foreign object or drain an abscess.

Bronchography

Bronchography is an X-ray procedure conducted in the radiology laboratory, using a radiopaque liquid to illuminate the bronchial tree. It can then be seen by X-ray. When the radiopaque liquid is injected into the circulatory system, the patient often feels a hot flush through the entire body, and may feel waves of nausea.

In both bronchoscopy and bronchography, the patient is usually NPO for at least 6 hours prior to the procedure. Following the bronchography, the patient must be placed in a semi-Fowler's position to prevent aspiration, since the gag reflex has been blocked. Vital signs must be monitored. The patient should be encouraged to cough up any secretions. Food and beverages are restricted until the patient's gag reflex returns, usually 1–1½ hours. The PCT's role is to assist in assuring patient compliance, provide mouth care as needed, and to report any deviations to the RN.

Thoracentesis

Aspiration of air or fluid from the pleural space by a needle is known as thoracentesis. This procedure is performed for diagnostic purposes, to relieve pulmonary congestion, or to instill medication into the pleural space.

The patient is usually positioned on the side of the bed leaning forward over the bedside table. The PCT's role in this procedure may be to obtain vital signs prior to the procedure and frequently after the procedure; assist with holding the patient in position; and observe the patient for any complaints of distress, drainage from the

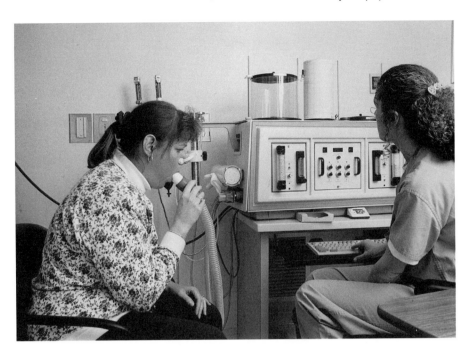

FIGURE 6-6
Pulmonary function test.

procedure site dressing, or coughing up of any blood. Report these to the RN immediately. If the patient suddenly experiences shortness of breath and chest pain, put pressure over the dressing site and put on the call light, but stay with the patient. Atelectasis, or collapse of the lung, may have occurred. The patient may also have a CXR to evaluate the results of the procedure.

Sputum Studies

These are the most common tests ordered for patients with suspected pulmonary disease. Sputum is secreted by the mucous membrane lining of the bronchioles, bronchi, and trachea and helps protect the respiratory tract from infection. When it is expelled it carries with it saliva, nasal and sinus secretions, dead cells, and normal oral bacteria. A culture of the sputum is obtained to indicate the presence of any specific organisms. This will help determine any disease process and type of antibiotic therapy indicated for the patient. A sputum culture usually is obtained prior to the start of any antibiotic therapy and following therapy to determine its effectiveness.

The PCT may be asked to obtain a sputum specimen from the patient. The equipment needed to obtain a sputum specimen is a sterile container with a tight-fitting lid, patient label, laboratory requisitions, facial tissues, emesis basin, and gloves.

Tell the patient you will need to collect a specimen of sputum, not saliva or spit. *The specimen should feel like it came up from the chest, will form a "glob" that sticks together, and will be opaque, not clear froth.* Instruct the patient to take a few deep breaths, then cough after a forced exhalation. The first sputum of the morning generally produces the most organisms. Provide the patient

with a sterile covered container at night and instruct him or her to cough immediately upon awakening if possible.

The patient is asked to cap the lid tightly when the specimen is obtained and to call for the PCT.

The PCT will then label the container with the patient's name, identification number, date, time, physician's name, and the initial diagnosis. The person sending the specimen should also put his or her initials on the label and document in the patient's chart that a sputum specimen was obtained and sent to the laboratory. Put the date/time on the requisition form with any relevant patient information, for instance, the patient had a fever or was taking antibiotics.

Place the specimen into a biohazardous bag for transport immediately to the laboratory.

Pulse Oximetry

Pulse oximetry is a noninvasive means of determining arterial oxyhemoglobin saturation. This measures the amount of functional oxygen saturated in the percentage of available hemoglobin in the red blood cells of the arterial blood circulation. It can be useful in the evaluation of sleep disorders, regulating oxygen therapy, and in clinical exercise testing.

The saturation is instantaneously measured optically by the sensing of color changes in hemoglobin in the area where the probe is placed. Pulse oximetry uses a probe placed over the index finger that passes light through a pulsating circulatory bed. The probe (Fig. 6–7) consists of two light sources and a photodetector. To obtain correct

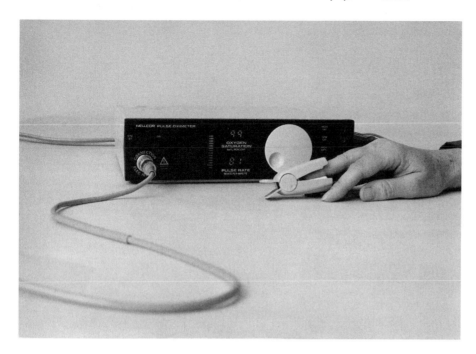

FIGURE 6 – 7
Pulse oximeter.

data, the probe must be correctly positioned so that the light sources and photodetector are directly opposite each other across the arteriolar bed. The probe must be placed to avoid light coming into it from another source such as the room light or sunshine. Care must be taken to avoid placement of opaque materials such as artificial nails or nail polish between the light source and photodetector. Constant motion or movement of the extremities with the probe attached may alter the reading.

Probes vary in sizes from those for newborns to adults. They can be placed on the fingers, toes, ears, nose, and foot. Either a disposable single-patient probe or a reusable permanent probe can be used.

STOP Always follow the manufacturer's instruction when using this machine. To prevent pressure necrosis, care must be taken to avoid excessive pressure to the probe site and to change the site daily.

The PCT should always determine that the probe is attached appropriately. When bathing the patient, always remove the probe from the site and observe the skin of the extremity for any breakdown. Some states require that the RN or Registered Respiratory Therapist (RRT) replace or move the probe. Always report any deviations and alarm sounds to the RN or RRT immediately.

 The RRT's responsibility is to assess the patient and place the pulse oximeter in place. The RN is responsible for checking the patient's response every hour. The PCT is responsible for reporting alarms and patient

changes in respiratory status or conditions affecting the pulse oximetry.

WORKING WITH RESPIRATORY THERAPISTS

Role of the Respiratory Therapist

The RRT is a licensed professional who has specialized education and training in the care of patients with respiratory problems. The RRT works under the direction of the physician who orders the specified oxygen or medication therapy for the patients. The RRT and RN collaborate to see that the patient receives the appropriate treatments. The RRT is responsible for assessment of the patient as it relates to the patient's respiratory therapy, applies the appropriate therapy, and documents care provided.

STOP Always report any problems with respiratory therapy equipment to the RRT or RN.

SPECIAL OBSERVATIONS OF PCT AND WHEN TO REPORT

The PCT can make important observations and report these to the RN regarding the patient's respiratory function. These can be accomplished by direct observation, noting the general appearance of the patient and the ability to breathe, rate and depth of respirations, breathing pattern, level of consciousness, and skin color.

It is the RN's responsibility to assess the patient, plan the care, provide the interventions, and evaluate the patient's response.

The PCT's observations and actions must be reported promptly for the RN to provide the appropriate treatment to the patient.

Report and document only facts and be objective in your observations.

A great deal of information can be gathered immediately about the patient's respiratory function by observing his or her general appearance. Observations can be made when meeting the patient for first time.

- What is the posture?
  If the patient's posture is stooped and the patient strains for each breath, this may indicate that the thoracic cavity is compressed and the lungs cannot inflate fully.

- Does the patient breathe easily or with effort and visible concentration on each breath?
  If the patient has to concentrate on each breath, this can drain energy and can produce anxiety if his or her care is hurried or he or she is asked to do too many new things.

- Can the patient change positions and still breathe comfortably?
  If the patient has difficulty changing from a sitting to standing position, this should be noted. The patient may fatigue easily and the pace of activities should be slowed.

- How many pillows does the patient use or does the head of the bed need to be raised?
  The patient may need to have the head of the bed raised at all times to breathe easily. He or she may need to sit leaned over a table with a pillow for support (orthopneic position).

- Can the patient breathe easily while speaking?
  If the patient has difficulty talking, or needs to talk in short phrases and take a few breaths with each phrase, his or her activity level must be slowed. This patient may also need to be on supplemental oxygen.

- What is the patient's mental status or level of consciousness?
  Patients who are confused and disoriented may be hypoxemic, with low levels of oxygen circulating to the brain. These patients need close observation for safety.

- What is the color of the patient's skin?
  Have a good lighting source to determine the patient's skin color or appearance.

 If the skin is dusky or gray or there is a bluish tinge to the lips, or if the patient is confused and disoriented, let the RN know immediately.

- What is the patient's general body size?
  Obese patients may breathe shallowly and pose difficult problems postoperatively. An extremely thin body in a respiratory patient often indicates chronic disease.

Pulmonary Surgical Patient

Once a surgical treatment has been identified, the PCT can assist the RN by gathering baseline vital sign data. Report observations related to the patient's respiratory status so that there is a comparison for measuring the postoperative respiratory state. These would include dyspnea, coughing, pain, and tolerance to activity. Encourage the patient to perform coughing and deep breathing exercises using splinting of the surgical site, and use of the incentive spirometer. Encourage arm and leg exercises to prevent postoperative stiffness and thrombi (blood clots) in the legs.

The most common postoperative complications are atelectasis (collapse of a lung), pneumonia, acute respiratory failure, and pulmonary embolism (blood clot in the lung). Table 6–2 shows what the PCT observations and interventions will include.

Maintaining pain control is always a balancing act for patients with respiratory problems. If a patient has pain, it interferes with respirations, since people tend to breathe more shallowly. On the other hand, many narcotic pain medications depress respirations. It is important for all team members to provide as much support of the patient as possible to decrease the amount of narcotics that may be required. Interventions that could be utilized are relaxation techniques like soft music with low noise and light levels, gentle muscle massage, and warmth and diversional activities such as television, radio, visitors, and conversation.

ROLE OF THE PCT IN SPECIFIC INTERVENTIONS

Counting respirations is the basis for the PCT's observations related to pulmonary conditions. The following are tips to increase the knowledge base for obtaining accurate readings.

STOP Respirations cannot be counted accurately if the patient is talking. Count respirations after taking the pulse while still holding the wrist or using your stethoscope to count an apical pulse. You may also put your hand over the abdomen or chest to count the rise and fall to determine the number of respirations.

Newborns, infants, and toddlers use abdominal muscles

T A B L E 6 – 2
Postoperative Complications and Interventions of PCT

NEEDS	OBSERVATIONS	INTERVENTIONS
Maintenance of patent airway	Dyspnea (difficulty breathing) Shortness of breath Increased secretions Decreased cough reflex	Assure that suction equipment is in place in room Maintain oxygen delivery device in place Raise head of bed to 45 degrees Report any deviations to RN immediately, by using call light; stay with patient
Stable vital signs (temperature, pulse, respirations, blood pressure)	Monitoring for abnormal result beyond accepted parameters Signs of respiratory depression (slow, shallow respirations, decreased levels of consciousness, low BP) Noisy respirations	Try to arouse patient and get him/her to respond with name, place, and time Maintain oxygen delivery device in place Raise head of bed to 45 degrees Have patient cough and deep breathe Report any deviations to RN immediately by using call light; stay with patient
Prevention of atelectasis	Maintaining position to assist with drainage from surgical site Chest tube dressing is intact and not draining Chest tube drainage device is patent	Utilize pillow or wedges to maintain and reinforce positioning with patient Turning patient q2h Report any drainage on the chest tube dressing to RN immediately Keep chest tube drainage device in upright position; report leakage from device to the RN immediately Coughing and deep breathing exercise qh Incentive spirometry qh
Pain control	Any complaints of pain during turning, coughing, deep breathing, ambulation, and any activity	Report to RN Assure that patient is using appropriate splinting techniques for coughing and deep breathing Log-roll patient to reduce any twisting that may cause pain
Control of anxiety	Patients' and/or significant others' concerns about treatment or diagnosis	Provide emotional support Meet patient needs as quickly, kindly, and completely as possible Report patient concerns to RN

for breathing. Look at the abdomen to count respirations for 1 full minute. Counting when a baby is asleep or quiet is desirable. Respiratory rates range from 30–80/min for infants and 20–40/min for infants and toddlers.

Count respirations of preschoolers and older children as you would an adult, but count for 1 full minute. Respiratory rates range from 15–25.

For adults, observe the rise and fall of the chest for each respiration. You should always note the depth and regularity of the respirations. The average rate of breathing for an adult is 14–20/min. Respiratory rates above 25 or less than 12 should be reported to the RN. Altered patterns of breathing often indicate underlying conditions and need to be reported (Table 6–3).

✔ Respiratory rates are given as guidelines. However, there is considerable individual variation at all ages.

The PCT will also need to be aware of the conditions listed in Table 6–4.

 The RN or RRT teaches the patient about his or her respiratory condition, treatments

T A B L E 6 – 3
Altered Patterns of Breathing

PATTERN	CHARACTERISTICS	POTENTIAL CAUSE
Tachypnea	Rapid, shallow	Fever, hyperventilation
Bradypnea	Slow but regular	Sleep, drugs
Hyperventilation	Increased depth, rate	Exercise, anxiety
Hypoventilation	Decreased depth, rate	Drugs
Ataxic breathing	Short bursts of irregular breathing interspersed with periods of apnea	Brain damage, respiratory depression
Cheyne-Stokes	Gradually deep and fast, then shallower and slower, alternating with periods of apnea	Sleep, heart failure, renal failure, stroke, drug overdose, brain damage

ordered, and any exercises prescribed. Your role is to reinforce these activities of the professional staff when working with patients.

Incentive Spirometry

Incentive therapy helps the lungs to expand fully. This prevents atelectasis and also helps prevent pneumonia. This procedure may be carried out with the patient in bed, with head and shoulders well supported, and fully sitting up if permitted. Also, the patient can be sitting with the feet on the floor and back straight to allow for full expansion of the lungs. The procedure should be taught before surgery when the patient is not stressed and in pain.

1. Ask the patient to take a few deep breaths and to cough.

2. Have the patient place his or her lips around the mouthpiece of the incentive spirometer then suck as if sucking on a straw with a deep breath to raise the balls in the chambers. Use the slide to mark the volume of air inhaled. Set that as a goal for the next effort.

3. The deep breath should be held as long as possible, keeping the ball suspended.

4. The patient then removes the mouthpiece and exhales in the normal manner.

5. The exercise is repeated as many as 3–6 times every 1–2 hours while the patient is awake.

6. Record the number of repetitions the patient is able to perform and to what volume and then how the patient tolerated the procedure.

 Observe for any complaint of dizziness, pain, or throat and airway irritation. When the

T A B L E 6 – 4
Observations by PCT

CONDITION	OBSERVATIONS
Productive cough	Is the sputum greenish or blood tinged? Save sputum that reflects a change in the patient for RN to observe.
Non-productive cough	Is cough dry or hacky?
Hemoptysis	Blood-tinged sputum. Note amount; report to the RN immediately if first time noted for patient.
Pain	When does pain occur, is it continuous or intermittent? Does it occur with respirations? Where is pain located; does it radiate? Is it sharp or dull? Have patient rate severity of pain on scale of 0–10. Is this pain new? Is patient requesting to be medicated? Call RN.
Breathlessness or shortness of breath	When does this occur? With activity or at rest? Is this new or usual pattern for patient? Raise the head of bed and slow patient's pace of activity. Report to RN if new.
Dyspnea	Patient may become anxious. Support patient emotionally and make sure oxygen delivery device is in place if indicated. Report any new changes to RN.
The patient has a sensation of not getting enough air and is conscious of breathing harder. Labored breathing	
Hypoxia (not getting adequate oxygen)	Patient may exhibit restlessness, personality changes, tachycardia, hyperpnea, dyspnea, and cyanosis. Support patient by ensuring open airway and oxygen delivery device in place if indicated. Report immediately to RN or RRT.

patient has completed the pulmonary exercise, the mouthpiece should be washed in warm water, dried, and replaced in the plastic bag and left at the bedside. Patients should be praised for efforts. Many times this encourages greater effort the next time the incentive spirometer is used.

Deep Breathing and Coughing

Deep breathing and coughing clear the air passages. This helps to prevent postoperative respiratory complications such as pneumonia and atelectasis. This may be an uncomfortable task when the patient has a new incision and feels fatigued. You can best assist the patient by:

1. Explaining the value of the exercise and carrying out the following procedure.

2. Check with the RN to see if medication for pain is to be administered before the exercise and how many coughing and deep breathing repetitions should be attempted. Wait for 15–30 minutes after the medication has been given before carrying out the exercise.

3. Use a pillow or binder to support the incision during the procedure. Have the patient place a hand on either side of the rib cage or over the pillow.

4. Ask the patient to take 4 deep breaths and hold for 3–5 seconds, and then cough deeply on the 4th breath exhalation.

5. Repeat this exercise as the RN indicated, or about 3–6 times unless the patient seems too tired. If so, stop the procedure and report to the RN.

6. Provide tissues to collect any secretions that are coughed up.

7. Put on disposable gloves to handle tissues.

8. Assist the patient to assume a new, comfortable position.

9. Clean the emesis basin.

10. Remember to wash your hands, report completion of the task, and document the time and patient response.

Positioning for Maximum Lung Expansion

Positioning of the patient to permit expansion of the lungs and a straightened airway is helpful in cases of respiratory distress. The position of choice is a high Fowler's position (Fig. 6–8). In the high Fowler's position, the patient is in a sitting position with the back of the bed elevated.

- Position pillows behind the patient's head and shoulders.

- Adjust the knee rest to keep the patient from slipping down in bed.

- The orthopneic position may be used as an alternative to the high Fowler's position. The position of the bed remains the same.

  - The bedside table is brought across the bed and one or two pillows are placed on top.

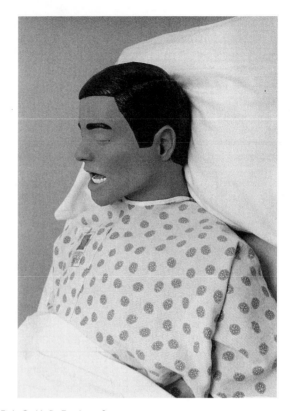

F I G U R E 6 – 8
High Fowler's position for maximum lung expansion.

- The patient leans forward across the table with arms on the bedside or on the pillows.

- Another pillow is placed low behind the patient's back for support.

Documentation

For any intervention there must be documentation that is objective with clear descriptive terms. There must always be a measurable outcome and a patient response. All documentation must be written clearly and legibly.

SPECIAL NEEDS FOR PATIENTS ON OXYGEN

Inspection of Skin

Pure oxygen is very drying to the skin. Dryness of the skin eventually can lead to damage of the tissues. Oxygen is usually humidified before entering the patient's body.

Be sure that the water level is adequate to create a misting effect in the oxygen delivery device. Report a lack of water to the RN or RRT. Also check to make sure there is not any pooling of water in the dependent loop of the humidification tubing. Always drain the water by backing up the tubes and letting the water pass back to the in-line water-collection bag. Drain water when the bag becomes half full.

 Never let the water in any respiratory tubing flow toward the patient. This may cause aspiration.

Always check the mucous membranes of the nose for any dryness; apply a water-based lubricant to the areas. Bleeding may occur from the dryness; report bleeding to the RN or RRT. Applying a warm moist washcloth to the areas when bathing tends to soothe the tissues.

Mouth Care

Since many respiratory patients breathe through their mouth, it is essential to inspect the patient's mouth every shift for mucosal dryness of the tongue, gums, and inner cheeks and for cracking of the lips. Apply non-petrolatum-based products as provided by the RN and ordered by the physician. Easy measures consist of application of moist washcloths to the affected area and frequent mouth care using foam toothettes or other swabs available in your setting.

Safety Hazards

Always remember that when oxygen is in use, special precautions are necessary to prevent fires and to administer the oxygen safely.

Fire Safety Measures

- No open flames and no smoking
- Call light within hand's reach
- Post *No Smoking* or *Oxygen in Use* signs
- Remove unneeded electrical equipment
- Use only specially grounded electrical equipment (no electric appliances, no razors or hair dryers).

DEALING WITH SPECIAL RESPIRATORY EQUIPMENT

It is always necessary to have a thorough understanding of all equipment to be used prior to their use on the patient. Always ask the RN or RRT if you have any questions.

Oxygen therapy consists of the addition of quantities of oxygen to the inspired air in an attempt to correct hypoxia. Because the body does not contain a reserve oxygen supply, supplemental inspired oxygen is required whenever the cardiorespiratory system is unable to supply adequate oxygen to the body's tissues.

Oxygen is delivered by many different types of devices. The source of the oxygen may be an oxygen tank that is taken everywhere with the patient, or oxygen may be piped into a wall unit in the patient's room.

Oxygen Tanks and Flowmeters

Oxygen is prescribed by a physician in a particular amount. The rate of flow is measured in liters. The flow rate is set by the RRT or the RN, since the delivery of oxygen is considered to be drug administration. As an unlicensed PCT you must be aware of the following:

- Be able to read the flow rate on a flowmeter gauge (Fig. 6–9).
- Notify the RN if you detect any change in the rate.
- Be able to inspect the tubing and unkink any obstructions noted in the tubing.

Note that all oxygen tanks are painted green.

- Be able to determine if the oxygen tank has adequate oxygen in it for your patient's therapy. A regulator that reads less than 500 pounds per square inch (psi) should be replaced with a full tank. The tank should be marked empty.
- Secure additional tanks if necessary for your patient's oxygen supply from the appropriate storage area.
- Properly mark empty tanks and return to the appropriate storage for refilling.
- Ensure that the tank is secured properly and cannot fall. All oxygen tanks must be secured appropriately in a holder with straps and never left standing freely.

Do not attach any device filled with water to the oxygen tank. Water may spill or splash back into the regulator and damage it beyond repair.

Oxygen Delivery Devices

Oxygen can be delivered by either a low-flow or high-flow system. Low-flow oxygen therapy systems provide part of the patient's inspiratory oxygen needs. The remainder of the oxygen the patient inhales comes from room air. Room air contains 21% oxygen.

High-flow oxygen therapy systems are designed to flood the patient's face or tracheostomy tube area with a high flow of oxygen at a constant rate.

As mentioned previously, most oxygen delivery devices are humidified to prevent drying of the mucosa that the oxygen comes in contact with. Always notify the RN or

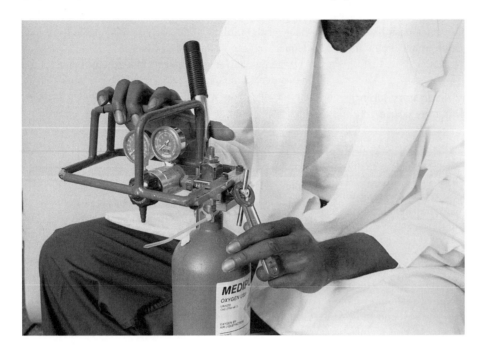

FIGURE 6-9
E cylinder (oxygen tank), regulator.
Note flowmeter gauge.

RRT whenever the bottles of water that humidify the oxygen are empty and need replacement.

Nasal Cannula

Oxygen delivery through a nasal cannula (Fig. 6–10) is the most common method used. It delivers 22–44% oxygen, which means that it is a low-flow delivery device.

The nasal cannula consists of tubing with two small prongs that fit into a patient's nostrils. The two short protruding prongs must be placed into the nares facing down. The tube circles behind the ears and then under the chin. Special attention must be paid daily to the condition of the skin under the tube, especially behind and on top of the ears and the nares. The oxygen can be drying to the nares, and care should be given to moisten this area.

Things to Observe

1. Make sure the strap is secure but not too tight. Place flattened cotton balls or split foam pieces around the tubing over the ears.

2. Check for signs of irritation where the prongs touch the patient's nose.

3. Check that mucus has not blocked the prong openings. Clean if necessary.

4. Attention must be given to the tubing to prevent twisting and kinks.

Oxygen Delivery by Mask

The following care needs apply to any oxygen delivered by mask. The flow rate can usually be regulated precisely provided the mask fits securely and is kept in place. Activities such as eating, taking medications, talking, and coughing tend to displace the mask. The PCT can assist by observing the following things:

1. Maintaining the mask over nose and mouth, unless otherwise indicated.

2. Be sure the straps are secure, but not too tight. Check areas that the straps come in contact with to observe for any skin breakdown. Place cotton balls under the strap if redness is noted. Report these to the RN.

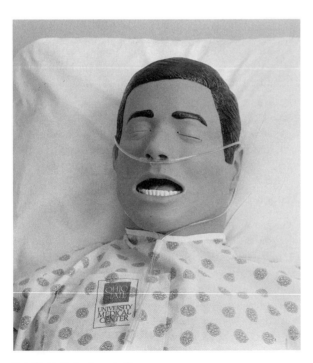

FIGURE 6-10

Nasal cannula.

3. Periodically remove the mask for skin care. Wash the areas under it. Dry carefully and replace.

Simple Face Mask

The simple face mask is another low-flow oxygen delivery device that is commonly used. It can deliver 30–50% oxygen. It is a cuplike mask held in place over the nose and mouth by an elasticized band that can be adjusted to fit the head securely (Fig. 6–11).

Venturi Mask

The Venturi mask (Fig. 6–12) was designed to limit oxygen delivery to a set percentage of 24–50%. It is a high-flow delivery system. The oxygen flow can be set to allow for a certain amount of room air to flow into the device.

Non-Rebreathing and Partial Rebreathing Masks

The non-rebreathing mask (Fig. 6–13) is a high-flow system that allows oxygen to be delivered into a reservoir bag. Then the oxygen goes through a one-way valve into the mask and to the patient. When the patient breathes out, the valve closes, and exhaled air flows out into the atmosphere through holes in the side of the mask. These masks can provide close to 100% oxygen if they fit snugly, but they can be uncomfortable to wear. The flow rate must be high enough to prevent the reservoir bag from collapsing. Non-rebreathing masks are generally used for only short periods.

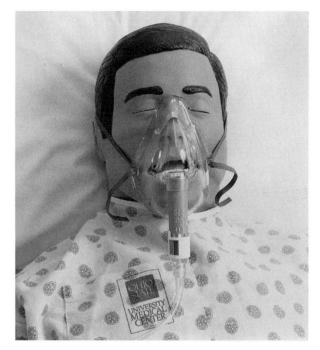

FIGURE 6–12
Venturi mask.

A partial rebreathing mask (Fig. 6–13) is the same as a non-rebreathing mask except that exhaled air is not prevented from entering the reservoir bag. It can deliver 50–70% oxygen as a high-flow device.

Continuous Positive Airway Pressure (CPAP) and Positive End-Expiratory Pressure (PEEP)

CPAP is an oxygen therapy system that maintains an airway pressure above atmospheric pressure during the inspiratory and expiratory cycle in patients breathing on their own.

CPAP is commonly used in the care of neonates with respiratory disease. This is most often delivered via nasal prongs. In adults, a nasal mask is used with nasal CPAP therapy to treat obstructive sleep apnea (airway collapses during sleep) and to treat chronic respiratory failure.

The PCT is responsible for reporting alarms to the RN or RRT. When providing hygiene, check for any skin breakdown where the strap and mask are located. Massage the bridge of the nose. Report any changes to the RN.

PEEP is used with mechanical ventilation. It is indicated for patient oxygenation problems associated with pneumonia, atelectasis, respiratory failure, and pulmonary edema and for treating patients with obstructive sleep apnea.

Intermittent Positive Pressure Breathing (IPPB) Machines

Oxygen is administered intermittently under pressure by the RRT or the RN. This technique is used to expand

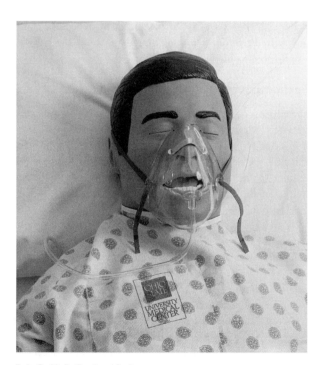

FIGURE 6–11
Simple face mask.

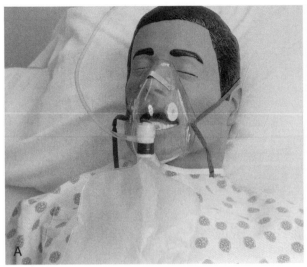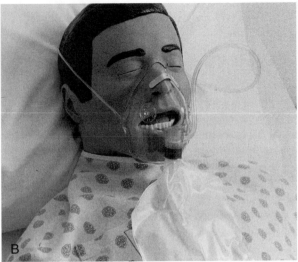

FIGURE 6-13
A, Non-rebreathing mask and *B*, partial rebreathing mask.

the lungs of a patient who has difficulty doing it himself or herself. These treatments are done several times a day.

Aerosol Therapy

Nebulizers deliver moisture or medication deep into the lungs. Drugs that thin the mucus (mucolytic) or dilate the bronchi are often prescribed. This medication can be delivered by a hand-held nebulizer or given in conjunction with an intermittent positive pressure breathing machine. After administration of the mucolytic, RNs and RRTs use various techniques to loosen the mucus and clear the air passageways. The PCT can help by providing an emesis basin for the patient to cough up secretions and sputum. Collection of a sputum sample may also be indicated and delegated to the PCT. Some medications can cause nausea and vomiting; always remember to place the patients on their side after completion of treatment.

Percussion and Postural Drainage

Percussion is accomplished by cupping the palms of the hands and striking the chest to loosen the secretions.

Postural drainage consists of positioning the patient on the bed or tilt table to encourage drainage from the respiratory tract by gravity. This requires close supervision to avoid injury to the patient as different positions are assumed. These procedures are performed by the RN or the RRT.

Airways: Oral and Nasal

An oropharyngeal or oral airway (Fig. 6–14) is a curved rubber or plastic device that is inserted into the patient's mouth by the RN to establish or maintain an airway. The airway is intended for short-term use, as in the

postanesthesia patient or in the recovery stage of the seizure patient.

The nasal airway is used to establish or maintain a patent nasal airway. This airway is the typical choice for patients who have had recent oral surgery or facial trauma in whom there may be a risk that edema will close off the airway and for the patient with loose teeth. It is also used to protect the nasal mucosa from injury when the patient needs frequent nasal suctioning. The PCT may be asked to clean the nasal airway to assist the RN in changing it. This is done by running hot water through the tube to remove any mucus or crustations and handing it back to the RN to replace. During hygiene care, note any skin breakdown around the nares from the airway. Report these changes to the RN.

Suction Equipment and Suctioning

Suctioning is used to remove loose secretions from the patient's airway. Nasotracheal and endotracheal suctioning must be performed by an RN or RRT. However, the PCT may set up the suction system and position the patient for airway clearance. The PCT can be of further help providing comfort to the patient as the procedure is carried out.

A suction system source may be from a piped system located in the walls or a portable pump (Fig. 6–15). The suction system has a vacuum source, a vacuum regulator, a trap bottle, a connecting tubing, and a suction catheter. The PCT can be responsible for setting up the appropriate equipment for suctioning.

A regulator is used to control the amount of pressure applied to the airway. The regulator that attaches to the wall vacuum or portable suction controls the suction by partially obstructing the flow through it.

A trap bottle is used to collect the secretions removed

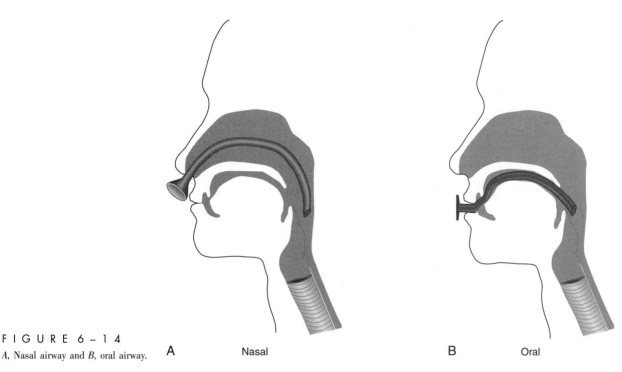

FIGURE 6–14

A, Nasal airway and *B*, oral airway.   **A**   Nasal   **B**   Oral

from the airway so they do not contaminate the vacuum regulator or suction machine. This attachment must be secure and free of air leaks.

The suction catheter is the part of the system that enters the airway of the patient. The RN or RRT should always test the suction tubing for correct connections prior to suctioning the patient. This is done by testing the suction with water through the tubing to ensure patency of the system.

When assisting with suctioning of the patient with a tracheostomy (trach), the PCT may be asked by the RN to remove the oxygen collar just prior to each suctioning episode and to replace it immediately after the suctioning episode to assist in the hyperoxygenation of the patient. In tracheostomy patients without supplemental oxygen, the PCT may be directed by the RN or RTT to hyperoxygenate the patient by using a manual resuscitator.

Other suction devices that can be used with patients

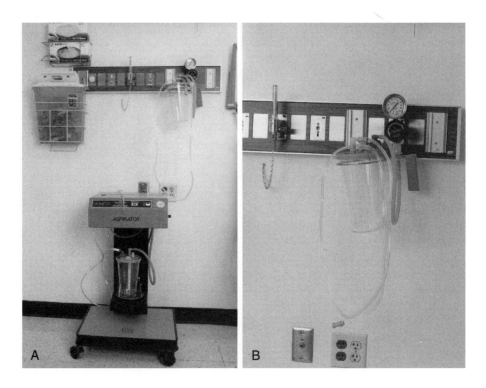

FIGURE 6–15

A, Wall suction and *B*, portable pump.   **A**   **B**

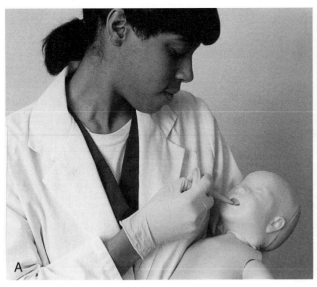
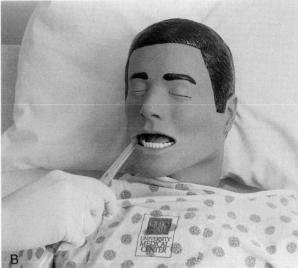

FIGURE 6–16

A, Bulb syringe and *B*, Yankauer-tip syringe.

are the bulb syringe and Yankauer suction (Fig. 6–16). These devices also assist in clearance of secretions from the airway.

The bulb syringe is used in a manual method for infants. The RN or RRT utilizes this to clear secretions from both the nostrils and mouth.

The Yankauer-tip suction device is useful in removal of secretions in patients after oral or maxillofacial surgery, after trauma to the mouth, in comatose patients, and with tracheostomy patients. Alert patients can use this device themselves to control secretions in the oral cavity. The RN or RRT will initially instruct the patient on its proper usage. The PCT can then reinforce its appropriate use by the patient or use it for patients as requested by the RN.

1. The device is inserted into the mouth along the gumline to the back of the mouth; it is moved until secretions are cleared.

2. The catheter should be rinsed with water. A cup filled with water should be provided.

3. Provide a damp washcloth for the patient for wiping the face. An emesis basin is needed at the patient's bedside for the Yankauer-tip suction catheter and the washcloth.

4. Care for the Yankauer-tip suction catheter consists of rinsing it with hot water to remove any crustations that may build up in the catheter. If this method does not remove the crustations, dispose of the catheter and obtain a new one.

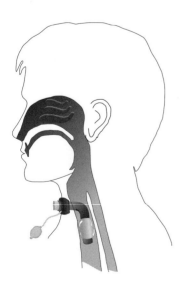
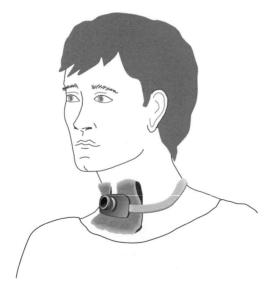

FIGURE 6–17

Tracheostomy in a patient.

Tracheostomy Equipment

Tracheostomy Tubes

A tracheostomy is the surgical creation of an opening through the neck into the trachea. A tracheostomy tube is placed to maintain the airway patency (Fig. 6–17).

The tube is held in place with a low-pressure cuff attached to the end of the tube that is in the trachea. This cuff helps to prevent aspiration of food and secretions. A tracheostomy tube may be plastic (most commonly used for acutely ill patients) or metal (common for long-term use), depending on the type and length of therapy.

The following equipment must be maintained at the bedside:

1. Suctioning equipment, because the patient may need the airway cleared at any time.

2. A sterile obturator to insert the tracheostomy tube, in case the tube is expelled (Fig. 6–18).

 Whenever a tracheostomy tube is expelled, call the RN or RRT immediately.

3. A sterile tracheostomy tube and an obturator the same size, in case the tube must be replaced quickly.

4. A spare, sterile inner cannula that can be used if the cannula is expelled.

Stoma and Outer Cannula Care

The PCT can provide stoma care to patients with a tracheostomy, but must be aware of the institution's policies and procedures regarding this care. The following is a general outline of how it can be done.

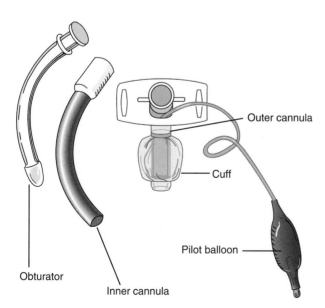

F I G U R E   6 – 1 8

Parts of tracheostomy tube (outer and inner cannula, and obturator).

1. Put on sterile gloves (for new stomas) and clean gloves for healed stomas.

2. With the dominant hand, saturate a sterile gauze pad with specified cleaning solution. Squeeze out the excess liquid to prevent accidental aspiration, and then wipe the patient's neck under the tracheostomy tube flanges and ties. Wipe only once with each pad, and then discard it to prevent contamination of a clean area with a soiled pad. Often manipulating the tracheostomy tube will stimulate the patient to cough. Make sure an RN is nearby to provide suctioning.

3. Saturate a second pad and gently wipe until the skin surrounding the tracheostomy is cleaned. Use additional pads or cotton-tipped applicators to clean the stoma site and the tube's flanges.

4. Rinse debris with specified solution with one or more sterile 4×4 gauze pads dampened in normal saline solution. Dry the area thoroughly with additional sterile gauze pads, then apply a new sterile tracheostomy dressing.

5. Remove and discard your gloves.

 The PCT caregiver never changes trach ties or inner cannula.

 Report care provided and any observations regarding the skin surrounding the stoma sites.

Changing Tracheostomy Ties

The RN may ask the PCT to assist with changing the tracheostomy ties because of the risk of accidental tube expulsion during this procedure. Patient movement or coughing can dislodge the tube while the change of ties occurs. The tracheostomy device should always be held in place when ties are being changed.

Closed-Chest Drainage System (CCDS)

The purpose of the CCDS or chest tubes is to restore the pressure necessary to keep the lungs inflated. Gravity is used to drain fluids. The water in the cannister allows the air and fluid to escape from the lungs and not re-enter. This is called a water seal (Fig. 6–19).

The PCT's role in chest tube drainage is to prepare the CCDS. To accomplish this:

1. Fill the suction control chamber to the prescribed level with sterile water, usually 20 cc.

2. Then add sterile water to the 2-cm level of the water seal chamber.

3. Keep the connector from the cannister to the patient sterile by leaving the cap on. The RN will connect the patient to the CCDS and suction device if indicated.

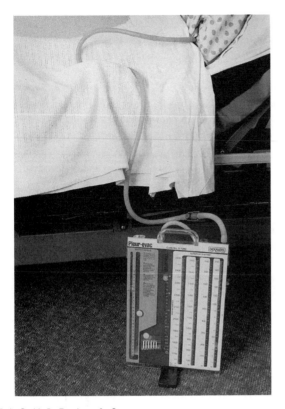

F I G U R E 6 – 1 9
Commercially prepared, disposable closed-chest drainage system (Pneumovac).

Precautions:

• Observe for kinks in the tubing, pooling of fluids, and leaks in the drainage system.

• Hang the CCDS on the bed frame or stand it on the floor. Keep it upright at all times. Avoid dependent loops.

• Note any complaint of pain, shortness of breath, change in vital signs, and increased apprehension in the patient.

• Assist the patient ambulating with the CCDS. Maintain it below chest level in an upright position.

• Encourage deep breathing and coughing, as well as use of the incentive spirometer.

• When providing personal hygiene, note whether the chest tube dressing contains drainage or is loose. Report these findings to the RN immediately.

CARING FOR PATIENTS ON VENTILATORS

A ventilator is a machine (Fig. 6–20) to augment or to act for the patient's muscles in performing the work of breathing. The patient who is on a ventilator cannot breathe on his or her own; thus this creates the need for the mechanical ventilation by the machine. The ventilator is connected to the endotracheal tube into the trachea. This makes it impossible for the patient to talk or eat while intubated. Ventilators are located in the home and extended care facilities, as well as acute care settings.

STOP Do not assume care for these patients unless you are educated regarding the equipment, the limits of your role, and how to respond to patient emergency situations.

Signs and symptoms of inadequate ventilation include restlessness, irritability, wakefulness, use of expiratory muscles, tachycardia, and anxious facial expressions.

These observations should be reported to the RN or RRT.

The PCT's care of the ventilator patient should:

1. Address the fear of patients by providing emotional support.

2. Provide an alternative means of communication for the patient, who cannot speak while intubated. This can be through a communication board or written notes. Remember: Just because the patient cannot speak does not mean he or she cannot hear.

3. All ventilators need an energy source to work. The PCT can help assure that the ventilators are plugged into the "red" emergency outlets. Also that the ventilator

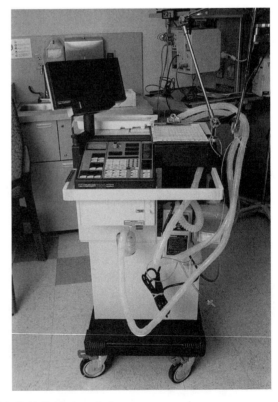

F I G U R E 6 – 2 0
Ventilator.

battery packs are in place when the patient needs to be transported. A manual resuscitator bag must be in the patient's room and during transport at all times in case there is a loss of both power sources.

4. Vital signs are obtained hourly to monitor for complications. Any abnormalities beyond the parameters indicated by a physician must be reported immediately to the RN.

5. Handwashing must be used as a measure of control to minimize the spread of nosocomial infections.

6. The PCT is responsible for helping with an every 2 hours (q2h) turn schedule to stimulate inflation of lungs. Use of pillows and wedges may be necessary. *Be sure to empty water from tubing prior to turning the patient. Check all tubings for free length to allow the patient to turn.*

7. Strict intake and output measurements (I & O) are essential to assist the RN in determining the patient's fluid-volume needs. The nutritional needs of these patients continue. Their body is in need of nourishment while they are NPO. This is usually accomplished by feedings called total parenteral nutrition (TPN) that are received through a central line.

8. Range of motion (ROM) exercise is indicated for the patient on a ventilator because of the immobility experienced while receiving this therapy. The PCT can provide passive range of motion exercises after instruction by the physical therapist.

9. Hygiene activities are indicated for the ventilator patient at least daily. Oral hygiene is needed every 2 hours. This can be done with a toothette.

10. The sleep/rest patterns are usually mixed up in the patient on a ventilator in the acute care setting because of the 24-hour environment. However, lights should be dimmed and the noise level lowered to stimulate natural rest/sleep patterns.

11. Endotracheal tubes have been placed to maintain a patent airway for attachment of the ventilator. The PCT's observations are essential to ascertain that the endotracheal tubes are patent and in place. During activity with the patient, take care not to interfere with the endotracheal tubes. During hygiene activities note whether there is any skin breakdown from the straps used to hold the tube in place.

12. Alarms need to be reported when the RN or RRT is not readily available to evaluate the problem associated with the particular alarm.

The PCT's Caregiver Role in Patient Education

Nursing care is directed toward assisting patients to breathe easier and reduce the transmission of respiratory infections. Patients with respiratory disease should be taught about their condition.

The RN is responsible for teaching the patient about his or her respiratory condition, treatments ordered, and any exercises prescribed. Your role is to reinforce these activities of the professional staff when working with patients.

All respiratory patients should be taught the following regardless of age—older children as well as adults:

1. Cover the nose and mouth when coughing or sneezing, and turn face away from others. An uncovered cough or sneeze can reach at least 3 feet from the point of the exit, which means anyone within that area may be contaminated by that person's germs.

2. Dispose of soiled tissues by placing them in a plastic or paper container to be burned or disposed of with biohazardous wastes. Germs can be reactivated from soiled tissues that are remoistened.

3. Wash hands after coughing or sneezing and handling soiled tissues. You may come in contact with others by shaking hands or handling common articles like telephones, doorknobs, BP cuffs.

Always wash your hands when you finish working with a patient to protect the other patients, staff, and yourself.

Respiratory Isolation

Visitors should report to the RN before visiting a patient. However, if they do not, as the PCT you need to inform them that the patient is in respiratory isolation and that they need to follow agency guidelines.

SUMMARY

All living organisms require a continual supply of oxygen. Chemical changes in tissue cells depend on it. Carbon dioxide is one end product of chemical changes in cells, and the excess needs to be eliminated. The exchange of these gases in the lungs and cells constitutes respiration.

Effective care for the respiratory patient involves communication and teamwork among the care providers to coordinate interventions appropriately. Having additional information about anatomy, illnesses, equipment, and treatments enables the PCT to provide more informed, safe, sensitive, patient-centered care. The PCT is an important part of the team.

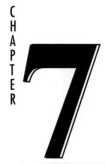

The Cardiovascular System

SUSAN JENKINS GALLOWAY, BA, BS

PREREQUISITE KNOWLEDGE AND SKILLS

- The body's response to stress
- Infectious process
- Concepts of comfort and pain
- Concepts of communication and patient education
- Function of the respiratory system
- Obtaining vital signs

OBJECTIVES

After you complete this chapter, you will be able to:

- Describe components of blood and the pathway of its circulation.
- List structures and functions of the cardiovascular system.
- Describe how the system works and relates to other body systems.
- Explain the relationship of blood flow to major organs of the body.
- Discuss common diseases and disorders of the system.
- Discuss common peripheral vascular problems.
- Explain function of Doppler ultrasonography.
- Explain function and safe use of intermittent pneumatic compression devices.
- Discuss the role and responsibilities of patient care technicians (PCTs) in implementing and documenting patient interventions.
- Identify special observations and know when to report them.
- Demonstrate how and when to take vital sign measurements.
- Discuss common hematological disorders.
- Discuss uses and means of blood transfusions.
- List actions and observations to take while monitoring a patient during a blood transfusion.
- Recognize adverse transfusion reactions.

KEY TERMS

Acute   A suddenly occurring phenomenon that usually has a short but severe course

Adhere   To stick or cling to another surface

Ambulate   To walk

Amputate   To cut off or remove a part of the body

Biconcave   Hollowed out on two sides

Carcinogen   A cancer-causing agent

Cardiac Output   The amount of blood expelled by the ventricles over a certain time

Chronic   A condition that has developed slowly over a long time

Coagulation   The process of forming a clot

Contractile   The ability to respond to a stimulus by shortening

Contraindicate   An existing condition or reason for not performing a procedure or doing a treatment to avoid harm to the patient

Debilitated   Weakened and feeble state of being

Dilate   To widen or enlarge

Distal   Farthest from the head or area to which one is referring

Embolus   A foreign body such as a clot, fat globule, or air bubble that is transported through the circulatory system until it lodges somewhere

Empathy   The refined ability to understand and appreciate another's feelings and emotions and what they may mean to that person

Gangrene   A large area of dead tissue usually due to decreased blood supply to tissues

Hemostasis   To stop blood flow by means of the body's clotting system or by physical or chemical means

Indwelling   Something, such as a catheter, left in a body space to promote drainage

Invasive   Penetration of the body tissue

Layman   A person who does not have expertise or extensive education in the field that is referred to

Mediastinum   An area of the body located in the chest from the sternum to the spine. All chest organs are found here except the lungs.

Necrosis   An area of tissue that has died

Nocturnal   A preference for activity during the night

Orthopnea   The need to sit upright to breathe

Orthostatic   Caused by taking an upright or standing position

Pacemaker   A natural or artificial means of initiating and maintaining a rhythmical electrical impulse whose purpose is to cause a muscular contraction

Palpate   To examine by feeling with the fingers and palms

Palpitation   The sensation of a pounding or rapidly beating heart

Patent   Open; not blocked

Perfusion   The infiltration of fluid throughout the body's tissues

Prominence   An outcropping or protrusion

Regurgitation   The backward flow of something previously passed

Somnolence   Extreme or unusual sleepiness or drowsiness

Synchronous   Happening at the same time or together

Syncope   A sudden loss of consciousness as in fainting

Thrombolytic Therapy   Medication used specifically to dissolve a clot that has caused a myocardial infarction

Thrombus   A stationary clot formed in a blood vessel

Throughout history man has written poetically about the heart. The heart epitomizes the very essence of a person's being. The dictionary carries as many as 31 definitions related to heart. Why do we have such reverence and fascination for the heart? Perhaps because a beating heart in any human represents life with all its hopes and dreams.

This chapter reviews the anatomy and pathophysiology of the heart with its related structures, diseases and disorders of the system, and medical and nursing personnel interventions.

BLOOD AND ITS CIRCULATION

Components of Blood

The human body is made up of an incredible number of cells. All these cells must take in nutrients and get rid of waste material to live. Blood and tissue fluid are mainly responsible for accomplishing this essential task. Blood is bright red to dark red, depending on which vessels it is in. It is thicker and heavier than water. The average-sized adult has approximately 4–5 liters of blood circulating within his or her body.

PLASMA. The watery component of blood is called plasma. Plasma suspends the red (erythrocytes) and white (leukocytes) cells as well as the platelets.

RED BLOOD CELLS (ERYTHROCYTES). A red blood cell (RBC) is a biconcave disk that is soft and bendable. An RBC is larger than a capillary, so it must be able to change shape to move into the capillary system. The most important part of an RBC is hemoglobin (Hb). Hemoglobin is a protein that has the ability to combine with and carry oxygen and carbon dioxide. When hemoglobin picks up 4 oxygen molecules a new compound called oxyhemoglobin is formed. Oxyhemoglobin is formed when the RBCs pass by the alveoli in the lungs. Oxyhemoglobin is what gives blood its bright red color. As oxygen is released to the body's tissues, the deoxygenated hemoglobin gives blood its dark red color in the venous blood system.

Another gas that hemoglobin easily combines with is carbon dioxide. The body's cells release carbon dioxide as a waste product that is picked up by hemoglobin and released in the lungs where it is exhaled. Iron is necessary for the manufacture of hemoglobin. If a person has an iron deficiency, the iron that is normally stored in the body will be used to make hemoglobin. If the deficiency continues, eventually there will be a shortage of iron in the hemoglobin. RBCs live about 120 days and then are destroyed by other cells.

WHITE BLOOD CELLS (LEUKOCYTES). White blood cells (WBCs) are cells of the immune system. WBCs are the body's weapons against infection and disease. Leukocytes are broken down into two main classifications; granular and nongranular.

Granular leukocytes consist of cells called neutrophils, eosinophils, and basophils. These cells contain chemicals that can kill and digest bacteria. The nongranular leukocytes are monocytes and lymphocytes. Monocytes rid the body of dead or injured cells. Lymphocytes start the body's immune response to fight disease.

PLATELETS. Platelets are cell fragments from giant cells found in the bone marrow. Platelets are necessary for hemostasis and coagulation. When platelets touch a disruption in the lining of a blood vessel, they become sticky and clump to mend the tear. If damage to the vessel is severe and bleeding is profuse, platelets will release coagulation factors to help form a clot.

Circulatory Pathway

A functioning and patent vascular system is necessary to maintain life. The vascular system is a closed circuit with blood leaving the left side of the heart rich with oxygen from the lungs, circulating throughout the body to distribute oxygen, collecting carbon dioxide, then returning to the right side of the heart and to the lungs to replenish itself with oxygen, and back to the left side of the heart, and on and on for the length of one's life. There are three main types of blood vessels in the vascular system: arteries, capillaries, and veins.

ARTERIES. Arteries transport oxygen-rich blood away from the heart via the aorta to the tissues and cells of the body. Arteries are thick-walled and strong vessels with elastic and contractive properties. Arteries become smaller and smaller as well as less elastic as they approach the tissues and interstitial fluid of the body. These tiny arteries are called arterioles.

CAPILLARIES. Capillaries are microscopic vessels whose walls are only one layer of cells thick. Because they have very thin walls, gases and chemicals can easily diffuse into the surrounding tissues and cells. It is in this way that the tissues and cells of the body are nourished and oxygenated. When capillaries constrict, blood pressure is raised. Conversely, when capillaries dilate, blood pressure is decreased. This is a very important concept and will be mentioned again when diseases of the vascular system are discussed. The capillaries link with the smallest veins, called venules (Fig. 7–1).

VENULES. Venules are the smallest veins. Venules have very thin walls that allow carbon dioxide and waste products from the body's tissues and cells to diffuse into them. Venules merge into larger and larger veins where deoxygenated blood and carbon dioxide are returned to the right side of the heart.

VEINS. Veins carry deoxygenated blood to the right side of the heart by way of a large vein called the superior vena cava. Vein walls are thinner, less elastic, and lie closer to the surface of the skin than arteries. Veins also have one-way valves that prevent the backflow of blood due to influence of gravity (Fig. 7–2).

Circulation of Major Organs of the Body

Categories of the Vascular System

The vascular system is divided into three main systems: (1) the pulmonary system, a short vascular network, which allows blood flow from the right side of the heart through the alveoli via capillaries and back to the left side of the heart; (2) the coronary system, which supplies the heart with blood; and (3) the systemic system, which is the longest system, to supply the rest of the body with blood.

Major Arteries (Fig. 7–3)

AORTA. The aorta is the largest and strongest vessel in the body. It rises from the left side of the heart, arching up slightly to the right and back. It then descends into the abdominal cavity. In the area of the small of the back, the aorta divides into the right and left branches of the common iliac arteries that supply blood to the legs.

CAROTID AND VERTEBRAL ARTERIES. These arteries supply the head and neck.

ARTERIES OF THE CHEST. These arteries arise from the thoracic portion of the aorta and supply the pericardium, bronchi, diaphragm, esophagus, and intercostal muscles as well as other structures located in the thorax.

ARTERIES OF THE UPPER EXTREMITIES. These include the right and left subclavian, axillary, brachial, ulnar, and radial arteries. Upper intercostal muscles, shoulders, arms, and hands are supplied by these arteries.

ARTERIES OF THE LOWER EXTREMITIES. Included are the popliteal, femoral, anterior and posterior tibials, and dorsalis pedis. These arteries supply the legs, genitalia, and feet.

Major Veins in the Systemic System (Fig. 7–4)

VEINS OF THE HEAD AND NECK. These include the internal and external jugular, which receive blood from the brain, face, and neck.

VEINS OF THE THORAX. The brachiocephalics and superior vena cava receive blood from the upper body, bronchioles, and thorax. The superior vena cava empties into the right atrium of the heart.

VEINS OF THE ABDOMEN AND PELVIS. These include the common iliacs and inferior vena cava and receive blood from structures in the pelvis and abdomen.

VEINS OF THE UPPER EXTREMITIES. The cephalic, basilics, axillaries, and subclavians receive blood from the upper extremities as well as the upper thoracic structures and neck.

VEINS OF THE LOWER EXTREMITIES. The great and small saphenous, popliteals, and femorals receive blood from deep and superficial veins of the legs and feet.

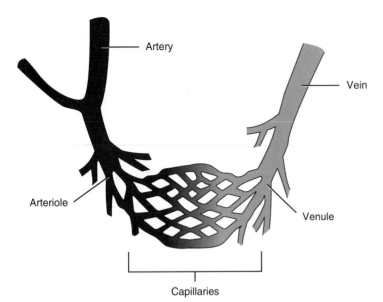

Artery

Vein

Arteriole

Venule

Capillaries

F I G U R E 7 – 1
Arterioles, capillaries, and venules.

CHARACTERISTICS OF THE HEART

Anatomy and Physiology

GENERAL DESCRIPTION. The heart functions as a pump to circulate blood throughout the body. It is a rather small organ that weighs about 11 ounces or 300 grams. It is approximately the size of one's fist. Small but powerful, the heart beats approximately 72 times/min, 100,000 times/day, and 22.5 billion times in an average lifetime. The heart is located in the mediastinum. It is a slightly cone-shaped muscle with the apex (tip) lying on the diaphragm and to the left of the midline. The base

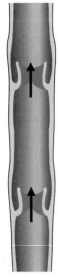
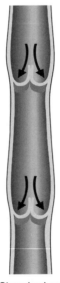

Open valves   Closed valves

F I G U R E 7 – 2
Venous valves.

(top) of the heart lies behind the sternum (Fig. 7–5). In Figure 7–5 the asterisk indicates placement of a stethoscope to take an apical pulse.

LAYERS OF THE HEART. The heart has three layers of tissue called the epicardium, myocardium, and endocardium. The epicardium is the outermost layer of tissue and is thin and transparent. The myocardium is made up of striated muscle that is responsible for the contractility of the heart. The endocardium is the innermost layer and consists of endothelial tissue that lines the heart's chambers and valves. The entire heart is enclosed in a sac of tissue called the pericardium. The pericardium is actually composed of two layers. The tough outer layer is called the parietal layer, while the inner layer, which closely adheres to the heart, is called the visceral pericardium. The pericardium functions to protect the heart from infection and trauma. The space between the two pericardial layers is called the pericardial space and contains 10–20 ml of fluid. This fluid serves to cushion the heart against blows and decreases friction between the layers created by the pumping heart.

CHAMBERS. The heart consists of four chambers with two on the left side and two on the right side. The left and right sides are separated by a muscular wall called the septum. The upper chambers are called atria, and the larger lower chambers are called ventricles. The right atrium collects deoxygenated blood returning from the body and heart muscle via the superior and inferior vena cava and coronary sinus. The blood pools in this chamber while the right ventricle is emptying (systole). During ventricular diastole (rest), the right atrioventricular (AV) valve, known as the tricuspid valve, opens, and blood from the right atrium pours into the right ventricle. After the right atrium contracts, sending the final squirt of blood into the right ventricle, the tricuspid valve closes,

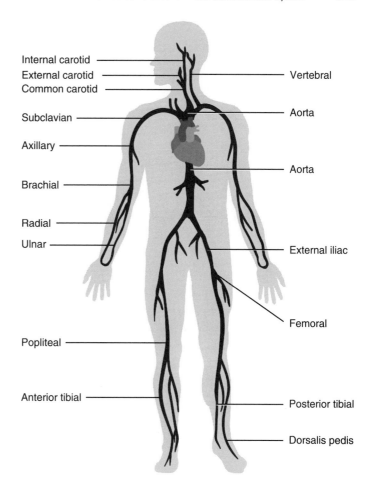

FIGURE 7-3
Arterial anatomy.

and it is the right ventricle's turn to contract. The pulmonic valve is forced open during contraction, and the right ventricle's supply of blood is sent to pulmonary circulation for reoxygenation.

The left atrium receives oxygen-rich blood from the pulmonary veins. This oxygenated blood accumulates in the left atrium during ventricular systole (contraction). During left ventricular diastole the left AV (mitral) valve opens, and blood flows into the left ventricle. After the left atrium contracts and sends the last of the reserved blood into the left ventricle, the mitral valve closes and the muscular and powerful left ventricle contracts. This contraction forces the aortic valve open, and the left ventricle's supply of blood rushes into the aorta for its journey to the rest of the body (Fig. 7–6).

CORONARY ARTERIES. The heart muscle itself must be supplied with oxygen and nutrients to live and function. This is accomplished through its own arterial circulatory system known as the coronary arteries. There are two main coronary arteries, the left and the right, which arise from the aorta. The left and right coronary arteries branch into many other arteries that supply the myocardium (Fig. 7–7). Disease of the coronary arteries is the leading cause of death in the United States and will be discussed later in this chapter.

CONDUCTION SYSTEM OF THE HEART

Some unique features of heart muscle allow it to contract and do the wondrous things we have discussed so far. Automaticity is the ability of heart muscle to initiate its own electrical impulses on a regular basis without aid from neurons or hormones outside the cardiac system. Conductivity is the ability of excited cardiac cells to move the electrical impulse along and across other cardiac cell membranes. Contractility is the ability of the stimulated cardiac cells to contract. The impulse and response take place very rapidly so that the heart muscle contracts rhythmically and synchronously. Only cardiac muscle cells have the ability to react so fast to a stimulus (Fig. 7–8).

SINOATRIAL NODE. Although most cardiac cells can initiate a cardiac impulse, the sinoatrial (SA) node has the most specialized cells in the heart to do this and so is the usual pacemaker of the heart. An electrical impulse is initiated here at a rate of 60–100 times per minute. The SA node is located adjacent to the superior vena cava in the right atrium.

ATRIOVENTRICULAR NODE. The electrical impulse leaves the SA node and travels via electrical tracts to the AV node. The AV node is located on the posterior

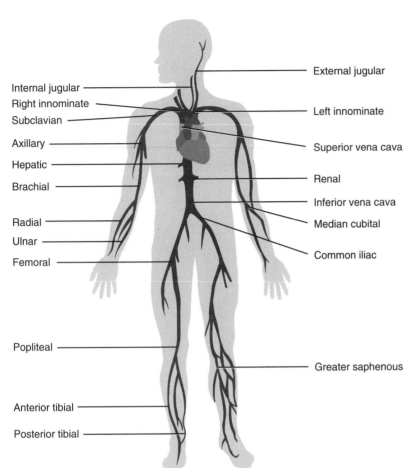

Internal jugular
Right innominate
Subclavian
Axillary
Hepatic
Brachial
Radial
Ulnar
Femoral
Popliteal
Anterior tibial
Posterior tibial

External jugular
Left innominate
Superior vena cava
Renal
Inferior vena cava
Median cubital
Common iliac
Greater saphenous

FIGURE 7–4

Venous anatomy.

floor of the right atrium. The electrical impulse is slowed down in the AV node to allow blood in the atrium to empty into the ventricles. The AV node has the ability to initiate electrical impulses at a rate of 40–60 times/min should the SA node fail.

BUNDLE OF HIS. The electrical impulse now travels through the Bundle of His, which is a short thick cable of fibers beginning at the tail of the AV node. The bundle of His branches off into the right and left bundle branches, which supply the septum and left and right ventricles.

PURKINJE FIBERS. The branches of the bundle of His merge into the Purkinje system, which is a network of fingerlike cardiac cells. The Purkinje cells spread into the myocardium of the ventricles where the electrical impulse is conducted to cause contraction. The final product of each impulse initiated in the SA node is a synchronous contraction of the heart muscle whose purpose is to distribute blood to the body.

CARDIOVASCULAR DISEASES AND DISORDERS

Epidemiology of Cardiovascular Disease

Cardiovascular disease in the United States is responsible for more deaths than all other diseases combined. In 1989 the American Heart Association reported nearly 1 million deaths due to cardiovascular disease. One in four people in the United States has some form of cardiovascular disease. The cost to the nation and taxpayers is staggering—hundreds of millions of dollars per year in prescriptions, doctor and nurse's fees, hospital and home care, and lost productivity. Despite the grim statistics,

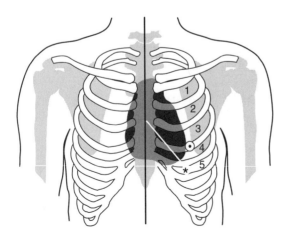

FIGURE 7–5

Anatomical location of the heart.

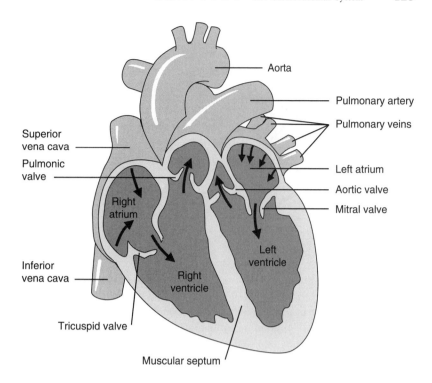

F I G U R E 7 – 6

Cross section of the heart to show chambers and
valves. Arrows indicate circulating blood.

death rates are declining. This reduction in mortality is
due in part to vast improvements in diagnostics and
treatment, and to prevention of heart disease through
education and adoption of healthier living habits.

Classification of Heart Disease

Cardiovascular disease is classified into two major areas, congenital and acquired. Congenital heart disease is
due to abnormal development of the heart during the
prenatal stage of life. Acquired heart disease develops
after birth and may suddenly or gradually affect the
cardiovascular system.

As health care providers it is important to be knowledgeable about the etiology of heart disease so we may
teach patients how to avoid disease or lessen the risks
associated with heart disease. It is also important to be
personally responsible in caring for our own hearts and
to be good examples of how to live healthier lives.

Arrhythmias: Effects on the Cardiovascular System

We have discussed the heart's unique ability to initiate
and conduct its own electrical impulses to produce a
contraction. Trauma, disease, or chemical imbalance can

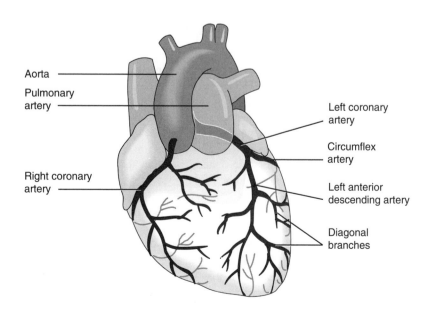

F I G U R E 7 – 7

Coronary arteries.

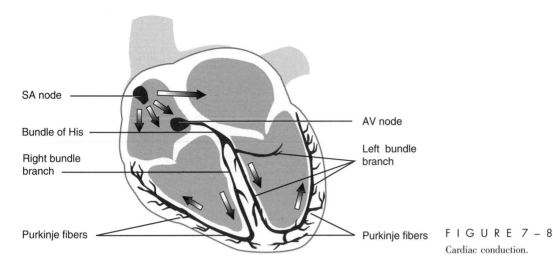

SA node

Bundle of His

Right bundle branch

AV node

Left bundle branch

Purkinje fibers

Purkinje fibers

F I G U R E 7 – 8
Cardiac conduction.

cause disruption in the impulse formation, conduction system, or both. This disruption in turn can cause irregular and/or abnormal heart rate and rhythms, or arrhythmias (also called dysrhythmias). Arrhythmias can be mild to severe. The most serious complication of arrhythmia is sudden death. There are approximately 300,000 deaths per year in the United States due to arrhythmias. This represents nearly one third of all cardiovascular deaths per year. It is vital that health care providers be able to recognize signs and symptoms of cardiac arrhythmias to promptly report them and obtain treatment for the patient.

CLINICAL OBSERVATIONS. A patient experiencing arrhythmias may complain of chest pain, palpitations, fainting, shortness of breath, edema in the extremities, or feelings of anxiety. These complaints from the patient are known as subjective data. The PCT must proceed to gather objective data.

✔ The PCT should observe and accurately measure the patient's respiratory rate and rhythm, blood pressure, rate and rhythm of pulse, color and temperature of skin, and mental status.

If the patient experiences one or more measurements not within normal limits, an ECG may be necessary.

MEDICAL INTERVENTIONS. Medical treatment could include such methods as medications, surgery, cardiac monitoring, diet restrictions and modification, and electrical countershock. The role of the PCT in these treatments includes patient monitoring, preparation for tests or surgery, and reinforcement of teaching.

NURSING INTERVENTIONS. Patient teaching is the task of all health care providers. The PCT can find this one of the most satisfying roles he or she performs. Many hospitals have preapproved and ready-made patient teaching materials. While the RN is responsible for patient education, the PCT may reinforce teaching about how to take a pulse; what, why, and when to report

symptoms; as well as precautions to take such as avoiding excess fatigue, overeating, smoking, and stress.

Remember to document subjective and objective data as well as any patient teaching you reinforce.

Coronary Artery Disease

DEFINITION. Coronary artery disease (CAD) is a disease of the coronary arteries. We have discussed the important role the coronary arteries play in supplying the myocardium with oxygen. Plaque buildup and lesions within the lining of the coronary arteries cause narrowing or even complete obstruction of the blood flow in the vessel. This process is known as atherosclerosis. Coronary atherosclerotic heart disease (CAHD) is the most common type of CAD. Atherosclerosis diminishes the supply of blood and oxygen to heart muscle and can lead to angina and myocardial infarction (Fig. 7–9).

EPIDEMIOLOGY. Studies have revealed that the incidence of CAD is higher in men than women of childbearing age, the wealthy in developing countries, and the elderly. Countries where diet is traditionally high in calories, fat, refined carbohydrates, and cholesterol have a higher incidence of CAD than do countries where the diet is lower in these compounds.

RISK FACTORS. Although not all of the causes of atherosclerosis are known, certain genetic, emotional, environmental, and personal factors that contribute to CAD have been identified. These risk factors can be classified as nonmodifiable and modifiable or risk factors that can be changed and those that cannot be altered.

Nonmodifiable risk factors include age, sex, race, and family history. Mortality due to CAHD increases with age; 40% of all deaths of men ages 55–64 are due to CAHD. Although the reasons are not clear, a strong family history of CAD, especially before the age of 50, puts one at greater risk for developing CAD. Genetics and environ-

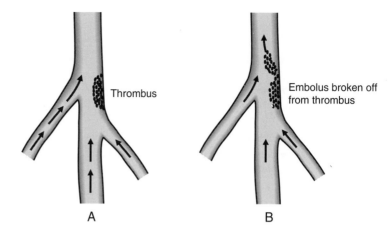

Thrombus

Embolus broken off
from thrombus

A   B

FIGURE 7-9
Thrombus development and thromboemboli.

mental factors probably work together in creating this risk factor.

Modifiable risk factors include diet, hypertension, obesity, cigarette smoking, diabetes, and elevated cholesterol levels. Elevated cholesterol levels have been positively linked to CAD. Persons with serum cholesterol levels greater than 260 mg/dl are at 3 times the risk for developing CAD than those with levels less than 200 mg/dl. Cholesterol is manufactured by the body in small amounts since it is a necessary chemical for normal bodily functions. The majority of cholesterol, however, is taken into the body through diet. Foods high in saturated fats increase the serum cholesterol level. The American Heart Association (AHA) recommends a modification in the diet of all Americans as 50% of our daily calories still come from fat. All persons should reduce the fat content of their diet and substitute polyunsaturated fat for saturated fat. Sources of polyunsaturated fat include corn, cottonseed, soy, olive, and safflower oils. Sources of saturated fat include animal fat, palm and coconut oils, and butterfat. Besides watching one's diet, one should also maintain body weight at normal.

Hypertension, or elevated blood pressure, may not always be preventable, but it is treatable. Persons with hypertension have a much greater risk of death due to CAD than those who maintain normal systolic and diastolic pressures. Patients need to be instructed to have their blood pressure monitored regularly, adhere to diet recommendations, and take their medication consistently.

Like hypertension, diabetes may or may not be preventable, but it is treatable. Diabetes increases the risk of developing early coronary atherosclerosis. Patients need to be taught to monitor their blood sugar levels and take their medications as directed by their physician.

Cigarette smoking is one of the three major risk factors involved in CAD. The death rate due to CAD is 70% higher in male smokers than in male nonsmokers. All smokers have more than two times the risk of developing heart attacks than nonsmokers. Tar, nicotine, and carbon monoxide found in cigarettes all contribute to CAD. Tar

contains carcinogens. Nicotine increases heart rate, myocardial oxygen demand, blood pressure, and the chance of lethal arrhythmias. Carbon monoxide decreases oxygen supply within the circulatory system.

Patient teaching is vital to help persons prevent or reduce their risk for CAD. Considering the incidence and extremely high cost to the nation, all persons need to take responsibility for preventing CAD when possible.

Angina Pectoris

Angina is a type of CAHD. Angina pectoris means chest pain. It occurs when there is a shortage of oxygen supply to the heart muscle. When there is an increased demand for oxygen by the heart muscle, the coronary arteries dilate and supply the myocardium with more blood and oxygen. Atherosclerotic plaque buildup decreases the coronary arteries' ability to do this, and a person experiences the chief symptom of angina—chest pain.

CLINICAL OBSERVATIONS. The patient will complain of chest pain, which may radiate to the left shoulder and arm. Less commonly, pain may radiate to the neck, jaw, or right shoulder.

Listen for patient complaints like "chest tightness," "heartburn," or "indigestion." Report these complaints immediately to the RN.

Pain is usually mild to moderate and lasts less than 5 minutes. Rest and/or the medication nitroglycerin will relieve pain. Angina may be brought on by exertion or emotions, or it may occur at rest.

Observe for clammy skin, dyspnea, anxiety, nausea, increased heart rate, and hypotension. Report immediately!

NURSING INTERVENTIONS. Nursing diagnoses might include activity intolerance, anxiety, knowledge deficit, pain, and alteration in tissue perfusion. Nursing staff interventions need to include eliminating or reducing factors contributing to pain.

 Observe for decreased pain tolerance, anxiety, fatigue, or lack of knowledge.

Encourage stress reduction activities during periods of increased life stressors. Promote a calm uncluttered environment in the patient's room. Ensure periods of rest during any physical activity.

Always obtain vital signs if patient has an episode of angina and prepare for obtaining an ECG.

PATIENT TEACHING. Patient teaching by the RN includes the cause of angina and ways to prevent it such as not overeating, avoidance of strenuous activity in cold or hot weather, avoidance of stressful situations, and stress-reducing activities such as meditation or guided imagery. Patients need to be taught what their medications are, their purpose, side effects, and method of administration.

While it is the responsibility of the RN to provide patient education, the PCT can reinforce this education.

Remind the patient to always carry his or her nitroglycerin tablets when leaving home; check the expiration date; and replace them immediately when empty or expired. Stress the importance of smoking cessation and give referral information to smoking cessation classes. Information regarding a "heart-smart" diet should be provided by nursing staff or a dietician. Teach the patient to avoid foods high in saturated fat, salt, and cholesterol.

Myocardial Infarction

CAUSE. Heart attack is the layman's term for myocardial infarction (MI). MI occurs when there is sudden blockage of one of the coronary arteries causing sudden death or eventual necrosis of the myocardium. MI is one of the possible consequences of CAHD. Necrosis is usually not immediate, but is the last event in a series of progressively worsening tissue changes. The absence of blood supply to the myocardium distal to the blockage results in ischemia due to lack of oxygen to the myocardium. If ischemia is not reversed within approximately 20 minutes, tissue death will occur and scar tissue forms. This area of scar tissue will never be able to contract again. Therefore, the larger the area of necrosis, the more serious the MI is.

CLINICAL OBSERVATIONS. Subjective findings may include complaints of severe chest pain, which can radiate to the arms, neck, or back. The patient may

describe the pain as crushing, burning, or sharp. However, in 15–20% of all MIs the patient may experience no pain at all. The patient may also exhibit and complain of confusion.

Objective findings may include severe pain lasting longer than 30 minutes and is unrelieved with rest or nitroglycerin tablets. The patient could also demonstrate anxiety, dyspnea, restlessness, nausea and vomiting, cold clammy skin, and elevated temperature. The physical examination may reveal decreased blood pressure, elevated pulse, coarse or fine crackles upon auscultation of breath sounds, and an irregular pulse.

 Report any combination of these symptoms immediately.

MEDICAL INTERVENTIONS. Relieving pain, giving oxygen, obtaining a 12-lead ECG, and assessing for possible thrombolytic therapy are the first and most important medical interventions for the patient with a possible MI.

NURSING INTERVENTIONS. Nursing diagnoses could include pain, dysrhythmia, decreased cardiac output related to decreased contractility of the myocardium, impaired gas exchange, anxiety/fear, and activity intolerance. The PCT can monitor the patient's response to pain medications, monitor vital signs, and prepare the patient for a 12-lead ECG.

Be alert for decreased responsiveness, urinary output less than 30 cc/hour, cyanosis, decreased strength in peripheral pulses, edema in the extremities, crackles in the breath sounds, and shortness of breath.

For acute symptoms, elevate HOB, put on call light, obtain vital signs, and stay with the patient. To reduce anxiety and feelings of powerlessness, provide the patient with a calm and quiet environment. Explain all procedures to the patient before instituting them. Encourage the patient and family to ask questions.

If you do not know the answer to questions, admit it. Tell the patient you will find the answer or ask the RN to speak to the patient. Make sure you follow up on your word, to instill patient confidence, trust, and quality of care.

The patient is at high risk for activity intolerance due to oxygen shortage caused by decreased cardiac output. The PCT should ascertain that the patient keeps his or her supplemental oxygen on at all times. The patient should be given plenty of time and assistance in the acute stage to perform activities of daily living, spreading them out over the course of the day if necessary. Finally, assist the patient with increased activity as prescribed by the cardiac rehabilitation nurse or physician.

Congestive Heart Failure

Congestive heart failure (CHF) is a condition in which the heart is unable to act effectively as a pump to supply the body with blood. Heart failure is the result of damaged myocardium. There are acute and chronic causes of CHF, including MI and hypertension.

CLINICAL OBSERVATIONS. All symptoms of CHF are related to an excess of fluid accumulation in the body. Heart failure may develop suddenly with the patient exhibiting symptoms of syncope, shock, and sudden death. Chronic CHF comes on gradually over time, and the hospitalized patient may exhibit dyspnea, anorexia, fatigue, heart murmur, pink frothy sputum, crackles in the breath sounds, and edema in the extremities.

MEDICAL INTERVENTIONS. Medical treatment is aimed at optimizing the heart's pumping ability and reducing the heart's work load. These goals are accomplished through oxygen therapy, medications, and diet management.

NURSING INTERVENTIONS. There are many possible nursing diagnoses for CHF, depending upon such factors as the patient's motivation, age, and cause of CHF. Generally, diagnoses would include decreased cardiac output, fluid volume excess, impaired gas exchange, and activity intolerance. Nursing staff interventions would include those covered under care of the patient with an MI. Interventions related to fluid excess would include carefully monitoring the patient's fluid intake and output, ensuring compliance with dietary restrictions by educating the patient and family on the need to restrict sodium and fluid intake, and keeping an accurate daily weight chart on the patient. Treatments for improving impaired gas exchange include ensuring compliance with use of oxygen. Humidified air and padding around the mask can increase patient comfort and compliance. The patient experiencing acute CHF is at risk for alterations in skin integrity related to bedrest, poor peripheral circulation, and activity intolerance.

Monitor areas over bony prominences frequently for signs of skin discoloration and breakdown. Have bed pan/urinal available, monitor dietary tray, and elevate patients' legs when they are seated in a chair.

Frequent changes in position and the use of protective coverings can help prevent decubiti from forming. Provide small but frequent meals that include a source of protein and complex carbohydrates.

Inflammatory Heart Disease

ETIOLOGY. Viruses, bacteria, toxins within the environment, cocaine use, and trauma are all possible causes of inflammatory heart disease. The causal agent can infect and inflame different parts of the heart, including the myocardium, the inner and outer layers of the heart, the valves, or the sac that surrounds the heart. The infectious agent can be severe enough to cause permanent structural damage to the heart and even death.

TYPES OF INFLAMMATORY HEART DISEASE. Rheumatic heart disease, pericarditis, myocarditis, endocarditis, alcoholic cardiomyopathy, and syphilitic cardiovascular disease are types of inflammatory heart disease.

CLINICAL OBSERVATIONS. Fever, fatigue, anorexia, dyspnea, and pain are complaints common to most types of inflammatory heart disease. The specific disease and cause are determined through such means as laboratory and radiographic studies, patient history and physical examination, ECG, echocardiography, and biopsy of infected tissue.

MEDICAL INTERVENTIONS. The disease may be treated with such measures as antibiotics, antiarrhythmics, cardiac monitoring, hospitalization, and surgery.

NURSING INTERVENTIONS. Prevention of disease is always preferable to having to treat a problem. It is important for health care providers to understand the ways infectious agents can be transmitted to avoid possible risk and harm to the patient. There are many procedures done within the hospital setting that can spread or make a patient susceptible to infection if the health care provider is not careful. Enemas, catheterizations, irrigations, IV therapy, and other invasive tests provide entry ways for infectious microbes.

STOP Always wash hands when finished with a patient, and just before procedures. Use sterile technique, when required, to reduce the risk of infection.

Valvular Heart Disease

The four heart valves—mitral, tricuspid, pulmonic, and aortic—help to maintain one-way flow of blood through the heart. If the valves are diseased they may restrict flow of blood through them, because of narrowing of the opening (stenosis), or allow back flow of blood into the previous chamber.

TYPES OF VALVULAR DISEASE. Mitral stenosis, mitral regurgitation, aortic stenosis, aortic regurgitation, and mitral valve prolapse are all diseases of the heart valves (Fig. 7–10).

CLINICAL OBSERVATIONS. Many of the subjective findings or complaints from the patient will not be voiced until years into the disease process. This is due to the heart's abilities to compensate for increased volume by expansion or to contract more forcefully to overcome resistant valves. When signs and symptoms do begin to emerge, the patient may complain of fatigue, dyspnea, chest pain, and orthopnea. Objective findings upon physical examination and diagnostic studies may reveal ECG changes, irregular pulse, resting tachycardia, heart mur-

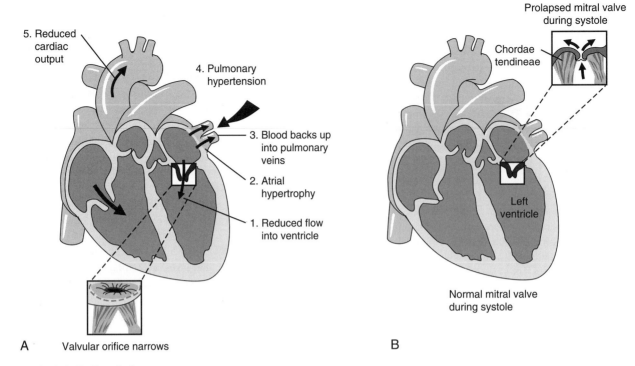

FIGURE 7-10
Cardiac valve disorders. *A,* Mitral valve stenosis. *B,* Mitral valve prolapse. Prolapse permits the valve leaflets to
billow back into the atrium during left ventricular systole. The billowing causes the leaflets to part slightly,
permitting regurgitation into the atrium.

murs and clicks, enlargement of heart and chambers, regurgitation of blood into the chambers, and flapping or stiffness of valve leaflets.

MEDICAL INTERVENTIONS. The initial intervention in mild to moderate disease may include limiting activity, medications, diet restriction, and oxygen therapy. As symptoms and disease progress, surgery will become necessary to repair or replace the diseased valves.

NURSING INTERVENTIONS. Nursing diagnoses related to valvular heart disease could include decreased cardiac output, activity intolerance, and knowledge deficit. PCT activities related to these diagnoses include accurate monitoring of vital signs, ensuring adherence to diet restrictions through teaching and monitoring of food delivered to the patient, assisting patient with activities of daily living, assisting with ECGs and other diagnostic procedures.

Aortic Aneurysms

An aneurysm is an enlargement or bulging of an artery somewhere along its length. Aneurysms are caused by atherosclerosis, infection, or trauma or are congenital in nature. Aneurysms can occur in any vessel, but are most commonly found in the abdominal aorta.

CLINICAL OBSERVATIONS. Abdominal aneurysms may be palpated at the level of the umbilicus and toward the epigastrium. Pain may be absent, intermittent,

or mild. Sudden severe pain may be due to rupture of the aneurysm. Aortic rupture can cause rapid and fatal hemorrhage into the peritoneal cavity.

MEDICAL INTERVENTIONS. Treatment will depend on the size of the aneurysm. Medication and a low sodium diet is the treatment of choice for persons with aortic aneurysms <4.5 cm in diameter. Surgery is usually performed for larger aneurysms.

NURSING INTERVENTIONS. Nursing diagnoses could include anxiety related to diagnosis and surgery, potential for decreased cardiac output secondary to aneurysm rupture or dissection, and potential for fluid volume deficit secondary to hemorrhage.

Watch and report any small change in vital signs. This can increase the patient's chances for survival. Also monitor changes in severity of pain and mental confusion.

Protect the patient's IV line. Monitor patient for compliance with diet restrictions, especially sodium intake. The patient needs to maintain normal blood pressure.

DISEASES OF PERIPHERAL CIRCULATION

Peripheral Vascular Disease

DEFINITION AND CAUSE. Diseases or abnormalities that impede blood flow through the upper and lower extremities causing tissue ischemia and/or necrosis are known collectively as peripheral vascular diseases (PVD). As we discussed in the section on angina pectoris and myocardial infarction, tissue that is deprived of oxygen and nutrients will suffer injury and eventual death if left untreated. During this process the danger of thrombus and embolus formation increases. Tissue damage may become so severe that the patient must have the limb amputated. In this section, PVD, risk factors, hypertension, types of PVD, prevention, and intervention are reviewed briefly.

RISK FACTORS IN PERIPHERAL VASCULAR DISEASE. Persons over age 65 are at risk for PVD, as are those who have hypertension, diabetes mellitus, atherosclerosis, smoke cigarettes, lead sedentary lives, and are obese.

Hypertension

Hypertension, or high blood pressure, is discussed here because it is a major risk factor in cardiovascular disease. Hypertension is defined as persistent elevation of systolic blood pressure >140 mm Hg and diastolic pressure >90 mm Hg. The precise causes of hypertension are not yet known, but there is evidence that the same risk factors for many of the cardiovascular diseases contribute also to hypertension. Hypertension can lead to CAD, stroke, renal disease, CHF, aortic aneurysm, PVD, and sudden death.

MEDICAL INTERVENTIONS. The first step in treatment involves educating the patient toward a healthy lifestyle by ceasing smoking, regular exercise, weight loss, diet management, blood pressure monitoring, and stress reductions. If blood pressure is not adequately controlled with these measures, then medication is used.

NURSING INTERVENTIONS. Patient education is probably the best tool in getting the patient to comply with the medical regimen.

 Use your resources throughout the organization to help with patient teaching.

Some hospitals have closed-circuit channels devoted to health care topics and education. The patient and staff education department may have regular classes on diet and stress management. Build a resource library on your unit.

Types of Peripheral Vascular Disease

Various arterial disorders and venous disorders come under the collective term *peripheral vascular disease.* A patient with an arterial disorder may experience such symptoms as pain described as cramping and that worsens with walking or elevation of the limb. Skin tends to be pale to cyanotic, thin, and shiny. Extremities are cool

and pulses decreased to absent. Patients with venous disorders may have symptoms of pain described as aching, improves with exercise, and complaints of nocturnal cramping. Their skin may have a brown discoloration, and large, generally painless, ulcers may develop in the lower extremities. Pulses are usually normal but difficult to palpate because of edema, which worsens by the end of the day.

MEDICAL INTERVENTIONS. Treatment is essentially the same as that for hypertension, but surgery may also be warranted for advanced disease.

NURSING INTERVENTIONS. Besides reinforcing patient education, PCTs can observe for edema in extremities, monitor peripheral pulses, and assist the postoperative patient with activities of daily living and exercise. Protect legs and feet from injury (See Chapter 12).

If elastic stockings have been ordered, be sure the correct size is being used. Help the patient put them on before he or she gets out of bed. Keep stockings wrinkle free and clean. Two pairs are handy to have so one can be worn while the other pair is being laundered.

Care of the Patient with an Amputation

Amputation is one of the oldest surgical procedures, dating back as far as 3500–1800 BC. It is often looked upon as failure to save a limb, but in fact may bring the patient welcome relief from severe chronic and debilitating pain. Many factors are taken into consideration before amputation is performed. The patient who has severe ischemic pain in the foot and toes may reach a point where rest, narcotics, and positioning cannot relieve the symptoms. Amputation can restore the patient to a productive and healthy lifestyle. Also, a patient with gangrene, uncontrolled infection, or large areas of muscle necrosis is a candidate for amputation.

Amputation Sites

The surgeon always tries to amputate as far distal on the limb as possible. The most common sites of amputation are the toe(s), metatarsal, below the knee, and above the knee (Fig. 7–11).

Types of Amputation

An open amputation is one in which the wound is left unsealed by skin flaps. The wound is packed with dressings, and traction is applied to the skin flaps that will eventually cover the stump. This procedure is used when there is severe infection in the tissue, which will need draining, care, and observation. A closed amputation is one in which the incision is made through healthy tissue and skin flaps cover the stump. This type of amputation is most often done for the patient with severe PVD rather than one who has experienced trauma or severe infection.

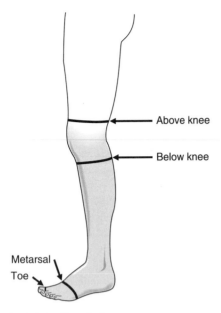

F I G U R E   7 – 1 1
Possible amputation sites in the lower extremities.

NURSING INTERVENTIONS

Rehabilitation, including physical therapy and counseling, is a vital component of the treatment plan for the patient undergoing amputation.

Nursing with its basic principles of holistic care, which focus on healing and caring for the patient as a whole person, plays a vital role in the rehabilitation of the patient. The nursing staff spends the most time with the patient and can continually assess the patient's needs and responses to therapy. Nursing diagnoses could include alteration in comfort, fluid volume excess, activity intolerance, grief, and altered body image.

The PCT monitors effects of pain control, gently helps position the patient to decrease pain, maintains the limb elevated for the first 24 hours after surgery, encourages and assists with range-of-motion exercises, measures limb size daily, observes the wound for color, odor, drainage, and intactness, and encourages the patient to express his or her feelings by being a patient and empathetic listener.

Praising and emphasizing gains made in independence and rehabilitation of the affected limb also serve to bolster the patient's confidence.

Intermittent Pneumatic Compression Devices

Patients with PVD are at risk for developing clots in the deep veins of their lower extremities. The intermittent pneumatic compression (IPC) device is a mechanical tool devised to promote circulation in the lower extremities of the patient who is confined to bedrest. The IPC device consists of a cuff with bladder similar to a blood pressure cuff except it is much longer. There are above- and below-the-knee devices. A pump with timer inflates the bladder to 40–50 mm Hg, which gently squeezes the muscles. It then deflates for about 45 seconds before pumping up again. The IPC device has proven to be very useful and has few side effects. The PCT should remove the cuff as directed to inspect the skin for signs of breakdown (See Chapter 12).

SPECIAL OBSERVATIONS REQUIRING MEASUREMENTS IN VITAL SIGNS

Because the PCT is in close and continuous contact with the patient, he or she may be the first to notice subtle changes in the patient's behavior or level of consciousness.

A patient who exhibits unusual or increased confusion, difficulty speaking, difficulty doing things he or she normally could do, has increased somnolence, complains of sudden severe pain, or expresses anxiety or feelings of impending doom needs to be immediately brought to the attention of the RN and vital signs immediately obtained.

Tips for Obtaining Accurate Measurements

Decisions about patient treatment may depend on data obtained and reported by the PCT. It is very important that measurements be taken accurately and reported promptly. Table 7–1 lists normal vital signs.

Pulse

If the patient is experiencing a change in status, the pulse should be taken for a whole minute and the rhythm and strength as well as the rate noted. A patient at rest with a pulse that is less than 60 beats/min, greater than 100 beats/min, irregular, very faint, very strong (bounding), or absent must be reported to the RN immediately.

T A B L E   7 – 1
Normal Vital Sign Parameters

VITAL SIGN	NORMAL RANGE FOR RESTING ADULT
Blood pressure	120/80 average for young adult; increases with age
Pulse	60–100 beats/min
Respirations	12–20 breaths/min

Respiratory Status

Respiratory status, including rate, rhythm, depth of respirations, ventilatory effort, and sound, needs to be assessed quickly in the patient with sudden change in health status. One respiration consists of inhalation and exhalation. The patient's respiratory rate can be calculated by counting the number of inspirations in 30 seconds and multiplying by 2. While observing inspiration, take note of increased effort to breathe, which may be demonstrated by using muscles in the abdomen and between the ribs, neck muscles, and flared nostrils. Note if the patient must sit bolt upright, appears anxious, cyanotic, pale, or diaphoretic. Listen for wheezing, grunting, or gurgling upon respiration. The normal adult respiratory rate is 12–20 breaths per minute. Normal respirations are regular in rhythm and depth.

Blood Pressure

An accurate blood pressure measurement is dependent upon many factors. It has become such a routine procedure that it is susceptible to poor technique. This section will review ways to reduce error and obtain an accurate reading.

CUFF SIZE. A cuff that is too small may yield a false high reading. Cuff size should be based on the arm size. The width of the cuff's bladder should be about 50% of the circumference of the patient's arm. A cuff that is too large for the patient's arm can yield a falsely low reading. Use a small adult or pediatric cuff for thin arms.

USE OF STETHOSCOPE. The bell of the stethoscope is designed to pick up low-frequency sounds and should be used if given a choice on your stethoscope.

POSITIONING PATIENT. The most important factor, whether the patient is supine, sitting, or standing, is that the cuff be placed on the arm at the level of the patient's heart. Be sure to position yourself so that you are reading the manometer at eye level. A reading taken with the arm dangling at the patient's side can give a reading 11–12 mm Hg higher than one taken at heart level. A reading taken above heart level may be falsely low.

OPTIMAL CONDITIONS FOR BP MEASUREMENT. The patient should rest for 5 minutes in the position in which the BP will be obtained before the measurement is actually determined. When possible, a BP measurement should be delayed 30 minutes after the last ingestion of caffeine or smoking of a cigarette. Studies show that BP is 5–6 mm Hg higher when the patient is talking during the reading than when he or she is silent. If more than one measurement needs to be taken consecutively, wait 1 to 2 minutes between readings. If you are checking for orthostatic changes, take the second reading 30 seconds after the patient stands up.

WHAT TO RECORD. The first sound of at least two consecutive sounds heard is recorded as the systolic pressure. The American Heart Association defines the diastolic sound as the last sound heard.

INFLATING AND DEFLATING THE CUFF. The cuff should be inflated no more than 30 mm Hg above the suspected systolic reading. Use the patient's normal BP as a guide or use normal BP parameters if you do not know the patient. The cuff should be deflated at 2–3 mm Hg per second. Deflating more slowly is uncomfortable, and at faster rates the mercury may fall 5–10 mm between sounds, giving a false low reading.

MEASURING BLOOD PRESSURE IN A LEG. A thigh or large cuff should be placed on the lower one third of the patient's thigh with the bladder centered over the posterior popliteal artery. Listen over the artery below the edge of the cuff. Expect the BP to be 20–30 mm Hg higher in the leg than in the arm.

 Be sure to document location of obtained reading as well as patient position.

OBTAINING MEASUREMENTS WITH PULSE OXIMETRY AND THE DOPPLER ULTRASONIC FLOWMETER

Pulse Oximetry

DEFINITION. A pulse oximeter is an electronic device that measures the amount of oxygen in the blood. The level of oxygen in the blood gives an indication of how efficiently the patient's respiratory system is functioning. Pulse oximetry is routinely used in many clinical settings, including intensive care units, the operating room, the postanesthesia care unit, and in areas where mechanical ventilation is used.

Oximetry is very useful in guiding oxygen therapy, evaluating effectiveness of pulmonary care, and monitoring a patient's oxygen saturation during invasive procedures such as airway suctioning. Pulse oximetry is cost-effective, as it helps reduce the number of arterial blood draws for measuring oxygen concentration. It is certainly more comfortable for the patient than a blood draw.

NURSING INTERVENTIONS. The sensor gently clips on or is fastened by Velcro onto the patient's finger, toe, or earlobe. The position of the sensor should be rotated periodically, as it is possible for pressure sores to develop with prolonged use. To get the most accurate reading possible, dark nail polish should be removed from the finger the sensor is attached to, and the probe should fit securely on the finger.

 Report an oxygen saturation reading of less than 92% to the patient's RN.

Doppler Ultrasonography

The Doppler is an electronic device that can detect the flow of blood through arterial and venous blood vessels.

Components of the Doppler include a transducer that "hears" the movement of red blood cells and an amplifier or stethoscope that allows the examiner to hear the pulse. Doppler ultrasonography is useful in determining patency of vessels following surgery, trauma, and suspected obstruction due to thrombosis. The PCT may be asked to evaluate lower extremity vessels by means of Doppler ultrasonography. The patient should be placed in a supine position with the head of the bed slightly elevated. The legs should be rotated externally and knees flexed. The probe is then placed at a 45–60-degree angle over the vessel to be examined. The examiner listens for a pulse with the stethoscope attached to the cord of the probe.

HEMATOLOGICAL DISORDERS

This section covers basic concepts of observation and intervention and general disorders of the blood, including the erythrocytes, leukocytes, and platelets and clotting disorders. Causes of blood disorders include hemorrhage, drug and chemical toxicity, genetic disease, dietary deficiencies, overproduction and underproduction of cells, infection, irradiation, and immunological disorders.

Diagnosis of the specific disorder is made through collection of data obtained from the patient by physical examination and interview and diagnostic studies, including blood studies and bone marrow aspiration and biopsy.

Anemias

Anemias are the major disorder associated with the erythrocytes or RBCs. Anemia indicates a less than normal amount of RBCs. There are different types of anemia: anemia related to blood loss, overdestruction of RBCs, poor production of RBCs, and anemia secondary to nutritional deficit.

CLINICAL OBSERVATIONS. A deficit in the number of RBCs means there will be a deficit in Hb. Hb is the protein in the RBC that carries oxygen. Hypoxia is the principal cause of all symptoms associated with anemia. Patient's with mild anemia usually do not have any symptoms. Those with moderate anemia complain of dyspnea, palpitations, diaphoresis, and fatigue. Persons with very severe anemia have pale skin, are sensitive to cold, are dyspneic, and complain of headaches, angina, tachycardia, and constant fatigue.

MEDICAL INTERVENTIONS. Oxygen therapy benefits patients with severe anemia. In cases of severe blood loss, blood transfusion is necessary. Medication and diet therapy are also important in treating anemia. Certain types of anemia may require radiation, chemotherapy, and bone marrow transplant.

NURSING INTERVENTIONS. Nursing diagnoses may include activity intolerance, potential for infection, ineffective coping, pain, and knowledge deficit. Stagger

activities of daily living throughout the day so the patient can have rest periods. Promote good nutritional intake by promoting a calm, clean environment at meal times. Assist the patient with eating as necessary.

Disorders Associated with Platelets and Coagulation

The normal blood clotting system of the body depends on an intact circulatory system, a normal number of platelets needed to seal a wound, and all of the clotting factors to form a clot over the platelets. To balance the clotting mechanism, enzymes, which break down clots, must exist, and anticoagulants, which prevent clot formation, are necessary.

CLINICAL OBSERVATIONS. The major signs and symptoms of disorders with less than normal amounts of platelets and clotting factors include small and large bruised looking areas on the skin. The patient may relate easy bruising, bleeding gums, black tarry stools, and hematuria.

MEDICAL INTERVENTIONS. Treatment may include blood product transfusion, medication, and surgery.

NURSING INTERVENTIONS. Nursing diagnoses include high risk for injury, potential of impaired skin integrity, pain, and knowledge deficit. The PCT must be alert for signs and symptoms of increased bleeding, such as spread of or new patches of bruises, mental confusion, and blood in the urine or stool. The patient should always wear shoes when ambulating to avoid injury to the feet. Grooming supplies should include a soft bristle or sponge toothbrush and electric razor. Frequent but gentle position changes can help decrease the chance of further tissue injury and breakdown.

Disorders Associated with White Blood Cells

WBCs, or leukocytes, are primarily responsible for fighting infection. Any disorder in this system leaves a person susceptible to infection.

Leukemia is the most commonly seen disorder of WBCs. Leukemia is distinguished by the overproduction of WBCs. This overproduction interferes with the production of other blood cells and results in immature and ineffective WBCs.

CLINICAL OBSERVATIONS. Signs and symptoms can include fever, swollen lymph nodes, paleness, and fatigue from anemia, anorexia, and weight loss.

MEDICAL INTERVENTIONS. The most common treatments for leukemias are chemotherapy and bone marrow transplant.

NURSING INTERVENTIONS. Nursing diagnoses and interventions include those discussed under disorders of platelets and coagulation. There is also a high risk for infection secondary to decreased WBCs. Meticulous handwashing by patient and health care providers is necessary.

Patients with indwelling catheters must be monitored closely for signs of infection. Any invasive procedures should be done using aseptic technique.

BLOOD TRANSFUSIONS

PURPOSE. The purpose for blood transfusion is to administer whole blood or one of its products to restore the quantity or quality of circulating blood. The RN administering the blood has a great deal of responsibility in preparing the patient, verifying the blood product, and administering the transfusion. The role of the PCT will depend on the institution's policy. The PCT may be called upon to monitor vital signs or take on added responsibility and tasks with other patients.

Transfusion Options

There are three transfusion options available to the patient. Homologous blood transfusion is from a random source. Autologous transfusion uses the patient's own blood. The third type, directed or designated blood, is blood donated for transfusion by a friend or relative. All donated blood undergoes extensive testing for typing and disease.

Types of Blood and Blood Components

The type of blood product a patient will receive depends on the deficiency that is to be corrected. To avoid wastefulness, whole blood is seldom given. A unit of whole blood can be separated to provide RBCs and one or two other components. It may be given in cases of massive blood loss. Packed RBCs may be given for acute or chronic blood loss. Platelets are administered to prevent bleeding or to control bleeding when platelet count is very low. Fresh frozen plasma is transfused in patients with severe clotting factor deficiencies.

Monitoring the Patient During Transfusion

The first 10–15 minutes of a transfusion are the most critical. The patient must be monitored closely during this time. Vital signs are recorded before the transfusion begins, after the first 15 minutes, and then every hour during the transfusion and the first hour after.

Although the RN will probably begin the transfusion and monitor the patient for the first 15 minutes, the PCT may be asked to obtain and record vital signs.

Signs and Symptoms of Transfusion Reaction

Observe for and teach the patient to report any back pain, chest pain, headache, apprehension or feelings of impending doom, and itching.

Monitor for fever, chills, dyspnea, rashes, itching, hives, hypertension, hypotension, tachycardia, bradycardia, wheezing, and nausea and vomiting. Report these signs and symptoms to the patient's RN immediately.

The RN will stop the transfusion, administer IV 0.9% saline solution, and contact the patient's doctor and blood bank for further instructions.

SUMMARY

The cardiovascular system transports vital products to the cells and carries away waste products. It performs many functions and is made up of the heart, vessels, and blood components. Diseases, disorders, and trauma that interrupt any part of this closed system interfere with its overall function. The PCT plays a vital role by providing assigned care and observing and reporting patient complaints and symptoms outside normal occurrences.

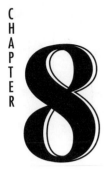

C
H
A
P
T
E
R

8

The Renal Urinary System

MICHELLE M. BUDZINSKI-BRAUNSCHEIDEL, BSN, RN,C

OUTLINE

Structures of the Renal System
Kidney
Ureters
Bladder
Urethra
Functions of the Renal System
How the Kidney Works
Disorders of the Genitourinary Tract
Congenital Anomalies
Urinary Incontinence/Voiding
 Dysfunction

Inflammation/Infections
Urinary Catheters
Management of Fluid Balance
Urine Testing
Urine Color Variations
Renal Failure
Dialysis
Hemodialysis
Summary

PREREQUISITE KNOWLEDGE AND SKILLS

- Assisting with activities of daily living (ADLs)
- Skin care principles, especially urinary incontinence skin care (Chapter 12)
- Basic hygiene
- Universal precautions
- Math skills
- General preoperative care (Chapter 3)
- General postoperative care (Chapter 3)
- Medical asepsis (Chapter 17)

OBJECTIVES

After you complete this chapter, you will be able to:

- List the structures and functions of the urinary system.
- Recognize signs and symptoms associated with urinary disorders.
- Describe procedures used to treat various renal problems.
- Discuss common disorders of the urinary tract.

- Describe the difference between hemodialysis and peritoneal dialysis.
- Describe the patient care technician's (PCT's) care with each type of dialysis.
- Discuss the various urinary drainage tubes.
- Explain how to collect tests specific for urine.

KEY TERMS

Acidosis pH in the acid range of 7.0 or below

Advocacy Being in support of; being a representative for someone or something

Alkalosis pH in the base range higher than 7.0

Aneurysm Abnormal bulging of a blood vessel, can be located in various areas of the body

Anomaly An abnormality of an organ or structure

Anuria Absence of or very little urine production for a 24-hour period

Ascites Abnormal accumulation of fluid in the abdomen

Bilateral Involving both sides, right and left

Calculus A stone, often in the renal system

Congenital Existing at or occurring at birth

Cystoscopy Procedure used to examine/visualize the inside of the bladder

Dialysis Therapy passage of a solute through a membrane; used to clean the body of wastes. There are 2 forms: hemodialysis and peritoneal

Emesis Vomiting

Enterostomal Therapist A certified person who cares for and instructs in the care of ostomies and sometimes wounds

ESWL Extracorporeal shock wave lithotripsy; crushing a kidney stone by means of shock waves transmitted through water

Extrinsic Originating outside a part

Filtrate That which is filtered out

Genitourinary Relating to the genital and urinary organs

Glomerulonephritis Inflammation of glomeruli of the kidney

Hematuria Blood in the urine

Hemodialysis Form of dialysis used to cleanse the blood; catheters placed directly into the blood vessels

Hesitancy Momentary delay

Hilus Part of kidney where the ureters enter

Homeostasis Balance of fluid, electrolytes, and chemicals in the body

Hydrometer Device used to measure the specific gravity of a fluid

Hypertension Blood pressure elevated above 140/90

Hypertrophy Increase in the size of component cells resulting in enlargement of a part

Hypospadias Developmental abnormality in the closure/formation of the (usually male) urethra

Incontinence Loss of control of function of the bladder or bowels

Intermittent Not continuous; at intervals

Intrinsic Situated within the body

Involuntary Not being in control or aware of the movement or function that is occurring

Malaise Vague feeling of general bodily weakness and discomfort

Meatus A body opening or passage

Micturition Urination

Necrosis Death of tissue

Nephrolithiasis   The formation of kidney stones

Nephron   The structural and functional unit of the kidney; the tiniest structure of the kidney

Nocturia   Frequent urination during the night

Nonpharmacological   Treatment that does not include the administration of medication, such as relaxation, music, or distraction techniques

Parenteral   Administration of medication other than through the intestine, for example, IV

Peristalsis   The alternating squeezing motion to aid in the forward movement of contents in tubular structures

Peritoneal   Pertaining to the peritoneum

Peritoneum   The thin membrane that covers the abdominal organs

Polycystic Kidney   A disorder in which the kidneys contain numerous cysts

Pruritus   Itching

Reflux   Regurgitation; flow of fluid or contents back toward the point of origin

Retroperitoneal   Behind the peritoneum

Sepsis   A toxic condition due to pathogenic microorganisms in blood stream

Sitz Bath   A treatment in which the patient sits in the tub while water is flushed on the perineal area

Sphincter   A ringlike muscle that contracts and closes a bodily opening

Stasis   Stagnant, not moving

Suprapubic   Located above the pubic region

Urinalysis   Examination of urine, usually microscopic

Urinometer   A device to determine the specific gravity of urine

Renal system disorders are recognized as major health care problems. Over 10 million adult Americans have disorders associated with the renal system, ranging from obstructions and infections to trauma. Structures of this system include kidney, ureters, bladder, and urethra (Fig. 8–1).

Assessment of the genitourinary tract is an important part of the overall physical assessment and observation of the patient. Included are information regarding voiding and renal function and questions or observations regarding the reproductive organs that may relate to potential problems such as impotence and uterine or prostate cancer.

STRUCTURES OF THE RENAL SYSTEM

Kidney

There are two bean-shaped kidneys. They are located on either side of the vertebral column between the 12th thoracic and 3rd lumbar vertebrae (at the small of the back). The right kidney is usually lower than the left because of the presence of the liver. Both are retroperitoneal (behind and below the abdominal cavity lining).

The inward curving section is where the renal arteries and veins, ureters, and nerves are attached. This region is called the renal sinus or hilum. Within the kidney there are three major areas: the cortex, the medulla, and the renal pelvis (Fig. 8–2). Connective tissue anchors the kidney to the surrounding structures, but allows the kidney to shift.

Each kidney contains more than 1 million tubular nephrons (the functional unit of the kidney, where urine is produced). The nephrons process approximately 180 liters of fluid a day from the blood stream. The nephrons filter out excess water, electrolytes, and waste products of metabolism. This filtrate is called urine. The balance of the fluid continues to circulate through the blood stream. Each nephron has 5 regions that carry out particular tasks:

• Bowman's capsule: Filtration

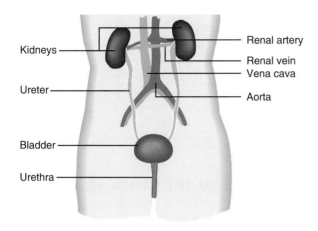

F I G U R E   8 – 1
Kidney structures.

- Proximal convoluted tubule: Reabsorption of sodium, potassium, chloride and tubular secretion
- Loop of Henle: Reabsorption of chloride, sodium, calcium, water, and urea
- Distal convoluted tubule: Reabsorption of sodium chloride and bicarbonate and secretion of potassium, hydrogen, and ammonia
- Collecting duct: Reabsorption of water and urea only

When one kidney ceases to function, the remaining kidney is capable of taking over. This is due to a large number of reserve nephrons that can hypertrophy (enlarge) and increase their function.

Ureters

The ureters are two continuous hollow tubes extending from the renal hilus to the base of the bladder. The primary function of the ureters is to carry urine from the kidneys to the bladder. They transport urine by means of muscle contraction or peristalsis. Each ureter extends slightly into the bladder to act as a valve, decreasing the chance of reflux or backflow of urine from the bladder back up the ureter. Reflux of urine can occur during bladder emptying (contracting) or bladder distention.

If urine is allowed to go back up (reflux) to the kidney, this could cause a severe infection.

Bladder

The bladder, the urethra, and pelvic floor muscles form what is called the urethrovesical unit or lower urinary tract. These organs allow the bladder to fill and store urine until the patient needs to urinate. This process is called micturition. The bladder is a flat, hollow muscular organ that is located in the pelvis. As the bladder fills with urine, it becomes distended and is easily palpated right above the pelvic bone at the lower abdomen. The nervous system acts on the lower urinary tract to allow micturition to occur.

Urethra

The final structure of the lower urinary tract and the final passage for urine is the urethra. The urethra resembles a tube-like structure and exits the base of the bladder. The urethra has a dual purpose by way of a sphincter mechanism that prevents leakage of urine and promotes nonobstructing urination. The adult female urethra is shorter than that of the adult male and exits the body just in front of the vaginal opening (Fig. 8–3A). The male urethra passes through the prostate gland and penile

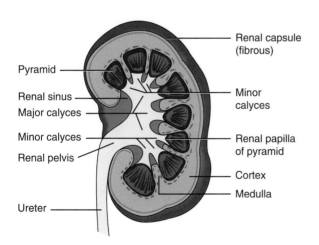

F I G U R E   8 – 2
Kidney areas.

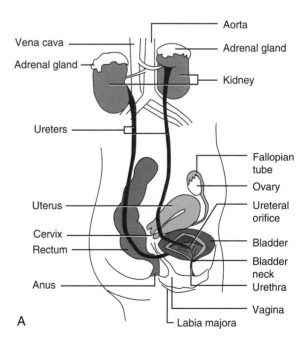

F I G U R E   8 – 3 A
Female anatomy.

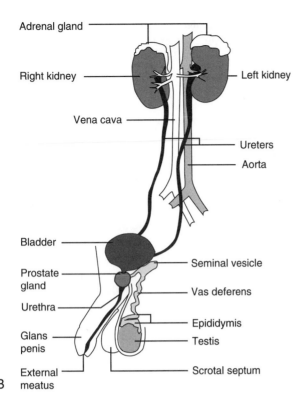

Adrenal gland

Right kidney

Vena cava

Left kidney

Ureters

Aorta

Bladder

Seminal vesicle

Prostate gland

Vas deferens

Urethra

Glans penis

Epididymis

Testis

External meatus

Scrotal septum

B

F I G U R E   8 – 3 B
Male anatomy.

shaft to the meatus (the opening at the tip of the penis) (Fig. 8–3B).

The renal system is very crucial to the housekeeping of the entire body. The two prime functions are elimination of waste products and toxic materials and maintenance of a stable internal fluid environment. The functional control of this system is the kidney. Its greatest responsibility is to maintain homeostasis, the delicate balance of all body systems.

FUNCTIONS OF THE RENAL SYSTEM

In addition to the prime functions of the renal system mentioned earlier, the renal system has the following functions:

• To rid the body of metabolic wastes

• To regulate fluid and electrolyte balance

• To help regulate blood pressure

• To aid in calcium metabolism

• To regulate red blood cell production

• To help maintain acid-base balance

How the Kidney Works

The kidneys filter all the fluid in the body. As blood enters the kidney through the renal artery, the artery

divides into millions of small vessels, each of which wraps around nephrons. The nephrons separate out the extra fluid and waste products from the blood. All these products create urine. The urine leaves the kidneys via the ureter and enters into the bladder. When the bladder is full, urine is excreted through the urethra. The clean blood leaves the kidney via the renal vein. This blood then circulates to other parts of the body.

DISORDERS OF THE GENITOURINARY TRACT

The patient care technician (PCT) needs to have a basic understanding of the renal structures, functions, and assessment/observation clues to recognize the abnormal signs and symptoms of common genitourinary disorders. Once the PCT is alerted to these abnormal findings, they should be reported immediately to the RN. These findings should be reported, documented, and monitored, to assure safety to the patient. Possible consults for other resources may be needed. Kidney diseases can attack anyone at any age. The 7 major warning signs identified by the American Kidney Foundation the PCT needs to know are:

1. Puffiness around the eyes
2. Gradual edema of various body parts, especially the ankles
3. Lower back pain just below the rib cage
4. Increased urination or changes in pattern of urination
5. Pain with urination
6. Blood or blood-tinged or tea-colored urine
7. Hypertension that is diagnosed by a physician.

The PCT can also reinforce the RN's instruction to the patient and the patient's significant other on these warning signs.

OBSTRUCTION. The first and most common disorder is obstruction. Obstructions could lead to infection or possible destruction/failure of the kidney. Obstructions can occur anywhere in the renal system—upper or lower urinary tract. The classification of the obstruction is determined by the location, its cause, the degree (partial or complete), and the duration or amount of time it has been present (chronic or acute). Urinary obstructions occur at all ages.

Causes. Obstructions can be acquired or congenital (from birth). Various obstructions are shown in (Figure 8–4).

Problems within the urinary tract (intrinsic):

| Renal calculi | Lesions |
| Blood clots | Infection |

Problems outside the urinary tract or putting pressure on a portion of the urinary tract (extrinsic):

Tumors/ Pregnancy
 cancer Gastrointestinal
Prostate disorders
 disorders Aneurysms
 Scar tissue

Signs and Symptoms. When an obstruction occurs in the urinary tract, the normal flow of urine is blocked. When the flow of urine is blocked the patient may show some signs and symptoms. Not all patients will have the same symptoms. Possible signs and symptoms that the PCT should observe for are:

- Difficult urination
- Pain, especially lower back or flank area
- Hematuria—blood in the urine either visible or a positive test on Hemostix or Chemstrip
- Increased or decreased urine volumes
- Anuria (minimal or no voiding of urine)

The PCT may ask the patient if he or she has any hesitancy, frequency, dribbling, or nocturia, or the PCT may be aware of it. The PCT must report any of these symptoms to the RN. It is crucial to have the obstruction relieved so that kidney function is not destroyed or severely damaged.

Extrinsic causes of urinary obstruction such as tumors or pregnancy may be due to compression of the ureters. Since the ureters are hollow tubes embedded in tissues and muscles and near many other organs, a change in the surrounding tissues could compress one or both. Pain is a frequent symptom.

 Any pain needs to be further investigated. Inquire where it is located and if it radiates

anywhere. The pain may be located in the flank region and be accompanied with pain on urination.

A change in voiding is the second frequent symptom to look for. Examples are:

- Decrease in the force of urine flow
- Urgency
- Incontinence
- Anuria with complete bilateral obstruction of the ureters or blockage of the urethra

If the patient has had no urine output (anuria) for the shift, the RN must be informed immediately. If anuria continues, renal failure could develop.

- Hematuria is a common symptom when renal stones cause obstructions.
- Hypertension, a blood pressure reading consistently above 140/90, may be another symptom.

Diagnosis. Tests used to diagnose renal obstruction are:

- Flat plate of the abdomen (plain abdominal X-ray)
- CT (computed tomography) to look closely at the collecting system of the kidney
- IVP (intravenous pyelography): An X-ray in which dye is injected into the blood stream to observe the urinary system
- Cystoscopy allows visualization of the entire urethra and bladder at the same time
- Kidney-ureter-bladder (KUB): X-ray obtained after

Causes of urinary tract obstruction

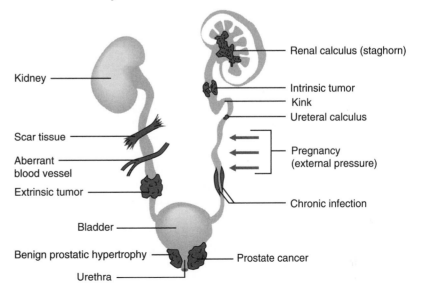

FIGURE 8-4
Various obstructions.

injection of radioactive dye into the blood stream and waiting for it to go through the urinary tract

- Serum electrolytes
- Urinalysis or 24-hour urine

Treatment. The treatment of urinary tract obstructions has both medical and surgical components. The site of obstruction determines the approach. The PCT's responsibilities include:

- Obtaining vital signs; especially blood pressure and temperature, every 6–8 hours
- Recording intake and output every shift
- Documenting/reporting urine color, or pain
- Preparing patient for any tests
- Obtaining any urine specimens

Check with your institution on what tests and specimens you are allowed to obtain. Generally the PCT can collect a voided specimen, including urine for culture and sensitivity test. The PCT does not collect specimens from urinary catheters.

RENAL CALCULI. Renal calculi (kidney stones), also called nephrolithiasis, are the leading cause of upper urinary tract intrinsic obstructions. The age group that tends to develop and form calculus is 30–50 years. Children rarely develop them. The stones are composed of many different substances that are normally soluble in urine.

Causes. The cause of calculus formation remains unclear. Certain risk factors and conditions could contribute to the formation of calculi:

- Chronic urinary tract infections (UTIs)
- Urine stasis
- Diet
- Heredity
- Specific medication
- Low urine pH
- Obesity

A urinary calculus is usually discovered when it becomes trapped as it is released from the kidney and blocks a ureter, resulting in acute renal pain. The stone may pass on its own or, more likely, it may become obstructive and could cause infection (see Fig. 8–4).

Signs and Symptoms. The renal pain is abrupt in onset and severe and tends to occur at night, awakening a patient from sleep. The severity and location of pain depend greatly on the stone location and size, degree of obstruction, and individual anatomy. Pain is usually the most predominant symptom. Other signs and symptoms associated with renal calculi are:

- Hematuria: urine may or may not be red; hematuria may be due to tissue trauma caused by movement of the calculus. Urinalysis helps to confirm the diagnosis and shows the presence of red blood cells.
- Nausea and vomiting: usually with upper-tract calculi
- Pyuria: Cloudy, foul-smelling urine from a urinary tract infection
- Abdominal distention, particularly bladder distention
- Urination changes such as burning during or after urination; pain with urination and/or frequency or urgency
- Possible fever

STOP Urinary stones associated with fever present a relative medical emergency because of the risk of clinical sepsis; thus any elevated temperature needs to be reported to the RN.

Diagnosis. The diagnostic studies used to confirm a renal calculus are numerous. The urinalysis, urine culture, urine pH, and 24-hour urine chemistries check for acidosis or alkalosis or abnormal levels of bacteria, electrolytes, and other solutes. Radiologic tests include a KUB X-ray, renal ultrasound, intravenous pyelography, retrograde pyelography, and voiding cystography.

These tests are used to determine stone location and provide detailed information on the extent of the obstruction. The laboratory chemistry tests of serum electrolytes, especially blood urea nitrogen (BUN) and creatinine, are used to determine the metabolism and function of the kidneys.

Management. Once the stone is diagnosed, treatment can be medical or surgical.

Any aggravated symptom (pain, vomiting, or hematuria) needs to be reported because it could indicate that the stone is moving, getting larger, or causing trauma.

Medical management of calculi includes encouraging high fluid intake, dietary modifications, medication to help dissolve the calculi, and/or exercise. There are several techniques to remove the stone surgically: extracorporeal shock wave lithotripsy (ESWL), pyelolithotomy, ureterolithotomy, percutaneous nephrostomy, lithotripsy, and endoscopic stone retrieval.

Patient care is aimed at keeping the patient comfortable while maintaining adequate kidney function until the renal calculi are removed. After consultation with the RN, the PCT can perform the following interventions:

1. Keep accurate record of intake and output. Documentation of specific fluid intake and urine output with accurate recording of time is extremely important, especially if associated with any type of pain or with urine

discoloration. Document and record all forms of output, including emesis.

Each form of output needs to be clearly identified separately, such as urine, emesis, nasogastric.

Report and document patient complaints of urinating difficulties such as burning, frequency, and pain to your RN.

2. Obtain specimens as ordered and directed—most likely for urinalysis, 24-hour urine, and urine for culture and sensitivity. See Chapter 21 on "Specimen Collection."

Obtain urine for culture and sensitivity test only after you have had training and returned demonstration competently.

3. Observe the patient for pain. Intensifying pain may indicate stone movement. Absence of pain may indicate passage of the stone or temporary lodging of the stone in the bladder. Provide nonpharmacological pain relief measures such as repositioning, back rubs, conversation, or using music as a distraction.

4. Obtain vital signs as ordered. Take special note of the temperature. If there is an increase in temperature or it exceeds (38° C) 101° F, report to your RN.

5. Encourage fluid intake of at lease 1500 ml/day (50 ounces). The patient will need continual encouragement to drink fluids. Adequate fluid intake may assist in passage of the stone.

You may want to consult a dietician to see what would be best for the patient. The dietician will be able to suggest the proper fluids and solids that would not cause further problems with stone formation. Offer the patient choices from fluids/foods suggested by the dietician.

6. Strain all urine. Strainers are provided and should be used to retrieve the stone. Urinary stones may be very small and difficult to see. Look carefully but do not touch the stone with your fingers. Once the stone is obtained, it will need to be sent to the laboratory for analysis so that proper medical management can be prescribed by the physician.

7. Tube care. Observe any drains or tubes for urinary output and/or signs of bleeding or infection. Foley care is a method to reduce infection. See section on Urinary Catheters for specifics on how to care for various catheters.

Congenital Anomalies

There is a wide variety of congenital anomalies related to the urinary system. The most common will be discussed

briefly. The anomalies can occur in any part of the renal tract. They occur more frequently in the *kidney* than in any other organ. Some anomalies create problems as the child grows; others are severe disorders that are obvious at birth and require immediate intervention.

In *hypoplasia* of the kidney, the organ is normal in structure, but the number of nephrons is fewer than normal. Some of these types of kidneys seem to be abnormal. Usually chronic renal failure and hypertension will develop.

In *adult polycystic kidney disease* (PKD) both kidneys are affected 95% of the time. The kidneys become larger than normal and contain various size cysts throughout. The cysts form grape-like clusters that block and destroy kidney tissue and cause deterioration of nephron functioning. The signs and symptoms associated with this disorder are pain, hypertension, and possibly fever. Radiologic diagnostic tests are used to confirm the disease. The treatment is usually medical support. The surgical approach has not been found to be particularly effective. These patients may be candidates for renal transplant after the kidneys are completely destroyed.

Under the direction of the RN, the PCT can do the following:

1. Force fluids if ordered; offer fluids of preference.
2. Assist patient in choosing and following a low-protein diet.

 Consult a dietician for meal planning.

3. Do not allow patient to participate in any strenuous exercise.

4. Monitor intake and output every 8 hours and weigh the patient daily. Document and report color of urine, urine output, and weight changes. Renal failure may develop.

5. Obtain vital signs, especially blood pressure because hypertension is a common complication.

6. Monitor for signs and symptoms of infections because the cysts are very prone to infection. Use good perineal care and handwashing techniques.

The second most common area for congenital anomalies is the *urethra*. Disorders of the male urethra include hypospadias and paraphimosis. In hypospadias, the urethra meatus opens on the ventral side (underside) of the penis. There are several forms of hypospadias, depending on the location of the penis (Fig. 8–5). The chief complaint may be difficulty in directing the stream of urine. The treatment is corrective surgery, usually before the age of 2 years.

Paraphimosis is an acquired condition in which the retracted foreskin cannot be replaced in its normal position. If not treated promptly, urethral occlusion and necrosis of penile tissue may occur.

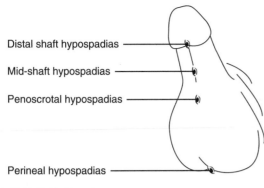

Distal shaft hypospadias

Mid-shaft hypospadias

Penoscrotal hypospadias

Perineal hypospadias

FIGURE 8 – 5
Hypospadias.

STOP Whenever pericare is completed, make sure that the foreskin of uncircumcised male patients is pulled back to its normal position over the head of the penis. If applying a condom catheter, never retract the foreskin; this will create a tourniquet effect on the penis and urethra. Make sure that the foreskin is forward at all times when care is not being directly provided.

In girls, the congenital anomaly of the urethra is fusion of the labia minora, which obstructs the flow of urine. Medical treatment to separate the labia consists of application of an estrogen cream to the area as directed.

Check with your institution whether the PCT may or may not apply an estrogen-based cream.

Urinary Incontinence/Voiding Dysfunction

Urinary incontinence is a major health issue that affects millions of people daily. Aging patients accept urinary incontinence as a sign of old age. In fact, it is not a disease, it is a symptom of another underlying disease. The disease that produces urinary incontinence could be a renal or neurological disorder. The normal voiding pattern is to urinate no more often than every 2 hours while awake.

Assessment of the patient's urinary elimination pattern is an important aspect in determining the type of incontinence and is the responsibility of the RN. This assessment is done primarily through interviewing, discussion, and observation. The PCT may help by reporting any of the following information that may be shared by the patient and/or family.

- How many times does the patient go to the bathroom during the day and night?

- Does the patient experience any particular sensation associated with voiding?

- Does the patient wear a diaper, pad, or some sort of shield in case of "accidents"?

- If the patient has an indwelling catheter, when was it placed and why?

- If the patient manages urinary elimination by intermittent catheterization, what is the schedule and who, if anyone, assists the patient?

- Find out how much and what type of fluid the patient drinks in a specified time frame, usually 24 hours.

- How does the patient describe the stream or flow of urine?

- Has the patient had any neurological injury such as a stroke?

- Does the patient have hypertension, diabetes, or cancer?

- What medications is the patient taking?

- If the patient is male, has benign prostatic hypertrophy (BPH) been diagnosed?

- All the information that is obtained will need to be reported to the RN and documented.

There are different forms and classifications of incontinence. The Agency for Health Care Policy and Research (AHCPR) has specific guidelines for urinary incontinence and definitions for the various forms of incontinence. The following definitions from the Urinary Incontinence Guideline Panel, March, 1992 describe the types of incontinence and their symptoms:

- Stress incontinence: A form of urinary incontinence characterized by involuntary loss of urine during physical exertion—laughing, for example, or coughing. The patient may need to go to the bathroom often to avoid accidents.

- Urge/reflux incontinence: Involuntary loss of urine associated with an abrupt and strong desire to void.

- Overflow/urinary retention: Involuntary loss of urine associated with overdistention of the bladder. Overflow incontinence results from urinary retention that causes the capacity of the bladder to be overwhelmed. Continuous or intermittent leakage of a small amount of urine results. The patient may make many bathroom trips during the night.

The diagnosis will include the following tests and procedures:

- Urinalysis and urine culture and sensitivity: To verify that there is an infection and to check the renal function

- KUB, intravenous pyelography (IVP), ultrasound of kidney: Diagnostic tests to determine renal anatomy and function

- Urodynamic tests: Various tests to measure functions of the urinary tract and micturition.

Medical management of incontinence includes medication, keeping a voiding diary, bladder-retraining program, catheterization (using intermittent, indwelling, and/or external catheters), and exercises. In some cases, surgery is necessary.

The PCT's role and interventions in caring for an incontinent patient include:

1. Obtain and record accurate intake and output, specifying what, when, and how much.

 Identify each form of intake and output with time, amount, and description.

2. Observe skin for any breakdown. Refer to Chapter 12 for signs and symptoms of breakdown.

3. Obtain specimens as ordered.

4. Assist patient in documenting a voiding diary if applicable. Figure 8–6 is an example of a voiding diary.

5. If ordered, apply an external collection device.

Consult an Enterostomal Therapist for more extensive and difficult cases or assistance with the application of a collection device.

6. Recommend a patient advocacy and support group for incontinence.

The AHCPR guidelines are free. The Patient Guide lists three national organizations to help support people with incontinence. To obtain a copy, call 1-800-358-9295.

7. Reinforce patient to do pelvic exercises if ordered.

8. If indwelling catheter is present, monitor catheter for patency, kinks, and tension.

Inflammation/Infections

Urinary tract infections (UTIs) is the common term used to describe various infections of the renal system. The different infections are named after the specific area of the urinary tract that is involved, for example, infection and inflammation involving the bladder is called *cystitis*. Infections of the kidney and its pelvis are termed pyelone-phritis. Inflammation of a specific part of the kidney called the glomerulus is known as glomerulonephritis. When an infection occurs, the immune system responds by trying to fight off the bacteria or other organisms causing the infection. The immune system releases fighter cell complexes that may become trapped in the glomeruli and obstruct blood flow. If blood flow is interrupted, complications can arise. One complication may be hypertension, and in severe cases of glomerulonephritis renal failure can develop.

The incidence of cystitis is higher in females than in males because of the anatomical location of the urethra. The meatus, located near the vagina, can be contaminated easily if care is not used when wiping after a bowel movement. In addition the urethra is short, and bacteria can migrate up it easily. The urethra in males is longer, which decreases the chances of organisms migrating up to the bladder (see Fig. 8–3B). This is why good technique is important in performance of pericare.

Inflammation of the prostate gland is called prostatitis. As the gland becomes inflamed, there is associated pain in the rectal suprapubic area. This inflammation can cause a change in the urinary pattern or a decrease in urination. There are different types of prostatitis.

Some risk factors are associated with UTIs: urinary obstructions, reflux of urine into the bladder, and invasive procedures such as catheterization. With all forms of inflammation and infections there are predominant signs and symptoms: pain (flank in pyelonephritis, or burning with voiding in prostatitis and cystitis), fever and chills, nausea and vomiting, and general weakness.

Tests used to confirm the diagnosis of UTI or inflammation are:

- KUB: For all UTIs, to see if an obstruction is the causative agent and to check renal function

- Urinalysis and urine culture and sensitivity: To identify the causative bacteria or other organisms

- Blood serum: Check laboratory values as they pertain to kidney function and perfusion.

The medical treatment combines many agents or procedures:

- Antibiotics

- Bedrest

- Forcing of fluids to keep bladder flushed

- Sitz bath or warm compresses for pain relief

- Patient education on good perineal care

- Patient follow-up care as directed by physician

The PCT interventions are to:

1. Obtain urine specimens

2. Monitor and document intake and output—to encourage intake of fluids as ordered; assure that fluids are the temperature that the patient desires and within reach.

DATE:				
TIME	AMT. VOIDED	LEAKAGE	FLUID INTAKE	OTHER SYMPTOMS

FIGURE 8–6

Voiding diary (See discussion in text).

3. Maintain bedrest if ordered.

4. Assist patient and instruct how to take a sitz bath, reinforce education on perineal care; assist with warm compresses as ordered.

5. Relate and document reports of pain to the RN—provide nonpharmacological pain relief measures.

6. Monitor and document vital signs, especially temperature and blood pressure.

URINARY CATHETERS

Various tubes (catheters) are used in catheterization. The purpose for their use, indications for their use, and the role of the PCT in their care are explained (Fig. 8–7).

INDWELLING FOLEY CATHETER

Purpose: To continuously drain the bladder into a closed urinary bag

Indications: Long-term use, incontinence, after surgery, neurological conditions, trauma

Role of PCT in care:

1. Empty bag whenever full or every 8 hours.
2. Document the amount of output.

3. Keep the bag below the level of the bladder at all times. This prevents urine from backing up into the bladder.

4. Provide plenty of fluids.

5. Do not have tubing pulled tightly. Never have any tension on catheter. Tension can be prevented by taping drainage tube on the midthigh or by use of an elastic tube holder that fits over thigh with a Velcro closure. Tension could cause bleeding/trauma or pull out the catheter. Tension also enlarges the bladder sphincter, and the incidence of incontinence is increased after removal of the catheter.

6. Pericare must be given every shift with soap and water to prevent possible infection. Peri-care should also be given after each bowel movement.

7. Observe for skin breakdown. Report any to the RN.

8. Observe for any leakage around the tube.

9. Never disconnect catheter from tubing or bag, which would lead to contamination.

 Catheterization should be done by a licensed person.

3-WAY FOLEY CATHETER

Purpose: to continuously irrigate the bladder with a solution, usually normal saline.

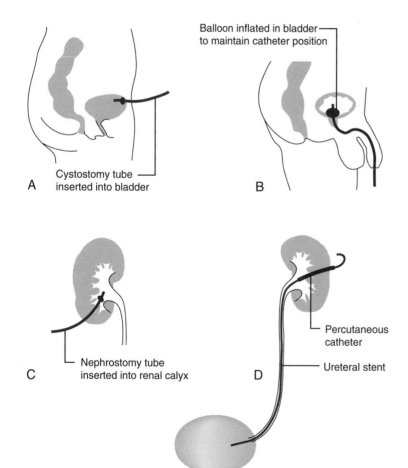

Balloon inflated in bladder to maintain catheter position

A   Cystostomy tube inserted into bladder

B

C   Nephrostomy tube inserted into renal calyx

D   Percutaneous catheter

Ureteral stent

F I G U R E 8 – 7

Various tubes. *A,* Suprapubic catheter; *B,* indwelling urinary catheter; *C,* nephrostomy tube; *D,* ureteral stent.

At the same time the solution is rapidly irrigating the bladder, the bladder is drained into an extra large bedside bag (usually 4-liter capacity).

Indications: Irrigation, postoperative, i.e., after a prostatectomy

Role of PCT in care:

1. The bag should be checked every 2 hours and emptied if necessary.

2. Document under a separate column the amount of output and the irrigation solution. The amount of the solution is subtracted from the volume of the drainage bag to give the true value of urine output.

3. Observe for blood clots.

4. Observe color of urine. While the irrigation is continuing, the urine should be amber to pink-tinged. If many clots are passing and the urine becomes a deeper red, there may be clot retention. Notify the RN of any color change.

Notify the RN if the urine output decreases or stops, or if the urine output is less than the amount of irrigation solution used. May indicate the catheter or bladder is blocked with a clot. RN needs to check and irrigate right away.

SUPRAPUBIC CATHETER (Cystostomy tube)

Purpose: To drain the bladder through the catheter, bypassing the urethra. The catheter is placed directly into the bladder, via an incision in the suprapubic area.

Indications: Urethral damage or trauma, bladder surgery, gynecological surgery, urethral blockage, neurological problem

Role of PCT in care:

1. Ensure that catheter is draining at all times.

2. Tape drainage tube to side of patient's abdomen to prevent dislocation.

3. Must maintain a closed system.

4. Observe that there are no kinks and no tension on the tubing.

5. Empty and document output at least every 8 hours.

6. Observe for leakage around suprapubic area. Observe that the dressing remains dry.

7. Catheter area must have a dressing on it at all times.

8. Observe for redness, warmth, edema, or drainage around catheter. Report any changes to the RN.

9. If checking residuals on a clamped suprapubic catheter:

- Have patient call you immediately after voiding.

- Unclamp catheter and drain.

- Measure urine (this is the residual).

- Document under a separate column the voided amount and the residual amount.

NEPHROSTOMY TUBE (Percutanous catheter)

Purpose: To drain the waste products and urine directly from the kidney. The nephrostomy tube is surgically placed into the renal pelvis and connected to a closed drainage system.

Indications: Obstructions, trauma, ureteral damage, infection

Role of PCT in care:

1. Maintain closed drainage system to prevent infection.

2. Never clamp tubing; keep tubing free of any kinks.

3. Drain/empty the drainage bag every 8 hours and record separate output for each kidney if there are two drains.

4. Observe for any leakage around insertion site and report to the RN.

5. Observe that the dressing stays dry and intact.

MANAGEMENT OF FLUID BALANCE

The two most important functions of the renal system are to rid the body of wastes and to regulate fluid and electrolyte balance. When there is fluid and electrolyte imbalance, there must be management of intake and output. The amounts of fluid the patient takes in (intake) are recorded and discharged/excreted fluids (output) are collected and the amount recorded.

Examples of different kinds of fluid intake:

- Oral fluids: Water, ice, beverages

- Semiliquid foods: Pudding, Jello, custards, yogurt

- Parenteral fluids: Intravenous fluids and medications, blood and blood products, total parenteral nutrition

- Any food that is liquid at room temperature: Popsicles, ice cream, frozen yogurt

The following are examples of various kinds of output:

- Urine: Normal voiding, diapers (wet), ostomies, ileal conduits, or indwelling catheters

- Vomitus

- Wound drainage

- Gastric drainage: from a nasogastric tube

- Liquid stools: diarrhea

- Perspiration

The body depends on a balance between intake and output to maintain normal functions of body systems. When the total intake does not equal the total output, there is an imbalance. This imbalance can be fluid volume excess or fluid volume loss. It can be represented as a teeter-totter. Figure 8–8 is a diagrammatic explanation of fluid balance.

Fluid excess may be due to kidney disease, liver disease, medication (steroids), abnormal fluid accumulation in body cavities, overinfusion of intravenous fluids, and pregnancy. Fluid loss may result from hypovolemic shock, excess body drainage, diarrhea, medications (diuretics), difficulty in swallowing or in feeding oneself, impaired physical mobility, postoperative factors, and fever.

Signs and symptoms and causes of fluid loss:

1. Concentrated urine: The body is retaining and excreting more solutes, less water.

2. Rapid weight loss: A large percentage of body weight is fluid.

3. Increased pulse rate: A cardiovascular adaptive mechanism to increase circulation.

4. Decreased skin turgor: Loss of resiliency of skin caused by decreased pressure of fluid on cells and skin.

5. Dry skin: Reflects fluid loss in skin cells.

6. Sticky mucous membranes: Reflect fluid loss in normally moist tissues.

7. Weakness or confusion: Fluid changes interfere with normal nerve conduction and decreased circulation to the brain.

Signs and symptoms and causes of fluid excess:

1. Edema or ascites: Abnormal accumulation of fluid in the spaces between cells (interstitial).

2. Rapid weight gain: Body tissues do not increase in size, but fluid accumulation will increase overall body weight.

3. Increased blood pressure: May indicate larger blood volume.

4. Taut skin: Excess fluid in the cells.

5. Increased venous filling: Possible circulation overload.

6. Shortness of breath: Excess fluid pools in the lungs.

The PCT will play a key role in the maintenance of fluid balance. Since you, the PCT, are a primary caregiver, most activities will occur in your presence. Some key points to remember with the responsibility of measuring and monitoring intake and output are:

1. Collect and record all intake/ output as it occurs. Do not rely on memory for later documentation and recall.

2. Measure contents in the appropriate containers and read at eye level. Record amounts separately.

3. Inform patients to call you when they have taken anything in or voided.

4. Usually totals are obtained toward the end of the shift, but may be ordered more frequently, depending on the patient's condition. Use a Foley drainage bag with a special adaptor to more easily measure small amounts of hourly output.

5. Document on the appropriate I & O flow sheet for your institution. Label the columns appropriately. Calculate the shift totals.

Not only does each shift need to have totals of intake and totals of output, but there should also be a 24-hour grand total for intake and for output.

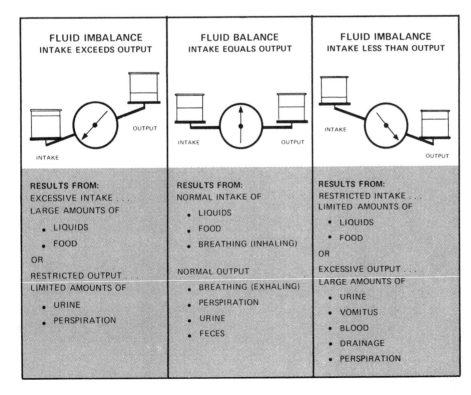

F I G U R E 8 – 8

Fluid volume balance. (From Schneidman, R. B., Lanbert, S. S., Wander, B. R.: Being a Nursing Assistant, 5/E. Chicago, The Hospital Research and Educational Trust, 1989, p 335. Reprinted with permission from the Hospital Research and Educational Trust.)

Rule of thumb for urine output is that a patient should have at least 30 cc of urine per hour or about 240 cc for an 8-hour shift. However, it depends on the patient's condition and total intake. If there is an unusually small amount, check the tubing for kinks or occlusions.

Check the urinary output at least halfway through the shift to see if it is at least 30 cc per hour. If not, inform the RN at this time.

URINE TESTING

As a PCT you will be relied upon to collect urine for specific tests. The most common will be for urinalysis, for culture and sensitivity (clean catch), for specific gravity, and for a 24-hour creatinine clearance.

Some general rules to be practiced when collecting urine specimens:

1. Wash your hands before and after collecting the sample.
2. Use universal precautions. Wear gloves.
3. Use a clean container for each specimen.
4. Use a container appropriate for the specimen. Make sure the lid is on firmly before labeling and transporting.
5. Label the container accurately with the requested information.

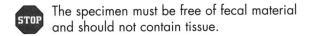 Complete label to include patient's full name, room and bed number, date and time the specimen was collected, and the name of the person who collected the specimen.

6. Do not touch the inside of the container or lid.
7. Collect the specimen at the time specified.
8. Instruct the patient to put toilet tissue in the toilet or wastebasket.

The specimen must be free of fecal material and should not contain tissue.

9. Place the specimen in a special biohazard materials transport bag. Take the specimen and the requisition to the designated storage place.

CLEAN-CATCH URINE SPECIMEN. The clean-catch urine specimen is also called a midstream specimen or clean-voided specimen. If possible, collect the first urine voided in the morning. The perineal area is cleaned before the specimen is collected. Perineal care reduces the number of microbes in the urethral area at the time the specimen is collected. The patient begins to void into the toilet, bedpan, urinal, or commode. Then the stream is stopped, and the specimen container is positioned. The

patient then voids into the container until the specimen is obtained.

Many people find it difficult to stop the stream of urine. The PCT may need to position and hold the specimen container in place after the patient has started to void. Be sure to wear gloves when collecting a clean-catch urine specimen. Clean-catch specimen kits are usually obtained from the materials handling departments or central supply area.

THE 24-HOUR URINE SPECIMEN. All urine voided during a 24-hour period is collected for a 24-hour urine specimen. Urine may be chilled on ice or refrigerated during the collection period to prevent the growth of microorganisms. (Check the institution's policy and procedure for specifications.) A preservative is added to the collection container for some tests. The patient voids to begin the test; this urine is discarded. All urine voided after that during the 24 hours is collected. The procedure and test period must be clearly understood by the patient and everyone involved in the patient's care.

URINE FOR DETERMINATION OF SPECIFIC GRAVITY. The measurement of urine specific gravity is important in determining the ability of the kidneys to concentrate or dilute the urine. Normal values for specific gravity of urine range from 1.003–1.030 for the adult. The procedure to determine specific gravity is as follows:

1. Make sure the hydrometer is thoroughly cleaned.
2. Fill the urinometer cylinder to about 1 inch from the top with the urine specimen. Remember to wear gloves when handling the specimen.
3. As the hydrometer is inserted into the specimen, a slight spin needs to be applied to the float as it is released.
4. Read the scale of the urinometer at the lowest portion.
5. Document the value and report to the RN.
6. Rinse out the cylinder with water and store in a clean, dry area.

URINE COLOR VARIATIONS

The color of urine is a very important characteristic. A change in color from the patient's normal color may indicate possible disease. The color variations and possible causes are shown in Table 8–1.

 Any change in urine color must be documented and reported to the RN.

RENAL FAILURE

Renal failure occurs when the normal demands of the body cannot be met by the kidneys. The kidney is very

T A B L E 8 – 1
Urine Color Variations and Possible Causes

COLOR	CAUSE
Pale yellow to dark amber	Normal
Straw color to colorless	Diabetes, overhydration
Cloudy to cloudy white (with or without sediment)	Infection
Red to red brown	Bleeding, drugs, dyes
Orange to orange red	Drugs, obstructive jaundice
Yellow brown to green brown	Presence of bilirubin, liver failure
Dark brown or black	Dehydration, melanoma, bleeding

resilient and can continue to function when there is damage to 75% of its tissue. There are two forms of renal failure: acute and chronic. Acute renal failure occurs when there is sudden damage to the kidneys. Acute renal failure can be defined as sudden, usually reversible, short-term loss of kidney function. Urine output less than 500 ml/day is called oliguria; less than 100 ml/day it is known as anuria. The causes for acute renal failure are numerous:

- Severe fluid loss without replacement (vomiting, diarrhea, burns, profuse sweating)
- Conditions that obstruct urine flow to the urethra or bladder
- Blood clots
- Trauma, hemorrhage
- Infection and acute inflammations
- Exposure to nephrotoxic agents
- Adverse effects from prescription and over-the-counter drugs
- Other medical conditions

The diagnosis is primarily made by means of urinalysis, blood studies, and radiology tests such as a KUB or CT. The treatment of the underlying cause consists of IV therapy or fluid replacement, possibly blood transfusions or dialysis, and nutritional support. The PCT's responsibilities are many and encompass the following:

1. Observe the following systems:

- Cardiac: any complaints of chest pain or irregular pulse

- Respiratory: rate and rhythm of breathing, changes in breath sounds, sputum, any odor to breath, especially a urine-like odor

- Gastrointestinal: nausea, vomiting, loss of appetite, mouth sores, metallic taste

- Skin: bruising, dry itching skin, pallor

- Neurological: change in behavior or level of consciousness

- Miscellaneous: weakness, fatigue, fever, any type of pain, i.e., headache, muscle cramps, or flank pain.

 Watch for these symptoms and report them to the RN.

2. Monitor and obtain:

- Urine output, possibly every hour or at least every 4 hours
- Specific gravity with each output
- Vital signs; include orthostatic blood pressure
- Daily weight
- Fluid intake and caloric count

RN may want to consult dietician for specific calorie requirements. Dietician can make recommendations and educate the patient or significant other regarding dietary restraints and substitutions.

3. Assist with activities of daily living, since patient will most likely be weak.

4. Encourage regular oral hygiene, handwashing, and adequate rest. This will help prevent infections.

5. If level of consciousness changes, provide a safe environment to prevent any injuries.

Chronic renal failure, also called end-stage renal disease (ESRD), occurs when the kidney function threatens the patient's life. It consists of permanent, slow, and irreversible damage to both kidneys. Damage may occur over a few months or several years. There are various causes for ESRD:

Congenital and hereditary: polycystic kidney disease
Connective tissue disorder
Hypertensive diseases
Infection: chronic pyelonephritis
Metabolic disorders: gout, diabetes
Obstructions

The diagnostic studies are the same as for acute renal failure. The role of the PCT with the patient who has ESRD is to:

1. Monitor and obtain vital signs every 4–8 hours, or more frequently if indicated. Take the blood pressure with the patient standing and sitting or lying. More than 80% of patients with ESRD have some form of hypertension.

2. Document vital signs.

3. Observe for changes in mental status.

4. Observe for any edema, especially in the neck and lower extremities.

5. Maintain fluid restrictions (possibly 1000 to 1500 ml/day).

6. Monitor intake and output every 8 hours and document.

7. Provide mouth care. Use standard mouthwash or half-strength peroxide.

8. Observe for nausea, vomiting, or anorexia.

9. Encourage food intake from types and amounts of dietary items permitted. Dietician will consult and explain choices and limitations.

10. Observe skin for dryness, itching, and color changes.

11. Observe for any blood in the urine and check mucous membranes.

12. Allow patient to talk about his or her illness.

13. Observe for signs and symptoms of infection and use good handwashing techniques.

14. Encourage and/or assist patient with activities of daily living.

The patient will most likely have some form of fluid restriction. The PCT can help the patient to deal with this restriction by allowing him or her to decide how the fluid intake should be divided up for the 24-hour period. Do not forget to leave some fluid allowance for taking any oral medication. Offer ice chips to help quench thirst. The ice chips must be included in the fluid restriction allotment and be documented. Remember that ice chips count as half the fluid volume of water or water and ice chips combined.

Dialysis

Dialysis is the treatment option used for patients with ESRD when medical treatment is no longer effective. It is a form of treatment to replace the work of failed kidneys. Long-term dialysis may be peritoneal dialysis or hemodialysis. Peritoneal dialysis is one type of dialysis used for patients with chronic renal failure. Peritoneal dialysis removes extra water, wastes, and chemicals from the body using the membrane lining of the abdomen, which is called the peritoneum.

There are three methods of performing peritoneal dialysis: intermittent peritoneal dialysis (IPD), continuous ambulatory peritoneal dialysis (CAPD), and continuous cyclic peritoneal dialysis (CCPD). The difference among the three types is how the treatment is done and the number of treatments (Fig. 8–9A).

Peritoneal dialysis works by instilling a cleansing solution, called dialysate, into the abdomen through a surgically placed tube. Waste products from the blood pass through the peritoneum and into the dialysate. After a specified time, the dialysate with the waste products is drained from the abdomen (Fig 8–9B). The advantage to peritoneal dialysis is that it is usually done at home and there are no needles to use. Depending on the type of peritoneal dialysis, the patient can fit it into his or her

own schedule and lifestyle. It is less costly than hemodialysis.

There are three important patient care issues with peritoneal dialysis: weight and fluid intake, prevention of infection, and daily activities of nutrition, elimination, and exercise. The PCT plays a crucial role in these patient care issues.

Weight and Fluid Intake. In renal failure, the ability to remove the excess fluid is lost. Dialysis provides this ability. All patients undergoing dialysis have an estimated dry weight (EDW) or target weight that is determined by the physician. This is the weight that the patient needs to attain. It is the patient's weight when free of any excess fluid. The following are crucial:

1. Weigh the patient every morning. (Patients undergoing CAPD should be weighed when the peritoneal fluid is drained.)

2. Monitor intake and output and record very accurately.

3. Monitor and document vital signs, especially blood pressure and temperature, every 8 hours.

4. May need to keep a calorie count diary.

5. Maintain fluid restriction.

6. Observe for chest pain and/or shortness of breath, which may indicate fluid overload.

PREVENTION OF INFECTION. The foremost complication, and the usual reason for admission to the hospital of patients receiving peritoneal dialysis, is peritonitis—infection of the peritoneum.

Peritonitis generally occurs when the catheter entering the abdomen becomes contaminated or disconnected. The catheter exit site could also become infected. The PCT needs to be familiar with signs and symptoms of peritonitis:

1. Redness or swelling around the catheter
2. Cloudy dialysate
3. Temperature greater than 99.5°F (37.5°C)
4. Abdominal pain
5. Nausea and/or vomiting
6. Diarrhea or constipation

 If any of these symptoms are observed, they must be reported to the RN immediately.

The care of the catheter site is usually done daily after a shower.

STOP The patient should never take a bath with a peritoneal dialysis catheter in place. Bath water is a combination of clean and dirty water. A shower provides continuous flow/flushing action of water.

No ointment, powder, or cream is to be used on the

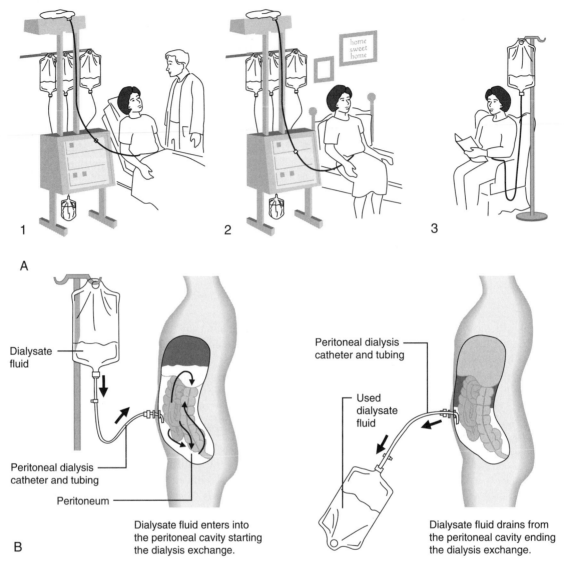

FIGURE 8 – 9

Types of peritoneal dialysis. *A*, Intermittent peritoneal dialysis (IPD); 2, continuous cyclic peritoneal dialysis (CCPD); 3, continuous ambulatory peritoneal dialysis (CAPD). *B*, Peritoneal dialysis.

exit site unless ordered by the physician. The responsibilities of the PCT with catheter care include:

1. Apply gloves. Remove old dressing and discard. Do not remove tape on peritoneal dialysis tubing.

2. Examine catheter site for possible signs and symptoms of infection (redness, swelling, tenderness, drainage).

3. Clean skin around catheter site with a 4 × 4 pad saturated with prescribed solution (i.e., Bactoshield). Clean in a circular motion from the catheter outward.

4. Assist patient with shower if applicable. Do not use a soiled washcloth around catheter site. Clean exit site first with clean washcloth and prescribed solution.

5. Rinse area with running water if patient is in shower, or with sterile water.

6. Wear gloves.

7. Dry skin with sterile 4 × 4 pad.

8. Place 4 × 4 over exit site and tape in a nonocclusive manner.

9. Remove old tape holding the peritoneal dialysis tubing to the abdomen and retape.

10. Document procedure and report findings to RN.

NUTRITION, ELIMINATION, AND EXERCISE.
Patients with chronic renal failure who undergo peritoneal dialysis may have difficulty with activities of daily living. The PCT's role with these activities includes:

1. Encourage ambulation or have patient up in chair 3 times a day, unless contraindicated. Make sure any activity occurs only for short periods. This will help prevent the patient from tiring.

2. Report complaints of constipation or diarrhea.

3. Promote independence. Encourage participation in care whenever possible.

4. Specifics regarding nutrition:

- Do not force the patient to eat; encourage slow eating.

- Provide 6 small meals a day. The patient may not feel like eating three full meals because there are about 2 liters of dialysate in the abdomen, creating a feeling of fullness.

- Encourage the patient to think of food as part of the medical care.

The RN may consult dietician for assistance in meal planning and physical therapist for activity and exercise regimen.

Hemodialysis

The second form of dialysis is hemodialysis. It is a procedure that filters the blood, controls blood pressure, and helps keep the proper balance of chemicals and fluid. The procedure uses a hemodialyzer, popularly known as an artificial kidney, to filter and clean the blood. It can be performed at a dialysis center or at home with special equipment and training and assistance of another person.

Access to the blood stream is necessary for this treatment. This is done by having a fistula or graft or an external catheter surgically placed. Hemodialysis treatments are performed 2–3 times a week, and require 3–5 hours per session. The blood travels through the artificial kidney machine and is filtered. Then the newly cleansed blood flows through another set of tubes back to the body (Fig. 8–10).

The PCT's responsibilities with hemodialysis occur at three separate times: if the patient needs to have a new graft/access, or revision of an old one, and preparation before and care after hemodialysis.

New Graft or Revision of Old

1. Prior to new graft, continue to monitor blood pressure and follow the responsibilities for the care of a preoperative patient.

2. Upon return, observe the dressing. Check for any bleeding or drainage.

3. Observe the capillary refill in the affected extremity.

4. Observe for any complications at site: warmth, redness, edema, pain, or numbness. If any of these are present, report immediately to the RN.

5. Keep affected extremity elevated and straight for the first 24 hours to help decrease the swelling. Check with the RN after the 24 hours to determine if the extremity still needs to be elevated.

6. Encourage the patient to use extremity during activities of daily living.

7. DO NOT take blood pressure in arm with the new fistula or graft.

STOP Some activities should be avoided: no blood draws, blood pressure determinations, or IV starts in the graft extremity. A sign may need to be posted above the patient's bed to alert other health care providers such as phlebotomists. The patient should not wear tight clothing or anything else that might constrict the arm.

8. Provide wound care as ordered.

9. Document all above findings each shift.

Preparation for Hemodialysis

The RN will have orders to follow on the day of scheduled hemodialysis. These particularly pertain to medications and laboratory tests. The PCT's role is also an integral part. The PCT needs to know and /or carry out the following:

1. Know the appointment time of dialysis. If for any reason it is delayed or postponed, the RN must be informed so that orders can be changed and the treatment is not delayed or altered.

2. Obtain patient's weight every morning at the same time in relation to meals.

3. Obtain vital signs, including orthostatic blood pressure.

4. Obtain a blood glucose level before meals, if ordered.

5. Order an early meal tray if needed for an early treatment appointment time.

6. Obtain and have available portable oxygen.

7. If time permits, the patient's bath should be completed.

8. Document all findings and events.

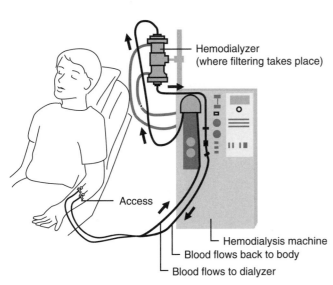

Hemodialyzer
(where filtering takes place)

Access

Hemodialysis machine
Blood flows back to body
Blood flows to dialyzer

FIGURE 8–10

Hemodialysis.

9. Complete the intake and output record thus far for the shift before the patient goes to therapy.

Care After Hemodialysis

Hemodialysis generally takes about 4 hours. Depending on how far the patient travels and if transportation is on time, the patient may be gone from the unit for a good portion of the shift. This is an excellent opportunity to make sure that all other duties and responsibilities are caught up. Prompt attention must be given when the patient arrives back to the unit. The responsibilities after hemodialysis include:

1. Obtain vital signs.

2. If the blood pressure drops more than 20 mm Hg from the supine to upright, the following interventions need to be implemented:

- Instruct patient to call for assistance when getting out of the bed or up from the chair because of the potential loss of balance or dizziness.
- The motion-related events or falls-prevention protocol needs to be followed.
- Check with the RN to see if the blood pressure needs to be taken more frequently.

Report to RN if systolic blood pressure is less than 100 mm Hg or much lower than the original baseline.

3. Observe sites for bleeding on shunt arm.

4. Check dialysis sheet for any pertinent information from the dialysis staff.

5. Observe for severe headache or sudden behavioral changes.

6. Order and set up meal tray if meals were missed.

SUMMARY

The urinary system has a very important twofold job: to keep the body clear of certain wastes and its fluid balanced. The various structures of the urinary system have specific functions to aid in this job. Many disorders can affect the structures, resulting in disruption of function. Treatment ranges from medical to surgical. The PCT plays an important role with each disorder and is an integral member of the health care team.

It is the RN's responsibility to assess and notify the physician of the patient's condition and/or changes. It is the PCT's responsibility to assist the RN with these assessments through observation and monitoring, gathering data, preparing the patient for tests or procedures, reinforcement of teaching, and documenting the findings. Having basic knowledge of the renal system enables the PCT to provide this type of quality of care.

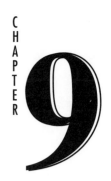

The Gastrointestinal System

CLAIRE R. ESSELMAN, EdD, RN,C

Upper Gastrointestinal Study
Small-Bowel Follow-Through
Barium Enema for Lower
 Gastrointestinal X-Ray
Computed Tomography

Magnetic Resonance Imaging
Liver Biopsy
**Your Role in Reinforcing
Education**

P R E R E Q U I S I T E
K N O W L E D G E A N D
S K I L L S

- Feeding of patients without swallowing difficulties
- CPR
- Personal hygiene for complete care patients
- Measuring accurate intake, output, and weight
- Giving enemas
- Universal precautions (Including blood and body fluids precaution)

O B J E C T I V E S

After you complete this chapter, you will be able to:

- List structures and functions of the gastrointestinal system.
- Describe normal observations associated with the gastrointestinal system.
- Discuss common disorders of the gastrointestinal system.
- Explain how to feed a patient with swallowing difficulties.

- Recognize signs and symptoms of gastrointestinal disorders that need to be reported to the RN.
- Select and implement treatment interventions with RN.
- Document observations and care given.
- Reinforce RN instructions in patient education.

K E Y T E R M S

Anorexia Lack of appetite; inability to eat

Aspiration Fluid escaping and becoming trapped in the lungs, causing choking and possible pneumonia

Bile A fluid produced in the liver, stored in the gallbladder, and secreted into the duodenum; essential to fat absorption

Colostomy An opening made surgically into the large intestine

Dehydration Loss of the normal fluid balance in the body, causing the patient to experience dry mouth, dry skin, low urine output, and possible constipation leading to fecal impaction

Duodenum First part of the small intestine, most important part in digestion; breaks down food into usable material

Dysphagia Difficulty in swallowing

Enzymes Complex proteins produced by living cells that induce specific biochemical changes without being changed themselves

Esophagus Collapsible, muscular tube 10 inches in length; conducts food from throat to stomach

Feces Waste products from the large intestine

Gallbladder Stores bile that is released into the small intestine to aid in the digestion of fats

Gavage Giving nutrients directly into the gastrointestinal tract

Ileum Third section of small intestine; also serves for absorption of food

Jaundice Yellow discoloration of the skin and white of the eyes

Jejunum Second section of small intestine; aids in absorption of food

Large intestine Five feet in length; made up of the cecum, colon, and rectum. The colon is divided into the ascending, transverse, and descending portions. The sigmoid or S-shaped part of the colon connects below to the rectum

Liver Largest organ in the body; produces bile, stores sugars, produces protein that aids in clotting of blood, stores vitamins, neutralizes toxins, and processes iron for the blood

Manifested Displayed

Ostomy Surgical formation of an artificial opening for bodily elimination

Pancreas Organ that secretes enzymes that aid in digestion

Peristalsis Involuntary contraction that propels contents of tubular organ, especially the digestive tract, forward

Pharynx Throat; provides a passageway for food, air, and swallowing

Rectum Pouchlike area, the terminal portion of the intestine. Waste products accumulate here until there is the urge to defecate

Resect To cut out a portion or all of a structure/organ

Resection Excision of part or all of a structure/organ

Salivary glands Located in the mouth; secrete saliva, which begins digestion

Small intestine Twenty feet in length; located in the abdominal cavity; connects stomach to large intestine divided into duodenum, jejunum, and ileum. Most digestion takes place here

Stoma The opening created in the abdominal wall by an ostomy

Stomach Muscular, pouchlike sac that prepares food for digestion

Strangulated Twisted, turned

Villi Tiny fingerlike projections found on membranous surfaces, specifically in the walls of the small intestine that absorb end products of digestion into the blood stream

The gastrointestinal (GI) tract or digestive tract is a hollow muscular tube that is lined with mucus and extends from the mouth to the anus (Fig. 9–1). It provides a means for food to be broken down mechanically and chemically into products that can enter the blood stream. The GI tract also disposes of the wastes from this digestive process.

A major activity of this system is to secrete substances that help break down the food we eat into proteins, carbohydrates, fats, vitamins, minerals, and water, which are then used by the cells in our body for energy, growth, maintenance, and healing. Other activities in this system move the food through the tract, digest it, and absorb the end products into the blood stream.

STRUCTURE/FUNCTION

The GI tract is about 30 feet long. The organs of this system are the mouth, pharynx, esophagus, stomach, small intestine, and large intestine. The accessory digestive organs are the teeth, tongue, salivary glands, liver, gallbladder, and pancreas.

Digestion begins in the mouth where food is chewed and mixed with saliva, which lubricates and softens the food mass and begins to break down carbohydrates. The teeth mechanically chop the food, and the tongue, which contains taste buds, aids in pushing the food back to the pharynx where it is swallowed. The food then enters the esophagus.

The esophagus serves as a passage for food from the mouth to the stomach. Its function is to move food from the pharynx to the stomach by muscular contractions called peristalsis. Peristalsis pushes a food mass ahead of a "wave" of muscular contractions. Peristalsis continues throughout the muscular GI tract.

The stomach, a muscular organ, is located just below and to the left of the diaphragm. It mechanically churns the food, mixing it with digestive enzymes that continue the digestion of carbohydrates. Here, only small quanti-

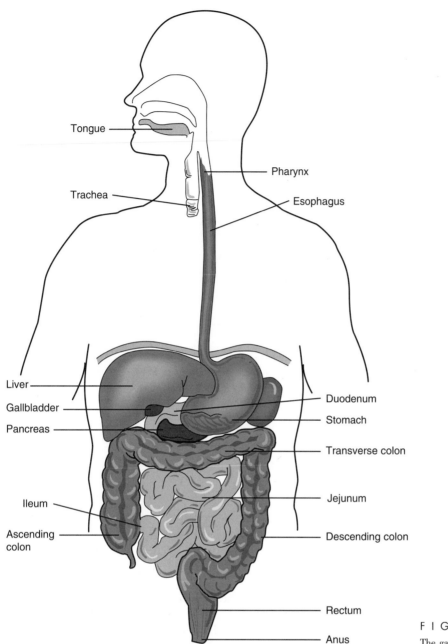

ties of water, alcohol, glucose, and drugs are absorbed into the blood stream, and most organisms are killed by the stomach's acid secretions. Food is changed to a semi-fluid material (chyme) and stored until it is sufficiently fluid to pass through a muscle at the end of the stomach called the pyloric sphincter. Chyme then enters the small intestine.

The small intestine is approximately 20 feet in length and coils within the abdominal cavity. It is divided into 3 main segments.

The *duodenum* is about 10 inches long and has two openings that receive additional digestive secretions. One opening, located under and to the right of the diaphragm, receives bile that is produced by the liver. Bile prepares

(emulsifies) fat for digestion. It is carried directly to the duodenum or stored in the gallbladder until it is needed to help digest a fatty meal. Bile also gives solid wastes the usual brown color. The second opening receives digestive juices from the pancreas to aid in digestion of protein and carbohydrates.

The *jejunum* is about 8 feet long and extends to the il-eum.

The *ileum*, about 12 feet long, is the end of the small intestine and joins the large intestine at a special valve (ileocecal valve). This valve controls the flow into the large intestine and prevents food from traveling backward into the small intestine.

Peristalic contractions move the semiliquid material

through the small intestine, and digestion is completed. The nutrients are absorbed into the blood stream by way of villi, which are fingerlike projections found in the walls of the small intestine (Fig. 9–2). Villi are in continuous motion stirring the intestinal contents and absorb end products of digestion into the blood stream. Most absorption of all nutrients takes place in the small intestine.

The large intestine extends from the ileocecal valve to the anus, is about 5 feet long and 2 inches in diameter. It is divided into 3 sections.

The *cecum* is the first 2 or 3 inches of the large intestine. Relaxation of this section allows contents from the small intestine to enter and continue through the GI tract. The appendix is attached here, but serves no useful purpose that we are aware of.

The *colon* is divided into 4 sections: ascending, transverse, descending, and sigmoid. No digestive enzymes are secreted in the colon. Mucus secreted in this section aids in the movement of wastes.

The *rectum* is the final section and extends from the sigmoid colon to the anal opening where sphincters control elimination of feces, or stool. This action is called *defecation.*

The major functions of the large intestines are to complete absorption of water and electrolytes, make and absorb vitamins including some vitamins B and K, form feces, and expel them from the body. In addition, organisms are present in the large intestine that break down remaining proteins and indigestible residue. This action causes the formation of gases, which provide bulk and help to propel the feces.

Disorders of the GI tract interfere with digestive activities, sometimes causing abdominal pain, nausea, vomiting, diarrhea, constipation, and weight loss, and interfere with other body systems. Disorders of this system cause more health problems than any other.

ORAL DISEASES

Thrush

Oral thrush is a fungal infection in the mouth, characterized by slightly raised, creamy, white, sore patches on the mucous membrane, the gums, and the tongue. It can be due to poor nutrition and hygiene. There may be decreased food intake because the lesions are painful. Patients who are NPO and taking antibiotics are prone to thrush, since antibiotics disrupt the balance of normal oral flora. Malnourished and diabetic patients are also prone to this condition.

Oral Maxillofacial Cancers

Cancer lesions can occur on the lips, the tongue, and the oral cavity. People who are heavy smokers and who consume high quantities of alcohol are more prone to develop this disease. White, patchy areas that are sore and fail to heal are signs of cancer.

Oral Surgery for Repair of Oral Diseases

Various types of surgical procedures may be performed that repair abnormalities, remove tumors, improve appearance, and repair lacerations and fractures. The discomfort and degree of care depend on the extent of the procedure, location of the incision, and whether the person can talk.

Maintaining the patient's airway is given first priority in the care of any oral disorder. In addition, giving gentle mouth care every 2 hours and offering bland foods and liquids as directed by the RN are helpful. Patients whose appearance is altered or who cannot talk need additional support to express their needs and feelings. Patient care technicians (PCTs) provide paper to write on, check on these patients frequently, and respond to the call light promptly. All caregivers must communicate acceptance, compassion, and caring through their manner.

SWALLOWING AND ESOPHAGEAL DISORDERS

Difficulty in swallowing is called dysphagia. It is caused by a disturbance in the normal transfer of food from the mouth, through the esophagus to the stomach. The most common cause of dysphagia is a cerebral vascular accident (CVA) or stroke. Other causes are obstructions and neurological disorders.

Hiatal Hernia

In this condition the upper part of the stomach and the esophagus "slide" into the chest cavity (Fig. 9–3). Heartburn is the major complaint. Sometimes patients bring up very sour-tasting gastric contents into their mouths. PCTs can encourage patients to remain in an elevated position with their head raised up at least 30 degrees, drink additional fluids with meals to assist food passage, and maintain regular bowel habits that avoid straining.

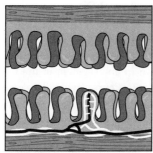

Villi

FIGURE 9 – 2
Villi.

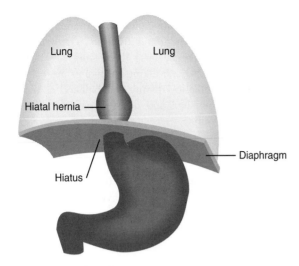

FIGURE 9 – 3
Hiatal hernia.

GASTRIC DISORDERS

Gastritis

Gastritis is inflammation of the lining of the stomach. It can be acute, which means severe or of short duration. It can be chronic, which means constant or occurring over a long period. Alcohol, drugs, or irritating foods can be causes of gastritis.

Ulcers

Peptic ulcers are caused by a break in the mucous lining of the GI tract. Recently recognized as a major cause of these ulcers is a bacterium, *Helicobacter pylori*. The breakdown may be in any part of the GI tract that comes in contact with gastric juices. A peptic ulcer may be found in the esophagus, stomach, or duodenum. *Gastric ulcers* generally occur at the base of the stomach and are also thought to be due to a break in the "mucosal barrier." Generally, patients who have ulcers should be encouraged to avoid alcohol, aspirin, and coffee, which tend to stimulate secretion of gastric acid.

Stress ulcers can occur after a medical crisis such as severe trauma or major illness, burns, head injury, drug ingestion (e.g., alcohol and aspirin), shock, or general body infections. These ulcers can occur within 72 hours. Unfortunately, few early symptoms accompany a stress ulcer.

✔ Patients who are seriously ill (especially with burns) are at risk for stress ulcers. Observe your patients closely for gastric pain, coffee-ground vomit (old blood), and vomiting of blood.

Bleeding

A major complication of gastric problems is hemorrhage. This is frequently due to perforation of a blood vessel. Older patients with gastric ulcers tend to have a high incidence of bleeding. Patients who are hemorrhaging vomit a large amount of blood and pass tarry (black) stools. They may experience dizziness, restlessness, and weakness.

Cancer

The signs and symptoms of stomach cancer are generally not present until the disease has spread to other organs of the body. The symptoms are usually vague. The patient may complain of gastric distress, loss of appetite, fatigue, and indigestion.

Patients should be encouraged to seek medical assistance when experiencing vague symptoms. Surgery is the treatment of choice if the cancer has not spread to other organs.

INTESTINAL DISORDERS

Inflammation

Inflammation occurs when there is some irritation, infection, or injury to a body part. The tissue response is usually demonstrated by pain, redness, heat, and swelling.

Appendicitis

The appendix is a small saclike attachment to the large intestine. It can become inflamed and cause severe pain. The main concern is that the appendix will rupture and cause serious infection. Surgery is the treatment of choice.

Diverticulitis

In the large bowel, diverticula, which are small outpouches of the bowel, may become inflamed. Elderly patients are more prone to develop this disease. Some causes are chronic constipation and lack of roughage and fiber in the diet. Patients complain of left lower quandrant pain, bloody stools, and flatulence (gas).

Inflammatory Bowel Disease
Crohn's Disease

Crohn's disease or regional enteritis is a chronic relapsing inflammation in any segment of the GI tract from the mouth to the anus. Sores typically develop in several separate segments of bowel. This causes edema and congestion, which bring about narrowing of the intestinal wall. The contents of the bowel cannot pass through the constricted area and therefore cause abdominal cramps, especially after meals. Other symptoms may be nausea, flatulence, weight loss, and chronic bloody diarrhea. Surgery of the diseased portion of the intestine is not curative, because there can be recurrence of the disease in other areas of the intestine.

Colitis

This disease is also referred to as ulcerative colitis. The mucous membrane of the left colon and rectum becomes inflamed, which can lead to ulcerations and bleeding. There is increased risk for developing cancer of the colon. Patients generally complain of rectal bleeding, weakness, anorexia, nausea and vomiting, and dehydration. Treatment is aimed at comfort measures and maintaining good nutrition. Possible surgical intervention would be removal of this section of the bowel.

Hernia

A hernia is a protrusion of the bowel through a weak area in the muscular wall of the abdomen. *Rupture* is another term to describe a hernia. The main concern with an abdominal hernia is the possibility of the hernia becoming strangulated or twisted so that circulation is disrupted. In addition to cell death, this strangulation could cause severe pain and intestinal obstruction. Emergency surgery would be required to resect or repair the bowel that was strangulated.

Intestinal Obstruction

Intestinal obstruction results when the contents of the intestines are blocked from going through the small or large intestines. Most obstructions occur in the small bowel. Obstruction can be caused by an adhesion (formed after surgery), twisting of the bowel, a hernia, tumor, fecal impaction, diverticulitis, or Crohn's disease. The obstruction can also be caused by lack of peristalsis due to surgery or certain narcotic drugs. Symptoms include cramping pain, nausea, elevated temperature, abdominal distention, and absence of or diminished bowel sounds.

A complete bowel obstruction is life threatening. The PCT observes for and reports signs of pain, vomiting, absence of bowel movements, and distention.

When there is a bowel obstruction, generally a gastric or intestinal tube is inserted to remove fluid and gas from the GI tract until bowel function returns. Because of the limited bowel function, oral intake is restricted. Mouth care should be given every 2 hours to prevent infection and provide comfort. Surgery is performed when there is a physical obstruction.

Tumors

A tumor is a new growth of tissue identified by uncontrolled growth of cells. The tumor can be benign or cancerous and occur in any portion of the bowel. How-

ever, malignant tumors are uncommon in the small bowel. Benign tumors of the large bowel are called polyps, which are small tissue masses. Malignant tumors generally occur in the last section of the large bowel (sigmoid to the anus). Patients may complain of abdominal pain, diarrhea or constipation, weakness, weight loss, rectal bleeding, and anorexia. The primary treatment is surgery.

Hemorrhoids

Hemorrhoids are veins in the rectum and anus that have become distended and congested. Development of hemorrhoids is due to chronic constipation, straining at stool, obesity, and pregnancy. Symptoms of hemorrhoids are pain upon defecation, itching, rectal bleeding, and protrusion of hemorrhoids. Treatment for hemorrhoids consists of high-fiber, low-roughage diet, analgesics, and stool softeners. Surgery is recommended in some cases.

DISORDERS OF THE LIVER, BILIARY TRACT, AND PANCREAS

Hepatitis

Hepatitis is inflammation of the liver. The major symptom is anorexia; liver tenderness and jaundice (a yellow color of the skin) usually develop. Patients complain of nausea and vomiting, fatigue, weight loss, and headache. Treatment includes rest periods, small, frequent meals, and general support to the patient.

Hepatitis Type A Virus

Type A virus is generally transmitted by the fecal-oral route, although transmission by other routes, such as urinary, and by other body fluids rarely do occur.

PROTECTION FROM TRANSMISSION. The PCT needs to know that type A virus can be transmitted by direct or indirect contact with feces. Gloves should be worn when touching any infective material.

Handwashing and universal precautions are the primary isolation measure.

Hepatitis Type B Virus

Type B virus is transmitted by blood and certain body fluids and by contaminated needles and other equipment that comes in contact with infected body fluids.

PROTECTION FROM TRANSMISSION. The PCT should wear gloves when touching blood and body fluids, mucous membranes, or nonintact skin of any patient. Masks, protective eyewear, and gowns should be worn by anyone coming in contact with any body fluids. Avoid needle stick injury. Needles should be disposed of immediately in a puncture-proof container and never recapped or used twice. Universal precautions and handwashing are to be consistently carried out.

Cirrhosis

Cirrhosis is a chronic disease of the liver. There is a breakdown of the liver that causes structural changes and vital loss of function. Symptoms may include nausea and vomiting, weakness, fatigue, anorexia, jaundice, weight loss, and pain in right upper quadrant. Treatment consists of diet management, bedrest, prevention of infections, and general support to the patient.

Gallstones

Gallstones are small, solid masses sometimes found in the gallbladder or in the bile duct. They are mostly composed of cholesterol and can block the flow of bile. When this occurs, patients generally complain of pain in the right upper abdomen, jaundice, and occasionally chills and fever.

Cholecystitis

Cholecystitis is inflammation of the gallbladder. It can be caused by gallstones blocking the exit of bile into the duodenum. Symptoms include indigestion after the eating of fried foods, nausea, vomiting, pain in the right upper abdomen that can radiate to the back and shoulder blades. Cholecystitis is treated by low-fat diet, bedrest, and analgesics. Often the gallbladder is removed—a procedure known as cholecystectomy.

Pancreatitis

Pancreatitis is inflammation of the pancreas. It can be acute or chronic. A particular enzyme, trypsinogen, which breaks down protein, becomes activated in the pancreas instead of the duodenum, therefore causing tissue damage. Causes of pancreatitis include alcoholism, bacterial or viral infection, and duodenal ulcer. Symptoms include nausea and vomiting, jaundice, pain upon eating, epigastric burning, severe pain, and weight loss. Treatment for pancreatitis is generally bedrest, low-fat diet, no caffeine or alcohol, and general support of the patient.

When caring for a patient with a GI disorder, the PCT observes for abnormal signs and symptoms, gathers accurate measurements and data from the patient, reports and documents carefully, and carries out interventions as directed by the RN.

SPECIAL OBSERVATIONS AND CARE OF GASTROINTESTINAL DISTURBANCES

Anorexia

A patient who has a GI disorder usually develops anorexia, which is loss of appetite for food. This can result from lack of gastric secretions or could be caused

by anxiety, unpleasant experiences, and the disease process.

The PCT should observe eating patterns of the patient who is experiencing anorexia. Keep the environment free from foul odors, confusion, and noise.

Nausea

Nausea is another symptom that occurs frequently with disorders of the GI tract. It is an irritating sensation that can cause the patient to experience tachycardia and profuse perspiration and the feeling that he or she may vomit. It is generally accompanied by weakness, low blood pressure, and paleness.

Vomiting

Because normal digestion is not occurring, the patient has sudden ejection of stomach contents through the mouth.

It is important that the PCT report nausea. If the patient vomits (has emesis), be sure to position for airway clearance. Turn the patient's head to one side. Stay with the patient and call for the RN.

It is important to record what you observed in relation to the emesis. The amount and color of the emesis are important data. Emesis may include fecal material, bright red blood, coffee-grounds material, or undigested food.

Save the emesis to show the RN what the patient vomited and perhaps to test for occult blood.

Difficulty in Chewing and Swallowing

The person with difficulty in chewing and swallowing may have problems when beginning to swallow, pain while swallowing, or a feeling that the food is meeting resistance.

Feeding a patient with swallowing difficulty should follow formal assessment and instruction by the designated professional.

The PCT should:

1. Check recommended positioning of patient.
2. Explain to patient what you are going to do.
3. Check the amount of food you are going to give the patient.
4. Check recommendations for proper food placement.

5. Check the temperature of the food.

✔ Foods that are too hot may burn the patient's mouth. Foods that are too cold may chill the patient.

6. The patient should not feel rushed. Allow sufficient time for the patient to chew and swallow the food.

7. Check to be sure the patient is allowed liquids.

8. Consider patient preferences in food choice when possible.

📢 Be alert for the following signs of choking: Partial obstruction: Wheezing or gurgling in airway, difficulty in breathing. *What to do.* Try to get patient to breathe through nose and cough out with mouth open.
Complete obstruction: Clutching the throat, unable to breathe or cough. *What to do.* American Heart Association recommends calling for help *first* then doing the Heimlich maneuver (abdominal thrusts) until the airway is open.

📓 The PCT needs to report and record any difficulty the patient has with eating or drinking.

Patterns in Diet Intake

A patient who has a GI disorder needs to be aware of the food and fluids that can be tolerated. The PCT should become aware of a patient's eating habits and cultural preferences. Attempt to talk to family members about the patient's diet intake. Prepare the patient and the environment for mealtime. Food is more palatable if the environment is free from foul odors and the patient is comfortable. Present the food in an attractive manner: warm foods served warm, cold foods served cold, and food served in small portions. Communicate with the patient during the meal and allow the patient time to talk if the person wishes to do so..

✔ The PCT needs to check that the meal that is served is the one that is ordered.

📓 The PCT needs to accurately measure and record the amount of food and fluids the patient consumes. If the amount of food consumed and fluid intake are poor (less than 50%), the RN should be notified.

Changes in Weight

A change in the patient's weight is important for the health team members to know since treatments are based on these data. For example, some patients are prescribed medications that cause them to lose water. A low-sodium diet could cause a loss of water from the patient's body. This fluid loss is reflected in the patient's weight loss, just as fluid retention may be identified by a weight gain. Medications are adjusted based on these data. When patients who are not eating well lose weight, additional nutritional supplements may be ordered.

📢 Report variations (increase or decrease) of more than 3 pounds in patient's weight to the RN.

OTHER COMMON MANIFESTATIONS OF GASTROINTESTINAL DISTURBANCES

Abdominal Pain

Pain is a very subjective feeling and a common symptom of GI disease. Abdominal pain generally alerts the patient to seek medical advice. The PCT can encourage the patient to describe specific information about the discomfort experienced, such as character (sharp, burning, dull, cramping, fullness), when discomfort began, whether it is constant or occurs at different times of the day, its location, severity, how long it lasts, what activities increase it, and what activities provide relief.

📢 If a patient who has a GI disease complains of severe abdominal pain, the PCT must immediately contact the RN. This could indicate an emergency. Avoid moving the patient until the RN assesses the situation.

📓 The PCT needs to report and record any type of pain that the patient experiences at any time of the day. Be very clear in stating what the patient describes to you concerning the pain.

Diarrhea

Diarrhea is the passage of liquid stool at frequent intervals. There are many causes of diarrhea. Generally the patients need treatments aimed at replacing fluid and nutrients and reducing the number, size, and frequency of stools. Besides giving care as directed by the RN, the PCT is helpful by:

• Immediately washing the anal area thoroughly to prevent any breakdown in the skin

• Protecting skin with moisture barrier cream or ointment

• Being aware of any reddened area around the rectum, because it could be a site for skin breakdown

• Reporting and recording the number of times the patient has expelled liquid stools.

Constipation

Constipation occurs when the stool stays in the GI tract as water is absorbed. Stool becomes very hard and difficult to expel from the rectum. Treatment is aimed at maintaining normal elimination habits by way of adequate fluids and diet, activity, and decreased use of laxatives. The PCT is helpful by:

- Encouraging liquids that are permitted
- Maintaining an elimination time, for example, after meals and at bedtime offering the patient a bedpan or use of a commode to encourage having a bowel movement
- Having patient sit in a natural position
- Providing privacy
- Not rushing the patient
- Using good communication skills, both verbal and nonverbal

Be aware of facial expression so that you do not display disgust or displeasure while assisting.

Report and record color, amount, consistency, and any abnormality of the stool. These data assist the medical team in making a diagnosis of the patient's condition.

Fecal Impaction

Fecal impaction occurs when the stool has become so hard that it has become lodged in the lower passage of the rectum. The patient may still expel a small amount of liquid from the rectum, since liquid can "leak" around the stool. Sometimes this leakage of liquid stool appears as diarrhea. If permitted, encourage patients to drink fluids and eat foods rich in fiber.

Be aware of any discomfort the patient has in the rectal area. If the patient has not had a bowel movement within 48 hours, it is important that you report this to the RN.

 You should record any time your patient has difficulty in passing stool from the rectum.

Change in Bowel Habits

A patient can experience a change in bowel habits from different types of food or medications that are consumed. Some foods, such as certain vegetables, cause a patient to have diarrhea. An example of this might be corn. Other foods can be very constipating for the patient. Some antibiotics can cause the patient to have diarrhea. Disorders of the GI tract, such as colitis, can cause

diarrhea. Regardless of the diagnosis, a PCT is aware of any change in the patient's bowel habits.

Change in Color or Consistency of Stool

Changes in color and consistency of stool could indicate a medical problem in the GI tract. Stool is usually medium brown and of a soft formed consistency.

Any change in color of stool or change in the consistency in the form of the stool needs to be reported and recorded as soon as possible.

Any stool specimen containing blood or that is black or tarry in appearance needs to be saved by the PCT to show the RN.

Bleeding

For a variety of reasons that are generally related to trauma, rectal bleeding may occur when the patient has a bowel movement. For example, when a patient has hemorrhoids, it is possible for bleeding to occur with a bowel movement.

As a PCT, you should remain calm when you observe any type of rectal bleeding. If you become upset, this may cause the patient additional anxiety.

Jaundice

Jaundice is a yellow discoloration of the skin and white part of the eyes (sclera). It usually occurs because of some blockage of the bile draining from the liver or the gallbladder.

In addition to the yellow of the skin and sclera, the PCT should observe and report a dark brown color of the urine, clay color of the stool, nausea, vomiting, and abdominal pain.

Check with the RN if you are unsure about questionable symptoms you observe in patients with jaundice.

COMMON ISSUES AND CARE NEEDS

Nothing by Mouth

Many patients who experience GI disorders are generally ordered nothing by mouth (NPO), that is, they are not permitted to take anything by mouth to "rest" the GI tract and decrease painful symptoms.

Mouth Care

Any patient who is NPO will experience a dry mouth because of mouth breathing and lack of oral fluids. The PCT should carry out oral hygiene measures every 2 hours.

Check with the RN about using mouth care products. Ask the RN if the patient may have ice chips or lozenges or chew sugarless gum.

Dehydration

Because of loss of fluid intake in instances of NPO and diarrhea, the patient with a GI tract disorder may develop dehydration. Signs to watch for are extreme thirst, drowsiness, dry tongue, poor skin turgor, and abdominal distention. The PCT needs to accurately measure the patient's intake and output. These data are as important as accurate weights for monitoring progress.

Obtain accurate weight of patient when ordered by using the same scale on the same patient with minimal clothing. Balance the scale to zero, and use a barrier to prevent patient contamination.

Monitoring Diets

It is important that the PCT monitor the diets of patients who have digestive disorders. Patients commonly in need of extra nutrition are those who are NPO and those who have cancer, Crohn's disease, or ulcers. Weight loss and poor healing will result from inadequate intake of calories.

The PCT must measure fluids and calculate the percentage of each meal that is eaten. Perform a calorie count when ordered.

Enteral Feeding

Enteral feeding is giving nutrients directly into the GI tract (Fig. 9–4). If the patient is unable to swallow or is unconscious, it may be necessary to administer an enteral feeding to provide nutrients. *Gavage* is another term for tube feeding. There should be normal functioning of the small bowel so that the nutrients can be absorbed. There are many different types of formulas for enteral tube feedings. A standard formula usually contains proteins, carbohydrates, and fat.

Nasogastric Tube

A nasogastric (NG) tube is a small tube that is passed through one nasal passage, through the esophagus, and down into the stomach (Fig. 9–4).

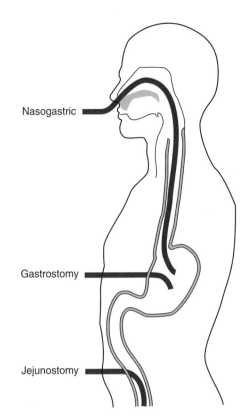

FIGURE 9–4
Insertion sites for nasogastric, gastrostomy, and jejunostomy tubes.

Observe the patient for any signs of distress such as continuous coughing, sneezing, nausea, emesis, or gagging. Contact the patient's RN at once. This could indicate that the tube is not in the proper position.

Gastrostomy

A gastrostomy tube or G tube is a tube surgically placed into the stomach (Fig. 9–4) that bypasses the pharynx and esophagus. Nutrients can be infused directly through a gastrostomy tube into the stomach.

Observe the skin around the gastrostomy tube. The gastric drainage around the stoma may contain enzymes that can be irritating to the skin. Report and record any drainage, skin breakdown, or redness around the site.

Jejunostomy Tube

A jejunostomy tube or J tube is a tube that is sutured into place in the jejunum. Patients whose swallowing reflexes are not present or who are unconscious are candidates for feedings through the small intestine. Jejunostomy tube feedings reduce the risk of aspiration (Fig. 9–4).

CONCERNS WITH TUBE FEEDINGS

Aspiration

The patient should always have the head of the bed elevated at least 30 degrees while receiving a tube feeding. This reduces the risk of aspiration of the fluid into the lungs. If a bolus type of feeding (about 200 cc at one time) is given, the patient should remain in an upright position for at least 20 minutes. The patient should be observed for any signs of gagging. The PCT should also notice if feeding tubes are stabilized and not in a different position (farther in or out of the original insertion site).

The RN routinely checks for proper tube placement. However, if you notice a change in tube length, notify the RN immediately.

Contamination

Tube feedings are usually given at room temperature. After a bottle or can of formula is opened, it should be used up within 8 hours or discarded. Any solution that has passed the expiration date should be discarded. Tube feedings may be given by gravity drip or a controller pump.

Clogging

 It is important that the tube be flushed with clear water after each feeding because the formula may tend to clog the tube. If a patient leaves the unit for a test and the feeding must be interrupted, notify the RN so that existing formula can be flushed through the tube with water before the patient leaves.

Diarrhea

Patients sometimes experience diarrhea because of the high concentration of formula being used. It is important to report how many times the patient experiences diarrhea, the color, the amount, and any other abnormalities.

Nasogastric Tubes to Low Wall Suction

To remove fluid and gas from the stomach, the RN will insert a nasogastric (NG) tube or Levin tube. A term for this is *decompression*. After the RN inserts the nasogastric tube for decompression, it is connected to low wall suction. This allows for the stomach contents to be removed rather than build up and cause distention. The contents are considered patient "output" and must be measured.

CONCERNS WITH ANY TUBE

Stability and Security

While caring for a patient with a tube in place, try to provide comfort and safety by stabilizing the tube. In some cases, you can pin the tube to the patient's gown to prevent pulling or dislodgment. Observe for redness and irritation of patient's nose when the tube is taped to the patient's nostril.

Drainage

A tube will not drain sufficiently if it is kinked in any way, so when moving the patient it is important that the PCT check that the tube is positioned correctly. The PCT needs to check if the tube is draining and if there is any abnormal color to the drainage.

Notify the RN if blood is coming from any drainage tube.

Labeling

A tube should be marked with the initials of the licensed person who inserted it. The label should also include the date and time the tube was inserted.

MAINTAINING ACCURATE INTAKE AND OUTPUT

It is important to maintain accurate intake and output (I & O) of your patients, since this helps determine the patient's fluid status. Intake includes fluids by oral, intravenous, or central lines and tube feeding routes. Output is measured from urine, stool, GI suction, wound drainage, vomiting, and sweating. I & O is a way to identify whether the patient is voiding sufficiently. Studies suggest that water intake actually exceeds the documented amount by as much as 30%. Failure to measure and record fluids accurately can result in a serious fluid overload. The PCT needs to be very accurate in measuring I & O by:

Communicating clearly the expectations of measuring I & O
Measuring fluids rather than guessing
Estimating and recording fluid loss from incontinence
Recording intensity of diaphoresis
Recording intake of ice chips. Water volume is about half the amount of the ice chips.

In addition, the PCT notices if a patient:

Drinks at least 1500 cc per day
Urinates at least once in an 8-hour shift
Has concentrated, foul-smelling urine
Has dry skin
Has a temperature above 99°F
Is perspiring excessively
Has excessive drainage from wounds

These observations produce valuable information about a patient's hydration status.

ACCURATE WEIGHING OF PATIENTS

Weighing the patient with a GI disorder is very important since it reflects nutritional and hydration status. It should be done accurately each day at the same time and with the same scale. The RN and physician need to have this information to follow the patient's progress.

SURGICAL INTERVENTION

Ostomies (Fig. 9–5)

An ostomy is the surgical formation of an artificial opening (stoma). This surgery is performed when there is some type of obstruction blocking the passage of stool. There are many types of ostomies (Fig. 9–5). Bowel ostomies are created to allow fecal passage. They can be classified as permanent or temporary and by their anatomical location. A colostomy is an opening into the large bowel. The location of the colostomy depends on the part of the bowel that is obstructed. If the opening is made at the beginning of the large bowel, the stool will be liquid.

If the colostomy is made at the end of the large intestine, the stool will be formed. An ileostomy is an opening into the small bowel. There is constant fecal drainage from the stoma.

POSTOPERATIVE CARE OF AN OSTOMY. In addition to the usual observations of any patient undergoing abdominal surgery (passage of gas, nasogastric suction, distention, drains) PCTs should also keep fecal contents away from the incision, provide emotional support while the patient adjusts to the body's change in elimination, and help reinforce the RN's instruction about caring for the ostomy.

In general, an appliance that is used to collect stool from an ostomy has three features: a pouch to collect the drainage, an outlet at the end, and a faceplate (Fig. 9–6) (See Chapter 12). The PCT ensures patient privacy and instruction prior to any procedure.

Record the amount of drainage that the patient expels. Note the color of the stool, the appearance of the stoma, and any abnormalities that you have observed such as dark coloring of the

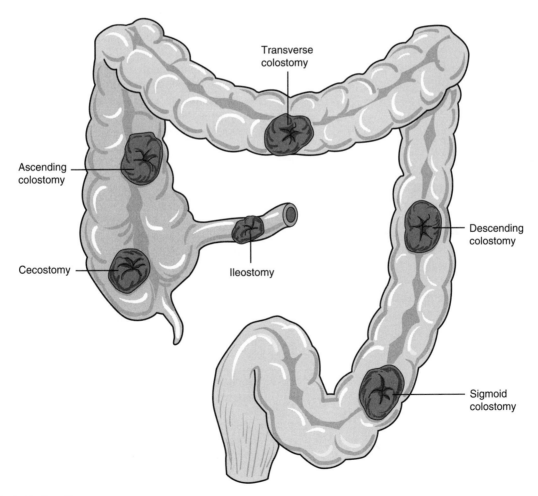

FIGURE 9–5
Stomas for ascending colostomy, transverse colostomy, descending colostomy, and ileostomy.

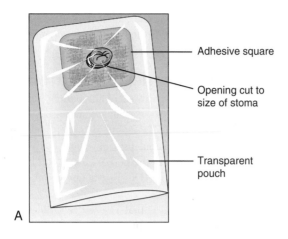

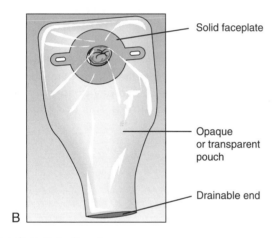

FIGURE 9 – 6
Ostomy appliance.

stoma, discoloration of the surrounding skin, or bleeding.

EMOTIONAL SUPPORT. A patient who is experiencing this type of surgery needs to have the opportunity to express his or her feelings. Patients experience a change in lifestyle. In addition to pain, postoperative patients typically feel that they have no control over body functions, which can be very embarrassing. It is important that the PCT be aware of nonverbal gestures when changing an appliance and attempt to offer as much emotional support as possible.

DIAGNOSTIC EVALUATIONS AND ROLE OF CAREGIVER

Since disorders can occur anywhere in the GI tract, many diagnostic tests are ordered to identify the exact location. Education and precautions are necessary to keep patients safe and informed.

Endoscopy

Esophagogastroduodenoscopy (EGD) allows the physician to visualize a patient's esophagus, stomach, and duodenum. A narrow, flexible tube called an endoscope is passed through the mouth into the patient's esophagus and stomach so that these areas can be visualized through a magnifying scope. Since the stomach must be completely empty for the best examination the patient is NPO before the test. Food or fluid should not be given for about 2 hours after the test since the patient will be drowsy and the gag reflex numbed for the procedure.

Colonoscopy

Colonoscopy is examination of the large intestine with the colonoscope. The patient will receive enemas and laxatives before the procedure so that the colon will be clear for inspection. A scope is passed via the rectum into the large intestine to observe for any abnormalities. After the procedure, the PCT should check for any bleeding from the rectum or abdominal discomfort.

Upper Gastrointestinal Study

An upper gastrointestinal (UGI) study is an X-ray study of the stomach, esophagus, and duodenum. The patient is given barium to swallow so that the esophagus, stomach, and duodenum can be examined via X-ray. The PCT gives special attention to eliminating the barium from the intestine, since it can become a hard mass that causes constipation. Stools will be white to light colored for 2 or 3 days, then return to normal. Encourage the patient to drink extra fluids and ambulate as soon as permitted after the X-ray.

Small-Bowel Follow-Through

A small bowel follow-through (SBFT) is an X-ray study of the small intestine. This test shows the lining of the small intestine and may identify problems such as ulcers, blockage, and general functioning of the small intestine. The patient is asked to drink several cups of a barium mixture that allows the small bowel to show up on an X-ray. The patient is encouraged to report any abdominal discomfort and to drink extra fluids to eliminate the barium.

Barium Enema for Lower Gastrointestinal X-ray

Barium is administered into the large intestine for its examination. Enemas and laxatives are given to the patient before the X-ray so that the bowel is clear. After the X-ray, encourage the patient to drink extra fluids if permitted. Monitor bowel movements for 2 to 3 days for signs of constipation. If the patient is unable to have a bowel movement, report this to the RN.

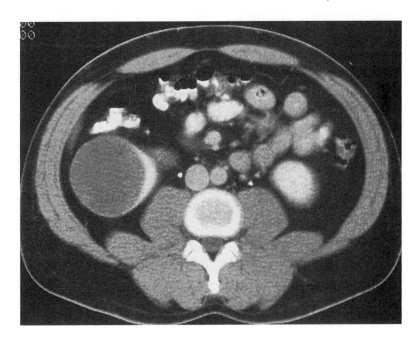

FIGURE 9-7

An example of a CT scan. (From Moss, A. A., Gamsu, G., and Genant, H.: Computed Tomography of the Body. 2nd ed. Philadelphia, W.B. Saunders Co., 1992, p. 964.)

Computed Tomography

Computed tomography (CT) or CAT scan is an X-ray procedure that uses a special scanner and computer to show cross-sectional pictures of parts of the body. The scan shows minor differences in the soft tissues (Fig. 9–7). Thick substances appear white, and soft substances appear dark. It gives a three-dimensional view of the organ that is viewed. Patients need to know that they must hold still during the procedure. Patients receiving abdominal scans are asked to drink a barium solution four times during the scan.

Magnetic Resonance Imaging

Magnetic resonance imaging (MRI) is one of the newest methods of diagnostic imaging. It provides clear detailed images of the internal organs and structures by using powerful magnetic fields and radio frequency waves rather than X-rays. The membranous organs plus the nerves and blood vessels can be viewed (Fig. 9–8). Prior to the procedure, remove any metal from the patient because of the strong magnetic field that develops in the machine. Examples are hairpins, jewelry, a watch, credit cards, electrode patches, and gowns that have metal snaps. Patients need to be reminded that they will be asked to hold still during the procedure, and they will hear noises similar to drumbeats or a jackhammer as the images are acquired.

Liver Biopsy

A liver biopsy is performed to identify the type of liver disease the patient has. A physician removes a small piece of liver tissue with a needle that is inserted through the skin. The patient should void just before the procedure, and baseline vital signs should be obtained. In caring for this patient after the procedure, you should position the patient on his right side. This provides pressure to the puncture site and guards against loss of blood from the liver. Vital signs are obtained frequently as directed.

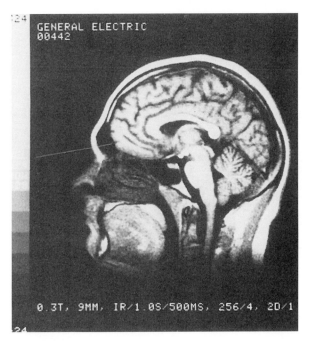

FIGURE 9-8

An example of magnetic resonance imaging. (From Putman, C. E., and Ravin, C. E.: Textbook of Diagnostic Imaging. 2nd ed. Philadelphia, W. B. Saunders Co., 1992, p. 5.)

Report any complaints of tenderness at the biopsy site, changes in vital signs, and evidence of bleeding to the RN immediately.

YOUR ROLE IN REINFORCING EDUCATION

While the RN assumes the responsibility for teaching the patient, the PCT plays an important role in education. Patients frequently tell the PCT rather than the RN when they are confused about instruction. As a PCT, it is important that you are able to reinforce what the RN has taught the patient and his or her family. For example, to encourage and assist the patient and the family to follow the correct diet or drink specific fluids, you must know exactly what the RN wants you to reinforce. While caring for any patient, you must report to the RN any time you believe that a patient needs to have additional teaching about the illness, treatment, and care.

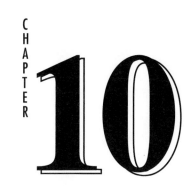

The Endocrine System

SUSAN M. BEJCIY-SPRING, MS, RN,C

P R E R E Q U I S I T E
K N O W L E D G E A N D
S K I L L S

- Blood glucose monitoring
- Urine collection and bedside testing for sugar, acetone, protein, blood, specific gravity, and urine stones (See Chapter 21)
- Vital signs
- Intake and output measurements
- Weights
- General skin and mouth care
- Therapeutic communication
- Venipuncture and blood specimen collection (See Chapter 21)
- Safe environment precautions
- Patient positioning
- Seizure precautions

O B J E C T I V E S

After you complete this chapter, you will be able to:

- List structures and functions of the endocrine system.
- Discuss common disorders of the endocrine system.
- Recognize signs and symptoms of endocrine disorders that need to be reported to the RN.

- Select and implement treatment interventions with the RN.
- Document observations and care given.
- Reinforce RN's instructions in patient education regarding management of endocrine disorders.

K E Y T E R M S

Bradycardia Slow heart rate

DKA Diabetic ketoacidosis; an emergency condition of high blood glucose levels and ketone production; typically seen in persons with IDDM

Exophthalmos Protrusion of the eyes, typically seen in persons with hyperthyroidism

GDM Gestational diabetes mellitus; diabetes that occurs during pregnancy

Hormones Substances produced by the endocrine glands that put into motion various processes in the body

Hyperfunction Increased function of an organ

Hyperglycemia High blood sugar level

Hypofunction Decreased function of an organ

Hypoglycemia Low blood sugar level

Hypotension Low blood pressure

IDDM Insulin-dependent diabetes mellitus or type 1 diabetes

Ketones The product of fat breakdown; also called acetone

Level of Consciousness The state of one's alertness or awareness

Metabolism The process by which the body converts substances into energy

NIDDM Non–insulin-dependent diabetes mellitus or type 2 diabetes

Tachycardia Fast heart rate

Tetany A state of severe tonic contractions of muscle groups

The endocrine system is a diverse system of glands and hormones that are responsible for regulating many of the body's functions. The important functions of these glands include physical and mental growth and development, production of energy, control of fluid and electrolyte balance, response to stress, and reproduction. The glands perform these various functions by secreting hormones. Hormones are chemical substances that are released into the blood stream and travel to specific organs where they put into motion those vital functions.

The endocrine glands work separately and together to regulate body functions. Collectively the glands of the endocrine system affect and are affected by all of the other body systems.

When there is an increase or decrease in the production of any hormone, special care needs to be given to the individual to prevent complications, promote rest and comfort, and provide emotional support. The disorders that occur when this system is not functioning appropriately affect growth and development, reproduction, the body's internal environment, and the body's response to stress.

STRUCTURES AND FUNCTIONS OF THE ENDOCRINE SYSTEM

The endocrine system consists of the pituitary gland, thyroid gland, parathyroid glands, adrenal glands, pancreas, gonads (ovaries in females and testes in males), and the hormones each gland produces. Figure 10–1 shows the locations of the glands within the body. Table 10–1 provides a summary of the functions of the endocrine glands.

Pituitary Gland

The pituitary gland is a small organ at the base of the brain consisting of two parts: the anterior lobe (the front part) and the posterior lobe (the back part) (Fig. 10–1). The anterior lobe produces hormones that affect growth of bones and muscles, promote milk production of the breasts, promote development of eggs and sperm, and stimulate production of hormones produced by other glands. The posterior lobe of the pituitary gland produces hormones that cause uterine contractions and control the fluid balance of the body.

Thyroid Gland

The thyroid gland is a butterfly-shaped organ in the neck (Fig. 10–1). This gland produces hormones that regulate metabolic activity, allow for growth and development during childhood, control calcium levels in the body, and assist with resistance to infection.

Parathyroid Glands

There are usually two pairs of parathyroid glands that are located on or near the back portion of the thyroid gland (Fig. 10–1). These glands produce a hormone that controls the levels of calcium and phosphate in the body.

Adrenal Glands

The adrenal glands are found on top of both kidneys (Fig. 10–1). These glands produce several hormones that

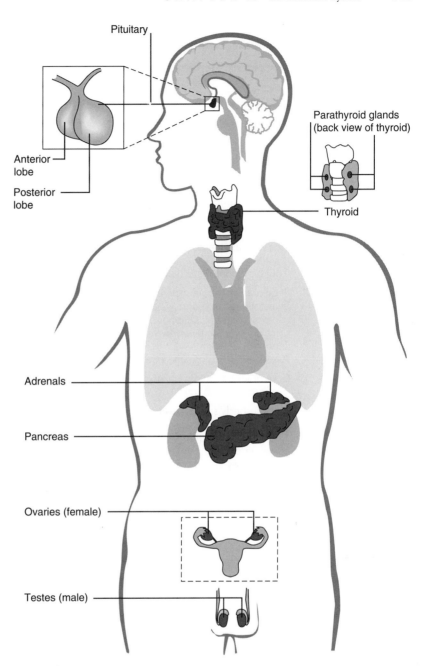

FIGURE 10–1
The endocrine system.

allow the body to adapt to stress and threatening or dangerous situations. The hormones they produce also assist with control of fluid and electrolyte balance. The adrenals also produce hormones that cause development of certain sex characteristics.

Pancreas

The pancreas is a fish-shaped organ located behind the stomach (Fig. 10–1). This gland produces enzymes to digest foods. Its endocrine functions include production and secretion of hormones that allow for metabolism of sugars, proteins, and fats and control of blood sugar (glucose) levels.

Gonads

The gonads consist of the ovaries in the female and testes in the male (Fig. 10–1). Their main function is in reproduction. Disorders of these glands will not be considered in this chapter.

DISORDERS OF THE ENDOCRINE SYSTEM

To be able to recognize the abnormal and intervene properly, the PCT needs to have an understanding of the endocrine system, the normal functions of the glands and

T A B L E 1 0 – 1
Structures and Functions of the Endocrine Glands

Structure	Function
Pituitary gland	
Anterior lobe	Affects growth of bones and muscles
	Promotes milk production of the breasts
	Promotes development of ova and sperm
	Stimulates production of hormones from endocrine glands
Posterior lobe	Produces uterine contractions at birth
	Controls body's fluid balance
Thyroid gland	Regulates metabolic activity
	Stimulates growth and development in childhood
	Controls calcium levels in the body
	Assists with resistance to infection
Parathyroid glands	Control levels of calcium and phosphate in body
Adrenal glands	Produce body's response to stress
	Control body's fluid and electrolyte balance
	Stimulate development of secondary sex characteristics
Pancreas	Produces enzymes that digest food
	Regulates metabolism of sugars, fats, and proteins
	Regulates body's blood sugar levels
Gonads	Reproduction. Responsible for secondary sex characteristics, e.g., facial hair, deep voice

hormones, and common disorders. The RN has ultimate accountability for the care of patients; however, the PCT is a valuable member of the team providing quality care to patients with disorders of the endocrine system. The PCT needs to monitor patients as well as promptly report important findings to the RN. Careful observations and complete documentation of patients' symptoms and interventions carried out are very important responsibilities of the PCT. Addressing patient safety and comfort needs are particular areas of concern and emphasis when working with patients who have disorders of the endocrine system.

Disturbances in the function of the endocrine system can usually be divided into two categories: hypofunction (not enough hormone produced) and hyperfunction (too much hormone produced). These problems can occur in any of the glands of the endocrine system. It is important to remember that hypofunction or hyperfunction of one

endocrine gland influences the other glands; therefore, multiple endocrine problems may occur in one patient.

Pituitary Gland

Diabetes Insipidus

Diabetes insipidus is a condition caused by decreased production or release of the hormone that controls water balance of the body. The causes of this pituitary disorder include damage to the pituitary and certain side effects of medication. Sometimes the cause is unknown.

Patients with diabetes insipidus complain of severe thirst. They also have large urine outputs (may be greater than 4 liters per day). The patient usually loses weight and has dry skin. The patient may also report constipation.

ROLE OF THE PCT. Because diabetes insipidus involves an imbalance of water in the body, accurate data collection and measurements by the PCT are important aspects in caring for these patients.

- Obtain and record vital signs, especially pulse and blood pressure.

Any increase in pulse rate or decrease in blood pressure needs to be reported immediately to the RN.

- Accurately measure and record urine output and fluid intake. Provide plenty of fluids and encourage patient to drink fluids frequently.
- Report to the nurse any difficulties the patient has in taking fluids orally.
- Measure and record urine specific gravity when ordered.
- Obtain and record accurate daily weights.

Weigh patient on same scale at same time of day with patient wearing the same clothing. Be sure to balance scale before each use.

- Moisturize dry skin as needed.
- Reinforce teaching to patient on how to measure and record intake and output and how to weigh self.

Syndrome of Inappropriate Antidiuretic Hormone

Syndrome of inappropriate antidiuretic hormone (SIADH) is a pituitary disorder in which the amounts of the hormone that controls water balance are increased. This disorder may be caused by an injury to the head, brain tumors, and infections and side effects of certain drugs. Early signs of this condition are confusion, disorientation, and uncooperativeness. The patient will have decreased urine output and weight gain. Specific gravity of urine will be increased. The patient may experience nausea and vomiting. There is also a risk for convulsions (seizures).

ROLE OF THE PCT

- Careful observations of the patient's level of consciousness by the PCT are extremely helpful in managing patients with SIADH. Patients may have very strict fluid restriction—possibly intake of only 500–600 cc/day. Maintaining this fluid restriction is an important part of the treatment for these patients.

- Observe any changes in patient's level of consciousness such as not knowing where he or she is or inappropriate or confusing conversation.

Since a change in the patient's mental status is an early sign of this condition, any change no matter how slight needs to be reported to the RN promptly.

- Maintain strict fluid intake limits.

- Obtain accurate intake and output measurements.

- Obtain accurate weight.

- Reinforce the RN's explanations for restricting fluid intake.

- Monitor patient's environment to control access to fluids.

Because of their severe thirst, patients with SIADH may drink water from bath basins, showers, and toilets. The PCT plays an important role in keeping the environment restricted to access to fluids. Since the fluid restriction can be very difficult for patients, providing emotional support is an important role of the PCT.

- Notify the RN immediately if the patient has any seizure activity (convulsions, uncontrolled twitching, unresponsiveness). Assist the RN in protecting the patient from injury during seizure activity; pad the siderails; remove dangerous objects from the area.

- Reinforce teaching to patient on how to measure and record intake and output and how to weigh self.

Thyroid Gland

Hypothyroidism

Hypothyroidism occurs when there is a decrease in production of the thyroid hormones. This is a common disorder that can occur when there is loss of thyroid tissue, injury to thyroid tissue, or dietary influences.

Patients with hypothyroidism are usually hypothermic, that is, they have a low body temperature. They may complain of feeling cold even when the environmental temperature of the room is warm. They have cool, dry, scaly skin. They also have a slow heart rate (bradycardia) and low blood pressure (hypotension). They may have an irregular pulse. These patients gain weight easily and are tired and sleepy. They may also become weak and forgetful. Patients with hypothyroidism tend to develop constipation and have low or decreased urine outputs.

ROLE OF THE PCT. The PCT has an important role in caring for patients with hypothyroidism. Patient care activities will include observations and interventions to maintain patient safety and promote recovery.

- Obtain accurate vital signs, weights, and intake and output measurements. Report any changes from the patient's baseline measurements to the RN.

- Observe for changes in the patient's level of consciousness—disorientation to person, place, or time; inappropriate conversation; or other signs of confusion. Report any changes promptly to the RN.

- Provide scheduled rest periods for the patient. Do not interrupt patient during rest/sleep times. These patients are very weak and tired and need plenty of rest.

- Provide care to decrease the work that the patient must do.

Because patients with hypothyroidism become tired easily and are weak, procedures should be spaced apart to allow for rest between activities. These patients need to save their energy.

- Explain procedures slowly and repeat explanations often, since these patients tend to forget easily.

- Observe for any swollen, bruised, or broken areas on the skin and report to the RN.

- Use warm blankets, robes, and socks to prevent further decreases in the patient's body temperature and to increase comfort level.

- Use lotions or moisturizers on dry skin to prevent skin breakdown. Turn bedridden patients frequently (every 1–2 hours). See Chapter 12 for other skin care interventions.

- Provide for safety in the patient's environment; remove clutter and provide assistance with patient's transfers and walking.

- Observe and document color, consistency, amount, and frequency of stool.

(Put time and date). Patient had small amount of hard black stool. Last BM was 2 days ago (7/26). Patient states she feels constipated and needs a laxative. Reinforced importance of drinking plenty of fluids. RN informed. *(Then sign your name.)*—B. Williams, PCT

- Encourage increased intake of fluids: 6–8 glasses of water per day.
- Use good handwashing techniques. Observe for and report any signs of infection.

✔ Patients with hypothyroidism are at increased risk for infection. Attention to universal precautions is essential.

- Provide reassurance and support to patients and family members.
- Notify the RN immediately if the patient has an increased heart rate, diarrhea, sweating, agitation, or shortness of breath.

📢 These symptoms may indicate a toxic condition if the patient is receiving thyroid medication. Prompt reporting of these signs and symptoms is an important role of the PCT.

Hyperthyroidism

Hyperthyroidism occurs when too much thyroid hormone is produced. It may be due to a tumor or to overfunctioning of the thyroid gland. Patients will usually have an enlarged neck and protruding eyes (exophthalmos) (Fig. 10–2). It may even be difficult for some patients to completely close their eyes. Patients with hyperthyroidism tend to be hyperactive, have mood swings, and have decreased attention spans. They also have loose bowel movements, increased sweating, intolerance to heat, and a fast heart rate (tachycardia).

ROLE OF THE PCT. The care of patients with hyperthyroidism requires careful observation, appropriate reporting of findings, and attention to their comfort, safety, and emotional needs. The PCT plays a major role in providing quality care.

- Obtain accurate vital signs; obtain sleeping pulse rate to obtain an accurate baseline.

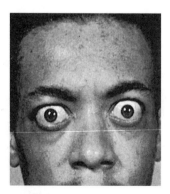

FIGURE 10-2

Exophthalmos. (From Delp, M. H., and Manning, R. T.: Major's Physical Diagnosis: An Introduction to the Clinical Process, 9th ed. Philadelphia, W.B. Saunders, 1981.)

📢 Promptly report any increase in temperature, pulse rate, irritability. These signs and symptoms may indicate increasing thyroid hyperactivity, called thyroid storm or thyrotoxicosis.

- Monitor and record color, character, consistency, frequency, and amount of stool.
- Obtain accurate daily weights; report loss of 2 kg or 4 pounds to the RN.

✔ Patients with hyperthyroidism have an increased metabolism rate and tend to lose weight. Major decreases in weight need to be reported so that necessary modifications can be made in the patient's diet.

- Monitor and record food intake; provide between-meal snacks.

🎓 Collaborate with the dietician and the RN to provide the patient with high calorie, high protein foods to meet increased metabolic needs.

- Provide a quiet environment—close the door, dim the lights—to promote rest.
- Keep room temperature cool; use light sheet for top cover; provide the patient with light, loose pajamas; assist the patient with clothing changes twice a day or more frequently to promote comfort.

✔ Because of the increased sweating, patients with hyperthyroidism may need frequent changes of bedsheets and clothes. Have linen and clothing/pajamas supplies ready for use.

- Be calm and supportive; be understanding of the agitation and hyperactivity, as this is a result of their condition.
- Have patient do as little work as possible and provide uninterrupted sleep to prevent fatigue.
- Observe patient's level of consciousness; report any changes to the RN.
- Avoid differences in the timing and method of doing procedures.

✔ Collaborate with other staff caring for the patient to set up plan of care and avoid differences and changes that may increase patient's irritability and agitation.

- Keep linens wrinkle free.
- Help patient to elevate legs to decrease or prevent swelling.

- Report any difficulties the patient has in closing their eyes.
- Reinforce the importance of scheduled rest periods and avoiding stress.
- Reinforce the importance of avoiding caffeine-containing foods and beverages (coffee, tea, colas, chocolate) to minimize irritability.

Patients with hyperthyroidism may need to have surgical removal of the thyroid gland (thyroidectomy). The responsibilities of the PCT who is caring for a thyroidectomy patient are many. The primary concerns are difficulties in breathing and bleeding.

- Obtain accurate vital signs and record.

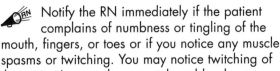 A decrease in blood pressure and increase in pulse rate may indicate bleeding and must be reported to the RN immediately.

- Observe respirations.

If the patient complains of difficulty breathing or you observe increased effort by the patient to breathe, immediately notify the RN. The patient may have an obstruction causing difficulty in breathing.

- Maintain Fowler's or semi-Fowler's position (Fig. 10–3) and keep the patient's neck and head supported with pillows, neck rolls, and sandbags. *Do not* flex or extend the patient's neck, as this puts stress on the suture line. Always support the patient's neck when repositioning.
- Assist the patient with oral intake as needed. Report any nausea, vomiting, or difficulty in swallowing to the RN.
- Observe the patient's neck dressing.

Any blood on the dressing or dressing tightness should be reported to RN promptly.

- Reinforce the importance of cough and deep breathing and incentive spirometry to prevent lung problems.

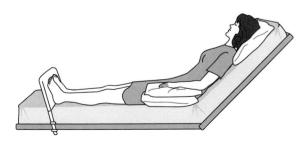

FIGURE 10–3
Fowler's positioning.

Notify the RN immediately if the patient complains of numbness or tingling of the mouth, fingers, or toes or if you notice any muscle spasms or twitching. You may notice twitching of the patient's arm when you take a blood pressure reading. This must be reported promptly to the RN. These can be signs of a serious complication of thyroid gland removal.

Parathyroid Glands

Hypoparathyroidism

Hypoparathyroidism is a condition that occurs when the parathyroid glands secrete too little of the hormone that controls the calcium level of the body. Usually this condition is caused by damage to the parathyroid glands during thyroid surgery. The patient who has hypoparathyroidism can experience muscle spasms, numbness of the fingers and mouth, tetany, and at times, seizures due to low calcium levels. The patient may be irritable and have headaches. The patient may also have nausea, vomiting, diarrhea, and abdominal pain. In addition, the patient may experience difficulties with swallowing and/or breathing.

ROLE OF THE PCT. The symptoms of hypoparathyroidism can range from numbness and twitching to seizures and obstruction of breathing. Careful observations and reporting, patient assistance and support, and patience are important responsibilities of the PCT.

- Obtain accurate vital signs and intake and output measurements and record.
- Provide assistance with ambulation and activities. Patients are at risk for falls.
- Maintain a safe and clutter-free environment.
- Provide high calcium foods to the patient and assist with intake. Observe as the patient eats to check for any difficulty in swallowing, which should be reported to the RN promptly.

Collaborate with the dietician regarding the best foods to offer the patient. Work closely with RN and dietary staff to consistently maintain a supply of calcium-rich foods at the patient's bedside.
Collaborate with the speech therapist and follow any guidelines made regarding how to feed or assist with feeding when the patient has difficulty swallowing.

- Be calm and reassuring to the patient—he or she is prone to agitation.
- Report any nausea, vomiting, or diarrhea to the RN.

Report changes in mood or level of orientation to the RN immediately.
Notify the RN immediately if the patient has difficulty breathing or has any seizure activity.

- Assist the RN in protecting the patient from injury during seizure activity (refer to Chapter 5 for further information about the PCT's role with patients who have seizures).

Hyperparathyroidism

Hyperparathyroidism is a disorder that results from oversecretion of the hormones from the parathyroid glands. Tumors are the primary cause of hyperparathyroidism. Symptoms of the disorder are caused by the increased calcium levels that occur. These symptoms include slow and irregular pulse rate, bone pain, increased urine output, formation of stones in the urine, nausea, vomiting, constipation, and weight loss. The patient may be drowsy and disoriented. This condition weakens the bones and places the patient at high risk for bone fractures.

ROLE OF THE PCT. The PCT plays an important role in keeping patients with hyperparathyroidism free from physical injury. Careful observations and patient support are necessary.

- Obtain accurate vital signs and record; report slow pulse rate to the nurse.
- Obtain accurate daily weights, intake and output measurements and record.
- Dipstick urine for blood and strain urine for stones—record and report findings.
- Provide the patient with plenty of fluids and encourage the patient to drink frequently.
- Assist the patient with ambulation and activities. Be sure patient wears nonskid footwear when out of bed.
- Keep the room free from clutter.
- Assist the patient in maintaining good body alignment.

Collaborate with the physical therapist on appropriate activities and assistive methods and devices to protect the patient from injury.

- Apply warm compresses to painful areas according to direction of the nurse.
- Assist the patient with splinting of ribs when turning and coughing to decrease stress on the ribs.
- Be calm and reassuring when working with the patient.
- Reinforce the importance of having the home environment free from hazards.
- Reinforce teaching on checking urine for stones and blood (Fig. 10–4).

- Reinforce teaching on maintaining proper body alignment.

Adrenal Glands

Adrenal Insufficiency

Adrenal insufficiency, or Addison's disease, is a disorder of decreased function of the adrenal glands. This disorder may be caused by adrenal tumors, fungal infections, and complications of tuberculosis. The onset of the disease is usually gradual with the patient feeling mildly weak and irritable. The patient may have nausea, vomiting, weight loss, and decreases in blood pressure. As the disorder progresses, the symptoms worsen. The patient may become confused and experience pain in the back, legs, and abdomen.

ROLE OF THE PCT. The treatment for patients with Addison's disease is life long. The PCT plays an important role in the treatment of these patients when hospitalization is necessary.

- Obtain accurate vital signs, usually every 4 hours, and record. Immediately notify the RN of any decrease in the blood pressure below the patient's baseline.

 Immediately report any irregularity in the patient's pulse to the RN.

- Measure intake and output accurately and record.
- Provide a calm, restful environment; patients need to avoid all stressors.
- Promptly report any complaint by the patient that might indicate an infection, for example, sore throat, burning with urination.
- Assist patient with slow changes in position (rising from lying to sitting to standing) to avoid drops in blood pressure.
- Take pulse and blood pressure with the patient in a lying, then sitting, then standing position and inform the RN of the measurements.
- Reinforce to patient the importance of reporting any lightheadedness or dizziness. If a patient reports these symptoms, have the patient lie down and rest and take the patient's pulse and blood pressure; then inform the RN.
- Provide for patient relaxation (darken the room, decrease noise level, give back rub) to help avoid stress.

Cushing's Disease

Cushing's disease or syndrome is a disorder of the adrenal gland in which there is increased production of the hormones that regulate blood glucose levels and the body's response to injury and stress. This condition may be caused by adrenal tumors, alcoholism, and therapeutic

TEACHING - LEARNING FLOW SHEET

Teaching method code*
A = audiovisual
R = role play
E = explanation
D = demonstration
H = handout
G = group class

No.	Date and Time	Intervention: Include content taught and identity of learner (if other than the patient)	Teaching method*	Response/Evaluation: States/ Identifies	Applies knowledge	Can return demonstrate	Routinely performs	No evidence of learning	Other	Revision: Reinforce content	Re-Teach	Needs practice	Other	Comments	Initials
	6/27	Instructed patient												Needs to practice	
	10^{A}	on urine dipstick for												with timing and	
		blood and straining												reading the	
		urine for stones. ——	E/D	✓						✓		✓		test strip.	K.L.-RN
	6/28	Patient demonstrated												Patient able to	
	9^{15} A	urine testing for blood;												read test strip	
		reinforced proper												result accurately.	
		timing of test. ——	E/D												P.R.-PCT

Initials	Signature and title	Initials	Signature and title	Initials	Signature and title
K.L.	K. Lipton RN				
P.R.	P. Reynolds PCT				

TEACHING - LEARNING FLOW SHEET

FIGURE 10–4
Documentation on reinforcement of teaching.

use of steroids. Patients with this condition experience increases in their blood pressure and blood glucose levels. They have weight gain, muscle weakness and wasting, and fatigue. These patients may have difficulty concentrating and remembering. They also have fragile skin that bruises easily and heals slowly. This disease may cause physical changes in patients that may alter body image. Figure 10–5 shows the typical body changes that occur in Cushing's disease.

ROLE OF THE PCT. The PCT will contribute to the care of patients with Cushing's disease in many ways. Special attention to the physical care of the patient's skin and emotional status will need to be given by the PCT.

- Accurately test urine for glucose, ketones, and protein as ordered and record the findings.
- Plan for rest periods to reduce fatigue.
- Observe skin for areas of thinning, bruising, and breakdown. Report any of these findings to the RN.
- Reinforce teaching of proper skin hygiene: washing skin gently, drying skin thoroughly, using lotion to moisturize dry areas.
- If drawing blood for testing, be sure to apply sufficient pressure to the venipuncture site to prevent formation of a hematoma (bruise).
- Keep the room free from clutter and sharp objects that could injure the patient.
- Provide socks, shoes, and slippers and encourage/assist the patient in wearing them when out of bed to prevent foot injuries.
- Provide emotional support to the patient and family.

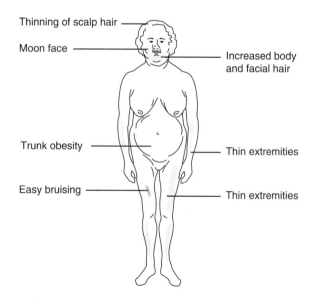

F I G U R E 1 0 – 5

Characteristics of Cushing's disease.

Patients with Cushing's disease are often irritable and depressed because of altered hormone levels and the physical changes that occur.

- Be sensitive and supportive in working with these patients.

Work closely with the mental health specialist. Follow recommendations on how to best work with the patient.

Pancreas

Diabetes Mellitus

Diabetes mellitus (sugar diabetes) is the most common disorder of the pancreas and the most common endocrine disorder. Diabetes is a disease in which the body cannot appropriately use food for energy because of a problem with insulin production or usage. Insulin is the hormone produced by the pancreas that helps move glucose (sugar) from the blood stream into the cells so that it can be used for energy and the work of the body. In diabetes, the insulin is either not present or not working, which results in large amounts of glucose in the blood stream (hyperglycemia).

Diabetes affects approximately 12–15 million Americans. One third of this number do not know they have diabetes. Together diabetes and its complications are the third leading cause of death by disease in the United States. No cause of diabetes is known at this time. However, research has found several factors that increase a person's risk of developing diabetes: a family history of diabetes, race (diabetes is more common in minorities—blacks, Hispanics, and Native Americans), overweight, stress, viruses, medications, and having diabetes during pregnancy.

There is more than one type of diabetes. The three most common types of diabetes are type I diabetes mellitus (insulin-dependent diabetes—IDDM); type II diabetes mellitus (non–insulin-dependent diabetes—NIDDM); and gestational diabetes mellitus (GDM) which is diabetes during pregnancy. Type I diabetes is usually diagnosed in patients below the age of 30. The pancreas of patients with type I diabetes produces no insulin, leading to high blood glucose levels; therefore, these patients must have insulin injections. These patients are usually underweight. Five to ten per cent of the total diabetes population has type I diabetes.

Type II diabetes usually develops in patients who are past the age of 40. In these patients insulin continues to be produced by the pancreas; however, the amount of insulin may be low, normal, or high. The problem is that the insulin is not used by the body as it should be, and this leads to high blood glucose levels. Type II diabetes is the most common type of diabetes; 80–90% of patients with diabetes have type II diabetes. Obesity is a major problem in type II diabetes with 80–90% of patients overweight at the time of diagnosis.

Gestational diabetes occurs during pregnancy. Women with gestational diabetes are typically overweight. The high glucose levels that occur during pregnancy usually go back to the normal range after the baby is born. Having gestational diabetes places the person at risk for developing type II diabetes later in life.

Symptoms of diabetes occur as a result of the increase in blood sugar levels (normal blood sugar level ranges from 60–120 mg/dl). Some of the common signs and symptoms of diabetes are delayed healing of wounds, blurred vision, excessive thirst and urination, fatigue, and skin infections.

There is no cure for diabetes. Diabetes can be controlled by diet, medications, and exercise. The three are held in a very careful balance and monitored by regular blood sugar testing as well as subjective feelings of the patient. The patient's diet order usually will be identified as a 1200 to 1800 calorie ADA (American Diabetes Association) diet, with the calories based on the individual's body size, regular activity level, and age. The meal plan is based on adequate servings from all food groups but does not contain any foods with refined sugar. A food exchange plan allows people to choose foods that they like from different exchange lists and sets the quantity of the food that will keep them within their calorie limit. The hospital dietitian works with patients to plan their diet in the hospital. The diet plan includes three regular meals plus an evening snack (possibly ½ sandwich and ½ cup milk). An afternoon snack may also be planned. For the patient who is diabetic, food is like medicine, and the quantity, content, and timing of meals and snacks are very important. They are all planned to keep an even, steady blood sugar level over 24 hours.

All activity of the body requires glucose (blood sugar), and situations such as increased activity, stress, increased body temperature, and infection increase the demand. Patients in the hospital may have less physical activity than they had at home, but glucose demands may increase because of other factors.

The insulin that is given to patients to allow their bodies to use glucose comes in different types. Some types of insulin are long acting and some are short acting; they are timed to be given so that peak insulin activity occurs during and after meal times. Frequently patients will receive several types of insulin. Often patients will receive Regular Insulin (short acting) on a "sling scale" before meals, based on blood sugar levels: The higher the blood sugar, the larger the dose of Regular Insulin that the nurse would give. This is usually given about 30 minutes before the meal.

Patients may be NPO for surgery or in preparation for a diagnostic examination. Others may be nauseated and have emesis, or just do not feel like eating. Physicians and nurses plan for patients being NPO; however, they rely on PCTs for accurate reporting of dietary intake, patient symptoms, and timely blood fingersticks.

The goals of treatment are to keep blood sugar levels within the desired range of 80–150 mg and to prevent or delay complications. Patients with diabetes can have large increases in their blood glucose levels leading to a condition known as diabetic ketoacidosis (DKA). In DKA, the body has too much glucose in the blood and not enough in the cells to use for energy. For energy, the body breaks down fats. Besides energy, fat breakdown produces ketones, which in large amounts can be toxic to the body. Dehydration and electrolyte imbalances are significant findings. DKA occurs in persons with IDDM. These are dangerous conditions requiring prompt treatment.

Diabetes causes an increased build-up of fatty deposits in the blood vessels, which can also lead to very serious long-term complications such as kidney damage, blindness, and foot ulcers (which can lead to amputations).

Patients with diabetes can have lower than normal blood sugar levels as a result of missing meals, taking too much of their medications, or exercising too much. This low blood sugar concentration is called hypoglycemia, and it can be a dangerous situation. Blood sugar levels below 55–60 mg/dl may produce symptoms of shakiness and lightheadedness and feelings of weakness and hunger. The patient may report a headache, blurred vision, or not being able to think clearly. When a patient has low blood sugar, he or she should eat something to raise the glucose level. When the patient is unconscious, no food or liquids should be given. Balance can be regained by the RN with IV glucose and IV insulin. Recommended snacks to correct hypoglycemia include 120–240 cc. of milk and 2 graham crackers, or 4 saltine crackers and cheese slices, or half a meat sandwich. These will raise the glucose level gradually. The patient's blood sugar level should be checked every 15–30 minutes after the snack to be sure that the glucose level is rising to about 100 mg/dl.

STOP Use caution when giving fruit juices, candies, or sugar for hypoglycemia. These foods can raise the glucose to a level too high too fast, which can later be a problem for the patient.

Tables 10–2 and 10–3 summarize the causes and symptoms of hyperglycemia and hypoglycemia.

ROLE OF THE PCT. The PCT is most likely to encounter patients with diabetes when it is first diagnosed, when they experience very high blood sugar levels (often referred to as diabetes out of control), or when serious complications arise. Care of patients with diabetes requires careful observations and accurate bedside testing of blood and urine.

• Obtain accurate vital signs and record.

✔️ In patients with very high glucose levels, vital signs may need to be obtained every 30–60 minutes.

- Observe respirations and level of consciousness of patients with very high blood sugar levels as in DKA.

📢RN Changes in the way the patient is breathing—slow, deep breathing—or disorientation need to be reported immediately to the RN. These symptoms may indicate worsening of the patient's condition.

- Obtain blood glucose levels by fingerstick and document results (Fig. 10–6).

✔️ Blood glucose levels may need to be obtained as frequently as every hour in cases in which patients have very high glucose levels.

- Blood glucose monitors allow for quick results at the bedside. Figure 10–7 shows a blood glucose meter that may be used for bedside testing. Proper technique is vital in obtaining accurate results. Table 10–4 gives tips on avoiding problems in blood glucose monitoring. Also, be prepared to take frequent blood samples by

T A B L E 1 0 – 2
High Blood Sugar (Hyperglycemia)

Common causes of high blood sugar in persons with diabetes:
  Not taking enough medication (insulin or oral medicines)
  Missing or delaying taking of medications
  Being under physical or mental stress
  Acute illness
  Eating more food than the meal plan allows
  Not exercising enough
  Having an infection or being ill
  Being pregnant
  Taking certain medications
  Sometimes no explanation

Common symptoms associated with high blood sugar levels in persons with diabetes:
  Being very thirsty
  Having to urinate frequently
  Having an increased appetite
  Experiencing weight changes (gain or loss)
  Having blurred vision
  Having numbness or tingling in the hands and/or feet
  Feeling tired, sleepy, fatigued
  Feeling moody
  Experiencing itchy skin
  Having delayed healing of any wounds
  Infections (skin, vaginal)
  Sometimes there are no symptoms

T A B L E 1 0 – 3
Low Blood Sugar (Hypoglycemia)

Common causes of low blood sugar in persons with diabetes
  Taking too much medication (insulin or oral medicine)
  Missing or delaying meals
  Doing too much exercise or increased activity
  Sometimes no explanation

Common symptoms associated with low blood sugar levels in persons with diabetes
  Feeling shaky
  Feeling dizzy or lightheaded
  Feeling like heart is racing
  Experiencing numbness or tingling around mouth
  Feeling nervous, irritable
  Having blurred vision
  Sweating
  Having a headache
  Not thinking clearly
  Feeling tired, weak, hungry
  Sometimes no symptoms (hypoglycemia unawareness; more common in persons with IDDM of more than 10–15 years)

venipuncture for additional laboratory tests or to verify low or high critical glucose levels.

- Fingerstick blood glucose testing should be performed 30–60 minutes before planned meal times to allow the RN time to prepare insulin if ordered and to approve the patient's getting a meal tray.

RN Report any blood glucose value out of the normal range to the RN immediately. For patients on a sliding scale insulin, report all values to the RN.

- Serve all diabetic patient their trays on time. Check with the nurse to see if any ordered insulin has been given.

- Check all meal trays and snacks against diet order. Monitor any extra food brought in for the patient by family or friends. Check with the RN if you are unsure about any food items. Encourage patients to eat all of their ordered food. Assist weak or confused patients to eat.

📢RN Inform the RN when a diabetic patient does not eat.

- Communicate clearly with the RN when a diabetic patient is NPO for surgery or tests. Hold the diet tray. Plan when food should be available after tests.

- Obtain accurate intakes and outputs and record.

- Check urine for glucose, ketones, and specific gravity as ordered. Document your results (Fig. 10–8). Table

Text continued on page 188

DIABETIC NOTES

Fingerstick method used   Accuchek III

Urine testing products used   Ketostix
                                    (glucose / ketones)

Date	Time	BLOOD GLUCOSE		URINE CHECK		INSULIN THERAPY		Other	COMMENTS / INTERVENTIONS- Include insulin reactions, treatment, symptoms, and diet changes	INITIALS
		Finger-stick	Serum	Glucose	Ketones	Type	Dosage			
3/7	11:00 am	48							Patient complains of feeling	
									"shaky and nervous";	C.J.-PCT
									RN notified. —————	
3/7	11:05 am								Patient given 120cc. of milk	
									and graham crackers at	
									RN direction. —————	C.J.-PCT
3/7	11:30 am	66							Patient states she feels	
									"better." —————	C.J.-PCT
3/7	1:00 pm								Patient ate 100% of lunch.	C.J.-PCT
									—————	
3/7	5:10 pm	308			trace				Patient states she ate	
									extra food after lunch and	
									feels "sluggish." —————	
									RN informed. —————	C.J.-PCT

FIGURE 10 – 6

Sample of documentation of blood glucose and urine ketone results.

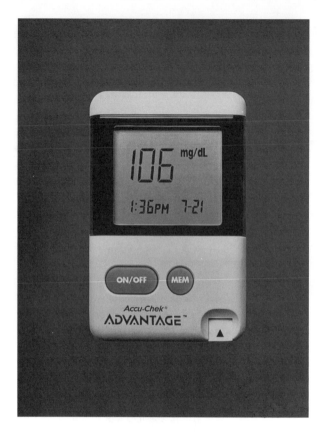

FIGURE 10-7

Example of a blood glucose meter. (Courtesy of Boehringer Mannheim Corp., Indianapolis, IN.)

TABLE 10-4
Avoiding Problems with Blood Glucose Monitoring

Tips for accurate results
  Be sure that the meter is calibrated appropriately; some meters use push-button coding while others have a coding strip.
  Perform required control testing before testing patient glucose levels; follow institution protocol on the frequency of control testing and for the corrective action if results fall out of the acceptable range.
  Obtain an adequate sample size; have the patient warm his/her hand with warm water or warm, wet cloth and hold the hand below the level of the heart—This can increase the blood flow to the fingertips; milking the finger until it turns bright pink can also be helpful.
  Use the sides of the fingers for the fingerstick because the side has more capillaries (more blood flow) and fewer nerves (less painful than using pad of finger).
  Always keep the cap of the bottle of testing strips on tightly to avoid exposure to light and moisture.
  Never use testing strips that are outdated or from a bottle that has been without its cap; sunlight and moisture can damage the testing strips and alter the results.
  Always time the test accurately with a watch or clock or by the timer on the meter.
  Clean the meter frequently to avoid buildup of residue that can affect the meter results; follow the institution's protocol for cleaning and document.
Important reminders with blood glucose monitoring:
  Always wear gloves when doing blood glucose testing to protect yourself from exposure to blood-borne infections.
  Be sure to remove the lancet from the lancet holder after use; to decrease your risk of needlestick injury, stick the exposed needle into its protective cap then remove the lancet by hand or use a hemostat to pull the lancet from the holder.
  Always discard the lancet into a sharps disposal container to prevent accidental needlesticks to yourself, the patient, or others.
  Use only the side of the fingers or the earlobes for the fingerstick; *never* use the toes or feet for the blood sample.

DIABETIC NOTES

Fingerstick method used   *Accuchek III*

Urine testing products used   *Ketostix*

(glucose / ketones)

Date	Time	BLOOD GLUCOSE		URINE CHECK		INSULIN THERAPY		Other	COMMENTS / INTERVENTIONS- Include insulin reactions, treatment, symptoms, and diet changes	INITIALS
		Finger-stick	Serum	Glucose	Ketones	Type	Dosage			
9/10	10:15 am	326			moderate				Patient states she	
									feels very tired and	
									vision is blurry.	
									RN notified of	
									patient's complaints	
									and + ketones.	C.J.- PCT

| Negative | Trace | Small | Moderate | Large |

F I G U R E   1 0 – 8

Urine ketone testing.

TEACHING - LEARNING FLOW SHEET

Teaching method code*   A = audiovisual
R = role play
E = explanation
D = demonstration
H = handout
G = group class

No.	Date and Time	Intervention — Include content taught and identity of learner (if other than the patient)	Teaching method*	States/ Identifies	Applies knowledge	Can return demonstrate	Routinely performs	No evidence of learning	Other	Reinforce content	Re-Teach	Needs practice	Other	Comments	Initials
	5/13 2¹⁵P	Instructed patient on foot care principles of inspection, washing, drying, and moisturizing. Also, instructed patient on foot safety practices. Provided patient with related handouts.—	E/H	✓	✓					✓		✓		Patient states she is eager to learn; asked appropriate questions; needs general reinforcement of information and practice.—	K.L.-RN
	5/14 10ᴬ	Reinforced with patient the importance of foot care. Provided patient with lanolin and reinforced proper application to feet. Also provided patient with a mirror to help with foot inspection.	E/D											Patient able to check feet with help of mirror; applied lanolin appropriately avoiding areas between the toes.	P.R.-PCT

Initials	Signature and title	Initials	Signature and title	Initials	Signature and title
K.L.	K. Lipton RN				
P.R.	P. Reynolds PCT				

TEACHING - LEARNING FLOW SHEET

F I G U R E   1 0 – 9

Documentation on reinforcement of teaching: diabetes.

PATIENT EDUCATION

Glucose record sheet

Name _____ **Phone** _____

Doctor's name _____ **Phone** _____

When to test _____

Target range _____

Special instructions: _____

Date	Glucose before breakfast	Glucose before lunch	Glucose before dinner	Glucose before bed	Insulin / Oral agent				Ketones	Comments
					Breakfast	Lunch	Dinner	Bed		

F I G U R E 1 0 – 1 0

Example of glucose record sheet.

10–5 presents guidelines for testing urine for ketones (acetone).

• Observe skin and especially feet daily for any areas of breakdown, discoloration, or apparent infection. Alert the RN to any of these areas. Patients with diabetes are at increased risk for infections and foot problems.

• Reinforce principles of proper hygiene and foot care. Table 10–6 gives foot care guidelines. See Figure 10–9 for sample documentation.

⚖ The RN is responsible for the comprehensive education that the person with diabetes requires. However, the PCT is an important partner in the diabetes education process. Appropriate reinforcement of essential information and practices by the PCT are valuable components of the overall instruction of proper diabetes management.

Reinforce to the patient the importance of maintaining a record of his or her blood glucose test results and medication regimen. Provide the patient with a record sheet to use for documentation while in the hospital and to take home after discharge. Figure 10–10 is an example of a glucose record sheet.

 Every patient with diabetes has a unique condition and lifestyle. Collaborate with the

T A B L E 1 0 – 5
Guidelines for Testing Urine for Ketones (Acetone)

Urine testing for ketones is important in patients with Type I diabetes who have:
    Glucose levels greater than 240 mg/dl
    Acute illness with nausea, vomiting, and/or diarrhea
    Pregnancy
To obtain accurate results:
    Test fresh urine.
    Use testing strips that are not outdated; expired testing strips need to be removed from supply area and not used for any testing.
    Do not use testing supplies that have been exposed to sunlight or moisture as this can damage the supplies and give inaccurate results.
    Time the test according to manufacturer directions; various manufacturers make ketone-testing products—timing of the test may vary; be sure to follow the directions.
    Match the color on the testing strip with the color chart on the bottle; be sure to be in an area of good lighting to make an accurate determination of the result.

T A B L E 1 0 – 6
Guidelines for Foot Care

Important information about foot care
    Daily foot care practices are vital for persons with diabetes, but also good general practices for others who have skin changes, bone changes, or other problems of the feet.
    The feet of persons with diabetes are at increased risk for problems such as nerve damage, ulcers, and infections; sometimes the problems are so severe that amputation of the foot may be necessary.
    Daily foot care can improve the condition of the feet and delay or prevent serious foot problems from developing.
Daily foot care includes
    Inspection of all aspects of the feet. Look closely for any areas of redness, dryness, cracks, blisters, ingrown toenails, and open sores—notify the RN if any of these signs is present.
    Gentle washing and drying of all aspects of the feet. Use a mild soap (no soaps with detergents) and warm water; be sure to rinse all soap residue from the feet; gently pat feet dry and carefully dry between each toe.
    Applying lotion or cream to the feet to moisturize. Use a lotion or cream with lanolin in it but not alcohol; do not put lotion between the toes.
    Placing lamb's wool between toes that have increased pressure or are overlapping.
    Preventing injury to the feet. Patients need to always wear footwear (socks/shoes, slippers); no heating devices should be applied to the feet; the feet should not be soaked (this dries the skin).

clinical nurse specialist (CNS), the diabetes nurse educator (DNE), the RN, and/or the dietitian to provide the essential aspects of patient education in diabetes management for each individual patient.

SUMMARY

Patients with disorders of the endocrine system experience many changes in their mental and physical health. Some patients must deal with mood and personality changes. They may experience feelings of depression, exhaustion, and debilitation. There is often the need to change their diet, activities, and lifestyle. With the coordinated efforts of the RN and the PCT, these patients can receive the necessary observations, monitoring, interventions, emotional support, and education to enable them to successfully live their lives and manage their conditions.

The Musculoskeletal System

NANCY R. NELSON, MS, BSN, RN,C

*P R E R E Q U I S I T E
K N O W L E D G E A N D
S K I L L S*

- Universal precautions/Body substance isolation
- Basic body mechanics
- One person stand and pivot transfer
- One person bending transfer with sliding board
- Two-person transfer
- Use of transfer/gait belt
- Moving a patient up in bed with use of trapeze; one-person assist and two-person assist
- Positioning of patient in bed with proper body alignment

- Use of mechanical assistive aids to include wheelchair, smooth mover, mechanical lift
- Working knowledge of the principles of range of motion and movement of major joints
- Knowledge of location and ability to palpate peripheral pulses

OBJECTIVES

After you complete this chapter, you will be able to:

- Define key terms.
- Describe the structure and function of the musculoskeletal system.
- Explain how the musculoskeletal system relates to other body systems.
- Describe how osteoporosis can contribute to bone fractures.
- Discuss the care of a patient with a sprain or strain.
- Describe procedure used to immobilize fractured limbs.
- State total hip replacement precautions.
- Explain the patient care technician's (PCT's) role in caring for a patient after joint replacement surgery.

- Describe normal observation of extremities in patients with musculoskeletal injury or disease.
- Describe two measures to help patients with inflammatory joint disease cope with pain.
- Describe range-of-motion exercises used to prevent contractures.
- Name three types of traction used on patients with injuries to the musculoskeletal system.
- Recognize signs and symptoms in an immobilized patient that need to be reported to the RN.
- Demonstrate how to document observations and treatments given to patients with musculoskeletal injuries or disease.
- Identify steps to prevent complications from immobility.

KEY TERMS

Articulating The surfaces of bones rubbing against each other as in a joint. These surfaces are covered by cartilage or fibrous material.

Atrophy To become smaller in size or wither away, as a muscle that is not used

Autonomic Self-regulating, able to control itself; the part of the nervous system that controls functions that cannot be consciously controlled, such as heart rate, digestion, and breathing.

Bursa A sac of fibrous tissue around tendons and joints. It is lined with a membrane that gives off fluid that lubricates and cushions the movement of the tendon over the bone.

Contract To shorten, as when a muscle is stimulated by a signal from nerves to shorten and pull on the bone to which it is attached to make that extremity move

Contracture Permanent shortening of a muscle due to spasm or paralysis that results in pulling up of the extremity and a fixed and immovable joint

Countertraction A pull or restricting force in the opposite direction of the pulling force of the traction to keep a patient from sliding down to the bottom of the bed. Often, just the patient's weight pushing down on the bed is enough resistance to prevent sliding down in bed.

Cyanosis A bluish, gray, or dark purple discoloration of the skin. It is a result of tissue not receiving enough blood or oxygen.

Dorsiflexion Flexing the foot so the toes point up and back

Flexion Bending of a body part, joint, or extremity; making the angle smaller between the two parts

Footdrop A complication of immobility from not supporting the foot in the dorsiflexion position. The muscles of the leg contract, the toes drop downward, and the foot is in plantar flexion. The patient is unable to raise the foot for normal heel-toe gait walking. A brace must be used to enable the patient to walk.

Fulcrum The point or support on which a lever pivots, turns, or rests

Hypostatic Pneumonia Inflammation of the lung caused by lung secretions that have pooled in the bronchial tubes and small lung sacs. This can happen to bedridden patients who do not move around enough and to patients who are too weak to cough up secretions. These pooled secretions can easily become infected.

Iliac Crest The upper, outer edge of the large bone of the pelvis or hip; the point where the pelvic traction belt goes around the patient, just below the waist. It is important to observe this area for skin irritation under the belt.

Joint Capsule A saclike enclosure around a joint. The membrane lining the capsule gives off a fluid that lubricates the joint.

Kyphosis An abnormal curvature of the upper spine that is commonly called dowager's hump. It is often seen in older people with osteoporosis.

Macerate Softening of the skin by constant exposure to moisture that makes it more likely to break down. This can happen to an incontinent patient who lies for a long time in a wet bed. The condition of the skin is similar to the prune-like appearance of wrinkled fingers that have been in water for a long time.

Neuropathy Inflammation of the nerves that causes numbness and tingling in the extremities. It can be caused by diseases like diabetes or multiple sclerosis or a vitamin deficiency.

Orthostatic Hypotension A condition in which blood pressure becomes very low when the patient stands too quickly from a lying position. The patient may feel dizzy and unstable and may actually lose consciousness.

Osteoporosis A disease causing the loss of bone tissue. Bones become thinner and full of holes; they are more brittle and are easily fractured.

Pathological Fracture A broken bone that happens because of a disease in the bone. The fracture can happen without any direct force or twisting.

Proprioception The sense of balance and the awareness of where the body is in space; the ability to judge weight and resistance of objects in relation to the body

Pronation To place the hand with palm down or to lay a patient face down

Serous Clear, watery fluid that may ooze from open areas of the skin; also, the watery part left after blood clots

Spastic A muscle that is tight and resists stretching or relaxation

Supination To place the hand with palm up or to position a patient lying flat on the back

Thrombus A clot that obstructs a blood vessel, especially a deep vein of the leg.

Traction To place a pulling force on an object

Urinary Retention Inability to empty the bladder of urine because of blockage from an enlarged prostate, poor bladder muscle tone, the bladder being too full for a long time, or nerve damage

Voluntary Able to be controlled as a person wishes. A voluntary muscle is one that a person can consciously control.

Mobility is an essential part of life and health. Disruptions in the musculoskeletal system, in the form of injuries and inflammation, affect mobility and limit a person's ability to enjoy life to its fullest. The study of this chapter will help the patient care technician (PCT) understand the musculoskeletal system. It will also provide nursing actions that can assist the patient to continue functioning as normally as possible and prevent complications or reinjury. PCTs can contribute much to caring for patients who are suffering from disorders of the musculoskeletal system through promoting independence, performing range of motion exercises, and reinforcing health teaching. The PCT must also be alert to signs and symptoms of complications that need to be reported to the RN. These roles are an important part of the care that is given to patients.

BASIC ANATOMY

The PCT needs to have a good understanding of the anatomy of bones and muscles to understand how they function and to recognize complications as they are developing. Muscles are a large part of the body and are what allow us to move. Muscles help the body stay upright, maintain posture, and produce heat. Muscles also give the body its shape as they soften and fill in areas of the bony skeleton to produce the contours we see.

Muscles

There are three types of muscle: skeletal, smooth, and cardiac. Skeletal muscles are attached to the bones of the body. They are considered *voluntary* muscles because they have nerves that allow them to be consciously controlled. Examples of skeletal muscles are the biceps muscle in the arm and the calf muscle in the leg. Skeletal muscles are involved in activities that we do every day like walking, talking, eating, and writing.

Smooth muscle is not attached to bones. Smooth muscles are not under voluntary or conscious control, but are controlled by the *autonomic* nervous system. Some examples of this type of muscle are the walls of the stomach, intestines, and blood vessels. These muscles help food move along the intestines and control the diameter of blood vessels, enlarging them to allow more blood to flow or making them smaller to restrict the flow of blood.

Cardiac muscle is found only in the heart. This type of muscle is not under conscious control, but is regulated by several mechanisms. Cardiac muscle is controlled by the autonomic nervous system in the same manner as smooth muscle. The nerves of the autonomic nervous system govern the rate the heart beats in response to the body's needs. When you exercise or run, the response is to increase the heart rate to supply the muscles with needed blood and oxygen. Cardiac muscle also responds to substances from the adrenal gland, like epinephrine, and to thyroid hormone. Substances from the adrenal gland increase the heart rate, as when a person is under stress or afraid. An abnormally high level of thyroid hormone will increase the heart rate also. Cardiac muscle is able to function throughout a person's lifetime, helping the heart to pump blood to the whole body. Cardiac muscle requires a continuous oxygen supply to function. If the muscle does not receive oxygen for as little as 30 seconds, the muscle begins to die and the heart will stop beating.

Muscles have only one action, they *contract* or pull. They cannot push. Muscles contract in response to a message from nerves in the brain or spinal cord and are attached to bone by tendons. The places where muscles are attached to the bone are called the origin and insertion. The end of the muscle that moves the least is called the origin; the end that moves the most with the bone is called the insertion. Because of where the muscles originate and insert, a lever action occurs when the muscles contract. A knowledge of levers helps promote an understanding of how muscles provide movement to the body. A simple lever is a hard, straight rod or shaft that is free to move about on some fixed point or support called the *fulcrum.* For example, to raise the forearm, the biceps muscle contracts and pulls on the insertion site on the ulna bone of the forearm. The fulcrum is the elbow joint. The action that results is *flexion* of the forearm. This principle is what makes all movement of the body possible. All the joints in the arms and legs move because of the action of muscles pulling around a fulcrum point and causing the joint to flex and the extremity to move (Fig. 11–1).

When a muscle is not used for an extended period, it begins to *atrophy* or waste away. This can happen when a cast is placed on an arm or leg or from other diseases like multiple sclerosis or stroke. If the muscle atrophies and the joint is not put through its range of motion over time, *contractures* can develop. The muscles become *spastic* and shorten and the joint becomes stiff.

Bones

Bones are hard, rigid structures made of living cells. Crystallized minerals give bone its rigid, hard quality. Bone is not solid as we may think of it, but filled with inner canals where bone marrow and blood vessels are present. Red blood cells are made in the bone marrow. Bone cells are rebuilt and the bones kept hard and solid by weight bearing and pull of muscles on the bones. *Osteoporosis* is a condition in which bones become thin

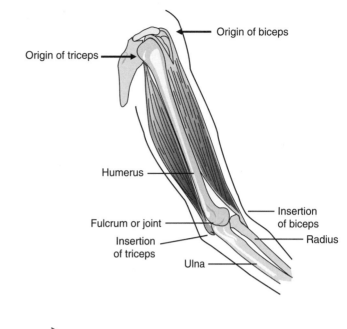

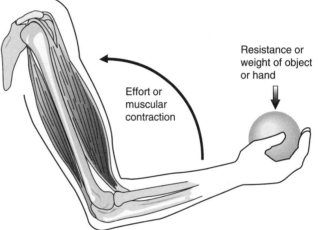

FIGURE 11-1
Lever/fulcrum principle.

and brittle and fracture easily. This can happen when a patient must be immobile or on bedrest for a long time. It is also common in older people, especially in women past middle age. Older people can even break a bone by coughing or turning over in bed. Exercise and weight-bearing activity help prevent osteoporosis.

Joints

Joints are classified according to how they are made and the amount and type of movement each joint can perform. Most joint surfaces are covered by membranes, cartilage, or other connective tissue to separate and cushion the *articulating* surfaces, or the surfaces that rub together. Ligaments extend over the joints or form capsules that surround them. Tendons of muscles may also extend around the joint.

There are several types of movable joints, and they are classified by the kind of motion permitted.

- Gliding joints permit only minimal movement such as the joints between the bones of the wrist, ankle, and the vertebrae in the spine.

- Hinge joints allow movement in one direction only, like a door hinge. Examples of this type of joint are the elbow and the knee.

- Pivot joints allow rotation such as the turning of the head. The radius and ulna form a pivot joint to allow *pronation* and *supination.*

- The thumb is actually classified as a saddle joint. This type of joint allows greater range of motion than the fingers.

- Ball-and-socket joints allow the greatest range of motion. Examples of this joint are the hip and shoulder (Fig. 11–2).

Range of motion (ROM) is the full movement that a joint can perform. The different types of joints allow a

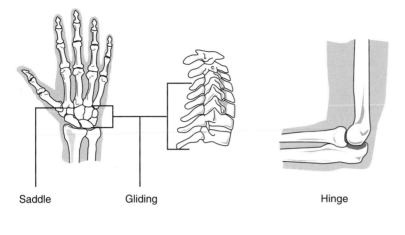

Saddle   Gliding   Hinge

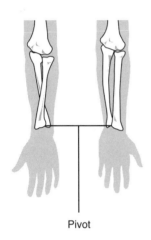

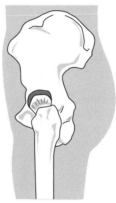

Pivot   Ball and socket

F I G U R E 1 1 – 2
Types of joints.

variety of movements that enable the body, trunk, and extremities to move. These movements are needed for activities of daily living such as brushing hair, brushing teeth, dressing, and walking. How to perform ROM will be addressed later in the chapter.

In addition to muscles and bones, the musculoskeletal system includes ligaments, tendons, and cartilage. Tendons are nonelastic cords that attach muscles to bone. Ligaments are strong bands of connective tissue that join bone to bone and support joints. Cartilage is a form of tissue that cushions the ends of bones so they do not rub together. Intervertebral discs are cartilage positioned between the vertebrae of the spinal column to absorb shock and give the spine and trunk flexibility. Freely movable joints have a *joint capsule* or *bursa* and a joint space that allow lubrication and cushioning of the joint. With age, these structures lose their elasticity and cushioning ability, and the bones may actually rub together, causing pain and stiffness. When an injury occurs, whether to the joint, a muscle, or bone, tissue surrounding the injured area is affected. When a bone is broken, muscles can be torn and swell or have such severe spasms that traction must be applied to relieve it. Swelling from an injury to a joint, such as a sprain, can put pressure

on blood vessels and nerves, endanger circulation, and cause numbness and tingling.

THE MUSCULOSKELETAL SYSTEM AND ITS RELATION TO OTHER BODY SYSTEMS

Structure

The musculoskeletal system provides a framework for the body and allows it to move. The skeletal system provides the bony framework for the body. It determines the size of the body frame and supports and gives protection to vital organs. Muscles are attached to bones, and when the muscle contracts the bones move. Muscles fill in the skeleton, and their size and shape provide the body curves. The muscles provide strength and flexibility to joints and extremities.

Function

Bones have several functions. The hard, rigid quality of bone serves to protect delicate internal organs. For example, the brain, inner ear, and parts of the eye are protected by the skull. The ribs and sternum protect the heart and lungs, and the spinal column protects the spinal cord. Bones are a storage area for minerals like calcium and phosphorus. In times of disease or malnutrition, the body is able to draw upon this reserve. For example, if the blood calcium level falls too low, calcium is released from bones into the blood stream. If the calcium level is too high, calcium release from bones is slowed or stopped, and the blood level becomes more normal. Bone marrow is also the place where red blood cells are formed.

Muscles make all motion possible. The muscles are composed of tissue that is able to contract (shorten) and relax (lengthen). When skeletal muscle contracts, the bone to which it is attached will move. Smooth muscle controls the dilation and contraction of blood vessels and regulates circulation. For example, blood vessels in extremities can contract when more blood is needed to protect vital organs such as the heart, brain, and lungs.

Nervous System

For muscles to contract and move the bones of the skeletal system, they must have a functioning nervous system. It is nerve impulses that signal the muscles to contract. Poor posture, poor body mechanics, fractures of bones, pressure on or loss of blood supply to a nerve can cause nerves to be pinched, severed, or damaged, and movement of the muscle or extremity will be lost. Pinched nerves can also cause pain so severe that a person can no longer work or enjoy life.

Other disease processes can cause disruption of the nerve impulses that affect a greater part of the body. Stroke, head injury, spinal cord injury, multiple sclerosis, and tumors of the brain are some examples of diseases that can affect more than one area of the musculoskeletal system and cause decreased ability to use extremities and perform daily activities.

Respiratory System

The musculoskeletal system provides support and protection for the lungs. The lungs are protected by the rib cage and short muscles that link the ribs together, called intercostal muscles. Muscles are involved with breathing by expanding and contracting the thoracic cavity to assist in inspiration and expiration. The respiratory system is lined with cells that produce a layer of mucus that catches particles such as dust and pollens that enter the lungs when a person breathes. There are also little hairlike projections that line the respiratory system that sweep particles trapped in the mucus up and out to be swallowed or coughed or sneezed out. Changing body positions also helps remove these mucous secretions from the lungs. Healthy persons are able to keep secretions mobilized because they spend much of their time in an upright position. During the day they move about, sit or walk uprightly, breathe deeply, and cough, which prevents lung

secretions from collecting in the small air pockets of the lung tissue. Patients who are not able to move normally and are confined to bed begin to suffer the effects of immobility. They breathe less deeply, and secretions pool in the dependent sections of the lungs, where they thicken and can cause *hypostatic pneumonia.* This condition decreases the ability of the lungs to use oxygen and can be life threatening.

Cardiovascular System

A definite connection exists between the ability to move or exercise and the cardiovascular system. When a person exercises, muscles require an increased supply of oxygen. The cardiovascular system meets this increased need for oxygen by increasing the heart rate and supplying blood and oxygen to the muscles. Over time, regular exercise produces fitness and cardiovascular conditioning. Some of the effects of this conditioning are increased efficiency of the heart, decreased heart rate and blood pressure, increased blood flow to all body parts, and increased circulating anticlotting factors in the blood. This fitness enables the cardiovascular system to more easily meet the oxygen demands of the muscles, and a person has less fatigue. This principle is one of the reasons patients who are immobilized by musculoskeletal injuries are given mild exercise.

Exercise and good muscle tone also improve venous return. No pump exists to return blood to the heart. The return of blood depends greatly on movement and pressure from muscles surrounding the veins, aided by a system of valves that maintain a one-way flow. Inactivity leads to slower movement of blood and pooling of blood in extremities, which can lead to blood clots.

Usually the body makes up for the effect of position changes on circulation by constricting and dilating blood vessels to keep an adequate blood supply to internal organs and extremities. With prolonged immobility, these mechanisms do not function adequately. If the person on prolonged bedrest tries to stand too quickly, the body is not able to make the adjustment to the change in position, and blood will pool in the extremities, which may cause less blood to flow to the brain. This results in dizziness, lightheadedness, and possible fainting. This is termed *orthostatic hypotension.*

Renal Urinary System

Mobility and activity are important in keeping the urinary system functioning efficiently. Regular exercise increases blood circulation and improves blood flow to the kidneys. This enables the kidney to filter wastes and maintain a proper balance of electrolytes in the blood. Patients who are immobile, or on bed rest for long periods, lose calcium from their bones. This calcium loss from the bone increases the calcium content in the blood that must be filtered by the kidneys. Kidneys drain normally when a person is upright, either sitting or standing. Immobility and bed rest make the urine pool in the kidney, and draining will occur more slowly. This sluggish activity and increased need to filter calcium leads to an increased chance of kidney stones.

It is normal for a person to urinate in the upright position. When a patient is on bedrest, it is more difficult to empty the bladder. This is especially true of men, who are used to urinating in a standing position. When a patient must remain supine, urine may pool in the kidney and lead to infection. When the bladder does not completely empty, it can lead to *urinary retention.* The over-distended bladder causes poor bladder muscle tone and incontinence. Urinary incontinence has many causes that can be worsened by bedrest and immobility. A person who does not have the strength to walk to the bathroom can have incontinent episodes if there is no one to assist with toileting. Poor perineal hygiene, incontinence, decreased fluid intake, or an indwelling Foley catheter can increase the risk of urinary tract infection for an immobile patient.

Gastrointestinal System

The proper functioning of the gastrointestinal system is directly related to mobility. With regular exercise and fitness a person has a better appetite, and the tone of the intestinal muscles is maintained, which aids digestion and elimination. On the other hand, immobility reduces appetite, food is not digested properly, and the body is unable to use it efficiently. Inactivity leads to a decrease in the tone of intestinal muscles, and food moves more slowly through the digestive tract. Because the food is moving more slowly, more liquid is removed from the stool. Constipation, impaction of dry, hard stool, and increased gas formation result. Incontinence can result from liquid stool oozing around hard retained stool. When a patient is unable to maintain normal mobility because of bedrest or weakness, incontinence can result from inability to get to the bathroom. If a patient must use the bedpan while bed bound, the unnatural position makes it difficult to evacuate the bowel.

Endocrine System

Endocrine diseases like diabetes mellitus, hyperthyroidism (Graves' disease), and adrenal gland disease have common symptoms of muscle wasting, weakness, and fatigue. Complications of diabetes mellitus affect the mobility of patients. Diabetic *neuropathy* is a disease of the nerves of the extremities that causes numbness and tingling in the hands, legs, and feet. Diabetic patients with this condition are often unable to feel the temperature of bath water and even step on pins or tacks and are unaware. Circulatory problems as a result of diabetes can lead to gangrene and amputation. Vision difficulties from diabetes limit a patient's ability to function independently.

Loss of *proprioception,* which is the sense of balance and a sense of where extremities are in space in relation to the rest of the body, makes a patient more prone to loss of balance and falling.

COMMON DISRUPTIONS IN THE MUSCULOSKELETAL SYSTEM

Strains and Sprains

A strain is a muscle pull that comes about because of overuse or excessive stress on the muscle. The patient will experience pain when trying to use the injured muscle. A sprain occurs when a ligament is twisted or torn. Ligaments provide support and flexibility to joints, and with injury there is an instability of the joint. With both strains and sprains there is bleeding into the tissue and pain and swelling. The care for both injuries is similar. A common acronym for this care is *RICE.*

*R*est: The affected part needs to be rested and not used until there is minimal pain. Often an immobilization device of some kind is placed on the extremity. An Ace wrap, splint, or soft cast may be used to prevent movement of the injured part and provide stability to a weakened joint.

*I*ce: Intermittent use of ice compresses helps reduce swelling. The physician may order ice for 20 minutes out of every hour for the first day, then alternating ice and heat, until pain and swelling are relieved. The ice causes vasoconstriction, which helps stop bleeding into the tissues and minimizes swelling.

*C*ompression: The joint or injured area is immobilized with a pressure bandage or Ace wrap. This serves to control edema and stabilize a weak joint.

*E*levation: Elevating the injured part helps to reduce swelling and edema.

These principles can be applied to the care of most patients who experience musculoskeletal injuries or disease. They are included in most therapy that a doctor may order for relief from pain and swelling of muscles and joints. It is important to understand the reason for treatments you will give to patients to help you notice abnormal signs that need to be reported to the RN.

Fractures

A fracture is a break in a bone. Fractures can be classified as open or closed. Open fractures are sometimes called compound fractures. In open fractures the bone protrudes through the overlying skin. With closed fractures the skin over the area of the broken bone is intact, and the ends of the bone may or may not be aligned. There are many types of fractures within these two classifications. The types of fractures (Fig. 11–3) are described in terms of what the break in the bone looks like.

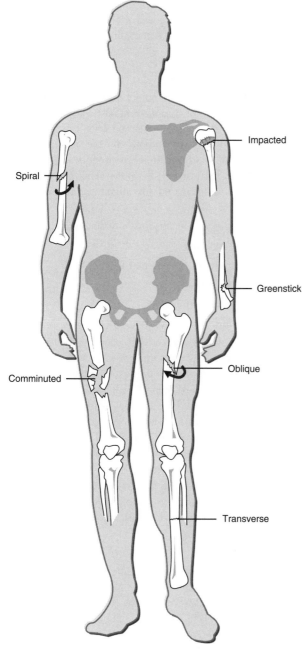

FIGURE 11-3
Types of fractures.

- Spiral fracture: The break coils around the bone.

A fracture can be caused by direct force, twisting, or strong contractions of a muscle, as when a heavy weight is lifted. Fractures that occur without some incidence of direct force or twisting are called *pathological fractures.* These spontaneous fractures happen because of a diseased or weakened area of bone. Pathological fractures can occur when metastatic cancer, tumors of the bone, or thinning of the bone, as in osteoporosis, is present.

One of the most common causes of fractures in the elderly is falls. Elderly are at great risk for falls because of decreased muscle strength, diminished coordination, changes in gait, and loss of sense of balance. Once an elderly person has fallen, he or she is often apprehensive and fearful of falling again. The elderly may lose their sense of security in ambulating up stairs and on familiar walking areas.

JOINT REPLACEMENT

Joint replacement is a common operation, especially in the elderly. Falls often result in a fracture of the hip that must be treated surgically. Hip fractures can be treated by placing a pin in the joint or bone, but often they require total joint replacement. Inflammatory and degenerative diseases like rheumatoid arthritis, osteoarthritis, and gout cause degeneration of such joints as knees, hips, and knuckles of fingers. Often the joints need replacement to relieve pain and restore mobility. Joint replacement surgery in the elderly is often complicated by the presence of other diseases. Frequently this results in a decline of both physical and mental function after the surgery and a long recovery period. Care of the patient after joint replacement is very important to prevent complications and help the patient to recover and return to his or her previous level of independence.*

As a PCT, your role in caring for patients who have had joint replacement surgery is crucial. If you are not sure of any part of the care you must give, there are many resources available to you. The physical therapist, occupational therapist, clinical nurse specialist, and experienced orthopedic nurses would all be willing and able to give you the information you need to deliver the proper and safe care to prevent injuries and complications for the patient.

Total Hip Replacement

The care of a patient after hip surgery and total hip replacement is very important. There are precautions that

- Greenstick fracture: The bone is partially bent and split on one side. It is not broken all the way through.
- Comminuted fracture: The bone is broken completely through and splintered into pieces with fragments causing injury to surrounding tissue.
- Impacted fracture: A fracture in which the bone is broken and one end forced into the other.
- Oblique fracture: A fracture in which the break in the bone runs in a slanting direction on the bone.
- Transverse fracture: The break runs across the bone.

Erickson, B., and Perkins, M.: Interdisciplinary team approach in the rehabilitation of hip and knee arthroplasties. American Journal of Occupational Therapy. May 1994; 48(5):439–441.

must be observed during the immediate recovery time. If they are not followed, the new hip can be displaced out of joint. Surgeons use different approaches to the hip during surgery. Some make the incision on the posterior or back of the hip and some use a side (lateral) or front (anterior) approach. The only differences in patient care between the two surgical approaches are:

Posterior approach (most common): Must not flex the hip greater than 90 degrees (a right angle)
Lateral or anterior approach: Must not slide the operative leg out to the side.

These are the only differences between the care of patients whose surgeons have used different approaches to the surgery. All of the following precautions apply to all total hip replacement patients and should be used when caring for a patient who has had total hip replacement. These precautions are usually observed for at least 6 weeks after surgery or until the doctor releases the patient to return to normal activity.

PRECAUTIONS IN CARING FOR HIP REPLACEMENT PATIENTS

- Keep the operated leg abducted at all times. When one is turning the patient, assisting the patient to dangle the legs at the bedside, or sitting the patient in a chair, the patient's legs should be slightly apart at all times. When turning a patient in bed, use an abductor pillow to keep the legs apart and the hip joint abducted. Use pillows to support the feet beyond the abductor pillow when positioning a patient on his or her side. When he or she is sitting in a chair place a pillow between the patient's legs to keep legs abducted (Fig. 11–4).
- Check the orders for your patient and your facility

policy to see if your patient may be turned to the operated side. Some surgeons prefer the patient to lie on the unoperated side, some allow the patient to lie on the operated side.

> **STOP** It is possible for the new hip replacement to become displaced out of the joint during turning of the patient. Caution must be exercised.

- When repositioning the patient, observe the circulation and sensation of the patient's extremities at regular intervals, at least every 2 hours. The leg and hip joint should be observed for alignment and signs of dislocation.
- Watch for signs of hip prosthesis dislocation
- Shortening of the leg
- External rotation of the leg and foot
- Bulging at the hip site
- Inability to move the leg
- Increased pain in the operated joint
- For patients whose surgeon has used the *posterior approach*: Never allow the hip joint to flex more than 90 degrees. Instruct/reinforce the teaching that the patient is not to lean forward to pull up the blanket or reach for bedside articles. Instruct the patient not to cross the legs, bend forward, or lie on a side with legs together. The head of the bed should never be raised more than 45 degrees. Instruct/remind the patient to use a chair with an elevated seat or to place 1 or 2 pillows in the seat of a chair before sitting down to prevent flexion of hip joint. The patient should also be reminded not to bend forward when getting out of a chair.

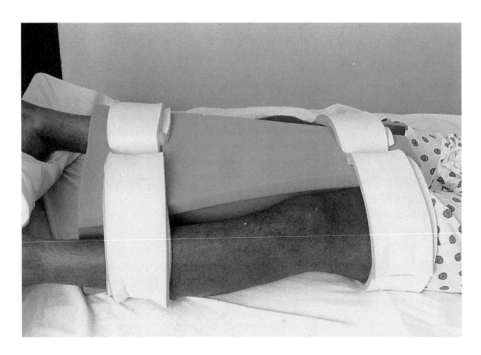

Abductor pillow.

• For patients whose surgeon has used the *lateral or anterior approach*: Do not allow the patient to try to slide the operated leg out to the side. Instruct/reinforce the need of the patient to obtain help to move the leg out to the side when attempting to sit at the side of the bed. A patient whose operation was done using the lateral/anterior approach does not have the restrictions about bending forward as in the posterior approach.

Check with your RN or physical therapist for the type of surgery done on your patient and the appropriate care and precautions needed for each patient.

• Keep the leg of the operated side in neutral position or slightly externally rotated. Internal rotation can also result in hip dislocation, and this movement can happen when a patient twists to reach for objects. Keep bedside supplies within reach for the patient.

• Observe weight-bearing guidelines when ambulating the patient after surgery. The physical therapy department will be working with the patient and will leave specific guidelines as to how much weight may be placed on the operated side. When offering the bedpan, instruct the patient to use the overhead trapeze and unaffected leg to raise the pelvis onto the fracture pan, making sure not to put any weight on the operated leg or hip.

(Put date and time.) Patient logrolled to unoperated side with three-person assist. Abductor pillow in place to keep operated hip abducted. Feet supported with extra pillows. No red areas noted on skin of patient's back. Dressing in place on operative site. No drainage noted. Patient able to move foot of operated side. No complaints of pain when turning. *(Then sign your name.)* J. Jones, PCT.

The patient should have a firm mattress and an overbed trapeze to assist with moving in bed. When one is making the bed, a turn sheet should be placed on the bed. Always make sure adequate pillows are available for positioning. The PCT should be aware of patient teaching that will help the patient's recovery process. Instructions that need to be reinforced are: deep breathing, use of incentive spirometer, positions to avoid, isometric exercises for the foot, ankle, calf, quadriceps and gluteal muscles that help to strengthen the legs for walking and prevent blood clots.

In most acute care facilities, physical therapists delegate many of the ongoing exercises and minor treatments to support personnel.* In Figure 11–5 are shown some of the exercises commonly used by physical therapists for

total hip replacement patients. You need to become familiar with the specific exercises prescribed for your patient so that you may be able to reinforce them while you are giving care.

Knee Replacement

Replacement of the knee joint helps relieve pain and restore motion to joints diseased by rheumatoid arthritis and osteoarthritis. Immediately after surgery the leg may be elevated to prevent swelling and enhance venous return to prevent blood clots. Pillows are used to prevent flexion of the knee. The patient may be turned while protecting the position of the knee. The doctor may order the patient's leg to be passively flexed and extended by a continuous passive movement (CPM) device. CPM devices are used after hip and knee surgery to provide slow, continual movement of the affected joint. It is used to limit the internal scarring that can prevent full movement after recovery. The patient's leg may be in the device when he or she returns from surgery or it may be placed in it a day or so later. The doctor and the physical therapist decide the amount of flexion allowed and the machine settings. The physical therapist will instruct the patient in the use of the CPM device and supervise the patient to be sure the limb is properly positioned in the appliance. As the joint heals from surgery, the flexion/extension allowed by the device will be adjusted by the doctor and the physical therapist. Transfer training and ambulation are usually begun on postoperative day 2.*

Check with the physical therapist or the RN if you have any questions about caring for the patient in a CPM.

The patient's leg should remain in the machine as long as tolerated. The leg may be removed from the CPM device for personal care. It is helpful to stop the CPM in the extended position (leg flat) and support the knee as the device is moved to the side of the bed. Often the patient will be taken out of the CPM for meals and to lie on the side for relief of pressure on sacral areas to prevent pressure sores.

(Put date and time.) Partial bath given. Patient able to assist with all except back and lower portion of legs. Replaced leg in CPM. Able to tolerate CPM for 2 hours at a time at 20 degrees flexion. No redness, swelling, or warmth at incision site. Pedal pulses present and equal on both feet. Toes warm. Reinforced teaching to do ankle pumps and gluteal and quadriceps sets as instructed by the

*Bashi, H.L., and Domholdt, E.: Use of support personnel for physical therapy treatment. Physical Therapy. July 1993; 73(7):421–436.

*Bahannon, R., and Cooper, J.: Total knee arthroplasy: Evaluation of an acute care rehabilitation program. Arch Phys Med Rehabile. Oct 1993; 74:1091–1994.

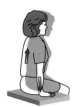

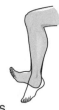

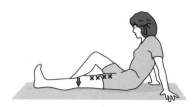

Sitting pushups

1. Sit on a firm chair.

2. Place your hands on the seat or armrest on either side of you.

3. Lift your buttocks off the chair.

4. Hold for five seconds, then relax.

Ankle pumps

1. Sit on a sturdy surface high enough that your feet don't touch the floor, or lie flat on the bed.

2. Pull the top of your foot back toward your knee as far as possible.

3. Hold for five seconds, then relax.

Quadriceps set

1. Sit on a firm, flat surface with the knee of your uninvolved leg bent.

2. Straighten your involved leg as much as possible, tightening the muscles on top of your thigh.

3. Hold for five seconds, then relax.

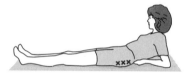

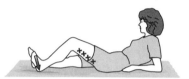

Gluteal sets

1. Recline on your back. Keep your legs straight.

2. Squeeze your buttocks together as tightly as possible.

3. Hold for five seconds, then relax.

Hamstring sets

1. Recline on your back.

2. Keep one leg straight, and bend the other to a height of about six inches.

3. Tighten the bent leg by digging down and back with the heel. Don't slide, just tighten the muscles behind your thigh.

4. Hold for five seconds, then relax.

F I G U R E 1 1 – 5

Exercises supplied by physical therapist: sitting pushups, ankle pumps, quadriceps sets, gluteal sets, hamstring sets. (From Adult Exercises I Exercise Instruction Sheets. Copyright © 1989 by Therapy Skill Builders, a division of the Psychological Corporation. Reproduced by permission. All rights reserved.)

physical therapist. Patient states is doing them every 2 hours. *(Then sign your name.)* J. Jones, PCT.

Role of Patient Care Technician in Caring for the Joint Replacement Patient

REINFORCE PATIENT TEACHING. The physical therapist will teach the patient exercises for the feet and quadriceps and gluteal muscles. It will be helpful to the patient's recovery if the PCT understands these exercises and encourages the patient to perform them (Fig. 11–5).

BASIC ORTHOPEDIC CARE PRINCIPLES. There are basic nursing observations and care common to all patients who have an operation on a joint. It is always important to observe the color of the toes or fingers, the patient's ability to move the tips of the extremities, and the patient's ability to feel you touch them. Also note the temperature of the fingers or toes on the extremity that has been operated on. Check for color, circulation, and sensation at least every 2 hours, as swelling of the joint can compress blood vessels and nerves.

PAIN MANAGEMENT. There are many helpful interventions to assist with pain management in the joint replacement patient. Immediate postoperative pain is controlled by patient controlled analgesia (PCA) or by pain medication given by the RN. PCA is a method of giving the patient pain medication by constant infusion either into a vein or the epidural space of the spinal column. A special pump is used with a control button that can be used to self-administer additional doses of medication when the patient is experiencing unrelieved pain. The patient is limited in the amount of extra doses he or she can self-administer to assure not receiving an overdose. Most patients experience good relief from pain and feel they have more control over their pain with PCA. In some facilities, patients may be restricted in their activity if they are receiving their PCA through the epidural route. When giving patient care, such as a bath, you must observe for any sign that the catheter is dislodged or leaking. Also observe for any redness or warmth at the site. As duties of the PCT keep you in close contact with the patient, you will have greater opportunities to see when the patient is in pain. This will enable you to alert the RN when the patient needs additional medication.

Some other techniques used to help the patient manage pain are distraction, therapeutic touch, imagery, and hot or cold therapy. These techniques will be explained in further detail under pain relief for inflammatory joint disease. These techniques are important for the PCT to learn and use in caring for patients in pain.

OBSERVE FOR SIGNS OF INFECTION. All incisions must be observed for signs of infection. Redness, swelling, warmth, drainage, and foul odor are signs of infection that must be reported promptly to the RN.

UNIVERSAL PRECAUTIONS USED WITH WOUND DRAINS. The patient will usually return from joint surgery with a wound drain. Some types of drains are the Jackson/Pratt (J/P), Hemovac, or a Surgidyne/Varidyne. These drains need to be emptied regularly. The J/P and Hemovac need the mechanical suction created when they are empty and compressed to provide the suction necessary to keep the bloody drainage from accumulating in the wound tissue. The edges of the incision will not heal properly, and abscesses may form if the drains are not managed correctly. The J/P and Hemovac need to be emptied when they begin filling and the suction is decreasing. This may mean emptying them several times a shift, depending on the amount of drainage. The Surgidyne and other brands are wound drains that are attached to controlled suction and need to be emptied only once a shift. Accurate intake and output are important as the surgeon uses these data to help determine when to remove the drain. If more than one drain is in place, be sure to record each one separately. Be sure to use gloves and universal precautions when doing this procedure as the drains contain bloody drainage.

GENERAL POSTOPERATIVE CARE

Surgical patients are at risk for blood clots. Report any complaints of calf pain, chest pain, or shortness of breath to the nurse immediately.

After surgery, all patients must regain activity and mobility as quickly as possible. This will help prevent complications of immobility. To prevent respiratory complications, patients must turn, cough, and deep breathe (TCDB) to keep lung secretions from collecting and causing hypostatic pneumonia. As a PCT you must encourage your postoperative patients to use their incentive spirometer as instructed by the respiratory therapist or RN.

In all postoperative and immobile patients, you must be aware of their tolerance of increased activity. Observe the patient for dizziness

upon arising, and teach the patient not to take any steps until he or she has balance. A good rule for beginning activity in an immobile patient is to use the "20 pulse beats" rule. Take the patient's resting pulse while he or she is lying in the supine position. Then assist the patient to dangle. Take the pulse again after 2 to 3 minutes. If it has increased more than 20 beats, the patient cannot tolerate that activity and must return to the supine position. Use the 20 pulse beats rule as the patient's activity is increased to sitting at the bedside and ambulating.

INFLAMMATORY JOINT DISEASE

Inflammatory and degenerative joint diseases like rheumatoid arthritis, osteoarthritis, and gout can cause pain and crippling changes in joints. Patients with fibromyalgia, a disease affecting the muscles, also experience pain and stiffness, but do not have the crippling changes in joints seen in the other degenerative diseases. They also experience difficulty sleeping and may experience some relief using relaxation exercises. The main goal of treatment for any of these patients is maintaining mobility, muscle strength, and pain control. The suggestions mentioned for mobility and mild exercises throughout this chapter should be used with arthritis patients to help them maintain as much muscle strength, joint mobility, and independence as possible. Several types of therapy are useful to assist the arthritis patient with pain control. Hot and cold treatments, rest, adaptive devices (such as reacher bars, sock aids, and built-up handles on eating utensils), relaxation exercises, and medication are used in combination to help the patient cope with chronic symptoms.

Heat and cold applications are often ordered for patients with joint disease. They have opposite effects on blood flow, but both are used to help relieve pain, stiffness, and muscle spasm. One difference in the effect of hot and cold treatments is that heat increases circulation and can increase swelling. Cold reduces circulation to the area and can reduce swelling. Complications can occur from both hot and cold treatments. As a PCT you may be asked to perform these therapeutic procedures.

Follow the guidelines carefully for any hot or cold therapy and observe the patient's skin closely for any burns, redness, blisters, and change in skin color or texture. Remove the treatment immediately and report the findings to the RN if any of these changes occur.

Patients with circulatory problems, unconscious patients, and those with loss of sensation to any body part are at greater risk for complications. Patients who have a loss of sensation must be protected from burns and injury to the skin from hot or cold treatments. If the patient is alert, ask if there is any numbness or tingling in the arms or legs before you administer any hot or cold treatment. It is the RN's responsibility to perform this assessment, but it is a good habit to double check with the patient before you proceed.

STOP Do not apply any hot or cold treatment if you notice any discoloration of skin or if the patient has any problems with circulation.

The following are general guidelines for both hot and cold therapy:

- Check with the RN for the exact type of hot or cold therapy to be used and verify the correct temperature of the material to be used.
- Check with the RN to know how long to leave any treatment in place and be sure to return to remove it promptly, checking the skin frequently during the treatment.
- Understand how to operate any electrical equipment used in hot or cold therapy and follow the directions carefully.
- Never put a hot or cold therapeutic pad directly on a patient's skin. Cover the pad with a cloth cover before applying to the skin.
- Report any patient complaints of pain, numbness, or burning to the RN immediately. Also report any changes in the skin such as blisters, burns, or color change and immediately remove the hot or cold treatment if these changes occur.
- Never apply heat to an inflamed or "hot" joint.

Hot Dry Treatments

Hot water bottles and electric heating pads are often used by individuals at home for dry heat. Usually in the hospital the aquamatic pad is used. An aquamatic pad is a rubber pad made of tubes filled with water that can be kept at an even temperature as it circulates through the coils of the pad. The unit is electrically controlled and maintained at a preset temperature that cannot be changed by the patient. The pad should be covered with a cloth to protect the patient's skin; it must not be placed under the patient, as burns may occur.

Hot Moist Treatments

Hot, moist compresses are the most common type of hot treatment. This could be in the form of a hot, moist towel or a commercially prepared compress. The compress is usually applied to a small area to bring relief from pain or as a treatment for skin irritations. Hot treatments are usually left on for 20 minutes and then removed.

The heat supplied by the aquamatic pad is dry heat, but it can also be used as a form of moist heat by placing the pad over a moist dressing. If applied to the skin too long, it may *macerate* the skin or cause it to become wrinkled like a prune. Follow the doctor's order for length of application. Examine skin carefully between treatments and allow to dry.

Cold Dry Treatments

An ice bag or ice collar is a dry cold treatment and should be covered with a cloth before being placed on the skin. If the cloth cover becomes moist, it should be replaced. Ice bags can be filled with ice chips, leaving enough room in the bag to be able to mold the bag to the body part to be treated. Commercially prepared ice packs are available and are frozen by placing them in the freezer section of a refrigerator. The frozen solution in the pack remains flexible and can be molded easily to fit a body part. This type of ice pack also needs a cloth cover before it is placed on the patient's skin. Ice bags are usually left on for only 10–20 minutes out of each hour to allow the skin and underlying tissues to recover from the cold.

Cold Moist Treatments

A cold compress is similar to a hot compress. It may be used for pain relief after minor surgery, for an injured area to reduce swelling, or to relieve a headache. It consists of a washcloth or gauze that is moistened with ice water and placed on the skin. A clean basin is filled with a small amount of water and some pieces of ice. The clean cloth or gauze is saturated with the cold water and wrung thoroughly before it is placed on the skin. Care should be taken to protect the bed linen, as a cold, wet bed would be very uncomfortable for the patient. The cold compress will pick up the body heat from the skin and need to be changed frequently. The treatment is usually continued for 20 minutes every hour as ordered by the doctor.

(Put date and time.) Hot, moist compress applied to right knee for 20 minutes as ordered. Skin checked every 5 minutes during treatment. No redness or broken skin seen. Patient states that treatment felt good and pain is decreased. *(Then sign your name.)* J. Jones, PCT.

Other Measures for Pain Relief

Relaxation exercises, guided imagery, and distraction techniques are types of therapy used to help arthritis patients cope with pain and stiffness of joints. Stimulation from touch is another means of reducing pain. These therapeutic measures may not be as effective against acute pain right after surgery, but for some they may give additional relief along with pain medication. There are tapes and books that can be obtained about these measures, but a simple explanation is included here.

RELAXATION EXERCISES. The patient should assume a comfortable position and begin deep and regular breathing while counting backward with each breath. As the patient begins to relax, he or she should visualize each number as the breaths are counted. By concentrating on these images the patient is taking his or her mind off the pain and helping begin the relaxation process.

GUIDED IMAGERY. The patient should assume a comfortable position and begin regular, relaxed, deep breathing. The patient should then picture a place he or she enjoys and pretend actually to be in that place, sensing all the pleasant feelings of the imaginary location. These are also good techniques to help a patient fall asleep.

DISTRACTION. Radio, television, and music or talking on the phone often can distract a patient enough to give some relief from chronic pain.

STIMULATION FROM TOUCH. It has been shown that the stimulation from touch also helps to reduce the sensation of pain. According to the "gate control" theory of pain, stimulation of large-diameter nerve fibers in the skin may reduce the intensity of pain. Skin stimulation can be accomplished by various forms of therapeutic touch. Back rubs, vibration, and use of heat, cold, warm baths, whirlpool baths, lotion rub, and menthol cream are some of the measures that can be employed.

A unit that produces a tingling, vibrating sensation on the skin in the area of pain is called a TENS unit (transcutaneous electrical nerve stimulation). The unit has electrodes that are placed on the skin in the area of pain, and the patient is able to adjust the force of the stimulation until the sensation is strong but not uncomfortable. This method of stimulation is very effective for some patients.

Positioning the Patient

When resting or performing activities of daily living (ADLs) the patient should maintain proper body alignment and posture. Positioning in bed should include use of a firm mattress. When the head of the bed is elevated during the day, the patient's hips should be where the bed bends. The patient should lie flat for short periods during the day to prevent flexion contractures of the hip. The patient should sit as straight as possible in a straight chair, high enough to get out of easily. Pillows may need to be used to help maintain posture.

Range of Motion

When a joint is not put through its ROM for a time, contractures can develop. The joint becomes stiff, and the muscles become spastic and contract. ROM of all joints is very important and should be done for the patient

if he or she is unable to move the extremities. If joints are painful and inflamed, perform as much movement as the patient can tolerate and move each joint slowly and gently. It is often helpful to splint a joint when it is in the acute stage of inflammation. Resting the joint helps to relieve pain and swelling and allow healing to take place. However, the joint should not be immobilized for long periods without performing ROM exercises. For patients with joint disease, ROM exercise helps to maintain mobility of the joint and may relieve pain. ROM exercise programs have even been shown to improve the cognitive ability of nursing home patients.*

ROM is the full movement that a joint can perform. The different types of joints allow a variety of movement that enables the body, trunk, and extremities to perform ADLs and work. The actions allowed by joints are classified as:

Flexion: Bending an extremity or the body
Extension: Straightening an extremity or the body
Hyperextension: Moving a body part past straight
Adduction: Moving an extremity toward the body
Abduction: Moving an extremity away from the body
Rotation: Moving an extremity in a circle
Ulnar deviation: With wrist in extension, moving the hand laterally (little-finger side)
Radial deviation: With wrist in extension, moving the hand medially (thumb side)
Eversion: Turning the foot outward
Inversion: Turning the foot inward
Pronation: Having the palm facing up
Supination: Having the palm facing down
Dorsiflexion: Flexion of the foot so the toes point up
Plantar flexion: Extension of the foot so that the toes point down

To prevent contractures, these movements must be performed for patients who cannot move for themselves. If a patient is unable to move his or her joints through the ROM each joint is capable of, it must be done for the patient. Patients with inflammatory joint disease or in casts or traction, elderly people who are weak and do not move easily, and patients who have paralysis of one or more extremities, all need to have ROM performed for them. As a PCT, this should be one of the skills you learned in earlier training. However, because it is so important and *often not done*, a review is included here.

 Never neglect to do ROM exercise. The importance cannot be emphasized enough.

Passive ROM is performed by the PCT for a patient who cannot move the extremity. Active ROM is performed

---

*Dawe, D., and Moore-Orr, R.: Low-intensity, range-of-motion exercise: Invaluable nursing care for elderly patients. Journal of Advanced Nursing. 1995; 21:675–681.

by the patient, either during ADLs or in a specific exercise program. Both active ROM and passive ROM reduce edema, as the pumping action of the muscles helps return fluid accumulated in the tissues to the venous circulation.* By using the strong, unaffected extremity to move the weaker, affected one through its ROM, the patient is using active and passive ROM. For example, a patient who is paralyzed on one side can tuck the foot and toes of the strong leg under the weak leg to lift it to the side of the bed in preparation to sit up. ROM is usually performed at the time of the bath and at bedtime. An excellent opportunity to perform ROM on extremities of a bedridden patient is during the time the patient is turned and repositioned with pillows. ROM can and *should be* incorporated into *all* aspects of patient care.

(Put date and time.) Patient performed active-assistive ROM to left shoulder, elbow, hand, and fingers. Able to raise left arm to eye level without pain. PCT completed internal/external rotation of shoulder. Reinforced teaching of occupational therapist. Patient tolerated well with no complaints of pain. *(Then sign your name.)* J. Jones, PCT.

ROM can cause injury if not performed properly. See basic nursing texts for specific illustrations of ROM exercises. A summary guideline is included here. Use the following rules when performing or assisting with ROM:

- Never exercise a swollen, red, or inflamed joint. Always report these findings to the RN.

- Perform each exercise 3 to 5 times on each joint.

- Never exercise a joint to the point of pain.

- Give good support to the extremity being exercised, either at the joint or near the joint, and do not strain the joint or cause spasm of muscles.

- Keep each movement smooth and slow.

Remember, patients often recover from an acute illness or episode such as a stroke and are unable to perform daily tasks or walk normally because ROM was not done and contractures resulted.

Adaptive Devices

Often adaptive equipment is recommended by the occupational therapist to help the patient with inflammatory disease perform ADLs. These adaptive devices help reduce stress on joints and enable the patient to perform ADLs more independently. PCTs can be of great help in assisting and reminding patients to use these devices and to alert the physical and occupational therapists as to what the patient might benefit from. Some assistive devices include long-handled reacher bars, sock aids, built-up spoon handles, and plate guards. These aids are useful when incorporated into a total program to help the patient maintain self-care.

Physical therapy is important in assisting patients with inflammatory joint disease to maintain independence. Exercises given to the patient should be reinforced and encouraged. Canes and walkers may be needed to help the patient with ambulation. Make sure the patient has well-fitting shoes to prevent falls when ambulating.

ORTHOPEDIC DEVICES

Traction devices are used to treat many injuries and conditions of the musculoskeletal system. Traction is used to apply a pulling force on bones to immobilize and align fractures, to relieve pressure on nerves that may be pinched in a joint, and to relieve muscle strains or spasms. When traction is applied for the purpose of stabilizing a fracture, it must be continuous to be effective and cannot be disconnected unless ordered by the physician. Never remove the weights unless directed by the RN or doctor.

The patient needs to be positioned so there is *countertraction*. Countertraction is the force acting in the opposite direction of the pulling force of the traction. The patient's body usually provides the needed countertraction, but there will be times when other provisions need to be made. Countertraction can be obtained by tilting the bed so that the patient tends to slide away from the traction force.* Follow the RN's or doctor's guidelines for positioning the patient. The head of the patient's bed should not be raised more than 20 degrees when traction is on the lower extremities or pelvis, as this would cancel out the countertraction and the patient would slide down in bed. All traction equipment must be inspected regularly to assure that weights are hanging freely. If the patient slides down in bed, the weights may touch the floor and result in decreased pull on the fracture.

TRACTION GUIDELINES

- Do not disturb the weights or permit them to swing, drop, or rest on any surface.

- Keep the patient in good alignment.

- Make sure that the body is providing proper countertraction by keeping the head of the bed elevated less than 20 degrees.

- Check under the cervical collar or pelvic belt for areas of pressure or irritation.

---

*Dirette, D., and Hinojosa, J.: Effects of continuous passive motion on the edematous hands of two persons with flaccid hemiplegia. American Journal of Occupational Therapy. May 1994; 48(5):403–408.

*Styrcula, L.: Traction basics: Part I. Orthopaedic Nursing. March/April 1994; 13(2):71–74.

- Check straps of halters and belts to be sure they are smooth, straight, and properly secured.
- Keep covers off ropes and pulleys.

Positioning the Patient in Traction

The patient usually must remain supine or lying on the back while in traction. Proper positioning includes keeping the entire body in good alignment. This means you must adapt your patient care techniques. It will be easier to make the patient's bed from top to bottom when unable to turn a patient from side to side. Be sure to check with the RN for specific guidelines for each patient. The patient can use the overhead trapeze to help raise the body off the bed. All patients in traction are immobilized to some degree and are at risk for the many complications of immobility. Be sure to use nursing care measures to prevent complications of immobility. These measures include turn, cough, and deep breathing (TCDB), ROM, adequate fluids, having the patient participate in his or her own care as much as possible, reinforcing isometric exercises prescribed by the physical therapist, and having the patient use an overhead trapeze to help move in bed to maintain upper body strength.

Skin Traction

Skin traction uses harnesses, sponge rubber boots, and bandages or special wrapping that attach to the skin. Only limited traction can be used with this method. Less than 10 pounds of weight are used for short periods, usually less than 3 weeks. Skin traction is used to relieve muscle spasm and minor fractures and to temporarily immobilize a fractured hip before surgery. A doctor must order the type of skin traction to be used, but the RN or technician can apply it. If this is to be one of your duties as a PCT, you will be given special training to perform these tasks. Some general guidelines and precautions are presented here. Skin traction is sometimes intermittent, and the patient can be out of the traction for personal care activities.

STOP Never remove any traction unless you have specific instructions that the patient is allowed to have the traction removed. Also, be sure to get instructions on the amount of time the patient is allowed to be out of traction and any activity limitations when out of traction.

If the patient is allowed to be out of the traction for short periods, use the following steps to remove the weights:
- Raise the weights slowly and smoothly, without jerking. If two weights are on the traction device, raise them evenly at the same time.
- As the weight is relieved and the harness straps

slacken, lift the weights off while holding the harness. Place the weights on the floor and remove the harness from the patient.
- To replace the weights, place the harness on the patient and stabilize with one hand while replacing the weights.
- As the weights are lowered and begin to exert their force, remember never to drop or jerk them. Do not lower them too quickly or unevenly, as this will cause pain for the patient.

Pelvic Traction

Pelvic traction is used infrequently in the acute care hospital, but it is seen in some facilities. Pelvic traction is used to treat minor fractures of the lower spine, low back pain, and muscle spasm. The pelvic belt is placed snugly around the pelvic area so that the lower edge is at or just below the greater trochanter. The doctor may order the foot of the bed elevated on blocks or the foot of the bed gatched (Fig. 11–6).

 Check skin under belt frequently for irritation, especially over the *iliac crest.*

Provide skin care by rubbing with lotion around, not on, any irritated areas. Padding may need to be applied to prevent pressure. A footboard will prevent *footdrop* and keep bed linen off feet.

Assist the RN by reminding the patient to do exercises (ankle circles and plantar/dorsiflexion of feet) to maintain muscle tone and help prevent blood clots. If the patient is unable to have the traction removed for a short time, a fracture pan should be used for toileting as it is more comfortable for the patient and requires less movement of the pelvis.

Mild exercises are very important for bed-bound patients. These are usually given to the patient by physical therapists, occupational therapists, and RNs. Make it a point to ask these members of the health care team for accurate instruction on exercises they have given your patient so you can reinforce them correctly.

Buck's Traction

Buck's traction (Fig. 11–7) can be applied to one leg or both. It is used primarily for immobilizing fractures of the femur and hip and simple fractures of the lower spine. One of the most frequent uses is to temporarily maintain the alignment of the bones and relieve pain and muscle spasm in hip fractures before surgery.* The foot of the bed is sometimes elevated for countertraction.

---

*Styrcula, L.: Traction basics: Part IV. Traction for lower extremities. Orthopaedic Nursing. Sept/Oct; 1994; 13(5):59–68.

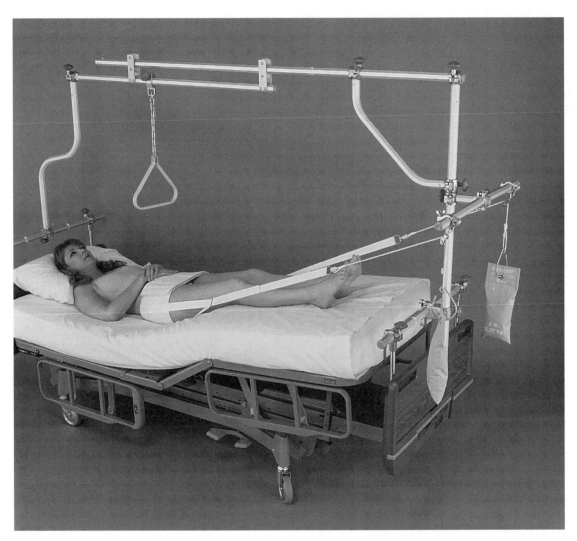

F I G U R E 1 1 – 6
Pelvic traction. (Courtesy of Zimmer, Inc., Dover, OH.)

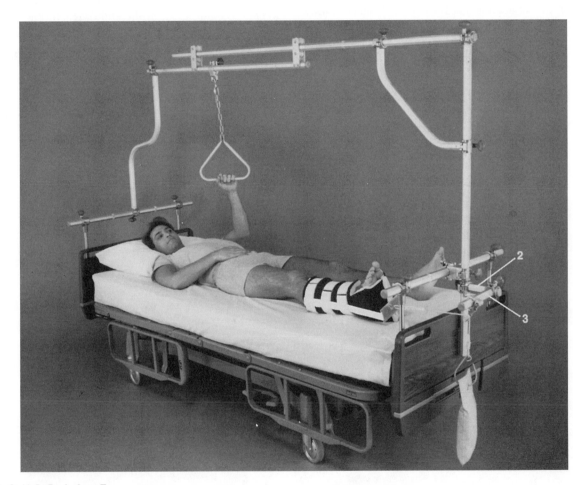

FIGURE 11–7
Buck's traction. (Courtesy of Zimmer, Inc., Dover, OH.)

Some specific precautions for patients in Buck's traction are:

- Observe for possible skin breakdown at the ankle and over the heel.

- Check circulation to assure that wrappings are not too tight by checking pedal pulses, color, temperature, and sensation of lower legs and feet at least every 2 hours.

- Maintain the foot in *dorsiflexion* by having foot at right angle to leg on a footboard to prevent footdrop (see Fig. 11–6). Do not allow any heavy linen or blanket to rest directly on the foot.

⚖ Only specially trained personnel can set up and adjust traction equipment. If you are specially trained and if permitted by the doctor's order, you may remove the wrapping on the leg for observation of the skin and for skin care.

Bryant's Traction

Some PCTs may work in the pediatric area and care for small children in Bryant's traction. This is a variation of Buck's traction and is used to treat fractures of the femur in children under the age of 3 years and weighing less than 30 pounds.* The legs are suspended at a 90-degree angle, and the buttocks should just clear the mattress when traction is in place. The child should be positioned supine with the bed flat. Traction cords and weights should be out of the child's reach (Fig. 11–8). *Note that the figure shows the crib with the siderails down so that the reader can see the traction. In practice, never leave a child alone with the siderails down.*

Styrcula L: Traction basics: Part IV. Traction for lower extremities. Orthopaedic Nursing. Sept/Oct; 1994; 13(5):59–68.

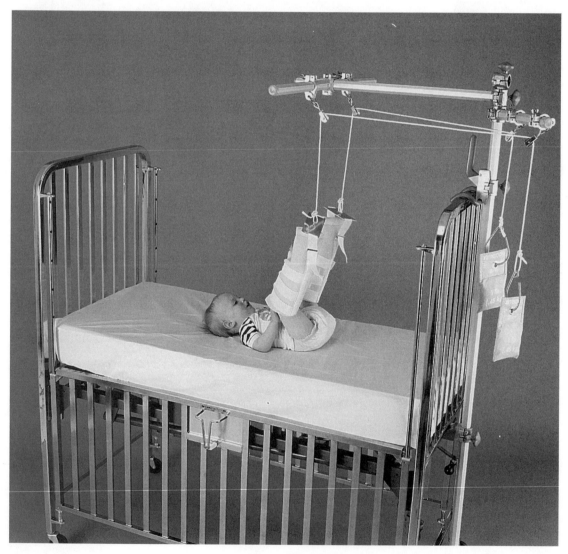

FIGURE 11–8

Bryant's traction. (Courtesy of Zimmer, Inc., Dover, OH.)

✔ Observe to make sure no pressure is on the back of the knee and the outer aspect of the fibula where the peroneal nerve is located (Fig. 11–9). Continued pressure over the peroneal nerve results in footdrop.

Check circulation in both feet at least every 2 hours by observing color, coolness, and pedal pulses. Also observe for motion and sensation. Observe the skin on the child's back and back of the head for any irritation. Report any abnormal or unusual findings to the RN. The child may need support and comfort when traction is first applied. The family should be encouraged to spend time with the child to help cope with the period of confinement.

⚖ A restraint may need to be used when the child is first placed in traction, but must be used according to facility policy and accrediting agency guidelines.

Skeletal Traction

Skeletal traction is accomplished by a pin or wire being surgically inserted through or attached to a bone. The traction apparatus is then attached to these pins or wires, and weights are applied. The pin is positioned so that it does not go through a joint, muscle, nerve, or artery. Many sites are used for skeletal traction. It can be placed on an arm, hand, wrist, leg, ankle, foot, finger, or toe.

Skeletal traction is most commonly used on the leg to immobilize femur fractures, and a balanced traction setup is used (Fig. 11–10). Countertraction is supplied by weights and not the patient's body. Balanced traction supports the extremity and exerts a pull in such a way that traction remains constant even when the patient moves. Balanced traction can be used with either skin or skeletal traction. This type of traction makes it easier to

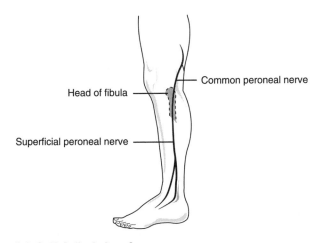

F I G U R E 1 1 – 9
Peroneal nerve drawing.

Head of fibula —
Superficial peroneal nerve —
— Common peroneal nerve

care for a patient and improves the patient's comfort. In many balanced traction setups, a ring is placed near the groin and may cause irritation of the skin. This area needs to be assessed every 2 hours and may need to be padded for protection from skin breakdown.

Skull tongs are used as part of devices to immobilize the cervical spine. The tongs are surgically implanted in the skull bones and traction applied. The head of the bed may be raised for countertraction. A variation of the skull tongs is the halo brace (Fig. 11–11). The brace is an external immobilization device worn by patients who have had injury to or surgery on the cervical spine. The patient can be fearful of moving and may not want to participate in ADLs. You need to establish a feeling of trust with the patient and provide encouragement and positive feedback. Remember that the patient's family will be affected by the stress of the halo, also.*

🎓 Check with the RN or social worker if the patient is depressed and not participating in normal activities. The patient may need counseling or a support group to help deal with the long-term psychological effects of confinement to the halo brace.

The brace is usually worn for 8–12 weeks, but may be worn longer.† During that time the patient can resume many of the activities he or she performed before surgery. Physical and occupational therapy can be performed to speed rehabilitation.‡ The brace has metal struts that are attached to pins inserted into the bone. These metal struts or bars are attached to a plastic brace or body vest that keeps the cervical area immobilized while allowing movement by the patient. To transfer a patient in a halo brace, never hold or pull on the rods or any part of the brace. You can safely use a stand-pivot transfer or a sliding board seated transfer. The brace or body vest is often lined with sheepskin that must be kept clean and dry. The sheepskin lining must be inspected frequently. When the lining needs to be changed it must be done by an expert technician or rehabilitation nurse.

🎓 Have your RN, physical therapist, or occupational therapist give you instruction and demonstrate the best way to transfer a patient in a halo brace.

 Never hold or pull on the rods or any part of a halo brace.

*Olson, B., Ustanko, L., and Warner, S.: The patient in a halo brace: Striving for normalcy in body image and self-concept. Orthopaedic Nursing. Jan/Feb 1991; 10(1):44–50.

†Mangum, S., and Sunderland, P.: A comprehensive guide to the halo brace. AORN Journal. Sept 1993; 58(1):534–546.

‡Styrcula, L.: Traction basics: Part III. Types of traction. Orthopaedic Nursing. July/Aug. 1994; 13(4):34–44.

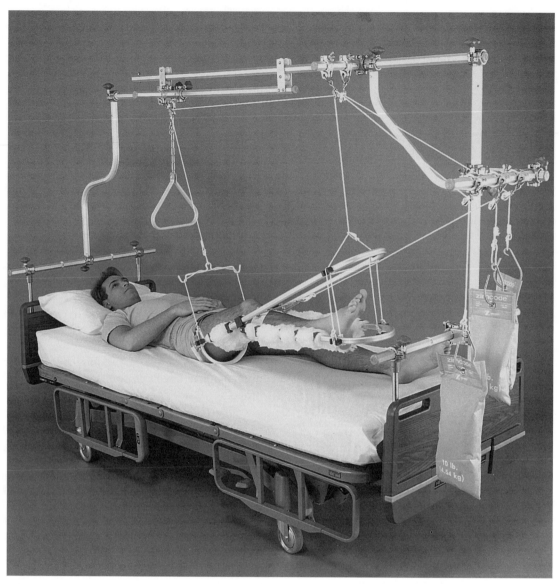

F I G U R E 1 1 – 1 0
Balanced skeletal traction. (Courtesy of Zimmer, Inc., Dover, OH.)

PIN CARE PRECAUTIONS. Because the skin barrier is broken where pins insert into the bone, there is very real danger of bone infection, which is difficult to treat successfully. Because of this, special care must be given to the pin sites. It is a good practice to observe the pin sites each time care is given and every 2 hours when turning the patient.

⚖️ In some facilities pin care may be one of the duties given to the PCT after special training. Be sure to check with your facility and follow procedures very carefully.

Take care that pin sites do not get wet when bathing the patient. Slight *serous* oozing of clear fluid that dries

and crusts at the site is often seen. Because of the chance of drainage, you should use gloves when bathing the patient in that area. The doctor may order the pin sites to be kept dry except for when the RN does pin care, usually every 8 hours, using hydrogen peroxide, Betadine, or alcohol, depending on the doctor's order. This removes any drainage that has dried around the pins. Doctors and facilities may have different methods of caring for the pin sites.* Some doctors may order gauze around the pins, in which case you would not be able to observe the skin directly around the site. However, you should observe for drainage on the dressing and other signs of infection like

---

Jones-Walton, P.: Clinical standards in skeletal traction pin site care. Orthopaedic Nursing. March/April, 1991; 10(2):12–16.

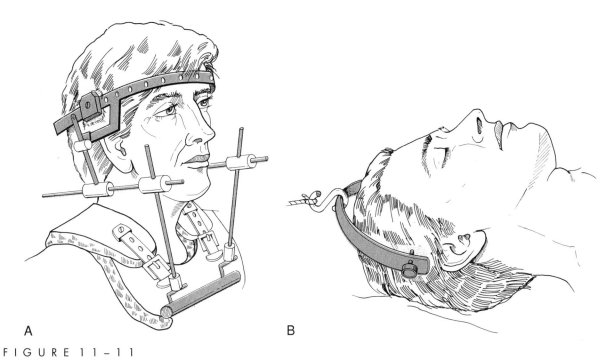

FIGURE 11–11

A, Halo vest and *B,* skull tongs. (From Linton, A., Matteson, M. A., Maebius, N. K.: Introductory Nursing Care of Adults. Philadelphia, W.B. Saunders, 1995.)

pain at the site or a fever. When dressings are not used, you can observe the actual pin site when you are giving care.

Indications of infection include redness, heat, drainage, odor, pain, or fever. These signs and symptoms should be reported immediately to the RN.

To prevent infection, instruct the patient not to touch the area around the pins. Observe for any loose pins and report them to the RN. After traction is discontinued and wires are removed, a small, sterile dressing may be applied over the site by the RN, and after special training you may be assigned this task. Be sure to observe for any drainage on the dressing and any swelling, heat, or pain at the site.

Complications of Immobility in the Traction Patient

All patients immobilized by any form of traction are at risk for the complications of immobility. Specific symptoms to watch for in the patient in traction are:

- Pressure sores: Pressure areas occur where any of the traction equipment comes in contact with the body, and where the body rests on the bed. Frequent inspection and good hygiene are important. If you cannot see the skin under the patient, use a flashlight and have the patient raise up slightly. You may also need to use a mirror to see certain areas. Always feel the skin under the patient to check the patient's sensation and feel for

any areas that may cause the patient irritation or pain. If there is a chance that the patient has broken skin or weeping sores, wear gloves when feeling the skin. Any wrinkles in the bedding should be eliminated. Crumbs that might be in the bedding should be removed. You may need to have traction devices adjusted or place padding on them to protect the skin. Inspect the sharp bars and clamps of the traction apparatus. There are foam balls, corks, plugs, and tape that can be used to cover any sharp areas to protect caregivers and visitors and to keep bed linen from catching on them.*

- Hypostatic pneumonia: Inability to turn and breathe deeply while lying in bed can lead to a slow, shallow respiratory pattern. This can lead to pooling of fluid in the lungs and hypostatic pneumonia. Emphasize the importance of deep breathing and frequent repositioning within the allowed activity for the patient.

- Contractures: Joint mobility, muscle strength, and circulation can decrease rapidly with the patient immobilized. This can lead to contractures and muscle wasting that will impair the rehabilitation process after the fracture is healed. Be sure to perform ROM exercises and teach the patient to do active ROM on any extremities that are able to be moved.

- Constipation: Patients undergoing traction are at risk of gastrointestinal complications. Many lose their appetite and suffer from constipation. Immobility slows the

---

*Styrcula, L.: Traction basics: Part II. Traction equipment. Orthopaedic Nursing. May/June 1994; 13(30):55–59.

movement of food through the digestive tract, causing more water to be resorbed. In addition, the pain medication prescribed for comfort can cause constipation. Many people have trouble using a bedpan, which can add to the problems with elimination. Food should be made as appealing and digestible as allowed. Under normal conditions, an adult should take in 2000–2400 ml (8–10 eight-ounce glasses) of water each 24 hours. The immobile patient should have an intake of at least 3000 ml of fluids to help prevent constipation. The RN may ask the dietician to consult with the patient and may ask the doctor for a laxative or medication to soften the stool. However, it is better for the patient if the constipation can be relieved by fluid, fiber, and activity, rather than by medication.

✔ Offer fluids frequently and help the patient choose foods from the menu that are high in fiber. Alert the RN if the patient is suffering from constipation.

- Deep-vein *thrombus*: A thrombus is a blood clot that can obstruct a blood vessel and can become detached and travel to other areas such as the lungs. When a blood clot travels to another part of the body it is called an embolism. It is a dangerous complication of immobility when a patient is in traction. It occurs from pooling of venous blood due to lack of muscle tone and lack of muscle contractions. Any complaint of pain in the calf is a serious problem and should be reported immediately to the RN. Pressure on areas behind the knee can cause obstruction of blood flow and increase the chance of clots. It is very important to observe the legs for any restriction of circulation and to change position frequently to relieve any pressure on blood vessels. The ankle and foot exercises mentioned earlier help to promote circulation and to prevent deep-vein thrombus.

Role of Patient Care Technician in Care of Patients in Traction

As a PCT caring for patients in traction, you have a very important role. There are specific guidelines for care and serious symptoms to observe for that need to be communicated to the RN promptly. The following are important considerations when caring for a patient in traction.

CARE GUIDELINES FOR PATIENTS IN TRACTION

- Maintain patient in proper body alignment to ensure the force or pull on the extremities is straight in line with the bones.
- Weights must hang freely from the bed. Check weights often to be sure they are not touching the floor.

- *Never* lift the weights of a patient who is in skeletal traction to relieve the pressure until the doctor orders traction discontinued.
- Question patients as to their understanding of the purpose of the traction and reinforce the need for them to maintain the bed position and body alignment.
- Instruct the patient how to use the overhead trapeze bar for self-movement and encourage the patient to use it to help you give patient care. Use of the overhead trapeze will also strengthen the upper body.
- Observe the condition of the traction cords, making sure they are not weakened or frayed.
- Observe for signs of decreased circulation or pressure on nerves and report them immediately to the RN. See the following section on the care of casts for specific signs of decreased circulation to observe for and report.
- Carefully observe the skin for signs of pressure ulcer formation. Sheepskin heel protectors and bed pads may be used for protection to reduce irritation of skin.
- Traction applied for the purpose of stabilizing a fracture will be continuous traction and must not be disconnected unless ordered by the physician.
- Skull tongs can become dislodged accidentally and press on soft tissue, causing severe pain. Be careful when giving patient care and report any unusual findings to the RN immediately.

CASTS

Casts are a form of immobilization of the trunk or a body part to enable a fractured bone to heal. They must be contoured to the body part to provide maximum immobilization and proper mending of the bone. When a patient is repositioned, the cast must be supported and the body kept in good alignment with pillows. Because a cast is heavy, assistance should be obtained when transferring a patient. A trapeze on the bed is helpful to assist the patient to move around in bed. If allowed by the RN, it is helpful to elevate the injured extremity slightly higher than the heart to help prevent swelling and tightness that might occlude circulation. There are often restrictions as to which side you may position the patient. Check with the RN for positioning guidelines. Often, the patient may not lie on the injured side. The cast should be checked for tightness or swelling every shift and more often if necessary. You should be able to easily slip one finger between the cast and the patient's skin.

PCTs may be asked to help with the application of a new cast. As a new cast is drying you may be asked to turn the patient frequently to permit air to circulate to all parts of the cast. Support the cast with the palm of your hand, not your fingers, when turning the patient. Do not cover the cast. That will hold heat in and prevent drying of the cast materials. In a newly casted extremity, it is important to observe the exposed parts, such as the fingers and toes, for signs of decreased circulation.

Report any coolness, *cyanosis* (dark, bluish gray discoloration of skin) swelling, pain, or numbness to the RN immediately.

When caring for a patient in a cast, observe for the following:

- Skin irritation around the cast edges: Rough edges may be padded with tape or soft material to prevent irritation.

- Odor or drainage that might signal an infection underneath the cast: There is usually an odor of unwashed skin and perspiration from under a cast, but a foul odor can be a signal of infection. Tell the patient not to put anything under the cast to scratch areas that itch, as that may lead to skin abrasions or tears that can become infected.

- Keep the cast dry: A wet cast will cause skin irritation underneath. Protect areas of the cast that might get wet or soiled when toileting by covering with plastic during those times.

Report any of the following signs of decreased circulation or pressure on nerves:

- *Color*: Toes or fingers that are pale, bluish gray, or white. Nailbeds should be pink.

- *Temperature*: Coolness of toes or fingers. Compare the temperature of the casted arm or leg with the extremities without a cast.

- *Capillary refill*: Slow capillary refill. Capillary refill is checked by squeezing and releasing the nail bed and observing for the pink color to return. Capillary refill should be brisk.

- *Sensation*: Any numbness, tingling or pain. If the patient is unable to feel you touching his or her toes or fingers, this should also be reported to the RN.

- *Edema*: Swelling that might restrict circulation.

- *Movement*: Inability to move fingers or toes or any weakness in the extremities, including fingers and toes.

- *Pulse*: No pulse (pedal or radial) in an extremity that has a cast. Compare the pulse rates of both feet or both wrists. Check to make sure they are equal. Report any abnormal findings to the RN. If a cast covers the area where you need to take a pulse, the other signs must be used to check for proper circulation (color, capillary refill, and warmth). Sometimes the doctor will cut a window in the cast to palpate the pulses.

The PCT should reinforce the teaching of the RN and physical therapist. Usually instructions for ankle exercises, quadriceps sets, and ROM exercises are given to the patient by the physical therapist to help prevent loss of muscle tone and strength and to retain joint flexibility. Using the overhead trapeze when moving in bed can help the patient to keep upper body strength.

ROLE OF PATIENT CARE TECHNICIAN IN CARING FOR PATIENTS WITH MUSCULOSKELETAL DISORDERS

The PCT has an important role to play in caring for the patient with musculoskeletal system disorders. Mobility and mild exercise help to maintain joint function, muscle strength, and coordination and prevent complications of immobility. The PCT spends a great deal of time at the bedside with the patient observing signs that need to be reported to the RN. This is a critical part of the role of a PCT. Patient education is another very important part of the PCT's role. Education is extremely important in helping patients return to independent functioning. It is important for the PCT to learn what the patient needs to know to return to the highest level of functioning and be able to reinforce that teaching. It is also important for the PCT to ask questions and clarify instructions given to the patient. When the patient has difficulty with new information and asks questions, the PCT must know when to seek the advice of experts and not try to clarify for the patient. *Wrong information can be as harmful as no information.*

Caring for patients with musculoskeletal disorders can involve assisting them to move while you are in an awkward position. Also, patient casts are very heavy, and you will need to obtain assistance when moving or transferring patients. Working with these patients can cause strains and back injuries for the PCT if proper body mechanics are not used.

Follow the basic principles of body mechanics when performing patient care.
1. Always have a wide base of support.
2. Use strong muscles in the legs by bending your knees to lift.
3. Avoid bending or twisting when lifting.
4. Hold the load close to your body and the center of gravity.
5. Obtain help if you will need to move more than half your own body weight.
6. Know the precautions for your patient.

REDUCING THE HAZARDS OF IMMOBILITY

Bedrest is meant to reduce physical activity so that tissues can heal and swelling and inflammation will be

COMPLICATIONS OF IMMOBILITY

Cardiovascular System
Increased work on heart
Orthostatic hypotension
Deep vein thrombosis

Respiratory System
Slow and shallow respirations
Pooling of respiratory secretions
Hypostatic pneumonia
Pulmonary embolism

Gastrointestinal System
Poor appetite
Poor nutrition
Constipation, fecal impaction

Urinary System
Urinary retention
Increased risk of kidney stones
Incontinence
Urinary tract infections

Musculoskeletal System
Muscle wasting
Stiff joints
Decreased balance
Loss of endurance
Osteoporosis
Contractures, foot drop

Metabolic System
Loss of stored protein
Fluid imbalance, dependent edema
Electrolyte imbalance

Integumentary System
Pressure on bony prominences
Impaired circulation to skin layers
Skin breakdown

Psychological Well-Being
Depression
Poor self-concept
Social isolation
Sleep disturbances
Confusion

EFFECTS OF EXERCISE

Cardiovascular System
Increased blood flow to body tissue
Slower heart rate
Heart works more efficiently
Lower blood pressure
Improved venous return

Respiratory System
Lungs fill more completely
More efficient carbon dioxide excretion
More efficient use of oxygen

Gastrointestinal System
Increased appetite
Better intestinal tone
Improved digestion and elimination

Urinary System
More efficient excretion of body wastes
Increased blood flow to kidneys
Better maintenance of body fluid balance

Musculoskeletal System
Stronger muscles
Stronger, more dense bones
Better coordination
Increased joint mobility
Improved balance

Metabolic System
More efficient use of energy and calories
Better body temperature regulation

Integumentary System
Healthy skin
Improved tone, color and moisture of skin

Psychological Well-Being
Energy, vitality, general well-being
Improved sleep
Improved appearance
Improved self-concept
Positive health behaviors

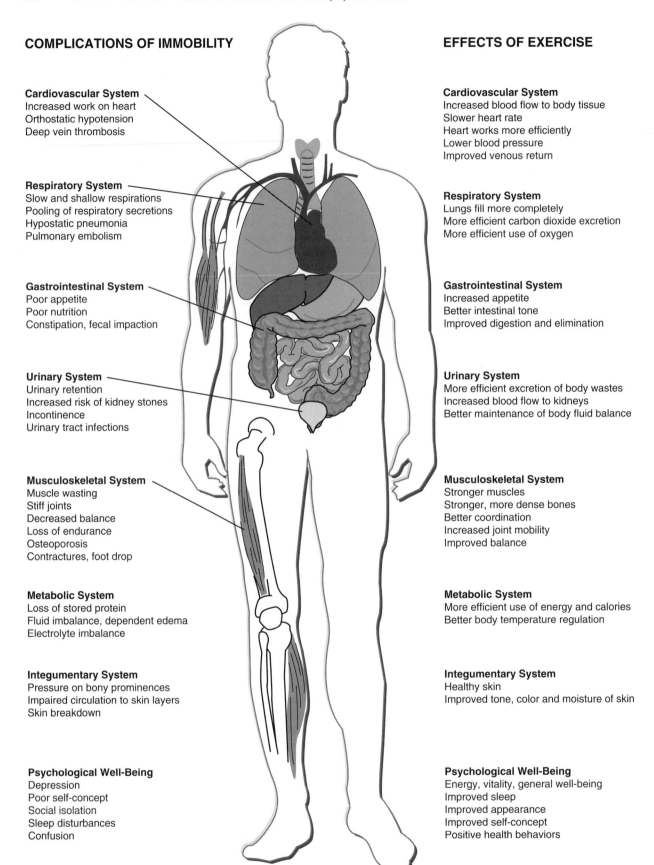

FIGURE 11-12

Complications of immobility and effects of exercise. (From Taylor, C., et al.: Fundamentals of Nursing: The Art and Science of Nursing Care, 2nd ed. Philadelphia, J.B. Lippincott, 1993.)

reduced in injured or diseased muscles and joints. When a person is sick and is required to spend time in bed, the intent is to have that rest period be helpful so the body can heal and be restored. Often there is a negative side to this immobility. The hazards of immobility (Fig. 11–12) and the interventions that the PCT should keep in mind when caring for patients follow.

- Cardiovascular complications of blood clots and orthostatic hypotension:
  - Remind patient to do exercises given by the physical and occupational therapist.
  - Encourage intake of adequate fluids to prevent dehydration.
  - Early ambulation as allowed
  - Proper positioning and avoidance of pressure on blood vessels
  - Do not massage the calf of the leg.
- Respiratory complications and hypostatic pneumonia
  - Remind patient to turn, cough, take deep breaths, and to use incentive spirometer.
  - Increase activity as soon as allowed by patient's condition.
  - Encourage fluids to keep lung secretions thinned.
- Gastrointestinal problems and constipation:
  - Offer adequate fluids.
  - Prevent incontinence by timely offering of the bedpan and early mobility for access to the bathroom.
  - Monitor patient's appetite and ask RN to assess for need of a dietician consult.
- Urinary incontinence and kidney stones:

- Keep accurate record of intake and output
- Observe for pain in the back and blood in the urine.
- Observe for signs of urinary tract infection: pain with urination, frequent urination of small amounts, feeling the need to urinate all the time, concentrated or cloudy urine.
- Muscle atrophy and contractures:
  - Perform passive ROM exercises for patients who are unable to do them and instruct patients who are able to do active or active-assistive ROM.
  - Position patients properly in bed, using good body alignment.
  - Remind/instruct patients to use good posture.
  - Remind and reinforce any exercises given to patient by physical or occupational therapists and RN.
- Skin breakdown
  - Observe for any sign of redness or sores on the skin.
  - Keep skin clean and dry.
  - Keep bedding free of wrinkles and crumbs.
  - Turn patient at least every 2 hours to reduce pressure on bony prominences.

SUMMARY

PCTs provide many valuable contributions to the care of patients who suffer from musculoskeletal disorders. PCTs are especially helpful when they recognize symptoms that need to be reported, provide care cautiously, ask questions when in doubt, promote patient independence, and reinforce the RN's patient education.

12

The Integumentary System

DONNA J. BRUST, MS, RN,C

PREREQUISITE KNOWLEDGE AND SKILLS

- AM and PM Care
- Personal hygiene for complete-care patient
- Assisting with partial-care patient's bath or shower
- Cleansing the perineal area
- Application of a condom catheter
- Giving back rub
- Assisting with oral hygiene
- Cleaning dentures
- Grooming hair
- Shaving a patient
- Giving nail care
- Bed making

OBJECTIVES

After you complete this chapter, you will be able to:

- List structures and functions of the integumentary system.
- Describe normal observations associated with the integumentary system.
- Discuss common disorders of the integumentary system.
- Identify causes of common integumentary disorders.

- Explain how to prevent pressure ulcers.
- Recognize signs and symptoms of disorders that need to be reported to the RN.
- Select and implement interventions with the RN.
- Document observations and care given.
- Reinforce RN's instructions in patient education.

KEY TERMS

Abdominal Binder   An apparatus that wraps and supports the area in front of the body below the breasts and above the pubic area

Bacteriostatic   Ability to halt the growth of microorganisms

Barrier Film   A type of dressing that prevents moisture from touching skin and damaging it. Generally used to prevent urine or feces from touching the skin, but also used to avoid the risk of abrasion and friction

Bony Prominence   Areas where bones are close to the thinnest skin and bear weight when one sits or lies down for a long time, such as hips, heels, lower back, elbows, and shoulders. Sores often form on these ''pressure points.''

Breakdown   An injury to the skin and the tissue under it, generally caused by unrelieved pressure

Colitis   Inflammation of the large intestine

Contracture   A condition of fixed tightened muscles due to nonuse

Débride   To remove dead tissue, blood clots, scabs, or dry crusts on a wound

Decubitus   Sometimes called bed sores; an injury to the skin and tissue under it usually caused by unrelieved pressure. Decubitus often happen to people who are bedridden and not very active.

Denuded   Severe injury leading to removal of the first layer of the skin

Diabetes Mellitus   A serious condition of the endocrine system in which the body is unable to use sugar to make energy. Poor circulation is sometimes a consequence of this condition.

Diaphoresis   Excessive sweating

Edema   Excessive fluid in body tissue causing swelling. This swelling interferes with good blood flow.

Electrolytes   Molecular substances that dissociate into ions when in solution and capable of conducting electricity

Excoriation   A severe abrasion or stripping off of the skin

Fissures   A split or crack in the skin surface

Fungus   A type of microorganism that can cause a spongy growth on the skin with excessive moisture, darkness, and warmth

Gangrene   Death of tissue that is caused by the lack of a good blood supply

Gastroenteritis   Inflammation of the stomach and intestines that causes discomfort

Granulation Formation of new skin granules

Impaction Tightly wedged stool in the intestine

Incontinence Inability to control urination and/or bowel movements

Knee Gatch A movable part on a bed that bends the knees and prevents a patient from sliding down

Maceration Wasting away of the skin due to soaking in moisture

Metabolism The changing of foodstuff into heat or energy; all the physical changes that go on in the body

Microbes Microorganisms such as bacteria, fungi, and viruses

NPO Abbreviation that means Nothing by Mouth

Ostomy A surgical opening

Perineum Area between the vulva and anus in the female and between the scrotum and anus in the male

Sebaceous Containing an oily, fatty matter secreted by a gland

Shearing Pulling or stretching of the skin that interrupts the blood supply to the skin and can cause pressure sores. This happens when a person confined to a bed slides slowly downward from a sitting position.

Stoma A small opening

Stripping A tearing away of the skin, usually by adhesive material

Supine Lying with the face upward

Topical Spray Medication applied to the skin's surface

Tunneling Passage under the skin

Wick The process of drawing solutions up and out of the source

The integument, or skin, is the natural covering of the body and is the largest body system. Sweat glands, hair follicles, oil, and nails are part of this system. In addition to helping form our self-image, the skin performs many physiological functions, including protection, temperature regulation, feeling of temperature and pressure, and vitamin creation and excretion. The skin is so extensive and performs such different functions that it affects, and is affected by, all other body systems. When any break in the skin occurs by tearing, pressure ulcers, burns, lesions, punctures, or cutting, steps need to be taken to prevent or control infection, promote new skin growth, control pain, and provide emotional support.

STRUCTURE AND FUNCTIONS OF THE INTEGUMENT

Structure

The skin has three layers: epidermal, dermal, and subcutaneous (Fig. 12–1). The epidermis is the outer skin layer in direct contact with the external environment and contains skin pigment that gives color to the skin. The cells of the epidermis constantly change and move forward as this layer regenerates itself. Specialized cells in this layer serve as touch receptors on the palms and soles and genital and oral areas. Other specialized epidermal cells also play a role in immune reactions of the skin. Glands that produce sweat, hair follicles, fat, and nails are also in this layer.

The dermis is a dense layer of tissue beneath the epidermis and gives the skin most of its substance and structure. The skin's lymphatic, vascular (blood supply), and nerve supplies are here. The dermis contains the body's major sensory (feeling) apparatus, with nerve fibers that form a complex network that registers pain, touch, cold, and warmth.

The subcutaneous layer, sometimes called the adipose layer because of its fat content, is connective tissue. The primary functions of this layer are insulation from extremes of heat and cold, a cushion to trauma, and a source of energy and hormone metabolism.

✓ Any disruption or damage to the integumentary structures or to the nerves or vessels that supply it alters its functions and puts patients at risk for infection, pain, disfigurement, and low self-esteem, since skin appearance is closely linked to self-image.

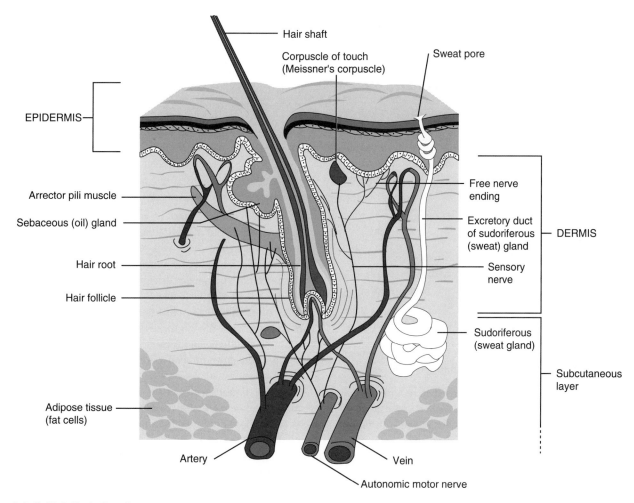

F I G U R E 1 2 – 1
The three layers of the skin.

Functions

The intact epidermal layer is a protective barrier against bacteria, foreign matter, and other organisms. The oily and acid secretions of the sebaceous glands protect the body further by limiting the growth of many organisms. Blockage of these glands is associated with acne and "pimples," occurring most commonly on the face and back.

The skin forms a barrier that prevents loss of water and electrolytes from the body and prevents the subcutaneous tissue from drying out. In general, it adjusts the body's metabolic heat production. The skin's blood flow determines the rate of heat loss. For example, either local or systemic (throughout the body) infection increases the metabolism (activity) of body cells. Heat is produced and blood flow increases. Localized skin infections appear red and warm to the touch. People with systemic infections have increased body temperatures, and the skin appears flushed (reddened) and warm to the touch as increased blood flows to the skin in an attempt to lose heat and

lower body temperature. If the skin is exposed to cold or the internal body temperature falls, the blood flow through the skin decreases and conserves body heat.

Nerve endings in the skin are responsible for responding to hot, cold, pain, light touch, and pressure. They have varying concentrations over the body. Nerves normally "tell" the body when to move to relieve pressure on the skin.

While not completely understood, itching is unique to the skin and mucous membrane. The skin also indicates emotion through color changes, as in the blush of embarrassment, pallor of fear, or the redness of anger.

The patient care technician (PCT) needs to understand the skin's basic structures, normal function, and common disorders to recognize the abnormal. While the RN is ultimately responsible for identifying and determining treatment for the patient's skin problems, the PCT is especially valuable because of close contact with patients during personal care. The PCT should be alert to abnormal signs and symptoms, prompt in reporting and documenting, cost-effective when initiating care, and sensitive to patient comfort, and should consult appropriate resources when needed.

DISORDERS OF THE INTEGUMENTARY SYSTEM

There are several types of disorders of the integumentary system:

Bacterial: Acne vulgaris, carbuncles (boils), impetigo, cellulitis
Viral: Herpes genitalia, anal herpes, herpes simplex, shingles, warts
Fungal: Ringworm, yeast infections
Parasites: Pediculosis (lice), scabies (mites)
Systemic: Diabetic ulcers, circulatory diseases leading to leg ulcers, or sores that will not heal, Kaposi's sarcoma in AIDS patients, cancer lesions, dry skin
Allergic reactions: Contact dermatitis, drug reactions, rashes, eczema, insect bites
Trauma: Pressure ulcers, burns, irritation, friction, shear, skin tears, bruising, excoriation from incontinence

This chapter focuses on disorders that require special care or hospitalization. Skin disorders that are especially painful or life threatening are given special attention. Other skin conditions that involve extensive treatment or those that could have been prevented if identified and treated early are emphasized.

PRESSURE ULCER

Pressure ulcer, also referred to as skin breakdown, bed sore, decubitus ulcer, or pressure sore, is a serious complication of immobility and debilitation.

Pressure ulcers form when the weight of the patient's body or limb presses against a firm surface, pressing tissue against bony areas, and circulation is cut off to these cells (Fig. 12–2A). Without circulation, cells die, and what is referred to as a pressure ulcer or sore begins

to form. If the pressure continues, more cells are damaged and the "sore" gets larger. If the pressure is relieved (by repositioning, for example) and circulation is stimulated (by movement and massaging around the reddened area), circulation is increased and the sore is allowed to heal.

Other factors that can cause pressure ulcers are sliding down in the bed or chair, which causes blood vessels to be stretched or bent. This is called shear (Fig. 12–2B). Even rubbing or friction on the skin may cause minor pressure ulcers.

Once a pressure ulcer forms, it can be difficult to treat. Therefore the best treatment for a pressure ulcer is prevention. The first step in prevention is to identify patients who are at risk. Patients who tend to develop pressure ulcers are those with paralysis, chronic illness that requires bedrest, incontinence of urine and stool, poor nutrition, and impaired feeling or sensation. In addition, others at risk are those having poor circulation, contracture, diabetes mellitus, dehydration, edema, or previous pressure ulcers; those of advanced age or taking certain medications; and those who are obese or very thin or who slide down in bed or chair, requiring frequent repositioning.

Because pressure ulcers are such a serious problem, caregivers in most health care facilities assess patients' risk factors for skin breakdown on admission and periodically throughout their stay (Fig. 12–3). Tools for pressure ulcer risk assessment generally measure immobility, activity, exposure to moisture, nutrition, consciousness, friction, and shear. The more risk factors identified, the more at risk a patient is for pressure ulcers.

Based on the results of this assessment, a plan for prevention and treatment is initiated for those patients who are identified to be at risk for pressure ulcers. Results of the treatments are documented, and the patient's status is reassessed on a regular basis.

Where Pressure Ulcers Form

Pressure ulcers form where tissue is under pressure and circulation is limited. This may be where bony parts of the body press against other body parts, a mattress, or

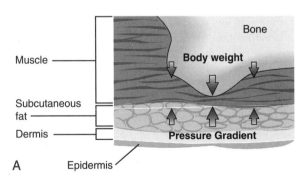
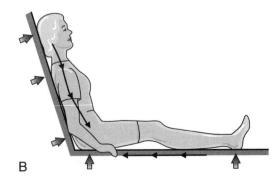

FIGURE 12-2

Pressure ulcers. *A*, "Tissue under pressure." *B*, Shear.

DERMAL/PRESSURE ULCER RISK ASSESSMENT TOOL

PARAMETERS	0	1	2	3	SCORE
General State of Health	good	fair	poor	critical	
Mental Status	alert	lethargic	semi-comatose	comatose	
Activity	ambulatory	needs help	chairfast (double score = DS)	bedfast (DS)	
Mobility	full	limited	very limited (DS)	immobile (DS)	
Incontinence	none	occasional	usually—urine or feces (DS)	total—urine & feces (DS)	
Oral Nutrition Intake	good	fair	poor	none	
Oral Fluid Intake	good	fair	poor	none	
Predisposing Disease/Treatment	absent	slight	moderate	severe	
Pre-existing Dermal Condition					Automatic 12
TOTAL SCORE					

GUIDELINES FOR USING TOOL

1. The higher the score, the greater is the potential for development of dermal/pressure ulcers.
2. Patients with scores of 12 or greater should be considered AT RISK and the protocol for the prevention and management of the patient with a dermal/pressure ulcer is initiated.
3. Documentation of risk assessment score
   a. Documentation of initial score with supporting rationale occurs in the original nursing assessment.
   b. Ongoing documentation of assessment score(s) with supporting rationale occurs in the Nursing Notes.
4. During the assessment, the nurse rates each parameter from 0–3 according to the following definitions:

General State of Health 0 = good (minor problem) 1 = fair (major but stable) 2 = poor (chronic/serious—not stable) 3 = critical	Incontinence 0 = none 1 = occasional (less than or 2/24 hours) 4 = usually—urine/feces (more than 2/24 hours) 6 = total—urine/feces (no control)
Mental Status 0 = alert (responds readily) 1 = lethargic (slow to respond) and/or inappropriate 2 = semi-comatose (responds only to verbal/painful stimulus) 3 = comatose (no response to stimulus)	Oral Nutrition Intake 0 = good (eats 75%–100% of meal) 1 = fair (eats 50%–74% of meal) 2 = poor (eats < 50% of meal) 3 = none and/or receives tube feeding
Activity 0 = ambulatory (without assistance) 1 = needs help 4 = chairfast 6 = bedfast	Oral Fluid Intake 0 = good (drinks 75%–100% of fluids offered) 1 = fair (drinks 50%–74% of fluids offered) 2 = poor (drinks < 50% of fluids offered) 3 = none and/or receives tube feeding
Mobility (Extremities) 0 = full (full active range of motion) 1 = limited (moves with limited assistance) 4 = very limited (moves only with assistance) 6 = immobile	Predisposing Disease/Treatment (DM. neuropathies, vasc. disease, anemia, vasoconstrictive drugs, hypothermia) 0 = absent 1 = slight (not altering health status) 2 = moderate (altering health status) 3 = severe (major alterations in health status) Pre-existing dermal condition—automatic 12

FIGURE 12–3

Dermal/pressure ulcer risk assessment tool. (Courtesy of the Department of Nursing, Ohio State University Medical Center, Columbus, Ohio. Modified with permission from the article "Validity and Reliability of an Assessment Tool for Pressure Ulcer Risk," from the May 1988 issue of *decubitus*, © Springhouse Corporation, Springhouse, PA.)

a chair. In persons who must stay in bed, most pressure ulcers form on the lower back below the waist (sacrum), the hip bone (trochanter), and on the heels. Other areas depend on sitting positions. Pressure ulcers can also form on the knees, ankles, shoulder blades, back of the head, and spine (Fig. 12–4).

Role of Patient Care Technician in Skin Care and Early Treatment

 The most important treatment of pressure ulcers is prevention.

Pressure ulcers may appear in a matter of hours. Therefore, interventions for skin care and early treatment are those that maintain and improve tissue tolerance to pressure and protect against pressure, friction, and shear. The following are interventions that are critical for prevention and early treatment of pressure ulcers. They are approved by the U.S. Department of Health and Human Services as practice guidelines and can be implemented by the PCT.

- Recognize those patients with whom pressure ulcers are likely to develop. Every shift, systematically (for example, head to toe) inspect the skin, paying close attention to common pressure areas.

⚖ While it is the RN's responsibility to collect thorough and accurate data by a formal assessment, your acute observations (listening, looking, touching, smelling) and prompt reporting are critical for an effective care plan.

- Keep the patient's skin clean and free from moisture. Make sure the skin is free of urine, feces, and perspiration. Wash the skin at the time soiling occurs.

📢 Any rashes, abrasions, blisters, drainage, foul odors, heat, redness, hardened areas, complaints of tenderness, discomfort, or feeling of burning should be reported immediately to the RN and documented in the patient's chart.

- Avoid hot water. Ask the patient or family if any soap is particularly irritating or drying to the patient and avoid using it. Apply moisturizers to dry skin and minimize situations that lead to dry skin such as exposure to cold and low humidity.
- Avoid massaging over bony prominences. Massage around them. When sources of moisture cannot be controlled, such as urine, perspiration, or wound drainage, use materials that absorb and present a quick-drying surface.
- Avoid using plastic incontinence pads directly against the patient's skin. Many specialty beds come with in-

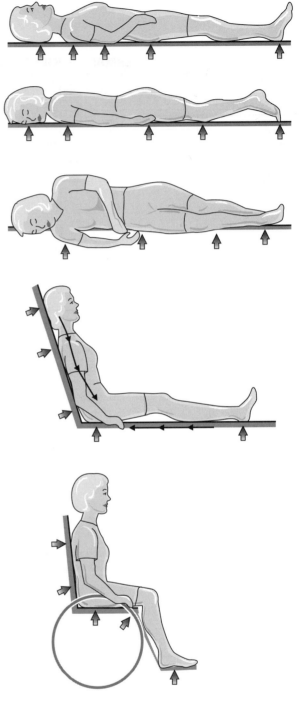

F I G U R E   1 2 – 4
Common pressure ulcer areas.

continence pads that wick away moisture without plastic backs. Reusable cloth pads may be used. Those that are not plastic may be placed directly under the skin.

- When any patient is immobile in bed, set up and adhere to a 2-hour minimum turning schedule. This shifting of weight allows blood to flow back into tissues for recovery from pressure.
- If a patient is able to help turn, put up a side rail so

he or she can assist. Ask about obtaining a trapeze bar or other assistive device.

- Encourage movement. With RN approval, get the patient out of bed whenever possible. Encourage active and initiate passive exercises to improve circulation. Gently massage areas around damaged skin to stimulate circulation. Maintain the patient's current activity level and mobility, since these reduce the effects of pressure on tissue.

Consult the RN, Clinical Nurse Specialist (CNS), Nurse Educators, Physical Therapist (PT), Occupational Therapist (OT), or Enterostomal Therapist (ET) to determine effective activity for patients with limited mobility.

- If additional activities are identified by these above resources, be responsible to carry them out throughout the day or as suggested.

- The majority of pressure ulcers occur over the bony pelvic area (sacrum, ischium and trochanter). Reposition the patient between supine position and 30-degree lateral position to avoid pressure on any bony prominence (Fig. 12–5). By limiting side-lying to 30 degrees, direct pressure on the trochanter is avoided.

- Reduce friction by applying lubricants (such as cornstarch and creams), protective films (such as transparent dressings and skin sealants), protective dressings (such as hydrocolloid), and protective padding (such as sheepskin, elbow or heel protectors). Apply moisturizers to dry skin. Apply powder where skin touches skin. Be careful when patient is using bedpan. Pressure from sitting on the rim and friction when putting the patient on and off the bedpan can create or worsen ulcers. Powdering the rim will minimize friction.

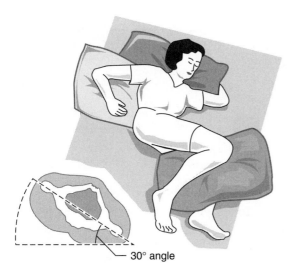

— 30° angle

FIGURE 12-5

Position the patient between supine position and 30-degree lateral position to avoid pressure on any bony prominence.

- Eliminate shear by elevating the head of bed no more than 30 degrees, which reduces the pull of gravity and sliding of tissues; position feet against a padded footboard, and use the knee gatch, which prevents sliding down in bed.

- Use a pull or draw sheet to move patients during transfers and position changes. This prevents dragging the patient's skin across the bed. If the patient is sitting, use a footstool and put a sheet behind the patient's back to keep the skin from sticking to the chair back.

- Use devices such as pillows, blankets, and foam that totally relieve pressure on the heels (Fig. 12–6). Ulcers on heels are among the most difficult to heal. Be aggressive with prevention strategies.

STOP Do not use donut-type devices on any area for pressure relief.

- Use pillows, wedges, or foam to keep bony prominences (knees or ankles) from direct contact with each other.

- When a patient is identified at risk for developing pressure ulcers, inquire about obtaining a pressure-reducing device, such as foam, air, gel, or water mattress (Fig. 12–7).

STOP When pressure-relief mattresses are used, avoid placing additional layers of linens, pads, and the like between the patient and mattress. This added material defeats the purpose of the mattress and adds potential for friction and shear.

- Keep linens clean, dry, and free of pressure-causing wrinkles. Watch for objects or equipment that can get under the patient while in the bed or chair such as needle caps, stopcocks, and IV, oxygen, or catheter tubing. Lying on these tubes can cause additional pressure.

- When a patient who is identified at risk for breakdown is in a chair (or wheelchair), set up and adhere to a strict 1-hour repositioning schedule. This shifting of pressure points is necessary to relieve the increased pressure caused by sitting. If a patient is able, encourage shifting of weight every 15 minutes. When at-risk

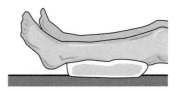

FIGURE 12-6

The heel is kept totally off the mattress.

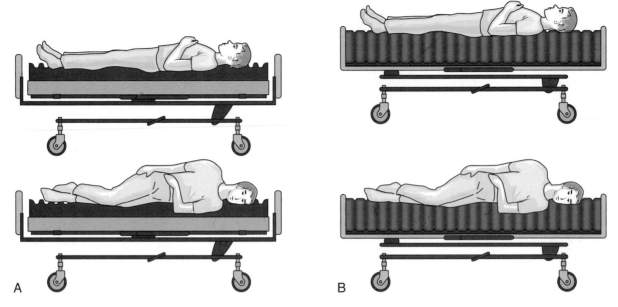

FIGURE 12-7

Pressure-reducing devices. *A*, Foam mattress (helps with the prevention of pressure sores). *B*, Air bed (generally used when pressure sores are established).

patients are in chairs, set them on foam, gel, or air pads, etc., that distribute weight evenly over the seating surface and reduce pressure (Fig. 12–8). Ask the RN if the at-risk patient may have foods that are high in protein, carbohydrates, and vitamin C and increased fluids. If permitted, encourage these through the shift. Pressure ulcers develop more quickly and are more resistant to treatment in patients with poor nutrition. Spend time with the patient to determine the reason for reduced intake and offer support during meals. Unless contraindicated, encourage fluids.

• Help keep instructions for patient care up to date and in plain site for all caregivers. These instructions should spell out exactly what to do, which staff member should do the task, how often it is to be done, what products are needed, and what the end goal should be (Fig. 12–9). Every caregiver can contribute appropriately when there is a well-defined plan of care.

• Post pictures that describe pressure-relieving positions, devices, and turning schedules so team members, the patient, and family members can help give consistent effective care (Fig. 12–10).

• Document the care that you provide and the patient's response. This information is necessary to re-evaluate the plan and change interventions when needed.

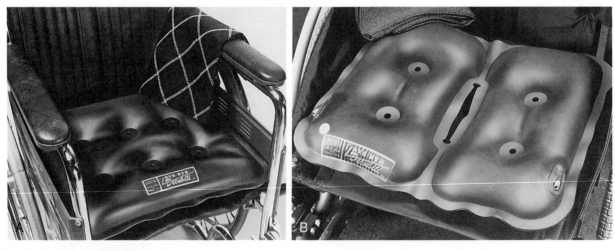

FIGURE 12-8

Devices that distribute weight evenly over the seating surface and reduce pressure. (Courtesy of Ken McRight Supplies, Inc., Tulsa, Oklahoma.)

PATIENT NURSING CARE PLAN		
Problem	**Expected Outcome**	**Plan for Care**
High risk for infection related to decubitus in pelvic area (coccyx) and patient diarrhea	Patient will be free of signs and symptoms of infection related to decubitus	1. Measure accurate vital signs every 4 hours (RN or PCT)
		2. RN assesses wound characteristics during dressing changes every shift 9 AM; 5 PM; 1 AM
		3. With assistance of PCT, RN will change wet-to-dry dressing and packing using sterile normal saline and gauze
		4. Follow posted 2-hour turning and activity schedule using pressure-relieving devices (RN, PCT, or family)
		5. If incontinence occurs, clean pelvic area with gentle soap and warm water; apply layer of moisture barrier cream; change damp linens and record (PCT, RN)
		6. Check hourly for incontinence (PCT, RN, family)

FIGURE 12-9
Instructions for care should be kept current and readily available to all caregivers.

 Example: *(Put date and time.)* Patient up in chair with one-person assist. Tolerated comfortably for *(total time).* Reddened area over coccyx reduced to size of lemon. Positioned on left side with pillow between knees. *(Then sign your name.)* T. Kraft, PCT.

Role of Patient Care Technician in Caring for Existing Pressure Ulcers

Sometimes a pressure ulcer develops despite all efforts for prevention. Pressure ulcers need to be treated quickly or they get larger and become painful and infected. They are made worse by continued pressure, moisture, heat, and lack of cleanliness. PCTs help when they carry out interventions aimed at reducing these situations and observe for changes in signs and symptoms such as new locations, increased redness, odor, drainage, and condition of the surrounding skin.

Licensed professionals are responsible for assessing existing wounds, identifying active ulcer stages, and determining treatment.

Changes of Tissue Damage in Formation of Pressure Ulcers

The changes of tissue damage in pressure ulcer formation generally develop through a series of four stages. Each stage progresses in severity, having different signs and symptoms that reflect a need for treatment.

STAGE I. Area of intact skin inflamed, reddened, blotched, or remains red for >5 minutes after removal of pressure (Fig. 12-11). A pressure ulcer begins as a small reddened area of intact skin over one of the pressure points of the body. This area remains reddened even when the patient's position is changed. If you press this area, you notice a lighter or paler color followed by a quick return to the red or dusky color.

Report this observation to the RN when first noticed.

Sometimes a reddened area is difficult to see on dark skin. It may appear dark blue or "purplish." Pay special attention to patients with dark skin who are at risk for skin breakdown.

Care You Can Give. Protect from additional insult or trauma. Keep the skin clean and dry. Initiate a plan for frequent turns or pressure-relieving devices. Many strategies for prevention and early treatment are appropriate for this stage and help remove the problem, such as getting the patient out of bed more often, increasing turns, putting up side rails or a trapeze over the bed so the patient can help in moving. Other choices are applying a protective film, moisture barrier, or nonadherent dressing as directed by the RN.

 Never put pressure on a reddened area or massage directly over it.

STAGE II. Area of skin blistered, superficially cracked, or broken through epidermis. You see the first sign of skin breakdown, a superficial skin loss or skin tear. The ulcer is superficial and looks like an abrasion, blister, or shallow crater (Fig. 12-12).

Care You Can Give. Notify the RN. With RN approval, wash the wound with a solution that stops or slows

TURNING / MOBILITY SCHEDULE

PATIENT: Frank Counts	**ROOM:** 1497 B
2400 Back - HOB↑ 30° pillow under ankles, knee gatched	1200 Bed R. side - peri care
0200 L. side, pillow betw. legs, buttocks open to air	1400 L. side - Blanket or pillow between knees, buttocks open to air
0400 R. side, pillow betw. legs, and under L. arm	1600 Back - HOB↑ 30° c̄ pillow under ankles to elevate heels
0600 Back - HOB↑ 30° pillow under calves to elevate heels	1800 Chair - cushion, footstool, arms on pillows
0800 L. side - pillow or blanket between knees	2000 R. side - pillow between knees, & under Ⓛ arm
1000 Chair - geomat cushion, footstool, arms on pillow	2200 L. side - pillow between knees, and under Ⓡ arm

FIGURE 12–10

Postings showing pressure-relieving positions, devices, and turning schedules.

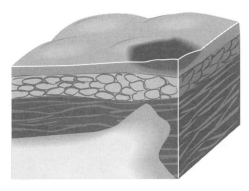

FIGURE 12-11
Stage I pressure ulcer.

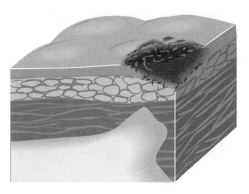

FIGURE 12-13
Stage III pressure ulcer.

the growth of bacteria. Depending upon the cause, a topical spray or barrier film without alcohol may be selected by the RN. Assist the RN by positioning the patient and observe for signs of wound healing.

 Never apply a dressing over a superficial wound without the RN observing it first.

STAGE III. Deep tissue involvement in skin break. You see full-thickness skin loss into subcutaneous tissue. You may see muscle and tendons (Fig. 12–13).

Care You Can Give. Observe characteristics of the dressing and surrounding skin. Remember that moisture and pressure are the biggest offenders of breakdown. Soiled or wet dressings need to be changed more frequently than dry, superficial ones. Dressings are soiled internally from drainage or externally from incontinence. Alert the RN when the dressing is damp and prepare to assist with the dressing change.

 Learn what dressings are being used and keep needed supplies readily available.

Carefully contain and dispose of the soiled dressing without contaminating yourself, the patient, or others.

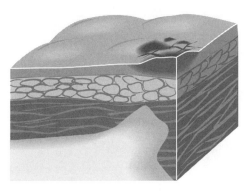

FIGURE 12-12
Stage II pressure ulcer.

With complicated dressings, your RN may consult an ET or a CNS for specific direction. When assisting the RN, maintain sterile technique.

When dressing changes increase in frequency, surrounded skin needs to be protected from the trauma of tape removal. Suggest the use of skin protective devices such as Montgomery straps or tape on top of solid wafer skin barriers (Fig. 12–14).

With your RN's approval, apply an abdominal binder to help hold a dressing on, or elastic net panties if the dressing is low on the abdomen or perineum.

STAGE IV. Deep tissue involvement exposing muscle and bone in skin break. You see full-thickness skin loss, extensive destruction, and tissue death. There may be tunneling of the wound, damage to bone and joint (Fig. 12–15).

 Stage IV is the most severe and life threatening.

Care You Can Give. The PCT closely observes for changes in the patient's condition such as elevated temperature, pulse, and respirations, decreased appetite, increased wound drainage and odor, decreased mental alertness, and additional complaints in this stage. When patients are unable to turn without putting pressure on another wound or are completely immobile, a pressure-relieving specialty bed should be considered. The PCT plays a key role in the successful use of special equipment by understanding their functions and how to operate them. Patients should float "like a pillow" on the mattress surface. Proper patient positioning and turning on this expensive bed is still necessary or the benefit of the specialty bed will not be realized. Know your specialty beds, chair cushions, and related equipment. Special slick turn or pull sheets are useful. Be alert for overinflated or underinflated cushions and high pressure alarms (Fig. 12–16).

Assist with and observe dressing changes. Help gather supplies to clean, treat, and dress the wound. Assist the RN in removal and containment of the soiled dressing.

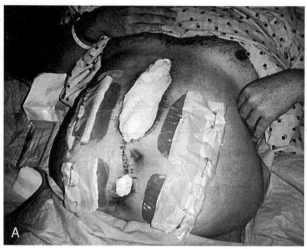
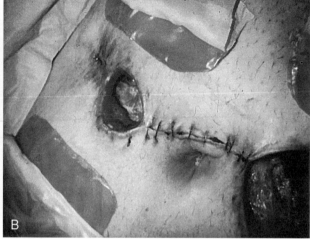

F I G U R E   1 2 – 1 4

Devices to protect against trauma of repeated tape removal. *A*, Montgomery straps. *B*, Wafer skin barriers.

Stage III and IV wounds are generally cleansed before being dressed. Therefore, protect the bedding and patient's gown from wound irrigation cleansing solutions. Assist with patient positioning for a gentle but thorough treatment.

Since the majority of stage III and IV ulcers are over the coccyx, trochanter, or gluteal folds, protection from stool and urine must be considered. Use strategies listed for urinary and fecal incontinence.

✓ If the treatment is painful to the patient, ask the RN about giving pain medication before the dressing change. Check the patient's level of comfort frequently throughout the treatment.

Wounds in stages III and IV require aggressive treatment that includes various products and pressure-relieving devices. While these are prescribed by licensed professional staff, the PCT is alert to when the prescribed treatment or special equipment is needed, restocks items, gathers supplies, and assists to provide consistent effective treatment.

GENERAL CARE FOR NONPRESSURE WOUNDS

For any wound in which skin is broken and tissue is damaged, including burns, leg ulcers, cancer lesions, and diabetic foot ulcers, the PCT can provide the following care:

- Implement strategies that are listed for prevention and early treatment of pressure ulcers.
- Protect the wound by using positioners, pillows, blan-

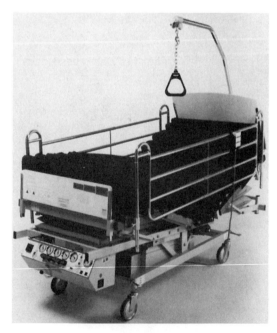

F I G U R E   1 2 – 1 6

A pressure-relieving specialty bed. (Courtesy of Mediscus Products, Inc.)

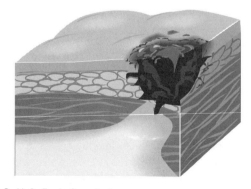

F I G U R E   1 2 – 1 5

Stage IV pressure ulcer.

kets, foam chair cushions, etc., to eliminate additional pressure, friction, shear, or trauma.

- Develop and post a specific turning/repositioning schedule with clear directions for staff so that the patient does not sit or lie on the wound for an extended period.

- Consistently follow activity orders such as ambulation, up in chair, range of motion, and gentle massaging around any bony prominence. These activities increase oxygenation and circulation and help the healing process.

✔ For efficient time management, notify the RN when the affected area is deliberately exposed, for example, during the bath. Prepare by coordinating this time with the RN's schedule for the RN to re-evaluate and medically treat the wound.

- Check with the RN for specific diet restrictions, then encourage the patient to eat and drink nourishing food and fluids with and between meals as permitted.

- Help control infection by good handwashing, observing changes in drainage characteristics such as amount, consistency, color, and odor. Drug-resistant microbes are on the increase and are most commonly found in areas where wounds are exposed. Therefore, in addition to gloving and handwashing, see that the patient's furniture, bed rails, blood pressure cuff, telephone, and other equipment are properly cleaned. Be prepared with appropriate attire such as personal protective equipment (PPE) before giving care. Be aware and cautious of moist areas where contamination can occur such as draining wounds, pelvic area (stool, urine, anal herpes, vaginal secretions), gastric tubes, oral secretions.

📢RN Any wound drainage with a foul odor generally needs additional evaluation. Alert the RN if a foul odor is present.

- Assist the RN to explore wounds for tracks that tunnel inward by positioning the patient. Help cleanse the wound and perform more frequent dressing changes. Soiled dressings with odors should be removed from the room.

✔ Exercise thorough handwashing, gloving, wearing a protective gown and mask when there is danger of splashing during dressing changes, and put contaminated material in plastic bags or wraps prior to disposal in designated infectious waste container.

- For all wounds, look at the surrounding skin for redness and other signs of involvement like rashes or allergic reactions.

✔ During care and treatments, observe your patient for signs of pain, discomfort, or stress. Alert the RN and help by responding with an appropriate comfort measure such as changing the patient's position, stopping treatment for a while to relieve pain, using a pillow to help support an extremity, or removing an unsightly or foul-smelling dressing.

- Document your observations and the care you gave on the appropriate form and sign your name. Using subjective (what the patient said) and objective (information gathered using the five senses) data, describe your observations and indicate that you notified the RN. Then sign your name.

📝 Example: (Put date and time.) Patient complained of tenderness in right foot during bath. Reddened area about size of nickel on side of foot and 1/2-inch "crack" between first and second toe with foul-smelling drainage noted. D. Brust, RN notified. Lanolin applied to feet and lambs' wool placed between toes. (Then sign your name.) B. Thomas, PCT.

SPECIFIC CARE FOR NONPRESSURE WOUNDS

Leg Ulcers

Many ulcers occur on the lower legs and feet because of poor circulation (Fig. 12–17). These are generally difficult to heal. Care and treatment of these wounds need to be consistent and specific.

ARTERIAL ULCERS. These ulcers are generally worse in patients who smoke, have diabetes, high cholesterol levels, and high blood pressure. Impaired circulation can be monitored through the quality of pulse. Therefore, accurately palpate lower extremity pulses as ordered. If a pulse cannot be palpated, use a Doppler (ultrasonic wave device) and report the results. Pain is the most common complaint by patients with arterial ulcers. Therefore, observe and report discomfort. Use precautions to prevent or identify early signs of infection. Observe for drainage, odor, color, and character of surrounding tissue. Use universal precautions and carefully dispose of wound dressings in biohazard boxes. Avoid heavy dressings and constricting clothing, socks, or footwear so that circulation is not further restricted and the wound can be closely observed.

🛑STOP Do not wrap the extremity with compression devices, stockings, dressings, or Ace wraps where an arterial ulcer exists.

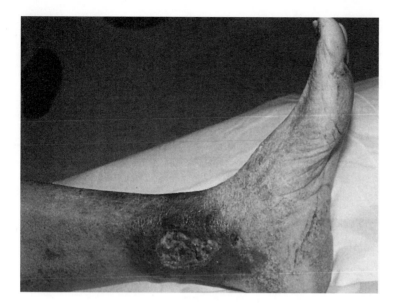

F I G U R E 1 2 – 1 7

A venous leg ulcer. (From McCarthy, W. J., Fahey V. A., Bergan, J. J., et al: The veins and venous disease. *In* James, E. C., Corry, R. J., Perry, J. F. (eds.): Principles of Basic Surgical Practice. Philadelphia, Hanley & Belfus, 1987, p. 463.)

Because edema (swelling) interferes with healing, help the patient avoid sitting for long periods or crossing the legs. Instead, slightly elevate the feet throughout the day, but not above the heart level. Weave lambs' wool or gauze between the toes to eliminate trapped moisture that can cause cracks.

VENOUS ULCERS. These ulcers result from disorders of deep veins. When venous pressure increases from conditions such as congestive heart failure, clots from pooling blood, inadequate valves, obesity, and muscle weakness, edema and ulceration occur. Treatment for venous ulcers centers around good nutrition, eliminating edema, and maintaining a moist wound environment.

Help reduce edema by elevating the legs as often as possible. Use elastic wraps on patients who are unable to tolerate elastic stockings. When ordered, graduated compression stockings should be applied before the patient gets out of bed and should be worn all day.

Intermittent pneumatic sequential compression devices (SCD) are frequently ordered to help reduce edema in the legs, assist blood return, and stimulate healing by inflating and deflating in a "milking" fashion up the leg. These leg wraps are generally worn while the patient is in bed or immobile in recliners.

✔ Unless ordered otherwise, remove compression devices for the bath, observe the skin's condition, apply lotion to dry skin, and reapply the device. Some SCDs have a cooling cycle that eliminates built-up heat and moisture. Turn this cycle on after SCDs are applied.

Diabetic Foot Ulcers

Diabetic persons often experience circulation problems that interfere with an adequate blood supply to the feet

(Fig. 12–18). They tend to experience decreased sensations in the feet and are not aware of injuries. High glucose levels in people with diabetes prevent normal healing. These patients are at risk for infections and gangrene, which can develop with absence of circulation. Amputation is frequently the result. Therefore, prevention and early treatment are essential.

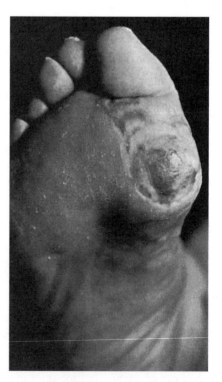

F I G U R E 1 2 – 1 8

A diabetic foot ulcer. (From Kozak, G. P., Campbell, D. R., Frykberg, R. G., Habershaw, G. M.: Management of Diabetic Foot Problems, 2nd ed. Philadelphia, W. B. Saunders Company, p. 71, 1995.)

Instructions for Care of the Diabetic Foot

1. Inspect the feet daily.

   Report any ulcers; red, white, or blue areas; warts; blisters; cuts; scratches; swelling and cracks between the toes to the RN.

2. Wash the feet with warm soapy water and dry thoroughly, especially between the toes.

3. If the feet are dry, rub a moisturizing lotion on them but not between the toes.

4. Keep feet safe by avoiding socks, slippers, or shoes that are tight and restrict circulation. Do not allow the patient to walk around barefoot.

5. Have the patient sit with both feet on the floor or footstool; discourage crossing of the legs.

6. If feet feel cold, put on socks. Avoid hot water bottles and hot water soaks.

7. Do not attempt to remove corns, calluses, or long toenails. Report these to the RN.

While it is well known that good foot care can prevent amputations, studies indicate that diabetics are not well educated about care of the feet. Reinforce this education with your diabetic patients.

If a diabetic foot ulcer exists, many interventions by the PCT are helpful:

- Help position the patient while the RN evaluates ulcers for size, depth, location, drainage, amount of black necrotic (dead) tissue, pink granulation tissue (new growth), and exposed bone and tendon. Observe the condition of the surrounding tissue for redness or heat.

- Assist with irrigating the ulcer to loosen surface debris and bacteria and thoroughly cleanse the wound.

- Apply a moisturizer to the dry, undamaged surrounding skin to keep it from drying or cracking further.

The selection of dressings depends on many variables, since wounds are different. There are dressings that débride (remove dead tissue) the wound, absorb drainage from it, retain moisture around it, and protect it from trauma. Generally a dressing is chosen that will keep the wound's surface clean and moist.

With regard to dressings, the PCT should remember to:

- Avoid using dry gauze dressings that stick to the wound and tear new tissue when the dressing is removed.

- Assist the RN to vigorously flush an infected wound that has yellow sticky drainage before applying the dressing. These dressings usually need to be changed more frequently than nondraining ones.

- Attach dressings without putting tape directly on the skin.

Cancer Lesions

Cancer is a condition in which certain cells of the body develop into nonfunctioning cells (see Chapter 13). They can grow rapidly and crowd out healthy functioning cells. Cancerous skin lesions can originate directly from types of skin cancer or develop from cancer that spreads from other parts of the body. Most strategies listed to care for other wounds apply to cancerous lesions. However, with cancer lesions, odors are often strong, and a thoughtful strategy must include control of offensive odors. Many products are available that absorb and cover odors. Effective strategies involve frequent dressing changes, containment of old dressing in a closed container, and removal of soiled dressings from the room.

Burns

Burns are a form of traumatic injury caused by thermal (heat), electrical, chemical, or radioactive agents. The severity of the burn depends on the depth, extent, age of the patient, part of the body burned, and condition of the patient. Whether partial- or full-skin thickness is involved, patients are at risk for infection. Apply strategies for comfort, wound protection, wound cleansing, and the principles of sterile technique while assisting with dressing changes.

Dry Skin

Dry skin is generally due to loss of natural moisture or inability to retain moisture. Wash with nondrying agents, avoiding soaps. Apply creams to restore moisture or ointments to protect the skin from loss of moisture. Inspect cracked areas for drainage or infection and report this to the RN. Protect dry skin from trauma and tearing, for example during transfers. Unless fluid is restricted, encourage increased fluids and nutritional supplements.

PROBLEMS ASSOCIATED WITH SPECIAL EQUIPMENT AND PRODUCTS

Pressure ulcers not only come from the weight of the body lying in one position for too long, they can come from splints, casts, restraints, dangling tubes, or bandages. Common examples of equipment that cause problems with skin breakdown are limb or body casts, Philadelphia collars, halos, condom catheters, tape, limb restraints, nasogastric tubes that pull tightly against the nose, tracheostomy tapes, oxygen masks that press on the nose and ears, catheters that pull, or attachment devices like stopcocks, clamps, and plugs.

The PCT is alert for potential problems with pressure from any external device.

 A properly fitting cast does not cause the patient pain or discoloration of a limb. Check patients with casts for discomfort, irritation, odors, drainage, or discoloration of tissue beyond the cast.

- The skin under or around any external supportive device must be inspected every shift for redness or signs of irritation. Skin under restraints must be checked at least hourly for signs of restriction, friction, or skin tears. The restrained extremity should be pink, warm to touch, and without swelling.

- Secure or stabilize all tubes not only to protect them from accidental pulling or migrating inward, but also from causing pressure near the exit site.

- Ask your RN or enterostomal therapist about devices other than tape, designed to secure tubes.

STOP Do not apply tape straight across a tube or skin crease. This maneuver applies pressure against the skin and places the patient at risk to develop a pressure ulcer or skin shear.

PROBLEMS RELATED TO MOISTURE

With pressure being first, moisture is the second biggest offender in skin breakdown. Urinary incontinence, diarrhea, and trapped moisture significantly contribute to disorders of the skin. PCTs perform tasks that address these situations in a prompt and efficient manner.

Urinary Incontinence

Incontinence as well as continual sweating (diaphoresis) are factors that can promote breakdown of superficial skin (Fig. 12–19).

The PCT is proactive with these prevention strategies and early interventions:

- Toileting is key in prevention. Provide the bedpan, urinal, or commode or help the incontinent patient to the bathroom on a 2-hour schedule or as soon as the request is made.

- Help the patient assume a normal position; give privacy and time to finish.

- With the patient's and RN's approval, apply a properly fitting condom catheter.

- Appliances for females are available.

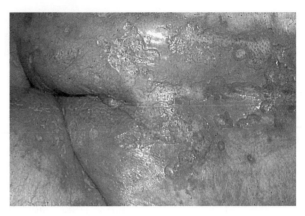

FIGURE 12–19
Maceration due to incontinence.

STOP Avoid propping urinals. Pressure and spillage lead to additional problems.

Once incontinence is apparent, skin protection must be initiated. Start with moisture barrier ointments.

Ask your RN or skin care specialist which moisture barrier ointment is appropriate for your patient.

After the skin has been cleansed, apply the moisture barrier. This ointment keeps the skin soft and lubricates the tissue.

After each incontinent episode, clean and dry the skin. A blower dryer on a cool setting may be used. Reapply the barrier ointment. Dry linens must be reapplied after each incontinent episode. Use incontinence pads or pants made of absorbent material that wick away urine from the patient. However, they must be checked frequently and changed immediately when moisture touches the patient's skin.

STOP Incontinence pants or "diapers" should be applied only for ambulating incontinent patients. They should be left unfastened and open for ventilation while the patient is in bed.

Most condom catheters need to be removed daily for hygiene and evaluation of the penis and reapplied. Candidates for condom catheters are those who when sitting have a penis shaft greater than 1 inch in length. Generally, patients who are not candidates for condom catheters are those who pull at tubing, have existing ulcers or rash on the penis or perineum, and are not able to be bladder trained.

If urine leakage is continuous or skin irritation develops, the skin must be further protected. Pretreated incontinence sprays or special wipes may be used, since they are gentle to the skin and generally more comfortable for the patient than washcloths, soap, and water. With the RN's approval, a mineral oil wash may be alternated with soap and water. It is not necessary to remove all the barrier ointment with each wash.

Trapped Moisture

Patients tend to develop excoriation and denuded skin where body parts rub or lie against each other causing increased moisture and maceration. Many skin rashes or ulcers occur around wounds or areas where moisture and heat are trapped, such as dressings over draining wounds, surgically placed feeding tubes, ostomy appliances, and deep skin folds where perspiration collects.

Candidiasis (a yeast infection) tends to grow in warm dark and moist areas of the body and is a common cause of skin rashes. This fungus is a normal inhabitant of the intestinal tract and a frequent contaminant of the vagina where discharge becomes thick and irritating (Fig. 12–20). When it is allowed to accumulate and grow on skin surfaces, however, breakdown and infection can occur.

Patient care is aimed at eliminating or controlling the causes of problems related to moisture and yeast. After consulting with the RN, the PCT can help solve problems related to trapped moisture with these suggestions:

- Check for trapped moisture around areas of the body where skin touches skin, such as under the breasts, between the folds of the buttocks, and between the thighs. In obese patients, look under "fat folds" on the abdomen, sides, legs, and back.

- Separate deep skin folds with soft material to absorb moisture. For example, pillow cases, abdominal pads, and other cotton material are effective moisture absorbers. Tuck them in the folds until you "hit bottom."

- Give perineal care to bedridden patients every 4 hours. Perineal care includes cleansing with a nondrying soap, applying a moisturizer where skin is dry, and applying

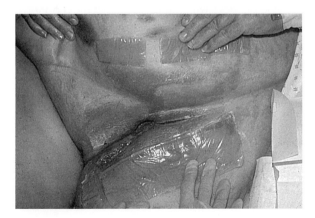

FIGURE 12-20
Yeast infection.

an ointment to prevent shearing and friction as well as to protect from the chemical effects of stool and urine.

- Inspect the skin under saturated or damp dressings, the groin, tube sites, breast and inguinal skin folds, and ostomy sites closely during bathing or times of contact.

✔ Secure all tubes. Do not allow them to "dangle" or pull against the surrounding skin or exit site. Closed-system drainage tubes and bags should also be attached securely to the bed or chair and not allowed to lie on the floor.

- Dust skin folds with absorbent powders such as cornstarch.

- Change dressings before the top layer becomes saturated. Avoid stacking dressings that just add more layers on top.

⚖ Wounds under the most routine dressings still need observation. RNs need to assess these wounds to determine healing progression and changes in treatment.

- Coordinate routine dressing changes and have supplies ready.

- Encourage the patient to take in nutritious foods and fluids as allowed. Frequent small feedings are helpful.

- Change an ostomy appliance that leaks or whose adhesive wafer is melting away from the stoma.

General Procedure for Changing an Ostomy Appliance

1. Gather equipment: soap, washcloths, towels, plastic container, scissors, pouch, wafer, stoma adhesive paste and powder, and if necessary a barrier film and adhesive remover.

2. Cut the stoma wafer the same shape as the patient's stoma and approximately 1/8 inch larger so that the wafer does not constrict the stoma after it is applied.

3. Remove the protective paper from the wafer.

4. Remove the old pouch while supporting the skin to prevent skin tearing. Dispose of the pouch in a biohazard bag.

5. Remove residue from skin by washing and wiping with a dry tissue. Wash around the stoma, rinse, and dry very well.

6. Treat reddened, excoriated areas around the stoma with a thin layer of stoma adhesive powder.

7. Have absorbent material ready to prevent any drainage from the stoma touching the skin until the new wafer is applied.

8. Apply a rim of stoma adhesive paste around the inner cut edge of the wafer or around the stoma.

9. Center and apply the wafer, pressing in and around the stoma and then out to the edge.

Most irritations around stomas are due to improperly fitting wafers. If leakage continues to occur after these steps, consult your RN or enterostomal therapist.

 Document your observations and the care you give.

Problems Related to Fecal Incontinence and Diarrhea

Fecal incontinence is the inability to control the passage of feces and gas through the anus. Diseases or injuries to the nervous system may cause anal incontinence, as well as delay in responding to the need to use the commode. During an acute episode of diarrhea, incontinence may result. Other causes of diarrhea include unrecognized impaction, viral or bacterial gastroenteritis, intestinal candidiasis, antibiotic therapy, ulcerative colitis, and enteral feedings, especially in the patient who is severely malnourished or who has been NPO for several days. Stool is an irritant and may result in rapid skin breakdown.

Generally the PCTs are the first to be aware of fecal incontinence and diarrhea in patients. Therefore, their preventive strategies, observations, prompt reporting, and early interventions are critical to prevent rapid skin breakdown. PCTs help when they:

- Respond quickly to a patient's request for the bedpan or assistance to the commode.
- Adhere to a toileting schedule.
- Encourage liquids and foods that contain fiber if the diet allows.
- Encourage activity as ordered.
- Monitor bowel movements every shift.

Alert the RN at the first episode of stool incontinence and report any sudden increase or decrease in fecal output or evidence of blood.

- Removing the cause is key to treatment. The information gathered from your observations and measurements helps the RN to determine the cause of incontinence and subsequent treatment.
- Clean and dry the skin immediately after an incontinence episode and apply moisture barrier ointments.
- Use a disposable or reusable bed protector. Be sure that plastic does not touch the skin, and change the protector immediately when it becomes wet or soiled.

Observe patients for signs of frustration, embarrassment, anger, and humiliation, since these are common emotions related to the psychological impact of incontinence. Be aware of your own nonverbal cues such as facial expressions that may communicate a negative feeling about cleaning an incontinent patient.

When incontinence cannot be controlled or managed by ordinary means, strategies to contain and measure stool are necessary until the underlying problem can be corrected. With the RN's and patient's approval an external collection device (fecal incontinence bag or pouch) can be used; it is a valuable early intervention to prevent rapid skin breakdown.

To apply a fecal incontinence pouch:

1. With assistance, position the patient on one side with knees bent for thorough exposure. Clean, rinse, and thoroughly dry a hair-free perianal area (careful shaving may be necessary).

2. Enlarge the opening in the wafer if necessary to about 1/4 inch larger than the anal area for effective coverage in folds or creases.

3. Remove the paper backing on the wafer section and apply stomahesive paste around the perimeter of the wafer opening.

4. To apply the bag, separate the buttocks, hold skin taut, and position the wafer opening over the anus. Start with the narrow portion and press against the perineal skin below the anal folds. Then press the widest portion onto the skin above the anal folds.

5. Remove paper backing from the lateral sections of the wafer and press them into place. Support the buttocks while applying the contact adhesive skin barrier with attached pouch, then release.

6. Check to make sure that sections are secure at all points.

7. Release the patient's buttocks and press the wafer firmly against the skin for 1 minute.

8. Tape the edges of the skin barrier with waterproof tape to seal the edges of the wafer against the skin.

9. To prevent bag leakage, logroll the patient and check tension on the tubing and leakage of the pouch every hour.

10. Change the pouch if leakage occurs.

When applied securely, this device adheres to the skin for at least 24 hours. If the fecal incontinence pouch is left intact or connected to a straight drain, be alert that the pouch does not fill with flatus (gas) or stool because it will pull off the perianal area. In situations in which diarrhea is copious, the fecal incontinence pouch needs to be connected to wall suction to prevent stool from coming in contact with skin. Ask your enterostomal therapist or clinical nurse specialist for assistance.

 Save specimens to help with early diagnosis of cause.

 Record daily bowel movements and the number of incontinent episodes. If the stool is liquid, measure and document the amount. Document your observations of color, consistency (hard, soft, liquid), amount, strange or different odor, and care that you gave.

SPECIAL PROBLEMS: SKIN TEARS AND BRUISING

Both immature and aging skin are fragile and at risk for skin tears or stripping (Fig. 12–21). People who have been undergoing long-term steroid therapy also are at risk for skin tears. It is important to recognize this fragile skin. Stripping and tearing can be prevented by careful transfer of patients to wheelchairs and carts. Keep rooms well lighted. Remove extending furniture and give assistance with activity. Avoid tape as much as possible, but when tape is necessary, apply and remove it carefully. When a tear is found on one area of the body, the patient is generally at risk for tears on other body parts.

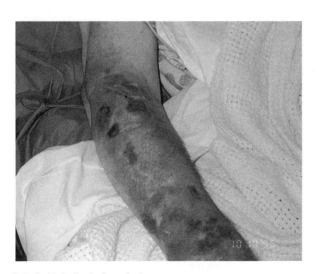

FIGURE 12-21
Skin tear.

After consultation with the RN or enterostomal therapist, the PCT may implement prevention or treatment strategies for skin stripping or tearing by the following:

• Cleanse the skin as ordered and gently pat dry.
• On patients who are at risk for tears, apply a skin-sealant liquid or wafer before applying tape.

STOP Do not stretch tape or film dressings when applying.

• Apply tape without tension. This prevents blistering or shearing of the skin under tape.

STOP Do not circle the extremity (wrist, for example) with selected tape or film dressing, since it may act as a tourniquet if there is swelling.

• Use porous tapes that are paper or cloth rather than adhesive. These allow moisture to evaporate.
• If available, use a dressing made of glycerin and water like elastogel over skin tears. Although expensive, this product eliminates the typical hazards of tape.
• Remove a film dressing by allowing it to "slough off." Trim the lifted areas for a neater dressing. It can be removed by slowly peeling tape away from anchored skin using adhesive remover to wipe simultaneously. Support the skin while lifting up the tape.
• Assist the RN to anchor dressings with roll gauze, tubular stockinette, or self-adhering tape when possible to avoid unnecessary tape on the skin. Secure dressings with Montgomery straps to prevent repeated tape applications. Solid-wafer skin barriers can be applied around a wound; wound dressings are then secured by anchoring tape to the solid-wafer skin barrier.

ROLE OF PATIENT CARE TECHNICIAN IN REINFORCING EDUCATION

It is the RN's responsibility to educate patients and families about treatments. The RN also explains patients' responsibility in their care and treatment. However, PCTs can reinforce this education at appropriate times. For example, remind patients with paralysis, and their families, of the importance of repositioning the patient at least every 2 hours and to avoid extremes in temperature. Paraplegics can use a trapeze to be more independent. Encourage patients to shift their weight frequently and inspect, adjust, and pad casts, braces, splints, and compression bandages. Emphasize the importance of diet, fluid intake, hygiene, and alerting caregivers immediately after incontinence has occurred. Reinforce diabetic foot care since good foot care can prevent further problems.

13

Challenges of the Cancer Patient

FRANCIE WOLGIN, MSN, RN, CNA

P R E R E Q U I S I T E K N O W L E D G E A N D S K I L L S

- Universal precautions
- Meticulous patient hygiene
- Sensitivity to emotional needs
- Concepts of teamwork and communication skills

O B J E C T I V E S

After you complete this chapter, you will be able to:

- Name common types of cancer.
- Identify factors that can predispose people to cancer.
- Recognize early warning signs of cancer.
- Discuss ways you can reduce risks of developing cancer.
- Identify common types of cancer treatment and related precautions.

- Name ways you can emotionally support cancer patients and their families.
- Describe the role of the patient care technician (PCT) when caring for patients with cancer.
- Recognize signs and symptoms that need to be reported to the RN.
- Implement precautions of treatment.

TERMS

Benign   Not cancerous; does not invade nearby tissues or spread to other parts of the body

Biological Therapy   Treatment to stimulate or restore the body's immune system's ability to fight disease and infection

Biopsy   Removal of a tissue sample, which is then or later examined under a microscope to check for cancer cells. Removing tissue or fluid with a needle is called a needle biopsy

Carcinogen   A substance producing cancer

Cervix   The neck of the uterus or womb

Chemotherapy   Treatment with chemical agents

Computed Tomography (CT)/Computerized Axial Tomography (CAT Scan)   An X-ray picture that shows a cross section of the body

Hormone   A natural substance that carries chemical messages from one part of the body to another

Hormone Therapy   A treatment that prevents certain cancer cells from getting the hormones they need to grow. Hormones control the actions of certain cells or organs

Immune System   The cells and chemicals of the body system that protect the body against foreign organisms or substances

Lymph   A clear fluid carried through the body in the lymphatic vessels. Lymph carries cells that help fight disease and infection

Lymph Nodes   Small organs that make up and store lymph cells. Bacteria or cancer cells that enter the lymphatic system may be found in the nodes or lymph glands

Mammography   X-ray examination of the breasts, used as screening test for breast cancer

Metastasize   To move from the primary site and spread via the blood stream or lymphatic vessels to other sites

Mutation   Change in a gene

Oncologist   A doctor who specializes in cancer treatment

Pap Smear   A simple screening test for detection of cancer from cells taken from the cervix. The test is named for Dr. George Papanicolaou, who developed it

Radiation Therapy   Treatment using high-energy rays to kill or damage cancer cells. It can be external, using a machine to aim high-energy rays at the cancer, or internal, placing radioactive material inside the body as close to the cancer as possible

Remission   The period during which symptoms abate; specifically, in cancer treatment, the time following when no cancer cells can be detected in the body

Risk Factor   Something that increases a person's chance of developing a disease

Stage   A phase in the course of a disease, life history of an organism, or a biological process; in cancer, its extent, particularly whether the disease has spread from the original site to other parts of the body

Systemic Treatment   Treatment that reaches cells all through the body by traveling through the blood stream. Chemotherapy is an example.

Tumor   A mass of diseased cells or excess tissue, sometimes but not always cancerous

X-rays A form of high-energy radiation that can make pictures of the inside of the body, damage cells, and either cause or be used to treat cancer

Cancer describes a group of diseases that exhibit uncontrolled cell growth. Cancer is an overall term/label used to designate any of a group of more than 250 diseases distinguished by abnormal cell growth occurring in various parts of the body. The cause of cancer is unknown, but a variety of factors have been identified that seem to increase the chances of acquiring cancer. Cancer has a high mortality (death) rate, and after cardiovascular disease, is the second leading cause of death within the United States.

Cancer is the mutation of cellular genes resulting in abnormal cells. While healthy cells replicate in predictable patterns and are replaced with new cells as they wear out, cancerous cells do not. Cancerous cells do not respond to the normal signals telling cells when to divide and when not to do so. Cancer cells grow in unpredictable and uncontrolled ways and serve no good purpose in the body. The cancer cells have a tendency to invade local tissues and then spread (metastasize) to other organs or sites in the body. They drain nutrition from the body and their growth damages other normal body tissues. Cancer may be caused by an inefficient immune system. When functioning correctly, the immune system can ward off or fight potentially cancerous mutant cells. When this defense breaks down or becomes less effective, the immune system no longer identifies these mutant cells as potentially dangerous, and they are allowed to grow and multi-

ply unchecked. The mutant cells may become cancerous when their growth is not stopped by the immune system.

Many people associate the word *cancer* with immediate death or with dying. They may have fears of experiencing a slow painful death, mental anguish, and feelings of hopelessness, depression, and/or despair. However, there are some effective treatments and many things a patient care technician (PCT) can do to help those cancer patients.

INCIDENCE. In 1995, more than 547,000 Americans died of cancer, and 1,252,000 new cases were detected. For 1996 it is estimated that cancer deaths will be 554,740 and new cases detected will be 1,359,150.

PROJECTION. The American Cancer Society is projecting that by the year 2000, as many as 40–50% of Americans will be affected by cancer or develop some form of cancer in their lifetime. There are projections that by the year 2030, virtually everyone will have or have had some form of cancer prior to their death. Figures 13–1A and 13–1B list the American Cancer Society's current statistics for incidence of cancer sites in men and women. Given these numbers, it is important to learn more about cancer.

TYPES OF CANCER. Numerous books and pamphlets have been written about cancer. In this chapter, there will be only a brief description of each of the common types of cancer. There are specific booklets available.

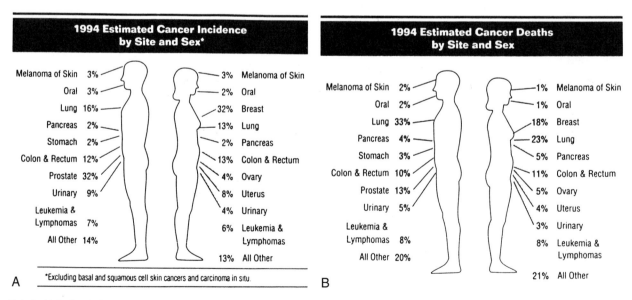

F I G U R E 1 3 – 1

A, Cancer incidence by site and sex. *B,* Cancer deaths by site and sex. (From A Cancer Source Book for Nurses, 6th ed. Atlanta, American Cancer Society, 1994, pp 12–13.)

In addition to local library resources, the National Cancer Institute publishes free booklets that are available by calling 1-800-422-6237. Spanish-speaking staff is available if needed. The American Cancer Society (1-800-227-2345) is another information and referral source. It will send published materials on cancer.

BLOOD CELL/LEUKEMIAS

Leukemias are diseases in which the malignant disease actually occurs in the white blood cell and results in overproduction of white blood cells or leukocytes. White blood cells are part of the body's immune system. While white blood cells help the body's ability to fight off colds or infections, the overproduction of white blood cells can cause an overcrowding in the blood stream, blocking growth and effectiveness of other blood cells such as red blood cells and platelets. Leukemias can be treated with chemotherapy or bone marrow transplant. Red blood cells (erythrocytes) are needed to carry oxygen. If there are too few red blood cells, a person can tire easily and feel exhausted because he or she is not getting enough oxygen for the body to work or function properly. Platelets are a type of blood cell needed to clot blood. Platelets may also become overcrowded by excessive white blood cells with leukemia. The inability to form clots after an injury or bump can lead to excessive bruising. Frequent nose bleeds are another sign of poor clotting.

AIDS (ACQUIRED IMMUNE DEFICIENCY SYNDROME)

Although AIDS is not a form of cancer, it is usually discussed in chapters on cancer because of the similarities in some of the symptoms and treatments. AIDS is a name given to a certain group of illnesses related to HIV (human immunodeficiency virus) infection. AIDS is acquired by exposure to HIV usually through high-risk behavior, including sexual promiscuity or having unprotected sex with an infected person. Persons who abuse drugs and share needles or syringes are also at a very high risk. Prior to 1985, blood transfusions were not screened, and some individuals acquired AIDS through transfusions. Infected mothers pass AIDS during pregnancy and birth to their babies. Many people are unaware they are carriers. Using universal precautions is an ideal way to avoid exposure and direct contact with blood and body fluids while caring for patients.

AIDS involves changes in the body's central nervous and immune systems. Usually several years into the course of AIDS, immunosuppression occurs, leading to increased susceptibility to cancer. The body's immune system is designed to fight infection, diseases, and foreign substances. A person with AIDS who experiences immunosuppression no longer has these natural defenses. Nearly 40% of AIDS patients develop Kaposi's sarcoma, a type of cancer distinguished by discrete skin lesions or bluish red nodules. These changes lead to a series of hard-to-treat infections, cancers, or neurological problems and may eventually cause death. AIDS patients also have a higher risk of developing non-Hodgkin's lymphoma, a malignant disease (cancer) of the immune system.

BRAIN

Tumors may begin in the brain, but more commonly in adults, they spread (metastasize) to the brain from cancerous tumors that began in other body sites. Cancers that originate in the brain are most common in children and young adults. Signs of brain cancer may include headache, speech difficulties, difficulty in walking, confusion, or occasionally, disturbances in vision. Usually the tumor will be quite large by the time these symptoms are noticeable. If the cancer is present only in the brain, a sample of the cells is removed in a procedure referred to as a biopsy. Treatment may include surgery, radiation, chemotherapy, and immunotherapy. Treatment can sometimes delay or arrest the tumor growth. If the cancer has spread from other locations, the prognosis is poor.

BREAST

The female breasts are milk-producing organs. Each breast has 15–20 sections, called lobes, and many smaller lobules. Milk-producing bulbs, lobules, and lobes are connected or linked together by ducts that lead to the nipple. After lung cancer, breast cancer is the second leading killer of women, affecting 1 in 9 women, and causing over 48,000 deaths each year in the United States. Breast cancer occurs most often in women over 50 years of age who have other family members with breast cancer. Women who have never been pregnant or who had their first child after age 30 are also at increased risk. If detected early, nearly 90% of breast cancers can be cured. Monthly breast self-examinations, regular checkups, and mammography every 1–2 years after age 40 are recommended. Mammography involves using a special machine to take top and side X-ray views of the breast. Any lumps or changes in breasts are signals to have the breast professionally examined. Treatment for breast cancer may include surgery, usually radiation and/or chemotherapy, and hormonal therapy using estrogen-blocking drugs. These combinations have demonstrated successful outcomes.

COLON/RECTUM

The risk of developing colon and rectal cancer is increased in those with a positive family history. Other risk factors include eating a diet high in fat and low in fiber. It is the second most deadly of cancers; however, early detection can result in an 86% cure rate. Treatment usually involves surgery. Depending on the location of the tumor and when reconstruction of the intestine is not possible, the diseased tissue is removed and a colostomy may be created. A colostomy involves an opening between the colon and body surface where a disposable pouch is attached to collect feces. Radiation and chemotherapy may be needed to prevent metastases.

BONE

Cancer that begins in the bone is primary bone cancer, most often appearing in the arms and legs of children or young adults. Primary bone cancer is referred to as sarcoma. Each type begins in a different kind of bone tissue. Osteosarcoma is the most common type, affecting the long bones of children. Chondrosarcoma is a type of bone cancer that occurs in the cartilage, the rubbery tissue around joints, in adults. In older adults it is rare for cancers to begin in the bones, and more often cancers of the bone are spread (metastasized) from other places in the body. Symptoms may develop slowly. Pain is most common, and occasionally a lump can be felt. Bones are likely to break more easily at the site of the tumor in patients with bone cancer. Treatment may include surgery, radiation, and chemotherapy. Amputation is sometimes necessary to effect a cure.

BLADDER

Blood in the urine is the most common sign of bladder cancer. Most bladder cancers develop in the inside lining of the bladder and may look like a mushroom attached to the bladder wall. An intravenous pyelogram (IVP) is obtained to view the kidneys, ureters, and bladder on X-ray, or a cystoscope can be used to directly view the bladder. A biopsy must be done to make a definite diagnosis. All or part of the tumor can be removed through a cystoscope. This is usually followed by intravenous chemotherapy or by instilling chemotherapeutic agents directly into the bladder. In some cases the entire bladder may be removed and the ureters brought out through the skin; a urostomy is created, and a disposable pouch is then required to collect the urine.

LIVER/BILE DUCT

Liver cancers are very hard to treat and probably develop in several stages. Primary liver cancer may be caused by infection from hepatitis B virus or exposure to other cancer-causing agents. An example of a cancer-causing agent is aflatoxin, a mold that grows on peanuts and corn that have started to spoil. Once a person has liver damage from the hepatitis B virus, the cells in the liver multiply faster than normal in an effort to correct the damage. The aflatoxin exposure causes the cells to mutate and plays a role in causing liver cancer. As with other cancer types, the most common cause of liver cancer is metastasis or spread from another site. Treatment may include radiation, chemotherapy, and surgery. Liver transplants may be tried in limited cases.

LUNG

Lung cancer is primarily caused by exposure of the lung tissue to smoke and environmental toxins; 85% of all lung cancer deaths can be attributed to smoking. Small-cell carcinomas and non–small-cell carcinomas are the two major categories. Of the non–small-cell carcinomas, adenocarcinomas start in the periphery of the lung beneath the lining. Small-cell tumors nearly always develop in smokers, usually in the central part of the lung, and are spread to the lymph glands and blood stream in the early stages of the disease. This type of cancer has often spread to other parts of the body by the time it is diagnosed. A more unusual type of lung cancer, mesothelioma, develops in the lining surrounding the lung and often is caused by asbestos exposure. Lung cancer may be treated with surgery if it is believed the lesion can be entirely removed. More commonly, treatment includes radiation and chemotherapy.

PROSTATE

The prostate gland is located between the bladder and the penis and surrounds the urethra. The prostate enlarges with age, and most men eventually experience symptoms of benign enlargements that usually cause difficulty in urination. Prostate cancer is the most common cancer among men in the United States. Cancerous tumors require treatment with surgery, radiation, and hormone therapy. Frequent complications and side effects of treatment include impotence and incontinence. The survival rate is over 57% following treatment. Often, treatment is not recommended in men over 75 years of age, as the tumor is generally slow growing, and the side effects of treatment may cause greater problems than the disease.

CONNECTIVE TISSUE/BONE/FAT

Sarcomas are tumors of connective tissue, bone, or fat and are frequently highly malignant. These tumors arise in cells other than those covering a tissue surface.

SKIN

Excessive exposure to invisible ultraviolet rays from the sun is a frequent cause of skin cancer. Skin cancers appear on the surface of the body and are easy to spot. They appear as pale, waxy lumps or scaly red patches. The most dangerous skin cancers, malignant melanomas, look like moles, or may begin to grow in an existing mole. Changes in warts or moles are early warning signs of skin cancer. Most skin cancers that are detected early remain localized and are easily treated by surgery, cautery (burning), or cryotherapy (freezing). Melanomas are the most dangerous type of skin cancer as they often metastasize and can be life threatening. Treatment includes surgery, radiation, and chemotherapy.

STOMACH

Stomach cancer is difficult to diagnose, as it often causes the same symptoms as stomach ulcers. Only 18% of stomach cancers are detected before they spread.

UTERUS/OVARY/CERVIX

Cancer of the female reproductive organs is the third most common cancer in women, after lung and breast cancer. Ovarian cancer occurs most often in women over 50 years of age who have a family history of a mother, sister, or daughter having the disease; women who have never been pregnant are more likely to develop ovarian cancer. Ovarian cancer occurs in either or both of the ovaries, the two female reproductive organs that produce eggs and hormones. It is very difficult to detect ovarian cancer early, as the symptoms are very subtle. When found, the cancer has frequently spread to the bowel or bladder. A woman may eventually feel bloated as the tumor grows and presses on nearby organs. By this time she may be experiencing loss of appetite, indigestion, nausea, diarrhea, constipation, or urinary frequency. The only definitive test for ovarian cancer is a biopsy in which tissue is removed for examination. Treatment usually includes a combination of surgery, chemotherapy, and radiation.

Uterine cancer has been increasing and is associated with the use of birth control pills and estrogen therapy in menopausal women over 50. Usual treatment is total hysterectomy and removal of the ovaries, fallopian tubes, and pelvic lymph nodes. This is followed by radiation, chemotherapy, and administration of large doses of progesterone. This combination has an 83% remission rate. Cancer of the cervix is common in women over 40 years, but there has been an increase in younger women who have had cervical dysplasia and/or herpes type II viral infections. Routine Pap smears are useful in early detection. A Pap smear is a medical test in which cells are taken from the cervix to be examined for evidence of possible cancer or precancer. When found, these abnormal cervical cells can be treated with cryosurgery, in which cells are frozen and killed using nitrous oxide. More advanced cases are treated with hysterectomy, radiation implants, or chemotherapy.

PREDISPOSING FACTORS

Cancer is a condition that develops gradually as a result of a very complex mix of factors related to an individual's lifestyle, environment, and heredity (see box below). Researchers have found that many risk factors increase one's chance of getting cancer. It is important to note that some people are more sensitive or responsive to various predisposing factors than others. Scientists have estimated that about 80% of all cancers are related to the use of tobacco products, what one eats or drinks, and exposure to cancer-causing agents or radiation in the environment. Routinely eating a diet high in fat and low in fiber may account for 60% of cancer cases in women and 40% of the cancer cases in men. While some factors can be avoided, others such as heredity cannot. Individuals who have had parents, grandparents, blood aunts and uncles, brothers or sisters who developed cancer need to be especially careful to reduce their risk. It is important to focus on those risk factors that can be controlled as well as to have regular medical checkups or examinations. Having been exposed to a risk factor does not mean that someone will develop cancer. It means that the chances of developing cancer are greater. It is best to avoid or

---

RISK FACTORS ASSOCIATED WITH CANCER

- Smoking/chewing tobacco
- Occupational—excessive exposure to:
  Cancer-causing chemicals: benzene, asbestos, nickel, vinyl chloride
  Sunlight
  Radiation/radon exposure
- Diet/eating habits: diet high in animal fat, low in fiber
- Alcohol
- Obesity/sedentary lifestyle
- Age >55 years
- Stress
- Hormones/particularly estrogen replacement
- Unprotected sex with multiple partners or one partner who has been exposed to AIDS
- Recreational or addicted IV drug use

eliminate factors such as smoking, which significantly increases risk. Regular checkups can help detect cancer in the early stages.

Determinations can be made concerning particular risks or benefits. For example, some postmenopausal women taking estrogen replacements who have a family history or other additional risk factors are found to have greater chances of developing cancer. Others whose cancer risk is low will benefit from the hormone.

EARLY WARNING SIGNS. Some cancers are not easily detected, or their symptoms are such that they are easily overlooked. Usually the sooner cancer is diagnosed and treatment begins, the better one's chances for recovery. The following signs may be associated with cancer and are signals to have a medical checkup (See box below). They can be remembered by the word CAUTION:

If a patient reports any of these to you be sure you document it and report it to the RN. Sometimes less serious conditions can have the same signs or symptoms. The American Cancer Society urges that if any symptom persists longer than several days, it should be evaluated.

The following are identified risk factors for cancer and related prevention strategies (See box below). Although these are frequently advertised in a variety of media, the PCT reinforces this education whenever appropriate.

TUMOR FORMATION AND GROWTH. Tumors begin as a new growth of cells somewhere in the body.

EARLY WARNING SIGNS OF CANCER

1. **C**hange in bowel or bladder habits
   - Bleeding from the rectum; black stools
   - Elderly men: difficulty in urination, blood in urine
   - Diarrhea alone, with no sign of flu
2. **A** sore or skin ulcer that does not heal
3. **U**nusual bleeding or discharge: bleeding from the rectum; fluid discharge from a woman's nipples
4. **T**hickening or lump in any part of the body: breast, neck, head, vulva, testicles
5. **I**ndigestion, or difficulty swallowing
6. **O**bvious change in the size, color, or shape of a wart or mole
7. **N**agging, persistent cough; cough producing blood in sputum; continuing hoarseness

Additional warning signs include pain that continues with no apparent cause and frequent infections.

Normal cells contain fluid (cytoplasm) surrounding the nucleus (central core). Normal cells divide in a controlled fashion, but cancerous cells divide in an uncontrolled, rapid manner. These abnormal cells multiply rapidly and form cancerous tumors. Tumors are referred to as localized, regional, or metastatic cancers.

Localized/Primary site refers to the original location of a malignant tumor. A tumor is considered localized when it has spread no further than the original place or organ in which it was discovered. There is no sign of cancer in nearby lymph nodes or other tissues.

Regional cancer means that there has been growth of a tumor in lymph nodes or tissues near the original site. There is, however, no evidence of growth or sign of cancer at distant sites. Cancer frequently spreads to secondary sites; for example, breast cancer that spreads to the lymph nodes of the armpit is considered regional.

Metastatic cancers describe those cancers that have spread or metastasized to organs or tissues located some distance from the original cancer site; examples include lung cancer that has spread to the bones or the brain or breast cancer that has metatasized to the liver.

STAGES OF CANCER. Stages of cancer are determined by tests and based on physical examination. For example, blood tests, CT, and X-ray examinations are done, and the results indicate the size of the primary tumor and extent of invasion to surrounding or distant areas. CT is a type of X-ray procedure that uses a computer to produce a detailed picture of a cross section of the body. The images can be reconstructed or put together to show the fine details of hard or bony surfaces. Oncologists have developed an elaborate system to precisely describe an individual's tumor progression (See box below). The system is designed to provide broad categories for estimating prognosis and determining treatment options. It is important to be aware of this system, as it communicates by a common rating method the extensiveness of a cancer. You will hear doctors, RNs, and patients talk about the stages. Clinical staging is based on evidence acquired before definitive treatment is started. Pathological staging is based on the clinical data plus the results of surgical exploration and examination of the resected specimen, tissue biopsy, or cytological study. Three variables make up the classification: (1) primary tumor (T); (2) the extent of lymph node involvement (N); and (3) the presence or absence of metastases (M). When this system is used to define the extent of malignant disease, it is called staging. The letter *T* is assigned a number from 1–4, describing the size of the tumor or level of invasion.

You may see others describe cancer in the following way:

Early

- Stage I: no spread
- Stage II: spread only to nearby lymph nodes

RISK FACTORS AND PREVENTION STRATEGIES

RISK FACTOR	PREVENTION STRATEGY
Tobacco	Quit smoking; avoid second-hand smoke; decrease smoking or smoke lower tar and nicotine cigarettes if you cannot stop smoking. Avoid use of snuff or chewing tobacco.
Diet	Decrease high-fat diet; reduce consumption of nitrates/nitrites found in cured meats, bacon, and pickled foods; increase fiber by eating more whole grains, cruciferous vegetables, i.e., broccoli, cauliflower; reduce weight if obese.
Sunlight	Use sunscreen of at least SFP 15; wear hat, protective clothing; avoid exposure 11AM–3PM; avoid tanning beds.
Alcohol	Avoid drinking and smoking in combination. Those who drink should limit alcoholic drinks (including beer) to 1–2 per day. More excessive drinking increases the risk of mouth, throat, esophageal, laryngeal, liver, and breast cancers.
Radiation	Avoid unnecessary X-rays; use protective shields when positioning patients.
Chemicals in Workplace	Use protective masks, gloves; follow safety rules; avoid contact with dangerous chemicals (benzene, asbestos, nickel, vinyl chloride); read/follow warning labels; report exposures in workplace; follow OSHA Guidelines/procedures.
Family Patterns	Be aware that environmental exposure could affect everyone exposed; follow doctor's advice about prevention; seek routine tests and checkups, especially since some cancers seem to have higher incidence in blood relatives.
Sedentary Lifestyle	Increase exercise.
Sexual Lifestyle	Use condoms; practice safe sex.
Stress	Seek support: social services, pastoral or mental health counseling.

Advanced—cancer in distant areas from original tumor

- Stage III: primary tumor very large; usually cannot be removed from body
- Stage IV: extremely advanced; primary tumor usually inoperable; has spread to multiple areas away from the original tumor.

PROGNOSIS. The prognosis is *good:* when there is a good chance that disease can be controlled/cured. It is considered *poor* when there is little chance of destroying the cancer. With cancer, the term "disease-free interval" is more commonly used to describe how long a patient has lived without recurrence of cancer. Although patients have certainly been "cured" of cancer, the fact is that cancer cells can be dormant for many years and then can begin growing again.

TYPES OF CANCER TREATMENT

The various methods used alone or in combination to treat cancer are described here very briefly. Many re-

sources are available through the American Cancer Society that give more detailed information about particular treatments.

Cancer treatment may be aimed at cure when it is thought that the disease can be completely eradicated, or it can be palliative, to reduce the pain and discomfort when a cure is not possible. Doctors have been aware of cancers for hundreds of years. Early treatments involved the application of arsenic paste or ground toads. With research and resulting treatments, up to 50% of patients survive 5 years without a return of the disease. The particular type of cancer influences both what treatment is most effective and the potential for long-term survival. Combining treatments may increase the possible overall outcome. Radiation and certain drugs fight cancer by damaging the genetic material of cells (DNA) keeping cells from reproducing, or killing the cells. Since cancer cells reproduce faster than other cells, they are harmed more by radiation treatment. The goal of cancer treatment is to prevent the spread of cancer cells by destroying them or interfering with their ability to reproduce.

TNM SYSTEM OF ANATOMICAL STAGING

T PRIMARY TUMOR

TX Primary tumor cannot be assessed
T 0 No evidence of primary tumor
T 1–4 Increasing numbers of tumors

N REGIONAL LYMPH NODES

N X Regional lymph nodes cannot be assessed
N 0 No evidence of lymph node involvement
N 1–4 Increasing involvement

M EVIDENCE OF METASTASIS

M X Presence of distant metastasis cannot be assessed
M 0 No evidence of metastasis
M 1–4 Increasing degrees of metastatic involvement

EXAMPLE
Breast Cancer Staging

Stage Tumor Size Metastasis
0 Confined to ducts/lobules No spread
Local area/few cells
1 <2 cm/less than 1 inch No spread beyond breast
2 2–5 cm/1 inch Spread to lymph nodes under arm
3 >5 cm/2 inches Spread to other lymph nodes or tissues near breast
4 Any larger size tumor Spread to other organs of the body—often bones, liver, lungs, or brain

Surgery

Surgery is a local treatment to remove a tumor, surrounding tissue, and often nearby lymph nodes. Laser surgery can be useful in treating premalignant cells or tumors that are localized. Laser surgery can be performed only on the types of tumors that can be seen directly or visualized with an instrument. Dermatologists frequently treat skin cancers with lasers to remove the cancer. Gynecologists can use lasers to treat cervical cancers or to remove precancerous cells from a woman's cervix. Some abdominal surgery is performed by using a laparoscope, an instrument inserted through a small incision. This allows visualization of the area and removal of the cancerous lesion.

Radiation Therapy

Radiation therapy uses high energy X-rays to destroy cancer cells or tumors. Radiation therapy is a useful way

to treat cancer because cancer cells grow and divide faster than normal cells, making them more sensitive to the radiation. Special equipment is used to aim the radiation beam at tumors or areas of the body where cancer cells are present. Radiation therapy can be external, using a machine, or internal, using implants. About 50% of cancer patients are treated with radiation therapy.

Chemotherapy

Chemotherapy destroys cancer cells by means of anti-cancer medications. Drugs may be administered intravenously (into the blood stream) to attack cancer cells in the area of the primary tumor and those that are in the blood stream or lymph nodes.

Frequently, IV catheters such as central venous catheters (CVC) or peripherally inserted central catheters (PIC) are inserted for long-term use when drugs will be given over several days or weeks. The catheters reduce the number of "sticks" that a patient receives and can also be used for the frequent blood draws that usually accompany treatment. Chemotherapy is given alone, in cycles, over a certain period, or in combination with other treatments. Drugs may be given in the home, in outpatient settings, or in the hospital. Patients and those caring for them are taught to care for the IV catheter and keep it clean. In most cases, patients who receive chemotherapy experience side effects, including suppression of the immune system. Therefore, they are prone to infections. Other common side effects of chemotherapy may include hair loss, fatigue, and loss of appetite. New medications to prevent nausea and vomiting have made chemotherapy easier to tolerate. During the months that patients receive chemotherapy, proper nutrition and rest are important to maintain their ability to fight infection and have strength or energy. Patients may get discouraged and need support of others during the months of treatment.

Diet/Nutrition

It is important to be well nourished to heal and tolerate the cancer treatments or therapy. The severity and number of side effects will be fewer and the patient will have more energy and be able to tolerate physical activity better when the body is well nourished. Patients are encouraged to maintain their weight. However, the nausea and loss of appetite that frequently accompany the treatments make this a continual challenge.

Hyperthermia

Hyperthermia is a technique in which a tumor in the body is heated up to 10–11 degrees Fahrenheit higher than the rest of the body, or the whole body temperature is heated no more than 8.6 degrees Fahrenheit, just before or after radiation therapy. Research has shown that if tumors can be heated for 1 hour, X-rays will kill twice as many cells as would occur in an unheated tumor. In the future it is likely this will become an increasingly used treatment. Most of the side effects, such as redness or feeling very warm or flushed, go away once the treatment has ended or the patient has recovered from the treatment.

Biological Therapy

Biological therapy, also referred to as immunotherapy, is treatment to stimulate or restore the ability of the body's immune system to fight infection and disease or to protect the body from some of the side effects of treatment. Examples of agents include monoclonal antibodies, interferon, interleukin-2, and colony stimulating factors. Short-term side effects include flu-like symptoms, loss of appetite, fever, nausea and vomiting, and diarrhea. Rashes, bleeding, and bruising easily can occur. Interleukin therapy also causes swelling.

SPECIAL EMOTIONAL NEEDS OF PATIENTS AND FAMILIES

Many patients, family members, significant others, and friends experience stages of grief reaction. When first hearing the diagnosis of cancer, even if the news was expected, initial shock and denial are common reactions. The reaction could range from anger to fear, uncertainty, feelings of hopelessness, shock, depression, or guilt. It is not uncommon for the initial anxiety and anger to be replaced with denial.

Denial is a defense that may help the individual cope as long as it does not interfere with seeking appropriate medical evaluation and treatment. Eventually most people work through their feelings and come to accept the reality that they have cancer. Support from family, friends, cancer support groups, and caregivers will help them cope. Do not be surprised that during your contacts with patients and families, they seem unable to focus or remember answers to questions or things you have told them. Most of the energy and attention of patients and families will be focused on their personal situation, fears, or pain. It is important to allow time to listen to their concerns and fears. Fear is a common feeling when patients do not know what the future holds. Encouragement, reassurance, hope, and emotional support are needed (Fig. 13–2).

Decisions need to be made regarding treatment options, and it is helpful for patients to have enough information to participate in planning their care. Occasionally family members or friends are afraid of or uncomfortable dealing with the side effects of treatment, the changes in their loved one, or the reality that death may be forthcoming. Extra support and encouragement help maintain hope. Focusing on the present and allowing people to verbalize their feelings and fears are useful ways to be supportive.

Religious Support

It is important to recognize that some patients may believe their cancer is a result of God's will, a deserved punishment from God, or a cross they have to bear. Others may find strength in their religion and find comfort through talking with a minister, priest, or rabbi.

Ask your RN about calling for religious support of preference. Your facility may have 24-hour pastoral services available for patients and others who need them.

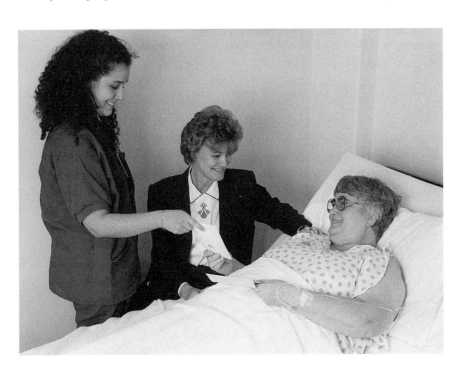

FIGURE 13–2
PCT giving emotional support.

Changed Self-Image

People want to feel good about themselves. Being sick with a potentially terminal disease may reduce their ability to feel good about who they are and how well they can care for themselves or other family members for whom they feel responsible (see Chapter 14: Self-Concept, Body Image, and Sexuality in Health Care).

The diagnosis of cancer usually adds pressure and stress so that family issues and problems that were previously manageable now become less so. Encourage relationships that promote recovery and add to the overall perception that one has good quality of life and hope.

Caregivers, significant others, and friends need to provide the patient and each other a sense of comfort and a chance to talk. They should not feel guilty about meeting their own needs and other obligations.

Role of the Patient Care Technician

Your primary role is to provide high-quality daily care, giving special attention to discomfort and emotional needs. Individuals will have different reactions or degrees of complications. It is important to stress that once the treatment has ended, many of the side effects gradually go away.

✔ Report all of the patient's complaints to the RN. Frequently, medications can be adjusted to reduce pain, nausea, or other discomforts.

ANTICIPATING AND DEALING WITH COMMON SIDE EFFECTS OF CHEMOTHERAPY AND RADIATION

FATIGUE. Fatigue occurs because a patient's body is working hard to get rid of destroyed cancer cells and toxins during and after treatment. Anemia results because red blood cells are harmed during treatment, leaving the patient feeling tired and weak. The body uses lots of energy healing itself.

✔ Plan rest periods during care. Anticipate that the patient may need extra help and offer it before being asked.

NAUSEA/LOSS OF APPETITE. Chemotherapy affects rapidly growing cells, and the mucous membranes lining the entire GI tract are particularly susceptible. Food does not taste good, it hurts to eat, and nausea and indigestion are continual problems. The PCT can help by:

- Reporting nausea and vomiting to the RN
- Reporting elevated temperature, signs of dehydration (dry mouth/lips) to the RN
- Recording accurate intake and output

- Providing distractions such as TV, reading material, movies, music
- Removing foul-smelling materials from room
- Having the patient rest with the head elevated or sitting up in a chair
- Offering small meals or snacks 5–6 times per day
- Encouraging the patient to rest after eating
- Avoiding liquids at mealtimes
- Offering drinks between meals (broth or Gatorade may be used to replace lost fluids and salt.)

CONSTIPATION. Constipation is a common side effect in patients taking pain medications. Decreased food and fluid intake may cause the constipation to worsen. The PCT can help decrease the severity of this complication by:

- Encouraging fluids and water as permitted
- Encouraging foods high in fiber such as bran, vegetables, and fruits
- Reporting absence of daily bowel movements
- Watching for signs of impaction such as no bowel movement for several days, leakage of diarrhea-type stools with coughing, abdominal distention and/or pain, foul-smelling breath, and complaints of back pain
- Encouraging mobility and ambulation of patients

DIARRHEA (See Chapter 12).
SORES IN MOUTH (STOMATITIS); THRUSH. Thrush is a fungal infection in the mouth. It occurs as white patches on the tongue or throat that look like cottage cheese. These sores or open lesions may develop as a result of some chemotherapy drugs. PCTs are encouraged to:

- Examine mouth during oral care at least daily (Fig. 13–3).

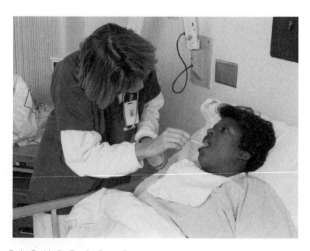

FIGURE 13–3
Gentle inspection and mouth care of patient with stomatitis.

Be gentle with mouth care. Most patients complain that their mouths are very sore.

- Report any white patches that look like pieces of cottage cheese on the tongue or throat.
- Document and report dry mouth, complaints of burning sensations, or increased sensitivity to hot or cold drinks or food.

FEVER, CHILLS, SWEATS. Fever, chills, and sweats are signs of possible infection. The PCT should:

- Take vital signs every 2 hours or as requested.
- Report and document patient's elevated temperature.
- Provide mouth care every 2 hours if sores are present or the patient is NPO.

A frequent side effect associated with chemotherapy is reduction in white blood cells. White blood cells are needed to fight infections. Therefore, special precautions need to be posted and carried out to reduce the risk of infection in patients who have low white blood cell counts (Fig. 13–4).

- Wash hands thoroughly before entering and leaving rooms.
- Avoid live plants and flowers in rooms, since they carry in organisms.
- Check fresh fruit and vegetable restrictions.
- Wear a mask before entering rooms if you have cold or flu symptoms.

BLEEDING PRECAUTIONS. Another condition occasionally associated with chemotherapy is reduction in the number of platelets. Platelets are needed to help clot blood (See Chapter 7). When reduction occurs there

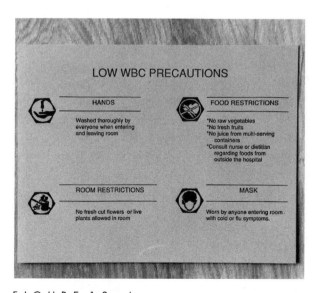

FIGURE 13–4
Low white blood cell precautions.

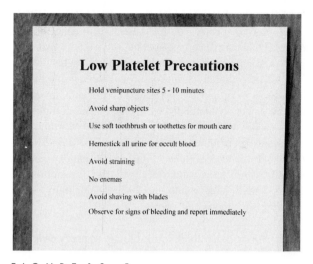

FIGURE 13–5
Low platelet precautions.

is a risk for bleeding. Precautions are needed to prevent bleeding (Fig. 13–5). The PCT is proactive with strategies to reduce risks for bleeding by:

- Holding venipuncture sites 5 minutes or until it is certain that bleeding has stopped
- Preventing bleeding from gums with gentle mouth care
- Reminding patients to avoid straining with bowel movements or lifting
- Shaving patients with electric razors rather than sharp blades
- Testing urine and stool for occult blood and observing for superficial bruising and petechiae

HAIR LOSS. Chemotherapy is effective in treating some types of cancers because it affects fast-growing cells. Hair loss occurs because the hair follicles are fast-growing cells. This means that patients may lose hair from their scalps, beard, legs, arms, pelvic regions, eyelashes, and eyebrows. This is an upsetting, but temporary condition. The usual onset is 2–3 weeks into treatment. The hair frequently falls out in clumps. Hair that grows during treatment is fragile and will break off easily. After chemotherapy is completed, the hair will grow back, but the color or texture may be different than before. Hair loss resulting from radiation to the head is generally more permanent. If hair returns it is often fine in texture. The PCT helps by:

- Using mild shampoo and conditioner when washing the patient's hair
- Reassuring the patient that hair will gradually grow back
- Suggesting a wig, cap, turban, or short haircut while hair is regrowing

SPECIFIC PRECAUTIONS FOR CAREGIVERS.

In addition to special care for patients with cancer treatments, PCTs must exercise specific precautions that prevent personal exposures to chemotherapy agents. Exposure to chemotherapy agents can occur through inhalation of aerosols or droplets, absorption into the skin, or ingestion by way of contaminated food, cigarettes, or cosmetics.

To ensure that all caregivers are aware of which patients are receiving chemotherapy, precautions and warning labels should be placed on doors, patient charts, utensils, and specimens (Fig. 13–6). Chemotherapy agents can be taken into the body accidentally when handling specimens and wastes.

STOP Wear extra thick latex gloves (or two pairs of regular gloves) when handling blood, stool, urine, vomitus, and contaminated linens. If the possibility of splashing or direct contact with skin or clothing exists, wear gowns, masks, and protective glasses.

When emptying vomitus, urine, and stool, empty the container close to the water in the commode and place a plastic-backed barrier over the commode bowl while flushing (Fig. 13–7). This helps prevent exposure through splashing and aerosolization. Accidental spills of urine, stool, or emesis or splashes of blood on the floor require special cleaning. Contaminated disposable items should be placed in biohazard wastebaskets. Avoid smoking, drinking, and applying cosmetics in chemotherapy preparation or administration area to reduce the risk of ingestion.

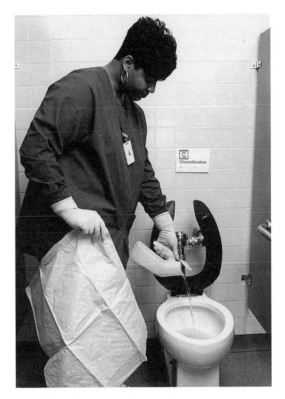

F I G U R E   1 3 – 7
Emptying body secretions using chemotherapy precautions.

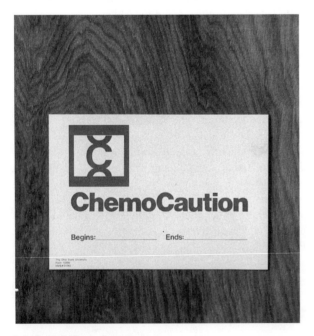

F I G U R E   1 3 – 6
Chemotherapy precautions.

Radiation is a special kind of energy carried by waves or streams. High levels of radiation can kill cells or keep them from growing and dividing. While radiation therapy is effective in treating half of all people with cancer, side effects also occur. The most common side effects are fatigue, loss of appetite, and skin changes. Patient care by the PCT for fatigue and loss of appetite have been discussed. Skin changes are caused when radiation passes through. Skin can look reddened, irritated, sunburned, or tanned. Since additional irritation to the skin increases discomfort, gentle skin care in the area of treatment is required. The PCT helps by:

- Using lukewarm water and mild soaps
- Avoiding putting anything hot or cold on the skin
- Not rubbing, scrubbing, or scratching sensitive spots or washing off skin markings
- Not applying any product on the skin unless ordered
- Reporting any complaints of discomfort to the RN

Other side effects of radiation occur, depending on the method or location of treatment.

RADIATION ENTERITIS. Radiation enteritis is inflammation of the intestine and small bowel caused by aggressive radiation to the abdomen, pelvis, or rectum. It may cause problems for several weeks after treatment is completed. PCT actions:

- Report cramping, nausea, loss of appetite, watery diarrhea.

- If permitted, offer and encourage fluids such as: Kool Aid, Gatorade, or Jell-O.

- Serve food/drinks at room temperature.

- Avoid greasy, fatty, or spicy foods; caffeinated beverages including tea, coffee, colas, and Mountain Dew.

SWELLING. The lymph nodes that drain fluid from the arms or legs can be injured by radiation therapy. They may also be removed from the axilla (armpit) or groin areas during surgery. Swelling occurs then in the hand, arm, armpit, groin, legs, or feet because the extra fluid is unable to drain normally. This extra fluid (lymphedema) collects in the tissues when lymph nodes are removed or blocked. Lymphedema occurs most often when lymph nodes have been removed for breast cancer, as well as advanced gynecological, prostate, and testicular cancers.

PCTs help to:

- Avoid injury to arms or legs as there is more likelihood of infection when swelling is already present.

- Avoid using blood pressure cuffs on the swollen arm (RNs will avoid starting IVs in swollen arms).

- Watch for skin appearing turgid/taut like a water balloon; report tightness in hands, feet, legs.

- Elevate the swollen extremity—do not allow it to "hang down."

- Document and report if patients cannot get rings on, if

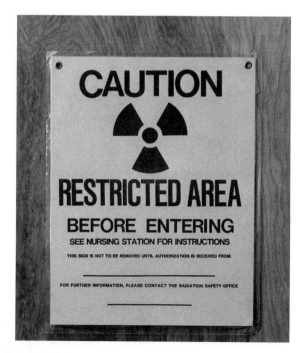

FIGURE 13–8
Radiation warning.

TABLE 13–1
Cancer Treatment and Side Effects

TREATMENT	INFLUENCED BY	SIDE EFFECTS
Surgery	Cancer site	Pain, weakness, tiredness, risk of infection; varying recovery time depending on other chronic diseases/ general health
Radiation	Dosage/site treated	Tiredness, rashes, red skin; loss of appetite may increase susceptibility to infection; lower WBC count
Chemotherapy	Drug(s) used/ dosage	Increased infections, nausea, vomiting, loss of appetite, mouth sores, hair loss, temporary or permanent loss of fertility
Biological therapy	Type of treatment	Flu-like symptoms, weakness, nausea, vomiting, decreased appetite, fever, diarrhea, rash, easy bruisability, swelling
Hyperthermia	Regional/local	Increased body, temperature, redness

their shoes do not fit, or they have aching or redness in an extremity.

- Position legs or arms at heart level whenever possible.

- Avoid tight bands around wrists or pant legs.

- Change body position frequently, keeping weight or pressure off the swollen area.

- Avoid exposing the area to heat or cold.

- Observe for return of swelling when fluid has been taken by needle aspiration or a drain has been recently removed. This happens frequently in women who have had recent breast cancer surgery.

As with chemotherapy, precautions should be taken to prevent radiation contamination to caregivers. Besides posting radiation signs (Fig. 13–8) and labels in the patient area, caregivers should follow their organization's specific protocols for staff exposure to patients' radiation therapy.

Pain

Pain is one of the common side effects of cancer. Cancer patients may experience pain for a variety of reasons as a result of the effects of the cancer itself or of the treatment. Psychological responses to illness, including depression, anxiety, and tension can make pain seem worse. The best way to manage pain is to treat the cause. Methods for controlling pain include pain medicines, operations on nerves, surgery to decrease the size or remove a tumor, nerve blocks, physical therapy, and techniques such as relaxation, humor, distraction, visualization, or imagery. Many factors will influence which approach or combination will best benefit each individual in pain. It is important to recognize that pain affects people differently, and patients have the right to receive the best pain control available to them.

It is not uncommon for patients to be concerned that taking strong pain medications will cause them to become addicted or dependent on the pain medication. Research has shown that health care providers often undermedicate patients because of the fear of addiction. However, patients with pain rarely become addicted. It is better to prevent pain before it starts or gets worse by using some regular pain relief schedule or method. People are different, and various methods will have different degrees of benefit to individual patients. Many patients benefit from evaluation by a pain specialist who can help them find the best relief for their specific pain and situation. As a PCT, there are several things you can do to assist patients in pain control.

- Ask the patient if he or she has pain. Some people with chronic pain are reluctant to complain, or fear they will become addicted to pain medications.

- Report pain to the RN.

- Observe the patient for mood changes.

- Report pain immediately that is described as "stabbing, penetrating, or excruciating."

- Have the patient rate the pain on a scale of 0–10 with 10 being the most severe.

- Inquire at least 30 minutes after pain medication has been given to determine if it has been effective in easing the pain. If there has been no relief, report this to the RN.

- When possible, wait 30 minutes after pain medication has been given before starting patient activity or treatment.

- Document the patient's response to pain medication.

- Provide comfort measures such as repositioning the patient, reducing environmental noise, and encouraging the use of relaxation techniques.

- Provide distractions such as movies, tapes, books, music, or TV; focusing on sporting events may help some patients cope with their pain.

Table 13–1 summarizes treatments for cancer and common side effects. The PCTs contribute valuable care when they reinforce education given by the RN, emotionally support the patient from diagnosis through treatment, observe and report side effects of treatment, and offer comfort measures to reduce pain. They also protect themselves and their teammates by following caregiver precautions related to cancer treatment.

Special Health Care Situations

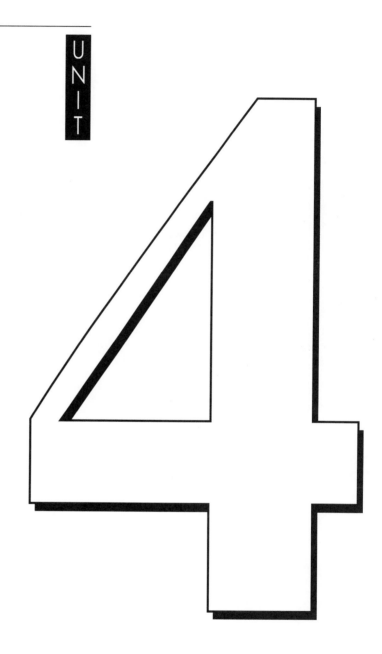

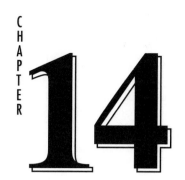

Self-Concept, Body Image, and Sexuality in Health Care

LINDA TERRY GODSON, MA, BSN

PREREQUISITE KNOWLEDGE AND SKILLS

- Basic communication skills with emphasis on listening in a nonjudgmental manner
- Acceptance of patient as an individual

OBJECTIVES

After you complete this chapter, you will be able to:

- Describe the four components of self-concept.
- Discuss the influence of culture and life experience on development of self-concept.
- Identify how injury, illness, or surgery can affect the self-concept and body image.
- Describe the role of the patient care technician (PCT) in responding to the patient's emotional needs.

- Explain three ways the patient care technician can assist the patient to rebuild his or her body image after illness, injury, or surgery.

- Identify sexuality as a key component to self-concept and personal identity.

- Recognize when to set limits on unwelcome sexual advances.

KEY TERMS

Body Image   What someone thinks his or her body looks like. This may not always be the same as the way others see it.

Personal Identity   All of the aspects of a person that make him or her different from someone else.

Role   A function or office assumed by someone. We all have a variety of roles we must respond to at one time. We have personal roles: mother, daughter, father; social roles: church member; job roles: patient care technician, RN; and position roles: member of a committee, president of an organization.

Role Performance   How individuals carry out their various roles and responsibilities. Are they good mothers, teachers, basketball players, etc.?

Self-Concept   What a person thinks about himself or herself. It includes the body image, self-esteem, role performance, and personal identity.

Self-Esteem   A person's belief about his or her own worth. It includes personal pride and self-respect.

Validate   To reinforce to someone that he or she is right, or important, or valuable.

The fast pace of our current health care environment demands that health care providers focus primarily on the technical and physical aspects of care. People enter the health care system needing that technical expertise; often their lives depend on it. When people are physically hurt, however, they also are hurt emotionally. A gash on the face from an auto accident, loss of a hand caught in machinery, or a stroke that results in speech difficulties and paralysis all result in major emotional as well as physical losses. An illness like heart disease may be invisible, but it still may make it impossible for the person to do all the activities he or she did before the illness or planned to do in the future.

Once peoples' basic needs for physical survival and safety are met, it is important to recognize and assist them in meeting their emotional needs. Every person needs to be respected, to be recognized for being valuable, in spite of whatever illness or injury they may be experiencing. They need to be loved, to have someone to love, and to have their loved ones with them and to support them during their illness. People need to feel included in discussions, decisions, and in fun. They need gentleness and kindness and a soft touch. People need the opportunity to have information, to make decisions, and to be assisted to reach their full potential—to be all they can be. They also need a sense of beauty and spirituality and may have a religious belief that supports them through difficult times.

People want to be seen as attractive to others. They want to be whole; they don't want to be different. People rely on their bodies to keep doing their job, but sometimes the body is disfigured or fails because of illness, injury, or surgery. This affects how people view themselves—their self-concept—as well as how they view their body—or body image. When people come to the hospital, there is an interference in their lives; their needs may not be recognized or met, and their body image is often changed.

This chapter will briefly discuss how self-concept is formed, how body image is affected by illness or injury, and the important role of patient care technicians (PCTs) in assisting people to feel better about their body and themselves.

FORMATION OF SELF-CONCEPT

Self-concept can be described as a picture of how individuals view themselves. People may view themselves as thin, bright, smart, handsome, a leader, a good father, and a capable health care worker; or they could think of themselves as ugly, not too bright, someone who never will amount to anything, a no-good father, and generally a loser. Actually, as we know, there are an endless variety and combination of characteristics that people of all ages use to describe themselves.

Self-concept builds up over time and is based on experiences with others. From infancy on, positive and negative reactions from others regarding appearance, responsiveness to others, personal successes or failures, individual recognition, success or difficulty in school or work, and the level of support of family members and others determines how people think of themselves—their self-concept.

The core of the self-concept has been formed by early childhood and affects how people approach new situations as children and as adults. Young children who feel good about themselves will be most likely to try new situations and have new opportunities to be successful. Their success brings more positive responses and increasing feelings of self-confidence.

Some young children, because of their social environment, appearance, or physical or mental ability, may have been less successful and had more negative experiences than others. They may approach new situations with more caution, and unless strongly encouraged, may not try new activities for fear of failure. This fear, and continued lack of successes, may continue into adulthood, and reinforces their already poor sense of self.

This pattern of reinforcement tends to continue when young people remain in the same environment, around the same people. Often, when a person moves and is put into a new social situation and has encouragement from others, he or she is able to gain new successes, get repeated positive reinforcement, and develop a more positive self-concept.

✔ PCTs can play a crucial role in patients' recovery and positive feelings about themselves by offering assistance and praise related to their efforts to recover.

Persons with a positive self-concept tend to be able to face new situations with more confidence. They feel they have been successful before, and therefore they will be successful again. They feel if they work hard they can take care of anything that comes along. That effort usually makes them successful.

Influence of Cultural Values

Many of the aspects of self-concept are based on cultural values. As people are raised, they are surrounded by a culture that describes the rules, roles, and norms of behavior, success, and appearance. People gain a sense of what is important, what is right, how people should act, and how they should look. They learn what is valued by those around them and tend to take on those same values for themselves. Part of their self-concept and body image is built on the cultural values in which they were raised.

People may be operating under several cultural value systems at the same time. They may be raised in an African-American, Hispanic, Asian, Appalachian, or Native American family and community that had a distinctive set of values. In the United States, they also are confronted by the values of the larger culture. As people get older and leave their community for more education or a job, they meet people and encounter values that may be quite different. This often is referred to as "culture shock" and may cause confusion for people as they figure out who they are and what is "right."

Other cultural values involve health and illness. For example, what does it mean to be sick? When do you go to the doctor? Do you go to bed and let your body heal or do you deny any illness and keep pushing, not letting it get you down? What does it mean to have a chronic illness, to have a stroke, or a disfiguring accident? What do you think about someone who is "different?" How should that person be treated?

The more closely people meet the ideals of the culture in which they are raised, the better they usually will think about themselves. In the larger United States cul-

ture, values of youth, physical attractiveness, being healthy, independent, and having a fully functioning body are reinforced in advertising, family and social interactions, and in expectations of others. Weight loss and fitness programs are multibillion dollar industries. Voluntary plastic surgery to make a person feel more attractive is on the increase and is big business. Models are young, attractive, exceptionally thin, with fully functioning bodies. It is only recently that some models have been shown in wheelchairs. Athletes are stars and often used in advertising. The message that all this sends is that people should somehow try to be like the models, stay young looking, hide any deformity or physical limitation, and stay healthy. This cultural value system has a major impact on people who are ill or suffer a traumatic or disfiguring accident. Other cultures often have other cultural values. These may cause an additional conflict for someone raised in two cultures.

Four Aspects of Self-Concept

Psychologists and sociologists generally identify four aspects of a person's self-concept:

- Body image—how persons view their own bodies
- Self-esteem—what individuals think of themselves and their capabilities
- Role performance—how people view themselves in relation to their various roles
- Personal identity—all the various aspects of persons that make them different from anyone else.

Self-Concept—Body Image

A person's body image is formed by reactions of others and comparison to cultural values regarding physical beauty. It includes the person's view of himself or herself as a sexual person. Is he or she considered beautiful or handsome, slender, muscular, or tall with attractive skin and hair? Persons who have always been recognized for being attractive may not have had to fully develop other aspects of themselves. Their physical appearance made relating to others easier. If they had an illness or injury that affected their appearance, others would react differently to them, they would feel worse about themselves, and their self-concept would be weakened.

Self-Concept—Self-Esteem

People who have developed a strong sense of self-esteem and a positive view of themselves may be able to handle bodily changes or changes in capability due to accident, illness, or injury more easily than others. They may have developed a variety of skills and interests on which to draw during their rehabilitation or recovery. They are more likely to separate the physical changes from whom they are as people, and keep a perspective about the changes. The changes may affect the way they look or what they can do, but not who they are as people.

Self-Concept—Role Performance

The aspect of self-concept having to do with role performance—how people view themselves in all of their personal roles—is always affected in some way by illness or hospitalization. A role can be described as a person's responsibilities in a particular setting. Usually people have many roles. Each of a person's roles has responsibilities associated with it at different times. People often carry out many roles at one time. They may be a mother, spouse or partner, or daughter caring for a parent, or they may have a job or a position in organizations or provide leadership in their communities—each role with different responsibilities. Most people will have some or all of their roles disrupted by illness or hospitalization. Caregivers can listen to comments of patients and family members and encourage them to talk together. They can also offer support for looking at ways to adjust their roles to the reality of the patient's present situation.

One of the cultural values that people learn early in life is how people "should" act when they are sick. This learned "sick role" will be viewed differently by many people, including individual patients, families, and caregivers. Cultural values also influence how people respond to the illness or injury of loved ones. In a number of cultures, the entire family believes they should be with their loved one at all times. Hospital rules, and the reality that often adult family members have jobs that do not allow them the freedom to be at the bedside, cause great personal strain and a conflict of role responsibilities (Fig. 14–1). Other families may believe that when a person is

in the hospital everything should be done for him or her—That's what the caregivers are hired for. This may result in a conflict of expectations in providing care. Often different learned experience and differing cultural value systems are at the root of conflicts between what the treatment team thinks should be done and what patients or their families want.

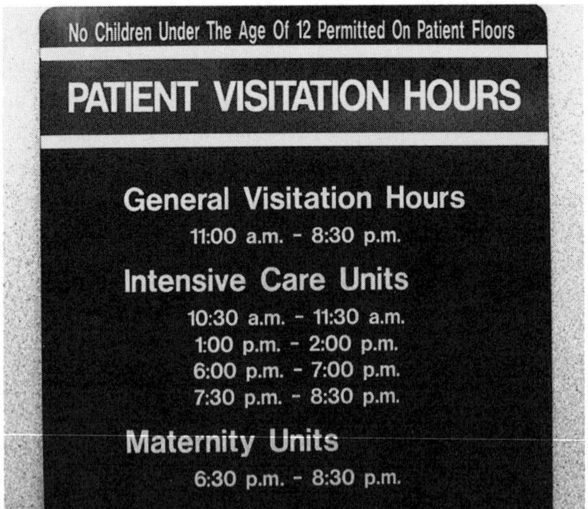

Self-Concept—Personal Identity

The fourth aspect of self-concept that may be affected by illness is the person's personal identity—What makes the person different from others? Personal identity includes physical description, special skills and special attributes, individual experiences, as well as sexual identity. Personal identity is affected by major physical or psychological changes. For people who feel their entire identity is tied up with what job they do, role performance and personal identity are inseparable. For example, an athlete, physician, or secretary who has put all of his or her identity into the performance role, would have great difficulty seeing any other positive options in his or her life, if illness or injury made it impossible to continue those primary roles. In other cases, a physician or an RN whose training and long-term experience had been as a caregiver may find great difficulty giving up some of the control that is necessary in the patient role. PCTs should recognize that the patient may experience anger and frustration as a result of the situation. This may be expressed in inappropriate ways against the patient's family and hospital staff.

In summary, people's self-concept and body image are built over time through interactions with others. Some people have a very strong self-concept that includes positive feelings about themselves in all four areas. Others are content with strengths in some areas and are comfortable with themselves the way they are. For many other people, their identity continues to be reflected in the reactions of others. How they feel about themselves is closely tied in with how people respond to them.

> PCTs must be sensitive to nonverbal as well as verbal responses to the patient. Patience and understanding are critical.

Times of illness and injury always put people's identity to the test. Will their self-concept be strong enough to give them the strength to work at positive recovery or rehabilitation? Will they feel overwhelmed, give up, and need strong support and intervention from caregivers? Although people have varying needs for validation from others, what is clear, is that no matter what happens to people, the reaction of caregivers and loved ones is critical to successful recovery. The positive reactions, acceptance and encouragement of others, allow people opportunities to remain *whole*, to still see themselves as valuable,

No Children Under The Age Of 12 Permitted On Patient Floors

PATIENT VISITATION HOURS

General Visitation Hours
11:00 a.m. - 8:30 p.m.

Intensive Care Units
10:30 a.m. - 11:30 a.m.
1:00 p.m. - 2:00 p.m.
6:00 p.m. - 7:00 p.m.
7:30 p.m. - 8:30 p.m.

Maternity Units
6:30 p.m. - 8:30 p.m.

FIGURE 14-1
Visiting hours.

and respected and lovable, in spite of the illness or trauma they might have experienced.

CHANGED BODY FUNCTION OR STRUCTURE

Some of the most basic changes in body function or structure occur during adolescence, pregnancy, and aging. These are all normal processes of life, but often cause major adjustments to self-concept: body image, self-esteem, role performance, and personal identity. Some individuals face major adjustment problems related to personal capability, appearance, attractiveness to others, and sexuality. Certainly their adjustment can be worsened by teasing or negative reactions of others. We can also identify people in our experience who sailed through those transitional life changes through the support and encouragement of others. As caregivers, it is important to recognize that people going through these normal stages of life are faced with many stresses and need extra support and nonjudgmental acceptance.

Process of Hospitalization and Diagnosis

The hospital experience can be difficult for patients and their families. Patients and caregivers often have different ideas of what will or should happen in the hospital. Patients and families may complain about the room, the view (or lack of it), the food, the staff, or any number of things. For some, the problem is a reality. For others, the complaints may come out of fear and uncertainty about what will happen to them, and what they will find out in the hospital. Loss of control, invasion of

privacy, disruption of their daily routine, different food, unusual or frightening sounds, and being confronted with the reality of the pain or suffering that other people go through are all part of what they experience coming to the hospital.

The process of diagnosis often is a difficult and painful experience.

> PCTs should learn what happens to patients during the tests usually ordered on their unit. They will be better prepared to support teaching and provide adequate post-test care.

Many people may enter the patient's room unannounced. Patients may be transported to other departments, wheeled through hallways and in elevators, visible to all. They arrive at each new test wearing only a hospital gown, are surrounded by frightening equipment and are poked, rolled, slid, and positioned to carry out the test carefully (Fig. 14–2). They may be given medication to put them asleep during the test and may fear what will happen to them. Diagnostic tests usually involve use of invasive tubes and needles. Patients need to discuss their history over and over again with people they do not know. The person may be in pain, nauseated, confused about treatments or tests, and fearful of the results. It requires submission to the rules and dictates of the health care system, and in itself puts people and their loved ones on an emotional roller coaster. Each new test brings new possibilities and diagnoses. A diagnosis made on one day may be rejected the next after results of new tests. The physician may believe the patient does not need all the information, and the patient may think the worst if he or she does not have it. It is a constantly changing environ-

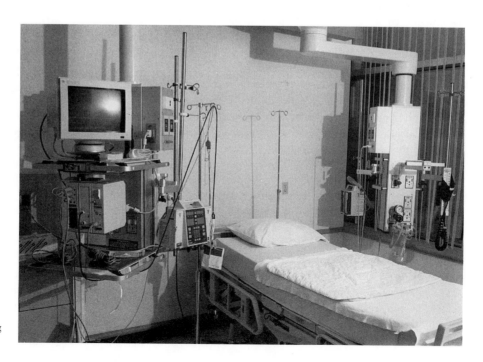

FIGURE 14–2

Equipment that may seem frightening to a patient.

ment. All come with their own hopes and fears and experiences. The cultural values and beliefs of the caregiving staff and the patient and family may be quite different. For caregivers, knowledge of what people need, willingness to listen, to be flexible and nonjudgmental, determination, and a desire to make a difference are keys to being effective.

✓ After diagnosis, patients tend to focus on personal issues and fears. Allow unrushed time to listen. Help provide or reinforce information.

Loss Related to Injury, Illness, or Surgery

Loss of function or structure may also be due to an injury, disease process, or surgery. Loss of function refers to the inability of a bodily organ or bodily system to perform the way it is normally expected to perform. Illnesses like heart disease, diabetes, Alzheimer's disease, and multiple sclerosis are examples. They may occur gradually with small changes or gradual loss of function and capability. These are not visible diseases, but they can be progressive and get worse over time, and there is no known cure. The impact on the person, on body image, and the potential to interfere with work, recreation, and sexuality are high. This often causes frustration because of the more frequent need to explain why the patient cannot do things. Because other people cannot "see" the problem, the patient may be seen as lazy or making excuses. Family members may deny or minimize the illness. This response may cause discouragement or continued denial in the patient. A new diagnosis adds pressures and stress. Problems that were previously handled easily are now unmanageable. PCTs should learn about the illnesses commonly seen in the patients they care for. That will enable them to more easily reinforce the teaching of the RN.

Loss of structure is the change or loss of a body part, often resulting in disfigurement or unusual appearance. This may often occur suddenly as the result of a traumatic accident. It may result in both internal and external (visible) damage and may involve structural changes such as major burns, scarring, an amputation, a colostomy, loss of vision, or spinal cord injury and paraplegia (paralysis of the part of the body below the injury). Some illnesses like cancer or skin diseases may cause deformities or changes that are visible to others. Visible bodily changes bring on a new set of issues for people. These kinds of bodily changes may cause others to respond with pity or distaste and may result in avoidance. For all who experience these major illnesses, there is an effect on their body image as well as a decrease in their ability to function.

Most people feel uncomfortable about needing others to help them take care of their bodily functions. An indication of disgust by a caregiver makes this situation even more uncomfortable and embarrassing. Your job as a PCT is to increase your patient's level of comfort. A calm, matter-of-fact attitude while performing duties related to bodily functions helps patients feel accepted and more comfortable with the status of their body.

✓ Watch nonverbal gestures when performing tasks related to skin diseases, stool, vomitus, mucus, and infected or draining wounds.

Depending on the extent of the illness or surgery, hospitalization, rehabilitation, and other community services may be a part of the patient's life for a time. The goal for the patient is to be as independent and productive as possible given the realities of the new situation. Physical healing depends on the extent of injury or surgery, the patient's general health prior to the illness, and the physical care, treatments, and emotional support received during the hospitalization. To adjust to changes caused by the illness or injury, the patient and family have to learn to live with the physical care required; the limitations to physical activity and recreation; acceptance of any changes in appearance; and recognition that the changes may interfere with personal or professional roles (Fig. 14–3).

Acceptance and an open friendly manner while performing care duties assist patients in feeling free to discuss their concerns. They also are more likely to ask questions regarding the changes they are experiencing in their view of themselves, as well as in the functioning of their bodies. Patients may also make negative "jokes" about their body. For example, when a patient says "Did you come in to see the freak show"? in response to a radical neck dissection, this often reflects concern about the changes he or she is going through.

✓ Discuss a patient's negative comments or jokes about the body with the RN. They may serve as an opportunity to discuss the patient's feelings about their experience.

The Grief Process—Response to a Loss

Emotional recovery from a traumatic injury, a disfiguring operation, or a chronic devastating disease is difficult to understand and to help. The person's ability to cope or manage the feelings and frustrations of living with the physical changes will be a key to successful recovery. It is important for the caregiver to recognize that the loss may cause a change in self-concept and observable behavior. From day to day, the patient's behaviors may change or seem irrational and unpredictable. These behavioral changes are a response to that loss.

Patients' initial response to a changed appearance or bodily function will vary and will be influenced by a

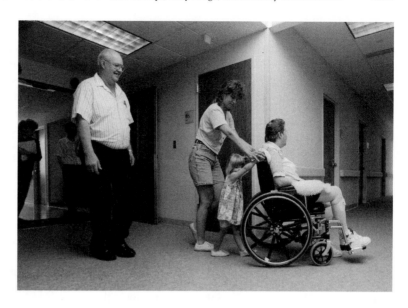

FIGURE 14-3
Family assisting patient in a wheelchair.

variety of factors, including their self-concept—body image, their individual coping skills, and support systems they have in place. The individual will often proceed through a grief process similar to that which occurs at the death of a loved one. The initial response may include such actions as:

- Denial that anything is really wrong: Refusal to look at or touch the changed area
- Anger: At the change, at family, God, doctor, or other caregivers
- Bargaining: Recognizing that there is a problem, but that it will not be too bad
- Depression or anxiety expressed by:
  - Feelings of helplessness or hopelessness
  - Fear of rejection by others
  - Preoccupation with bodily functions
- Understanding and acceptance

The grief process continues back and forth through the stages and may be characterized by continued anger, withdrawal and social isolation, depression, and negative feelings about their bodies or themselves. It is the role of all caregivers to understand that the grief process is normal, to accept people wherever they are in the process, and to continue to offer reassurance.

It is also important for caregivers to offer hope. Hope doesn't mean false reassurance that everything will be all right. Hope means possibility for the future. Hope is a step-by-step process and can be found in conversations with people who have faced similar problems, staff who have seen and can describe new possibilities, and families who offer love and a reason to try. When patients see new possibility for their lives in spite of the changes, they are able to move toward acceptance in the grief process.

 The PCT can help patients through the grieving process by:

- Recognizing their feelings and their need to work through the stages of their grief
- Supporting the patient in the grieving process
- Helping patients break tasks down into small steps that may be easily achievable and encouraging their efforts
- Offering possibility by focusing on the present and celebrating small steps in the healing process

A person with a new spinal cord injury and paralysis who has believed in the past that to ask for help with anything would mean he or she was weak and inadequate would probably have a hard time reaching acceptance. Offering praise for simple activities that serve as steps in the total process encourages people to try again. Recovery is always a series of small steps and repeated efforts.

The effect of self-concept body image on behavior must be recognized by the caregiver to assist the patient to adapt to necessary changes. The staff can also better predict potential problems the patient may have adapting to temporary or permanent bodily changes.

Communication—A Key Factor

A patient with a new diagnosis of multiple sclerosis refuses a meal tray and states to the caregiver, "I'd rather die than live in a wheelchair." The caregiver should recognize that this patient may need some help adjusting to the diagnosis and its accompanying problems. An appropriate response from the PCT, such as, "It sounds like this new information is pretty difficult for you to deal with; I'll let the RN know. Is there anything I can do for you while I'm here?," recognizes the patient's fear. This must be documented and reported to the RN.

A patient who requests that the room door remain closed may want to keep the noise out or may be withdrawing as a reaction to surgical removal of a cancerous breast. The PCT will be able to consider both possibilities and take appropriate steps, such as asking some leading questions about the noisiness of the hospital unit.

 The PCT should document patient quotes that reflect the patient response to the illness.

Report patient's verbal or emotional responses to the illness or treatment to the RN. The RN will assess the patient's responses before deciding on the next action.

With the information from the caregiver and after talking with the patient, the RN will develop a plan of care and discuss roles of each team member in the plan.

Understanding some of the individual's beliefs and values will increase the caregiver's success with patient care. The PCT who has developed the ability to talk with patients in a caring manner may spend a significant amount of time with a patient. This increases the opportunity for the patient to share information and emotions that he or she may not share with other staff. The caregiver will know how to communicate in a genuine, thoughtful, nonthreatening manner that encourages patients to express their feelings.

A patient may express negative feelings about the changed body, for example, "They made a freak out of me," stated a woman after a mastectomy. It is important that the caregiver does not say, "You shouldn't feel that way." Expressing feelings about a change in the body can be a first step in acceptance. A supportive comment that would allow the patient to continue talking would be, "It sounds like it's pretty hard to go through all of the changes you're facing."

The PCT should listen carefully to what the patient says, offering genuine concern. Sharing the conversations with the RN will enable the RN to offer suggestions or support as the PCT continues the relationship with the patient. Discuss documentation of the patient's progress.

Some reactions are helped by the passage of time—time for the individual to see and hear caregiving staff provide care; time to cleanse or dress the surgical or trauma site; time to see positive responses from others; time to accept the reality of the diagnosis; and time to begin to see alternative possibilities for their lives.

When patients begin to feel they are a part of the healing process, they begin to feel a sense of control over some aspects of the changes. This feeling of having some control of their destiny allows them to begin to integrate the change into a new, revised body image. During the integration or reorganization phase, the individual begins to recognize and deal with the limitations imposed by the changes to develop new interests, and to restructure his

or her lifestyle. Integration is a very slow process and there is no effective way to hurry it.

Acceptance is a goal for most people to attain. Whether or not they successfully reach acceptance depends on such factors as coping skills, support systems, and personal strengths. People progress toward acceptance at different rates. For example, some women may accept a mastectomy in a few days, but others will take months or years to adjust to the changes in their bodies. The caregiver needs to discuss problems with the RN, but must always keep a nonjudgmental, accepting attitude toward the patient.

Acceptance and support from caregivers help patients take the first steps toward acceptance and adjustment to changes in bodily functioning and appearance.

Role of the Patient Care Technician

The PCT will be able to give the patient the physical care that the condition requires. Much of the earlier chapters of this book focus on specific care that is necessary to recover from a particular illness or surgical event.

Emotional support or encouragement should be offered throughout the recovery process. Brief moments are just as important as longer conversations. For example, when the patient says, "The occupational therapist showed me a weird spoon yesterday," the caregiver can encourage interest in the adaptive equipment. "Even though the spoon looks different, I've seen people use it and it works really well."

PCTs should be familiar with, validate, support, and encourage other team members' work with their patients.

The first attempts to adjust to a new body image may occur immediately before a planned surgical procedure or be delayed until after the surgical dressings are removed. In the case of a traumatic event, such as a car accident, the work will begin afterward. Caregivers should be attuned to respond to a patient's needs for validation and support from admission through to discharge.

Because of the delicate nature of the emotional aspects of care, the PCT is encouraged to seek the support and guidance of the RN or social worker who is working with the patient. All team members need to provide the patient and family with a consistent message.

Following are some suggestions to support the self-concept and individuality of all patients:

- Provide for patients' basic need for recognition. Ask if the patient has been in this hospital or another hospital before. Provide a thorough orientation to the room, the unit, and the usual daily routine. Discuss meal schedules and visiting hours. Ask if they have any particular needs or concerns that you could help with. Ask patients about their family, spouse, significant other. Who do they expect will be visiting? How could you help? Encourage patients to talk about their jobs, hobbies, and family, as appropriate.

- Meet peoples' needs for inclusion. Involve them in discussions and ask for their input into decisions about their care. Give them choices. Never carry on a conversation with a family member or caregiver in the presence of the patient, without involving the patient.

- Be sensitive to everyone's body image issues—adolescence through aging. Maintain privacy when providing all personal care, dressing changes, and performing diagnostic tests like electrocardiography. Provide a matter-of-fact approach when dealing with elimination issues, ostomy care, amputations, and other forms of disfigurement. Provide glasses, dentures, prosthesis, hair pieces or other personal items to increase the comfort level around others. Make efforts to wash and style the hair, shave the beard, allow patients to wear their own gown or pajamas if appropriate.

- Provide a gentle touch or an occasional pat for all, from very thin to obese, from young to old, and from the friendly to the quiet or depressed. Wear gloves only when you expect contact with blood or body fluids.

- Use people-first language when addressing or talking about a person who has a disability. Identify the person first, and then the disability. For example, "Mrs. Jones in room 228 is having difficulty sleeping," or "Mrs. Jones in room 228 is diabetic; I just checked her blood sugar and it's 365."

- Support the person's spirituality or religious belief system. Do not make judgments about the patient's beliefs or pass your belief system on to others. Accept that for some, religion may not be important.

- Understand your own values, beliefs, and attitudes regarding illness, disability, disfigurement, sexuality, sexual identity, and people who are different. As a caregiver, you may have different views, but you must not try to pass them on to patients or families. It is essential that you be able to accept people as they present themselves.

- Focus the caregiver–patient relationship on what the patients' needs are, what is affecting them, how they feel, and what they want to talk about. It is not appropriate for the caregiver to focus on his or her own problems or illness or on staff, unit, or hospital problems or concerns. This differs from the social relationship you would have with a friend or neighbor. In the social relationship, both people in the relationship are free to discuss their own issues and problems and to seek understanding and support from each other.

Following are some suggestions for dealing with patients who may be experiencing illnesses or surgical procedures that are a direct assault on their body image:

- Encourage the patient to verbalize his or her feeling of anger, anxiety, fear, and loss. The caregiver must be open and ready to see and hear emotions that are unsettling, unpleasant, or difficult. The caregiver will need to be accepting of whatever emotions are expressed, while being careful not to agree with expressions of hatred or self-violence (if they occur). It is important to accept where the patient is in his or her reactions to the changed body.

STOP Do not use cliches, such as, "It's not really that bad" or "You should be glad to be alive," to minimize the impact of the diagnosis or event on the patient.

- Encourage, but do not force, the patient to touch or look at the changed body part. It may take some time before the patient is willing to do this.

- Reinforce the reality of the changed body part and recognition that the patient will have to provide care after going home; for example, "Yes, it will take some practice to learn to care for your colostomy. The RN and enterostomal therapist will teach you the easiest and best ways."

- Encourage the patient to go to physical therapy or other rehabilitation services and to practice what is learned to improve functioning of the affected part or area. Talk about changes you have seen and improvements patients have talked about after their series of physical therapy measures.

- If ordered by the physician, encourage and assist the patient to use cosmetic devices or services available for disfiguring surgery and mechanical devices for improved functioning. If a device is available, but not being used, work with the RN and the patient to determine why it is not being used (Fig. 14–4).

- Encourage the patient to use the support services or groups in the community. If the caregiver is not aware of services for support or rehabilitation, a referral to the social services department can help link patients with hospital or community resources.

To reinforce the information, it is important for the caregiver to know what resources have been suggested to the patient or family.

- Reinforce ways to improve the patient's body image, such as dress, applying makeup, and performing simple exercises to foster feelings of success.

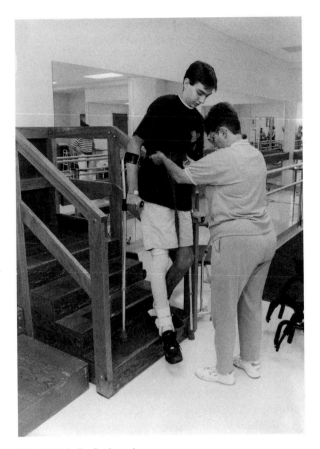

FIGURE 14-4
Practicing using the stairs in physical therapy.

• Acknowledge and reinforce the patient's attempts to improve the appearance, such as wearing different clothes and shaving.

• Help the family focus on what the patient can do, instead of what he or she cannot do. Consistently offer *hope* and help the family concentrate on developing ways they can be helpful in their loved one's recovery.

SEXUALITY

Sexuality is an aspect of health, identity, and humanity that is frequently avoided during an illness or following an injury or surgical intervention. Sexuality is part of how a person feels about himself or herself. It does not refer only to the genitals, which define a person as male or female, it refers to all of the aspects of the person and the person's identity as a man or a woman. Sexuality is deeply rooted in self-concept, body image, self-esteem, and personal identity. Besides the hereditary aspects, sexuality is a cultural phenomenon and is influenced by family, social influences, and religious values.

Sexual Identity

Sexual identity could be described as one's sexual self-concept. It involves whether or not the person perceives himself or herself to be attractive and sexually desirable. Whether an individual identifies himself or herself as heterosexual (attracted to the opposite sex), homosexual (attracted to the same sex), or bisexual (interested in relations with either sex) depends on a number of life factors. Those factors may include genetic predisposition, socialization, reaction to life events, and/or in some cases, personal choice. The exact reasons that determine a person's sexual identity or preference are not known at this time.

Caregiving staff should expect no difference in caring for patients whether they are homosexual or heterosexual. In most cases, it is not their sexuality that brought them to the hospital. It is important, however, to recognize that whoever shares a person's life can be of primary importance in healing, well-being, and overall health. Regardless of the sexual identity involved, loving relationships are key to the patient's comfort and recovery. All relationships must be treated with respect and dignity. Long-term homosexual relationships or heterosexual relationships that do not involve legal marriage are as important to the participants as is the spousal relationship between husband and wife. Your support of the primary relationship or partner is very important and should be handled with the same tact and consideration that would be offered to any patient in the hospital.

If staff find they are overly uncomfortable or embarrassed about dealing with patients whose sexual identity is different from their own, they should seek assistance from the RN, a trusted friend, clergyman, or counselor to help deal with their feelings or biases in a positive manner. Both the caregiver's verbal communication and nonverbal facial expressions or body postures must reflect a nonjudgmental, supportive attitude.

Hospitalization and Illness

Sexuality is an important aspect of health, identity, and basic humanity. However, discussion of sexuality with patients is too often avoided or ignored as a crucial element in patients' ultimate recovery from an illness, injury, or surgical intervention. Although sexuality may be a low priority for the caregiving staff's attention during the initial phases of illness, this key issue in patients' lives does not disappear because they experience a change in their health status and personal routine.

Many people fear that a major illness or a change in body function or structure will adversely impact their sexual attractiveness, interest, ability, performance, and enjoyment. Many factors influence whether the patient will initiate a discussion of sexuality with caregivers. These include how the patient perceives that the topic of sexuality will be received by caregivers; the degree of rapport that has been built among the patient, family members, and caregivers; and the patient's individual comfort level with his or her own sexuality and sexual identity.

Often, patients do not approach the topic of sexuality with their physicians because of embarrassment or fear that their concerns about their functioning will be confirmed. Likewise, physicians, who are involved in healing patients' primary disease or injury, may not think to adequately inform patients and their loved ones that restricting sexual activity may not be necessary, or to explain modifications that can assist them in regaining confidence in themselves as sexual beings and resuming satisfactory sexual functioning.

If patients ask questions or make comments or jokes related to their sexuality after experiencing an illness, injury, or surgery, inform the RN or physician so that options can be discussed with patients and their families.

Without frank discussion and education about sexuality and sexual activity, patients may unnecessarily withdraw from sexual activity or try to reassure themselves of their continued sexual abilities by unwisely increasing their activities. The topic of sexuality should be addressed by professionals as an integral part of the ongoing, individualized education and plan of care for patients and their families.

When a patient experiences lengthy hospitalization, physical needs may lead to masturbation. This is a normal response, and a caregiver who interrupts should excuse himself or herself, leave, close the door, and allow the patient some privacy. The issues of sexuality and intimacy for the patient and significant other also need to be discussed. The RN will probably build that into the patient's plan of care. The PCT should check with the RN about offering the patient an opportunity for some private uninterrupted time with his or her spouse/partner.

Sexually Transmitted Diseases

Sexually transmitted diseases (STDs) are infections that are transmitted or received during unprotected sexual contact with a person who has the disease. There are many: Chlamydia infection, gonorrhea, and genital herpes are examples. Several others like hepatitis B and the human immunodeficiency virus (HIV), the virus that can cause AIDS (acquired immune deficiency syndrome), have also been passed on in a variety of other ways associated with contact with the blood or body fluids of an infected person. People who are hospitalized with sexually transmitted diseases face a variety of physical as well as emotional problems.

The HIV virus attacks the body's immune system and it may be 8–10 years before a person develops AIDS. The weakened immune system makes it difficult for the body to fight infections and that makes the person susceptible to many serious infections. A person is said to have AIDS when he or she has developed some of the AIDS-related illnesses like pneumocyctis pneumonia, an unusual type of pneumonia; Kaposi's sarcoma, a type of skin cancer; or neurological problems.

It is important to prevent the patient infected with the HIV virus from being exposed to other harmful organisms. Be especially careful of colds, flu, herpes, and chickenpox.

A person cannot get AIDS through casual contact. The PCT should use gloves, gown, or mask as needed to prevent exposure to infected blood or body fluids. Exposure could occur through a break in the caregiver's skin or splashing into the mucous membranes of the eyes, nose, or mouth. In addition all possible care should be used to prevent needlestick injuries.

Do not share razors, or other implements that may come in contact with blood or body fluids, from one person with anyone else.

Anyone exposed to blood or body fluid through a needlestick injury or a break in the skin *must* report it to the RN immediately.

Since having one of these diseases usually indicates that the person has been sexually active, it may bring out new issues for relationships with spouses or families. For spouses, issues of infidelity and fears that they could have also been exposed to the disease may interfere with their ability to be supportive. For families, it may have come as a surprise that their child had been sexually active. Hospitalization with an AIDS-related illness like Kaposi's sarcoma, a type of skin cancer, may trigger a discussion with loved ones for the first time about being gay. It also could bring on accusations or suspicions about being gay that are not true. Although AIDS does have a high incidence in the gay community, it affects men, women, and children of all ages. Since there is no known cure at this time for HIV or AIDS, fears related to having an incurable illness affect both patients and families. Fear, and avoidance by others, place additional strains on self-concept and body image. Some actions that would be very helpful, include:

- Encourage the person with AIDS to be involved in his or her own care.

- Do not avoid the person with AIDS. You do not always have to talk. Offering some company or quiet time when you have the opportunity is very supportive.

- Let the person talk about the disease if desired.

Do not be afraid to touch the person with AIDS. Holding a hand or giving a back rub can be very supportive. However, be sensitive when people do not wish to accept physical closeness.

It is important that you are fully aware of your hospital's rules and regulations regarding patient confidentiality and that you diligently observe and practice these rules. Sexuality is perhaps the most intimate, personal aspect of self-concept, and the patient's trust, dignity, and privacy must be protected in this sensitive area at all times.

Sexually Aggressive Patients

According to B. F. Skinner, behavioral scientist, all behavior is rational and motivated. However, when a patient becomes sexually aggressive in either a verbal or a physical manner, the rationale behind the behavior is not the immediate concern. Inappropriate touching or suggestive, sexual comments are not acceptable at any time.

Often a situation involving sexual aggression on the part of a patient can be defused by setting firm limits: removing the patient's hand and telling the patient calmly but firmly that the behavior or language is unacceptable.

If the PCT is successful in defusing a situation by setting limits with the patient, it may be reasonable to explore the motivation for the patient's behavior. A patient who has not been able to ask appropriate questions about the ability to perform sexually after an illness or injury, or is questioning his or her sexual desirability, may act out fear and frustration in inappropriate ways such as making sexually explicit comments or suggestions or attempting to touch the caregiver's body in an improper and sexual manner. Although this does not in any way excuse the behavior, it presents an opportunity to discuss the patient's concerns and fears about sexuality in more detail.

Inform the RN when a patient acts out in a sexual way. The RN may use the opportunity to discuss the patient's sexual needs or fears in more detail.

Should, however, a patient continue to make inappropriate advances to the caregiver and refuse to respect firm limits on his or her behavior, the caregiver should report the problem to the nursing staff. The RN can advise you of your hospital's rules and procedures regarding unacceptable, sexually aggressive behavior and can assist you in documenting the situation and reporting it through appropriate procedural channels.

SUMMARY

People want to feel good about themselves and their appearance. They have developed an image of their body, which is a part of how they view themselves. Body image is attacked and tested with a new diagnosis such as diabetes, a new disease such as cancer, side effects of treatment such as hair loss, disfiguring surgery, or loss of a limb through trauma. While body image is personal, and invisible to others, attacks to body image affect recovery and quality of life. Sexuality, a part of body image as well as personal identity, often is affected by illness or injury.

PCTs play a major role in helping patients heal emotionally as well as physically after illness or injury. They validate the patient's experience by accepting him or her, offering support and encouragement for small steps in the recovery process, and celebrating small as well as large successes. Maintaining open communication and working cooperatively with other team members sends a clear message of support to patients and their families.

Organizing Your Work Assignment

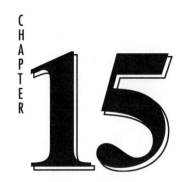

DOROTHY H. MUNDY, MN, RN, BSN
JANICE M. CRABILL, MSN, RN

OUTLINE

Assessing the Assignment
Planning Your Workday
Time Management and Setting Priorities
Estimating Time Frames

Adapting the Work Assignment Throughout the Day
Summary

PREREQUISITE KNOWLEDGE AND SKILLS

- Report process
- Concept of teamwork
- Job description and scope of practice
- Recognition of emergency patient situations
- Operation of bedside and emergency equipment

OBJECTIVES

After you complete this chapter, you will be able to:

- Identify sources of information that help to plan a work assignment.
- Describe the use of a patient assignment worksheet as a tool to organize patient care.
- Explain how to organize patient care using the "What, Who, When" plan.

- Identify situations that need to be reported immediately to the RN.
- Develop a flexible time plan that accommodates changes in patient care priorities.
- Evaluate work for quality, accuracy, and completeness.

KEY TERMS

Nurse Practice Acts   The nurse practice acts define what each level of nursing staff is allowed to do within a particular state. Each state may define different tasks as acceptable for the patient care technician (PCT). Your job description is an excellent source for finding out what patient care tasks have been identified as acceptable by your agency and as lawful by your state for a PCT to carry out.

Delegation   Delegation is an informal contract between two individuals. One of the individuals is given the authority to act in the place of the other individual. The delegator has the responsibility to assign tasks appropriately and to follow up on the outcome of the delegated function. The individual who received the delegated task has the responsibility to be self-directed and to complete the assigned task in a reasonable time and report completion to the delegator, who maintains overall responsibility for safe completion of the task.

It is 7:30 AM and you have just received a report on your patients for this shift. You have a "full load" and are wondering how you will provide all the needed care for your patients in a timely and complete manner. You must deliver this care during hectic times, keeping in mind that each patient is your number 1 customer (Chapter 1), demonstrate leadership in organization (Chapter 2), and continually communicate relevant information efficiently to team members (Chapter 3). All this work needs to be done without any patient sensing the demands of your total assignment.

This chapter presents suggestions to the patient care technician (PCT) for organizing time, setting priorities, and adjusting to unexpected situations so that the work flows smoothly and is completed by the end of the shift. While the RN is responsible for identifying and delegating patient care tasks, PCTs must organize their delegated tasks to ensure that patients receive all assigned care in an efficient and safe manner.

ASSESSING THE ASSIGNMENT

The first step in organizing your work is to identify what you have to do throughout the shift. This work begins as soon as you receive your assignment from the RN.

⚖️ The RN has the legal responsibility of delegating tasks to other team members based on their job description, educational background, competency, and specific state nurse practice acts. The RN and PCT remain responsible for safe completion of delegated tasks.

Although you may receive information about your patients from staff who worked on previous shifts, there are three main sources of patient information:

• Shift report
• Kardex and patient chart
• RN responsible for your assigned patient

This exchange of information is passed from staff members of one shift to the next and describes the most current concerns for each patient.

The shift report is typically a review of patient status, description of unusual patient events during the shift, tests, follow-up activities, or special needs for the next shift. The shift report usually does not review the detailed activities of daily living (ADLs) or the routine components

of a patient's day, but focuses attention on the extraordinary or unusual events.

🛑 *Always* receive a current report before starting patient care. Patient status, especially that of patients in acute care situations, may deteriorate quickly. For example, a patient care activity such as walking to the bathroom that was appropriate one day may be contraindicated the next after surgery, seizure activity, or a blood clot discovered in the leg.

The Kardex is a useful tool for the PCT to identify routine as well as specific patient care tasks that are ordered by physicians, RNs, or other care providers (Fig. 15–1). In contrast to the shift report, the Kardex offers a detailed examination of the activities to be completed for each individual patient. The patient chart, especially the flow sheet, further outlines the specific plan of care and additional interventions to be carried out for the patient (Fig. 15–2). PCTs must recognize which interventions are within their job description and be responsible to carry them out. When kept up to date, the Kardex and flow sheet usually include information about:

• Frequency of vital signs
• Special checks
• Measurements that need to be reported
• State of alertness
• Amount of assistance needed for ADLs
• Special precautions
• Diet and needed assistance with meals
• Activity level
• Skin and tube care
• Elimination pattern
• Specimens to collect and test
• Respiratory assistance
• Treatments
• Diagnostic tests
• Consultations
• Special equipment used in the care of each specific patient.

Critical Pathways or Care Maps (Fig. 15–3) are a recent multidisciplinary adaptation of the nursing care plan or Kardex. These care plans identify typical progressive interventions for specific medical conditions. A new "goal" is set for each day during a patient's hospitaliza-

Text continued on page 271

Nursing Kardex

University Medical Center
Department of Nursing

ALLERGIES:

Room 920	Bed A	Name *Jane Doe*		(preferred name)	Hospital No.		Primary Nurse
Adm. Date 11/20	Age 72	Current medical problem/ surgical procedure	⒧ CVA, S/P G tube placed		Serv. M1		Physicians
Family name/relation to patient and phone numbers		*Son – Henry ph 614-293-8000 (work)*				Religion *Cath*	Sacr. of Sick *Yes*

PATIENT PROFILE (Perceptions, expectations, family, customs, previous medical and nursing care)

70 yo female admitted through ER after son found unconscious at home. Hx of ⒧ CVA, has not regained complete alertness since stroke. G tube placed p̄3 wk of refusing po intake. Pt is alert to name only.
Supportive son.

DISCHARGE PLANS (destination, referrals, travel, learning needs, length of stay, anticipated date of discharge)

Possible N H placement social serv contacted - will need C.O.C. Clergy, PT, OT, Speech.

DATE		DATE	
11/20	**WT** *qd (bed)* **TPR** *q 4 h* **BP** *q 4 h*		**DIET** - *Full liquids (encourage)* Calorie counts
			Tube feeding *osmolite @ 25 ml/hr per G-tube*
	SPECIAL CHECK		**NPO** why
	CS ac & hs		⒤&O) Total daily fluid *2000* ml.
	HAU, GAS		Dietary *1000* Unit *1000* IV *∅*
			7-3 *400* 3-11 *400* 11-7 *200*
	CALL *HO* if		**EATING** (feed), assist
	SBP > 180, DBP > 90		special needs √ *aspiration*
	P > 100		⒨OUTH CARE⒠ Dentures: full partial √
	R > 28		
	⒮AFETY PRECAUTION) *seizure prec*		**BATH**
	restraints *- soft wrist* siderails *X1* ↑		tub shower bed sitz self assist (total)
	bed position *Hob* ↑ *30°*		
	⒤SOLATION⟩ *MRSA – G tube site*		**SKIN CARE** *nystatin to groin p̄ peri-care.*
	MENTAL STATUS alert unconscious		*On specialty bed for pressure*
	⒞onfused/disoriented⟩		*relief*
			TUBE CARE –
	SENSORY DEFICITS ⒨ ⒧ ⊖		*GT site care c̄ soap & H₂O*
			Foley care.
	IMMOBILITY partial (complete)		
	why ⒧ *CVA*		**DRESS/GROOM** self assist (total)
	ACTIVITY UAL (Up with assist) BRP BR		
	ambulation		
	chair *– OOB bid*		**PROSTHETICS/ORTHOTICS** *∅*
	exercises *ROM*		
			ELIMINATION Bowel *– uses Bed pan*
	TRAVEL BY *cart*		
	self assist need _3_ people		last BM
	⒫OSITIONING⟩		Bladder *– Foley to SD*
	turn *q 2 hr* √ bony prom -		(over)

FIGURE 15–1
Front and back of Kardex.

Date	MEDICATIONS	Dose	Rt	Freq	Hours	Notes	Name:		
							Date	SPECIMENS	Done
							11/20	CC urine for C & S	
							11/20	Sputum C & S	

Date	IV THERAPY		Date	RESPIRATORY THERAPY
			11/20	O$_2$ 2L N/C
			11/20	Incentive spirometer
				q 1 hr while awake

Date	OTHER		Date	MEDICAL TREATMENTS	Hours
11/20	Sequential Compression				
	Devices (SCD's) on both				
	legs A T C				

Date	BLOODWORK	4-digit no.	Freq.	Hours	Date	TESTS/CONSULTS/APPOINTMENTS	Done
11/20	chem 7		qd		11/20	chest x - ray	
11/20	C B C D and P		qd		11/21	E G D	
11/20	P T and P T T		qd				

F I G U R E   1 5 – 1

Continued

NURSING FLOW SHEET

DATE					
SIGNATURE — 11-7					
SIGNATURE — 7-3					
SIGNATURE — 3-11					
Temperature/ — 12M					
4A					
Pulse/ — 8A					
Respirations/ — 12N					
4P					
Blood pressure — 8P					

Weight	kg	lbs	kg	lbs	kg	lbs	kg	lbs
Bath/shower								
Back care								
Oral hygiene								
Activity								
Diet								

Appetite — B = breakfast, L = lunch, D = dinner	B	L	D	B	L	D	B	L	D	B	L	D

Bowel movement

Nighttime Rest/sleep — S = sleeping, A = awake, R = resting	11PM	12M	1A	2A	11PM	12M	1A	2A	11PM	12M	1A	2A	11PM	12M	1A	2A
	3A	4A	5A	6A	3A	4A	5A	6A	3A	4A	5A	6A	3A	4A	5A	6A

SPECIMENS

Diagnostic tests

NURSING INTERVENTIONS — IV tubing change					
IV site care					

NURSING FLOW SHEET

FIGURE 15–2

Nursing Flow Sheet.

VR on _____ (date)

University Medical Center
Critical Path for Valve Patients

NEEDS	KEY INDICATOR	DAY 1		DAY 2		DAY 3	
Maintain Tissue Perfusion	1. Vital Signs	VS Q 4 Hrs. T < 101 P 60 – 100 R 12 – 20 BP $\frac{90-150}{60-95}$		VS Q 4 Hrs. T < 100.5 P 60 – 100 R 12 – 20 BP $\frac{90-150}{60-95}$		VS Q shift T < 100 P 60 – 100 R 12 – 20 BP $\frac{90-150}{60-95}$	
	2. Diagnostic Tests	CBC, Lytes, BUN, Cr, PT, PTT CXR ECG if pacer off		PT if on coumadin		CBC, Lytes, BUN, Cr, PT	
	3. Cardiac Rhythm	NSR Pacer ON if arrhythmias Telemetry		NSR Pacer wires Telemetry		NSR Pacer wires Telemetry	
Maintain Gas Exchange	4. Oxygen	O_2 Wean per RT protocol		Wean O_2		RA	
	5. Pulse Ox	$O_2 \geq 92\%$		$O_2 \geq 92\%$		$O_2 \geq 92\%$	
	6. Incentive Spirometer Goal=baseline	Level > 500 x 10 q 2 hrs. ATC Resp. Tx consult		Level > 500 x 10 q 2 hrs. W/A		Level > 750 x 10 q 2 hrs. W/A	
	7. Chest Tubes	DC if drainage < 50 cc/shift		None		None	
Progress Activity	8. Activity	Up in chair BID Walk in room		Amb 50 ft. TID PT consult if > 1 person assist		Amb 100 ft. TID	
	9. Pain Scale	< 5 with po meds.		< 4 with po meds		< 3 with po meds	
Maintain Nutritional Intake	10. Diet	Clear liquids		Advance to 4 gm Na, ↓ chol, NCS diet after BM		4 gm Na, ↓ chol, NCS diet	
	11. Weight Pre-op	Wt QD		Wt QD		Wt QD	
	12. I & O	Q shift Fluid Restriction		Q shift Fluid Restriction		Q shift Fluid Restriction	
	13. Medications	Begin Coumadin if indicated Lasix K supplement DC antibiotics unless indicated		Coumadin Lasix K supplement		Coumadin Lasix K supplement	
	14. Bowel Movement	Bowel Sounds x 4 quads; Adb soft		Same Bowel movement or LOC			
Maintain Skin Integrity	15. Incisions and insertion sites	S/L approx, drsg D&I, 0 inflammation		S/L approx, OTA, 0 inflammation; Pacer wire/CT site, drsg D&I		S/L approx, OTA, 0 inflammation; Pacer wire/CT site, drsg D&I	
Provide Post-Op Teaching	16. Teaching	Reorient to unit Instruct on C&DB, splinting, incentive spirometer		Instruct activity progression; Reinforce pulmonary techniques		Instruct diet and heart A & P; Reinforce activity progression	
Assess Home Needs	17. DC Planning	Consult CRP		Identity support system and home		Identity location for laboratory tests	

F I G U R E 1 5 – 3
Critical pathway.

tion, and interventions to meet each goal are outlined. Many interventions are delegated to the PCT.

✔ It is important to begin each shift with a careful review of the Kardex and flow sheet for each patient. Although this consumes time at the beginning of a shift, it saves time later by identifying priorities and preventing inefficiencies such as:

• Missed or delayed appointments for required tests or procedures that could extend the patient's stay and increase cost
• A patient not receiving ordered care activities
• A patient receiving care activities that have been cancelled

The RN responsible for overseeing the care of patients is the most valuable source of information in planning work assignments. At the start of a shift, the PCT communicates with the RN. This initial communication should include:

• Discussion about the information received in the RN shift report
• Clarification of major patient needs for the shift
• Symptoms and responses that need to be reported to the RN
• Review of pertinent information concerning patient outcomes and expectations
• Expected time frames for completion of tasks
• Preferred methods and times of reporting patient responses to interventions

✔ If your assignment overlaps patients of two RNs, it is important that all three of you discuss any conflicting priorities or expectations.

In addition, the PCT independently checks for overbed signs that list precautions for bleeding, blood pressure, blood draws, swallowing, positioning, sensory deficits, etc.

Worksheets (Figs. 15–4 to 15–6) are excellent tools to efficiently organize patient data that has been collected from various sources. Worksheets can be started when assignments are made by entering the patients' names and room numbers. As you receive the shift report, begin to fill in the blanks about each patient's anticipated shift activities. The PCT's review of the Kardex for each patient will provide additional details of the anticipated tasks of the shift to be added to the worksheet.

📓 Use different colored inks or pencils on the worksheet to quickly identify various classes of activities, for example:

• RED to identify stat or extremely important activities
• BLACK to list specific situations that require immediate feedback to the RN
• PENCIL to describe routine ADLs

This tool will help you track care and patient outcomes, provide data for documentation on the patient's chart, and assist in reporting progress to the RN.

After completing the worksheet for each patient, review your entire assignment to identify unfamiliar interventions, equipment, tests, abbreviations, terminology, or questions about the Kardex. As the report from the RN is received, clarify the questions. If tasks that are outside of the PCT's job description are delegated, remind the RN that these tasks cannot be performed by you, but that you will be willing to help. Evaluate if it is reasonable for the RN to expect you to complete the assigned patient care activities within the allotted time frame.

⚖ The unlicensed PCT has the responsibility to communicate to the RN when:

• An assigned task is new or unfamiliar.
• The RN's expectations are unclear.
• Necessary resources are not available.
• The delegated task is outside your position description.

PLANNING YOUR WORKDAY

Efficient planning of your workday is key in providing all care for your patients in a timely manner. PCTs need to know the roles of other team members, be skilled in time management, setting priorities, estimating time frames for giving care, and in using worksheets and charts in planning daily patient care. Additionally, the PCT needs to be flexible to include spontaneous tasks such as new admissions, STAT blood draws, ECGs, or covering the desk at the patient care station.

Flexibility also is very important when it becomes necessary to respond to an emergency with an assigned patient or with another patient on the unit. When emergencies arise, it is often necessary to reprioritize care to meet the needs of additional patients while increased numbers of staff respond to the emergency.

TIME MANAGEMENT AND SETTING PRIORITIES

Various tools and worksheets have been identified in the previous section of this chapter to assist in pulling together the information needed to plan and provide pa-

Patient Care Associate Assignment Worksheet

PCA	Date	RN	Phone	Charge RN	PSA	Meal Time	Break	Report to RN Q	hrs.	Feedback/Comments

Pt Information	Priorities	Measurements	Activity	Special Needs	Respiratory	Dressing/Tube	Personal Care	Dietary	Spec. Collect	Elimination
Room # Name Dx Problem	Test OR Procedure ECG Teaching	Vital signs Weight AccuChek	UAL Ambulate BRP Chair BSC BR/Turn Other	Isolation Prisoner Seizures DNR Restraint Suicide Other	Oxygen Inc Spir C & DB Pulse OX Other	Types:	AM Hygiene bath oral shave hair skin PM Hygiene Foley care	I & O NPO Restrictions Tube Feeding IV/CVC Special diet Encourage	Blood Draw Stool UA/C&S Sputum GAS HAU	

NOTES:

Pt Information	Priorities	Measurements	Activity	Special Needs	Respiratory	Dressing/Tube	Personal Care	Dietary	Spec. Collect	Elimination
Room # Name Dx Problem	Test OR Procedure ECG Teaching	Vital signs Weight AccuChek	UAL Ambulate BRP Chair BSC BR/Turn Other	Isolation Prisoner Seizures DNR Restraint Suicide Other	Oxygen Inc Spir C & DB Pulse OX Other	Types:	AM Hygiene bath oral shave hair skin PM Hygiene Foley care	I & O NPO Restrictions Tube Feeding IV/CVC Special diet Encourage	Blood Draw Stool UA/C&S Sputum GAS HAU	

NOTES:

Pt Information	Priorities	Measurements	Activity	Special Needs	Respiratory	Dressing/Tube	Personal Care	Dietary	Spec. Collect	Elimination
Room # Name Dx Problem	Test OR Procedure ECG Teaching	Vital signs Weight Accuchek	UAL Ambulate BRP Chair BSC BR/Turn Other	Isolation Prisoner Seizures DNR Restraint Suicide Other	Oxygen Inc Spir C & DB Pulse OX Other	Types:	AM Hygiene bath oral shave hair skin PM Hygiene Foley care	I & O NPO Restrictions Tube Feeding IV/CVC Special diet Encourage	Blood Draw Stool UA/C&S Sputum GAS HAU	

NOTES:

Pt Information	Priorities	Measurements	Activity	Special Needs	Respiratory	Dressing/Tube	Personal Care	Dietary	Spec. Collect	Elimination
Room # Name Dx Problem	Test OR Procedure ECG Teaching	Vital signs Weight AccuChek	UAL Ambulate BRP Chair BSC BR/Turn Other	Isolation Prisoner Seizures DNR Restraint Suicide Other	Oxygen Inc Spir C & DB Pulse OX Other	Types:	AM Hygiene bath oral shave hair skin PM Hygiene Foley care	I & O NPO Restrictions Tube Feeding IV/CVC Special diet Encourage	Blood Draw Stool UA/C&S Sputum GAS HAU	

FIGURE 15–4
Worksheet.

PCA WORK PLAN

Room _____ Patient _____
Report to RN " _____ "
Problem _____
Safety Needs _____
Activity/Turns _____

🖐 WASH HANDS 🖐

Vital Signs _____
ASK: Is there anything you need? _____
Vital Signs _____
Weight _____
AccuChek _____
IV: Yes _____ No _____ I & O _____
Diet _____
Appt _____
Incentive Spirometry _____ O$_2$ _____
ECG _____
Blood Draw _____
Bath _____ Bed _____
Dressing/Tube _____
Elimination _____
Pain/Comfort _____
Tubes/Drains _____
Special Care Area _____
Specimens: _____
Isolation/Other _____
Documentation _____
Precautions _____
Restrictions _____

PCA WORK PLAN

Room _____ Patient _____
Report to RN " _____ "
Problem _____
Safety Needs _____
Activity/Turns _____

🖐 WASH HANDS 🖐

Vital Signs _____
ASK: Is there anything you need? _____
Vital Signs _____
Weight _____
AccuChek _____
IV: Yes _____ No _____ I & O _____
Diet _____
Appt _____
Incentive Spirometry _____ O$_2$ _____
ECG _____
Blood Draw _____
Bath _____ Bed _____
Dressing/Tube _____
Elimination _____
Pain/Comfort _____
Tubes/Drains _____
Special Care Area _____
Specimens: _____
Isolation/Other _____
Documentation _____
Precautions _____
Restrictions _____

PCA WORK PLAN

Room _____ Patient _____
Report to RN " _____ "
Problem _____
Safety Needs _____
Activity/Turns _____

🖐 WASH HANDS 🖐

Vital Signs _____
ASK: Is there anything you need? _____
Vital Signs _____
Weight _____
AccuChek _____
IV: Yes _____ No _____ I & O _____
Diet _____
Appt _____
Incentive Spirometry _____ O$_2$ _____
ECG _____
Blood Draw _____
Bath _____ Bed _____
Dressing/Tube _____
Elimination _____
Pain/Comfort _____
Tubes/Drains _____
Special Care Area _____
Specimens: _____
Isolation/Other _____
Documentation _____
Precautions _____
Restrictions _____

F I G U R E   1 5 – 5
Worksheet.

NURSING ASSISTANT ASSIGNMENT

Team Leader: _____

Team Members: _____

Date: _____

Shift: _____

Room	Patient Name	Special Comments	TPR	B/P	NPO	IV'S	I & O	Foley	Keto Diast	Wt.	Pre Op	Post Op	TCDB	TEDS	SPECIMEN Time Collected						Activities
															Urine	Sputum	Stool	Emesis	24 hr. Collect		

AM or PM Care	Feed	Discharges	Other

F I G U R E 1 5 – 6

Worksheet.

tient care. The next step in the process is to identify the most effective use of time to provide high-quality patient care.

M. Lynch in her writings on time management makes the following statement: Managing time effectively isn't a simple skill. It's a whole way of approaching each day. It involves planning, organizing . . . and prioritizing. And no matter how adept you are at time management, the human element that makes each day unique can upset the best of plans.*

The PCT needs to be prepared for "human elements" that change each day and learn to organize and set priorities for patient assignment. A helpful strategy is to utilize a "What, Who, When" approach to plan.

- *What*: What needs to be done? What equipment and supplies are needed?

- *Who*: To whom does the care need to be given? Who will provide the care? Are there tasks that require more than one person?

- *When*: When does the care need to be given?

Answering "what" is accomplished as the report is given and the worksheet is filled in from the Kardex. Initial priorities may be set by the RN for early operations, transport, or unstable patients, for example. Specific tasks assigned to you for the day, such as blood draws and routine ECGs, will also affect early prioritization.

To plan and begin prioritizing, identify *what* patient care must be done, including all of the following:

- Handwashing between patients and announcing yourself before entering each room
- ADLs
- Vital signs
- Weights
- Treatments
- Tube/drain care
- Incentive spirometer or reminders to cough and breathe deeply
- Linen changes
- Meal assistance
- Fluid encouragement or restrictions
- Dressing changes
- Ambulation or get up to chair
- Position changes/turns
- Assistance with elimination
- Specimen collection and testing
- Blood draws
- ECGs

- Transporting to scheduled appointments, tests, or procedures
- Intake and output
- Accuchecks
- Special precautions/isolation/restraint checks
- Comfort measures
- Room checks
- Documentation
- Reporting
- Responding to pages, calls, patient and visitor requests

Once you have identified *what* care needs to be given to whom, identify *when* care or treatments need to be completed. For example, Mr. Jones may be going to surgery at 8:30 AM and needs his bath given and documented by 8:00 AM, while the rest of your patients do not need AM care completed until later. Therefore, you will need to plan the care of Mr. Jones to make sure that his bath and other required care are completed prior to 8:00 AM.

Taking time to think through and answer the following questions will aid in identifying other factors needed to prioritize work schedules: Are there activities, tasks, or measurements that must be done first or by a specific time? In other words, *when* should activities be performed? Situations to be considered are:

- Patients who require special preparation for a test or surgery
- Patients who leave the unit early for a test or procedure
- Patients who need to be weighed before breakfast
- Patients who need blood drawn before meals
- Patients who need specimens tested before or after meals

Will other staff members be needed to help with any care activities such as lifting a heavy bed-bound patient? If so, *who* will assist? After considering the roles of other staff on the unit, coordinate the best time with team members who are able to help.

Are there hospital routines or policies that need to be considered? Do those routines or policies influence *when* care is provided? For example:

- Visiting hours
- Meal times
- Feeding times for newborns
- Shift-specific tasks
- Physician team rounds so that vital measurements are available at the time of rounds

How many patients will need assistance or total care for ADLs? Answering this question will help decide *when* to provide the care, because more time will be spent with

---

Lynch, M. P-A-C-E yourself: Tips on time management. Nursing, Vol. 21, No. 3, 1991, 104, 106, 108.

these patients. Extra help may also be needed to position patients or to get them up to a chair after the bed bath.

Are there special patient needs that will determine *when* activities, tasks, or measurements are performed? For example, a postoperative patient has an order to ambulate. Coordinate with the RN a time to ambulate after appropriate pain relief medication or measures are administered.

What equipment and supplies will be needed to give care? The PCT should gather all equipment and supplies needed to provide care to save time and money.

Once the PCT has determined what, who, and when, priorities for care will emerge, and establishing a work plan within a time frame becomes easier.

ESTIMATING TIME FRAMES

Most units have unofficial patient care schedules with expectations for completion of specific tasks within a particular time frame. Sometimes it is based on patient meal times, physicians making rounds, or laboratory or radiology schedules. The following is an example of a unit time schedule. Prioritize patient care assignments with the unit time frame. A first-shift assignment might look like this:

0700:

- Write down assigned patient's room number, name, and assigned RN on worksheet
- Pick up beeper/pager (if available)
- Go to your patient's chart, Kardex, flow sheet, and other forms and begin filling out your worksheet
- Begin vital signs, weights, Accucheks, and document them on the patient's flow sheet

Report any measurement not within normal limits as outlined in hospital policies to your RN immediately.

0800:

- Contact the RN assigned to your patients for a report before proceeding with meals, baths, and beds. Find out which patients are leaving the unit early for appointments so they can receive care first. Ask about patients' special care needs.
- Assist patients to get ready for breakfast.
- Collect all prebreakfast specimens and perform blood glucose testing.

Any patient on sliding scale insulin should have blood glucose test results reported to the RN.

- Help patients needing minimal assistance start their breakfast.
- Place clean linen and bath supplies in the room.

0900:

- Pick up breakfast trays, calculate intake and caloric counts, and document.
- Complete unfinished vital signs and record on all patients.
- Assist patients who need help with eating.
- Pick up breakfast trays and calculate intake.
- Bring linens and bath supplies for those patients needing minimal assistance.
- Begin baths and linen changes on complete care patients.

1000–1100:

- Return to patients needing minimal assistance and offer help with their back and feet; change linen.
- Be sure oral care is completed for all patients.
- Chart all portions of the bath and amount of assistance needed on the patient flow sheet.
- Assist with patient activity; ambulation, up in chair, turn, or other needs.
- Begin blood glucose testing and vital signs.

1200:

- Check incontinent patients; bathrooms; clean up rooms, finish morning activities.
- Set up patients for lunch and assist as needed.
- Arrange to take your own break.
- Ask if any admissions are expected.

1400–1530:

- Pass fresh drinking water.
- Empty all drainage containers.
- Calculate intake and output and document on chart.
- Check all charting against assignment sheet and sign off all charts.
- Check all incontinent patients.
- Provide special care requests.
- Report to RN and turn in your beeper.

Once you have identified a plan and time frame, there are some "helpful hints" you can utilize to further guide your day:

- Since medications and treatments are frequently based on your accurate measurements (blood pressure, pulse, blood glucose), chart and report them as soon as they are obtained.
- When completing care or a task with the patient ask,

"Is there anything else I can do for you before I leave?" This saves time for both the RN and PCT.

- Immediately report changes noted in patient's behavior or condition to the RN.
- Take stock periodically to assess progress and plans; reassess priorities as needed and report back to the RN for any change in plans.
- Use a highlighter to mark off tasks on the assignment sheet as they are done.
- Ask "What is the best use of my time right now?" to help focus on priority care.
- Check rooms hourly for patient assistance and urine and stool collection, and restock supplies.
- Volunteer to help other team members.

 Document care as it is given rather than waiting until later in the shift. This decreases the chance of forgetting valuable information or having to rush at the end of the shift.

ADAPTING THE WORK ASSIGNMENT THROUGHOUT THE DAY

Despite accurate assessments of the anticipated work to be completed and well-founded plans to meet the needs of your patients, adjustments must be made when:

- New patients are admitted to the unit.
- Patients are unexpectedly transferred or discharged.
- Unexpected diagnostic tests are ordered.
- A patient's condition deteriorates quickly.
- Unanticipated staffing changes occur.

The best way to prevent these adjustments from disrupting the work flow is to coordinate care with the other members of your nursing staff throughout the shift. Frequent communication lessens the impact of changes by allowing the team to anticipate needed adjustments and to facilitate requests for help from other staff members. The positive results of this teamwork include:

- Increased unit morale
- Improved patient care and satisfaction
- Smooth transitions and continuity of care during break times and change of shifts
- A relaxed atmosphere in the department despite unanticipated events
- Completion of all assigned tasks
- More group members who get meal breaks and go home on time

Throughout the day, periodically communicate with other staff members. Every 1 or 2 hours is an ideal time frame to evaluate the effectiveness of the original plan for the shift and to anticipate adjustments to the plan. At these informal meetings, patient updates of vital signs or wound conditions can be given to the RN by the PCT. Additionally, the RN can explain needed changes in interventions, newly ordered activities, or special patient observations to be reported, based on results of diagnostic tests.

 During these periodic communications the following questions should be asked:

- What has been completed since the original plan was made?
- What remains to be completed during the rest of the shift?
- What new unit events (such as admissions or changes in patient status) have occurred to change priorities?
- Who will complete each part of the new plan?
- How have the patients responded to their care?
- Are there any changes in the patient's condition?

The answers to these questions will help the RN and PCT to decide if additional staff is needed to complete specific patient care tasks, if adjustments in the assignments should be made to accommodate changes in patient status, and who should complete which part of the new plan. Although it may be difficult to meet periodically, it is necessary in order to accomplish all tasks efficiently.

In addition to the routine communication throughout the shift, the PCT should report immediately any unusual or unexpected patient symptoms, behavior, complaints, or response to treatment.

 Specific clinical situations to report immediately include:

- Abnormally high, low, or changed vital signs
- Abnormal glucose levels
- Changes in skin color
- Reddened, puffy, foul smelling, or draining wounds
- Abrupt changes in mood, memory, or consciousness
- Abnormal weakness or change in gait
- Complaints of pain or injury
- Any complaints of chest pain, shortness of breath, itching, or rash
- Weight changes of 2 pounds or more per day

Nonclinical situations involving a patient that should be reported immediately include:

- Threats of violence
- Threats to leave the hospital before the physician writes a discharge order (Against Medical Advice—AMA)
- Threats to sue the hospital or any individual
- Violation of the rights of other patients
- Requests to read the medical record (This usually is not wrong, but most agencies want the physician to review the chart with the patient to explain test results or terminology the patient may not understand.)

At the conclusion of the shift the PCT will need to present an accurate and objective report to the RN and/or the next shift. An accurate report describes the patient's care as it happened. An objective report describes the patient responses in specific terms so that comparisons can be made with prior treatment and prior responses. For example, it is more useful to describe skin breakdown or dressing drainage in terms of actual size in centimeters of length and width than to say it is big and red. This helps the RN identify the extent of a particular patient problem.

✔ The end-of-shift report should include:

- A "head-to-toe" review of the patient care activities completed
- Identification of those tasks that were not completed
- Patient responses to treatments.

⚖ In some agencies the reporting mechanism may include review of written documentation of the care provided in the patient's chart. The patient's chart is the medical record and is considered a legal document. Information should be written clearly in black or blue ink and all entries dated, timed, and signed.

🛑 *Never* cross out, write over, or white-out information that has been written incorrectly in the medical record. If an error is made, draw one line through the mistake, write *error* over it, and sign your name and title.

SUMMARY

This chapter has provided the PCT with the tools to organize a workday. It is important to begin to organize the workday as soon as the initial assignments are posted and supplement the data as the report is received from the previous shift. The Kardex or multidisciplinary critical pathway is an excellent source of specific information about the care needed by each patient.

Communication with other members of the team throughout the shift is critical. As soon as possible after the report is finished, the PCT should meet with all appropriate RNs to identify priorities and expected outcomes of the assignment. Throughout the day, the team should meet to identify new priorities and rearrange the work assigned to meet any unexpected needs. At the end of the shift the PCT should review with the RNs all care provided throughout the day as well as patient responses to treatments.

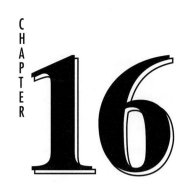

Emergency Care

SANDRA L. WALDEN, MS, RN,C
ELLA SCHULZ, BSN, RN

OUTLINE

PREREQUISITE KNOWLEDGE AND SKILLS

- Basic anatomy of the respiratory and cardiovascular systems
- Measuring vital signs
- Basic life support
- Use of bag-valve resuscitation device

OBJECTIVES

After you complete this chapter, you will be able to:

- Identify possible causes, patient descriptions, and actions that the PCT should take for potential life-threatening situations.

- Describe the role of the PCT with the patient who is experiencing cardiac arrest.

- Identify poor quality cardiac rhythm tracings and how to correct problems.

- Provide a safe environment for a patient with a temporary cardiac pacemaker.

- Demonstrate correct actions in response to equipment alarms.

KEY TERMS

Apnea   Absence of breathing

Artificial Pacemaker   Device that can deliver an electric shock to the heart causing it to contract (heart beat)

Bradycardia   Pulse rate less than 60/minute

Electrocardiogram   Electrical "picture" of the heart beat; the heart tracing

Electrode   Small piece of metal or conducting material in contact with a body organ or skin surface

Epiglottis   Fold of tissue that covers the entrance into the trachea during swallowing; prevents food from going into the lungs

Hypertension   Blood pressure of 140/90 mm Hg is considered borderline; blood pressure exceeding 160/95 mm Hg is considered hypertensive

Hypotension   Systolic blood pressure less than 90 mm Hg

Lead   An electrocardiographic view of the heart. Also refers to the lead wire connecting the cardiac monitor to the patient's electrode on the chest.

Luer-Lok   Type of connection for intravenous lines that holds the pieces of tubing and needles together, preventing accidental separation

Myocardial Infarction   Heart attack; muscle tissue in the heart, called myocardium, dies because of lack of oxygen supply

Myocardium   Heart muscle; sandwiched between two thin layers of tissue: the epicardium covers and the endocardium forms the lining of the heart

Orientation   Mental state consisting of a patient's ability to identify person, place, time

Pace   To deliver an electric shock to the heart muscle that causes it to contract and produces a QRS complex on the ECG

Precordial   Across the left chest wall from sternum to midaxilla in the area over the heart

Premature Beat   A heart beat that occurs earlier than one would expect based on the rate of heart beats per minute

Pulse Generator   Main part of an artificial pacemaker system; contains the circuits, controls, and energy source (battery)

Syncope   Fainting spells; brief loss of consciousness

Tachycardia   Heart rate that exceeds 100/minute

Trachea   Tube through which air passes to and from the lungs

Ventricular Rhythm   The pacing site of the heart is in the ventricle instead of in the normal pacemaker (sinoatrial node)

The patient care technician (PCT) may be the first person to identify a potential patient emergency. Recognition of a potential life-threatening situation can be the most important action that occurs during the patient's hospitalization. Think about the patient with cardiac arrest. Cardiopulmonary resuscitation (CPR) is usually effective only if begun within the first 4–6 minutes of the cardiac arrest, after which irreversible brain damage occurs. In this clinical situation as well as many others, the first person to identify the emergency has the extraordinary opportunity to make the difference. When the PCT is the first person to identify the emergency and knows what to do, the appropriate medical response can be initiated.

This chapter will present potential life-threatening emergencies and appropriate actions that the PCT should initiate. In addition, the role of the PCT with cardiac monitoring, pacemakers, and response to equipment alarms will be introduced.

ANTICIPATING EMERGENCIES

Obstructed Airway

Airway obstruction is one of the most frequent life-threatening emergencies. The most common cause of airway obstruction is unconsciousness. When unconsciousness occurs, the tongue may fall backward into the *pharynx* causing obstruction to respiration. Other causes of obstructed airway include blockage of the entrance of the *trachea* by the *epiglottis*, vomitus, and more commonly foreign objects such as food. The most common foreign body that causes airway obstruction in adults is meat.*

American Heart Association, National Center, Dallas, 1993.

Steps that can be taken to prevent airway obstruction in patients:

- Cut food into small pieces.
- Place the patient in high Fowler's position prior to feeding.
- Feed slowly.
- Observe the swallowing ability of the patient prior to feeding.
- Position unconscious or heavily medicated patients on the left side or in semi-Fowler's position unless contraindicated.

Essential to a successful outcome in obstructed airway is early recognition and appropriate actions (Fig. 16–1). It is important, therefore, that the PCT be able to identify an obstructed airway.

When the patient is conscious with a completely obstructed airway, the patient will be unable to speak, breathe, or cough, often clutching hands at the throat (universal choking sign). If the patient becomes unconscious, death will result quickly if immediate action to relieve the obstruction is not taken by the PCT. The obstructed airway maneuver should be initiated quickly, using the American Heart Association (AHA) obstructed airway maneuver (Figs. 16–2 to 16–4).

Altered Vital Signs

Hypotension

Hypotension is defined as blood pressure below 90 mm Hg systolic. There are several causes of hypotension. Shock is an emergency situation caused by inadequate delivery of oxygen and nutrients to the cells by the cardiovascular system. One of the resulting symptoms frequently seen is hypotension. Shock may be caused by a variety of medical conditions or situations. Failure of the heart to function as a pump (from myocardial infarction), decrease of blood volume (from hemorrhage, vomiting, or diarrhea), general collapse of the circulatory system (from an overwhelming infection) may all cause shock.

Any time the body senses a decreased fluid loss in the circulatory system, because of actual blood loss or fluid shifts, the body compensates in an effort to maintain an adequate blood supply to the heart and brain. The peripheral blood vessels constrict to bring more fluid to the central circulation and the heart rate increases.

The signs and symptoms of shock include hypotension, tachycardia (pulse rate faster than 100/min), cool, moist, pale skin, increased rate of respirations, and decreased level of consciousness. The patient also may report feeling anxious and thirsty. Depending on the extent of the circulating volume loss and the cause of the shock, symptoms the patient experiences may vary (Table 16–1).

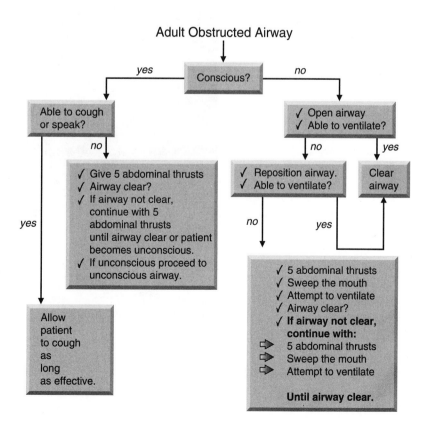

FIGURE 16–1
Adult obstructed airway action chart.

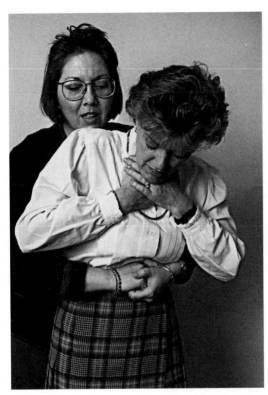

FIGURE 16-2
Abdominal thrusts in the conscious adult patient.

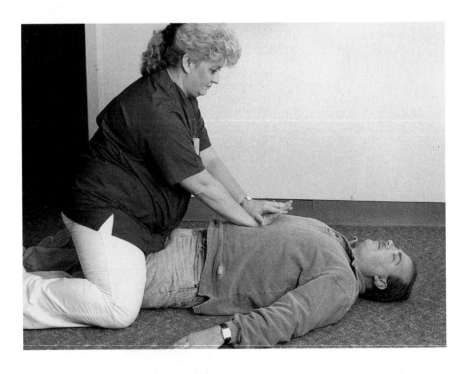

FIGURE 16-3
Abdominal thrusts in the unconscious
adult patient.

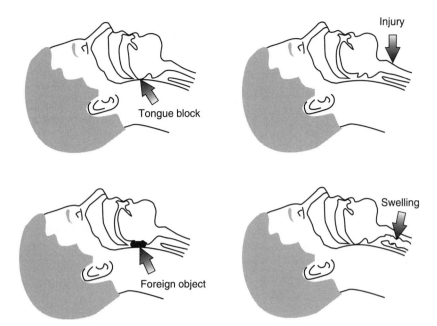

FIGURE 16–4
Causes of airway obstruction.

✔ The successful reversal of shock depends on the severity of the shock and how long it has existed.

Recognition of hypotension and notification of the RN by the PCT are crucial to the patient's survival. When the PCT obtains a BP that is 20 mm Hg lower than the prior blood pressure, the PCT should notify the RN. The RN may have the PCT monitor the patient and take the pressure again within 30 minutes, because moderate changes in blood pressure may occur with activity changes or in response to differing levels of stress. If the BP has become still lower, obtain a complete set of vital signs and note any increase in heart rate. Notify the RN of changes; treatment measure will be initiated to identify the cause and prevent shock.

✔ When the PCT obtains a systolic blood pressure reading that is less than 90 mm Hg, the RN should be summoned immediately.

Hypertension

Hypertension is intermittent or sustained elevation in systolic and/or diastolic blood pressure. The patient would be considered hypertensive if the systolic/diastolic blood pressure exceeded 160/95 mm Hg. Blood pressures less than 140/90 are considered to be normal. Blood pressures that fall between normal and hypertensive (140/90–160/95) are considered borderline hypertensive. Associated symptoms that might be seen with the hypertensive patient include headache and dizziness.

✔ When the PCT observes a patient's blood pressure to be unexpectedly elevated, the RN should be notified immediately.

Bradycardia

Bradycardia (a heart rate below 60/min) may be normal for certain patients or may be a sign of a potential

TABLE 16–1
Signs and Symptoms of Shock

VITAL SIGNS	UP TO 15% BLOOD LOSS	15–30% BLOOD LOSS	30–40% BLOOD LOSS	GREATER THAN 40% BLOOD LOSS
Blood pressure	⊗	Mild ↑ in diastolic	Systolic ↓ 90 mm Hg	Systolic ↓ 90 mm Hg
Pulse	Mild ↑ rate	↑ Rate	Rapid rate	Rapid rate
Respirations	⊗	Mild ↑ rate	Rapid rate	Rapid rate
Skin temperature	⊗	Mildly cool	Cool and clammy	Cool and clammy
Airway	⊗	⊗	Airway difficulties possible	Airway difficulties
Consciousness	⊗	⊗	Restlessness, anxiety, or decreased level of consciousness	Decreased level of consciousness

⊗ = no change (normal).
Data from Sheey, S. B., Lombardi, J. E.: Manual of Emergency Care. St. Louis, C. V. Mosby, 1995.

or impending emergency. In individuals who are highly athletic, bradycardia may be normal. As the result of physical fitness, the athlete's heart works more efficiently as a pump and therefore does not need to contract as many times per minute as the average heart. However, slow heart rates may also indicate coronary artery disease or drug intoxication.

Tachycardia

Tachycardia is a heart rate that exceeds 100 beats/min. Tachycardia may be due to fever, exercise, emotional stress or anxiety, or use of stimulants (caffeine or nicotine), or it may be a sign of more serious consequences such as shock or heart disease. The actions for tachycardia are the same. The effects are dangerous to the patient when they result in inadequate circulation of blood that is reflected in decreased blood pressure.

If the patient's systolic blood pressure is below 90 mm Hg, or the patient is experiencing confusion, dizziness, or chest pain, the PCT should take immediate action:

- Stay with the patient.
- Summon the RN immediately.
- Make the patient comfortable (often Fowler's or semi-Fowler's position).
- Continue to observe vital signs.
- The PCT should be alert to the possibility of cardiac arrest in the patient who exhibits these symptoms.

Altered Level of Consciousness

Alterations in level of consciousness may range from mild confusion to unconsciousness in which the patient does not respond to verbal or painful stimuli.

Confusion may be established by asking simple questions such as, "What is your name?" "Where are you?" "What is today's date?"

Stroke (cerebral vascular accident) occurs when the vessels in the brain become blocked by an embolus (blood clot) or cerebrovascular hemorrhage (blood vessel in the brain ruptures). Anything from confusion to unconsciousness can be seen with a stroke. Signs and symptoms seen with the patient experiencing a stroke depend on the area of the brain affected and the extent of the damage. Additional common symptoms include weakness or inability to move one side of the body, elevated blood pressure, slurred speech or inability to speak, visual disturbances, cool wet skin, pulse rate changes, decreased respirations, and seizures.

When caring for a patient who is unexpectedly confused or unconscious, the PCT should:

- Summon the RN immediately.
- In the unconscious patient, establish the airway by performing the jaw lift, head tilt immediately (AHA technique for opening the airway).
- Monitor the pulse and respirations until help arrives. The PCT should be alert to the possibility of cardiac arrest in the patient who is unconscious.

Shortness of Breath

Of primary importance to any health care worker is the patient's respiratory status. Patients will have typical descriptions of shortness of breath that the PCT should observe (Table 16–2). These symptoms include rapid shallow breathing; cool, wet, cyanotic skin; and noisy, wet respirations. The patient who is reporting difficulty in breathing or is noticeably short of breath may be having a critical emergency. The causes of labored breathing can be very serious. Possible causes include partial obstruction of the airway that may have been caused by foreign objects (most common is food), trauma, swelling, vomitus, and blood. Other causes include respiratory disease (emphysema and asthma), pneumonia, and pulmonary edema. When the left side of the heart fails to pump adequately, blood may back up into the tissues of the lungs causing a condition called *pulmonary edema*. Immediate treatment of pulmonary edema can mean the difference between survival and death for the patient. Patients who have pulmonary edema may exhibit any or all of the symptoms identified in Table 16–2.

 The onset of pink-tinged frothy (bubbly) sputum is a hallmark of pulmonary edema.

 The PCT should take immediate actions with any patient who is short of breath:

- Stay with the patient.
- Get the patient in a comfortable breathing position (Fowler's or semi-Fowler's).
- Summon the RN immediately.
- Talk with the patient quietly and calmly, offer reassurance, and ensure that oxygen is in place properly.
- Be prepared to perform CPR should the patient stop breathing and/or develop full cardiac arrest before help arrives.

Chest Pain—Myocardial Infarction (Heart Attack)?

Cardiovascular disease accounts for nearly 1 million deaths in the United States annually. Approximately

T A B L E 1 6 – 2
Shortness of Breath and Chest Pain Action Chart

PROBLEM	PATIENT DESCRIPTION	SIGNS AND SYMPTOMS	ACTION

Shortness of breath—pulmonary edema?	Difficulty breathing
	→*Cannot get adequate air*
	→*Inability to lie flat*
	→*Awakening in middle of night*
	Irritating dry or wet cough
		Rapid, shallow breathing
		Paleness; cyanotic skin
		Sweating
		Noisy, wet respirations
		Chest pain
		Cough; frothy pink sputum
			Stay with patient
			Call for help
			Get vital signs
			Comfortable position for patient
			Oxygen
			When help arrives get:
			  Emergency equipment
			  Monitor defibrillator
			  12-lead ECG
			  Crash cart

Chest pain—myocardial infarction?	Located middle or behind sternum and sometimes left arm and back →*Pressure* →*Tightness* →*Crushing* →*Squeezing* →*Choking* Feels like: *Band or belt around my chest* →*Elephant on my chest* →*Ton of bricks on my chest*	Chest pain Shortness of breath Weakness, looking ill Paleness Profuse sweating Anxiety, fear Confusion	(Same as above)

675,000 Americans are hospitalized every year for myocardial infarction (MI). Six million Americans have significant coronary artery disease and are at risk for MI; 45% of all MIs occur in persons under the age of 65 years. Sudden death related to coronary artery disease is the most frequent medical emergency in the United States today. It is possible that a large number of these deaths can be prevented by prompt action that provides rapid emergency medical intervention.*

It is imperative that the PCT understand that chest pain may develop into serious consequences if actions are not quick and decisive. The chest pain that is associated with MI (Table 16–2) has typical descriptions, including heavy, tight squeezing; choking; pressure; and crushing. Many RNs and doctors who have witnessed MIs have heard many patients say that it feels as if an elephant is sitting on their chest. In addition, the PCT may observe signs and symptoms associated with chest pain, including shortness of breath, weakness, profuse sweating, cold and clammy skin, anxiety, fear, cyanosis, and confusion.

American Heart Association, National Center, Dallas, 1993.

The status of any patient who is experiencing chest pain, regardless of other symptoms, should be evaluated by the RN immediately. In addition to MI there are many other causes of chest pain that can be just as life threatening.

When the patient reports chest pain, the PCT should:

- Stay with the patient.
- Call for help.
- Obtain vital signs.
- Get the patient in a comfortable position (usually Fowler's or semi-Fowler's).
- The PCT should be prepared to perform rescue breathing and/or CPR if the patient stops breathing or experiences cardiac arrest before help arrives.

Cardiac Arrest

Every year more than 1 million people with heart disease die because their hearts stop beating. In addition, metabolic disturbances, drowning, drug overdose, electrocution, trauma, stroke, and drug intoxication cause cardiac arrest. Clinical death occurs when the heart stops beating and breathing stops. The various cells and tissues in the body do not immediately die, but begin to deteriorate as the oxygen supply stops. To prevent cell and tissue death, CPR must be initiated within 4–6 minutes of the cardiac arrest.

✔ Most hospital-based caregivers are certified in basic cardiac life support. If these skills are not used routinely, CPR may not be performed satisfactorily. It is imperative, therefore, that periodic practice and review of CPR procedures be performed. Health care workers who are skilled in the correct methods of CPR help to provide the overall best possible outcome for patients.

STOP The American Heart Association has identified the steps and procedures to follow in determination of a possible cardiac or obstructed airway situation. The response is referred to as the ABCs of CPR, and describes the steps to check the Airway, Breathing, and Circulation of the victim (Fig. 16–5).

- Call for help.
- Begin CPR.
- Continue CPR until help arrives.
- Someone should bring emergency equipment including the crash cart and monitor/defibrillator. Oxygen supplies, intubation equipment, bag-valve mask, and suction equipment should also be brought if not kept on the crash cart.
- Once help arrives, the PCT may be relieved to get necessary equipment or supplies, take specimens to the laboratory, or care for other patients on the unit.

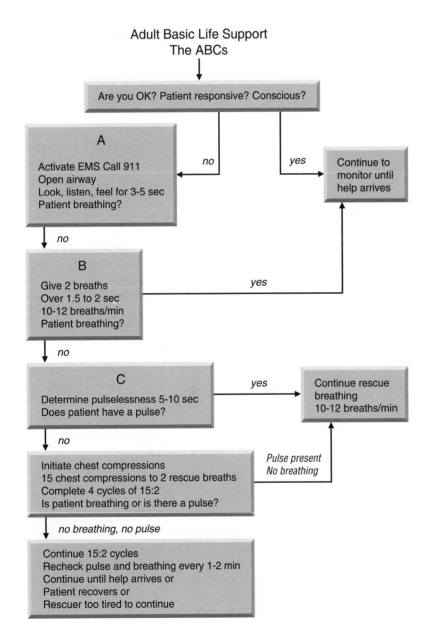

FIGURE 16–5

Cardiopulmonary resuscitation action chart.

CARDIAC MONITORING

Patients who have known cardiac problems are placed on cardiac monitoring to enable hospital staff to quickly identify any rate or rhythm changes and respond appropriately. This capability of viewing the heart rate and rhythm has saved many lives.

A cardiac monitor is a device that displays the electrical activity of the heart during the cardiac cycle. It displays the electrocardiogram (ECG) as well as various pressures of the heart and cardiovascular system. This provides information about the patient's cardiovascular status. Monitoring systems vary greatly, but all include a screen, heart rate indicator, modules for measuring pressure, and alarm systems. In the acute care setting, monitoring of the cardiac rhythm is most often accomplished by using two types of monitoring devices—hard wire and telemetry. Heart rate refers to how frequently the heart beats in a minute. Heart rhythm refers to how regular (or irregular) the heart rate is.

Both telemetry and hard-wire monitors have a screen that displays the ECG in much the same way as a TV displays a picture. A heart rate indicator averages the heart rate for each minute and displays this average rate on the screen and/or a digital readout. There is often an audible beep or a flashing light indicating each heart beat. The rate indicator connects to an alarm system that triggers an audible and visual alarm when preset limits are exceeded.

⚖️ Rate limits are determined by the RN according to the specific needs of the patient and unit routines. An initial rate limit might be 25 above or below the average heart rate; the RN may readjust as patient's need or heart rate changes.

✔️ Patients experiencing chills or tremors can create movement of the ECG screen that the machine falsely counts as heart rate. This may set off the alarm.

Hard-wire monitoring consists of a cable running from a wall-mounted monitoring unit to electrode patches placed on the patient's chest. The ECG is transmitted to the monitor through this cable, and a "picture" is created on the screen. This type of monitoring is most frequently used in intensive care units for monitoring the heart rate, heart rhythm, and blood pressure.

Telemetry is a wireless method of monitoring that sends the ECG to a monitor by a small transmitter similar in size to a pocket radio. The transmitter attaches to the patient's chest via small wires connected to electrodes. It is usually carried in a pocket or pouch. This type of system allows the patient to move around and ambulate, but restricts the distance a patient can move away from the receiver without going out of range. When a patient travels too far away from the receiver the signal "fades," similar to your car radio fading as you travel away from the station.

Both systems attach to a recorder so that periodic ECG tracings are obtained and placed in the patient's record for documentation of the heart rate and rhythm. The PCT can obtain the tracings from the recorder and notify the RN if a change in the heart rate or rhythm is noted. Always check a peripheral pulse with any change in the heart rhythm. Careful observation of the heart rate has an important role in the determination of patient need. The RN should be immediately notified of any change in heart rate or rhythm so that the rhythm changes can be evaluated when they occur.

✔️ When alarm limits are exceeded most systems will automatically trigger the recorder for a tracing. These tracings should be kept for the RN to evaluate.

Characteristics of the Tracing of the Electrocardiogram

The ECG will consist of several different waves moving across the monitor screen each minute. Each heart beat consists of a P, QRS, and T wave. The P wave represents electrical stimulation of the atria (the top chambers of the heart). The QRS represents electrical stimulation of the ventricles (the bottom chambers of the heart), and the T wave represents return to resting state of the ventricles. Normal P, QRS, and T waves are shown in Figure 16–6.

✔️ The baseline (the line where the P, QRS, and T waves all begin) of the ECG tracing should not wiggle or twist, and the tracing should move straight across the screen without drifting up or down.

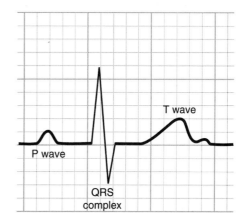

FIGURE 16-6
Normal ECG waveforms.

Electrode Placement and Selection of Lead

Electrodes are placed on the patient's chest. Monitoring systems will vary as to the number of electrodes needed, but the most common ones use 3 or 5 depending on what view of the heart they want to monitor. One electrode is attached to each lead wire, which is plugged into the monitoring cable or the transmitter.

A common type of electrode used for continuous monitoring consists of a small sponge that has conducting gel and is bonded to an adhesive sponge or porous tape. Most of the electrodes used for cardiac monitoring are disposable and are meant for one patient use only.

✔ Properly applied electrodes and skin preparation are the most important factors to obtaining a good electrocardiographic tracing.

Meticulous attention must be given to site selection and preparation. The site should be prepared by:

1. Clipping or shaving any excess hair that would interfere with adhesion of the electrode to the chest wall
2. Cleansing the skin with an alcohol prep pad/swab; acetone may be used to remove oils or residue
3. Gently rubbing the skin surface with a gauze pad to remove dead skin cells

After skin preparation the PCT should:

1. Remove protective backing from the electrode and press firmly in place.
2. Attach the lead wire to the appropriate electrode (according to the label on the wire).

Cardiac monitoring electrodes should be removed daily with bathing and relocated to an adjacent area of fleshy tissue on the chest. This can help ensure that the cardiac tracing has a clear pattern. Avoid placing electrodes directly over the ribs or clavicles. If a patient complains of itching around the electrode site, relocate it, and have the nurse check the skin. She may suggest that you substitute hypoallergenic electrodes, available at most agencies, in place of the ones causing skin irritation.

Monitors can interpret more than one view of the heart rhythm and often have a button for selection of the view that the physician wants to monitor. Monitors usually offer at least three lead selections and often as many as seven. Different leads pick up the heart's electrical activity from different directions and angles and look different on the monitor. Two common ways to set up electrodes to get different views of the heart are referred to as lead II and MCL₁ (Fig. 16–7).

The monitoring cable and telemetry system lead wires are labeled for right and left extremities and a chest or precordial lead. A three-lead system consists of right arm, left arm or left leg, and a ground or right leg wire. A five-lead system consists of a right and left arm, right and left leg, and a chest or precordial lead. The leads are color coded as follows: white = right arm (RA); black = left arm (LA); green = right leg (RL); red = left leg (LL); and brown = chest (C) or precordial lead. Electrodes for each lead are not placed on the extremities. They are placed on the appropriate areas of the chest. The arm leads are placed on the upper chest under the clavicles and the leg leads on the lower thorax. The V or precordial lead is usually placed in the fourth intercostal space, right sternal border.

Do not place electrodes on the ribs or the clavicles, but attach them to the fleshy surfaces. Rotate or shift the position to avoid skin irritation, but remember to place the electrodes in areas with limited muscle activity to prevent interference (artifact) on the tracing.

Troubleshooting

When an alarm sounds, remember to first observe the status of the patient, then decide the necessary action in response to the alarm. If the patient is less responsive than they were, do not silence the alarm. If the patient is not experiencing any apparent difficulty, check the monitor screen for the appropriate waves and palpate a pulse. If the pulse rate and waves are the same as they have been, reset the alarm and notify the RN or report as outlined by your institution's policy.

🛑 *Never turn off* a heart rate alarm; always use the alarm reset button to silence the alarm. If your institution has a policy regarding PCTs resetting alarms, be sure to follow those guidelines.

Eliminate tracing problems by giving careful attention to skin preparation and lead placement. Other factors that can affect the quality of the tracings include broken lead wires, agitated patient, improperly grounded electrical equipment, running electrical cords under the bed, and loose electrodes. Actions you can take to ensure quality tracings are:

- Set up the room so that cords are not under the bed.
- Check the condition of the plugs and cords; if frayed or faulty, do not use them.
- Replace loose electrode pads.
- Change all electrode pads when one needs replacing.
- Unmatched electrodes (different kinds) do not always work well together, so make sure you apply the same kind to all areas of the monitoring lead.
- Ensure that cables and lead wires are intact, with no cracks or breaks in the wire or insulated covering.
- Secure the cable wires to the bed or the patient in a way that provides slack and avoids tension on the electrodes attached to the patient.

4 lead system

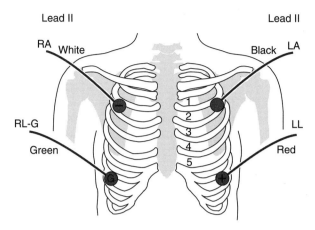

MCL, 3 or 5 wire system

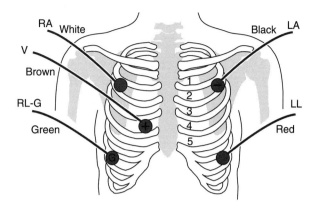

FIGURE 16-7
Leads II and MCL₁.

✔ Prevention is the best treatment for tracing problems. With selection of the proper site, skin preparation and attention to the environment will prevent many problems.

Documentation

You should document date, time, preparation of the electrode site, where you applied the electrodes, and obtain a rhythm strip for documenting the heart rhythm.

📝 Example: 7/25/96/0600/Areas under clavicles shaved and skin cleansed with alcohol swab. Skin on upper chest and lower thorax rubbed with a gauze pad, and disposable electrodes applied. S. Swift, PCT

Care of the Patient with an Artificial Pacemaker

An artificial pacemaker may be required for patients who have an irregular or slow pulse to restore a regular rhythm to the heart beat and improve cardiac output. An artificial pacemaker can be permanent or temporary. In a permanent pacemaker, all of the technological equipment is placed inside the patient's body.

A permanent pacemaker pulse generator may be seen and felt as a hard foreign body, placed under the skin on the chest. It may be in almost any location on the chest, and is connected to the heart by the pacing catheter. When caring for a patient with a new permanent pacemaker, it is important to keep the patient on complete bedrest for 24 hours to avoid displacing the catheter.

In a temporary pacemaking system, the pacing catheter is inside the body in contact with the heart. The pulse generator is outside the body and carried in a pocket or pouch, very similar to a telemetry monitoring unit. Most

of the information contained in this chapter refers to temporary pacemaker systems.

A pacemaker unit consists of 3 basic parts: a pulse generator, a pacing catheter, and electrodes. The pulse generator is the heart of the pacemaker unit, containing the circuits, controls, and the energy source or battery. The battery provides the energy for pacing the heart and the power for the circuits. The catheter and electrodes are placed directly on the myocardium (heart muscle) or guided through a vein into the right ventricle of the heart. Either application ensures that the electrodes on the pacing wires are in contact with the myocardial surface on the outside of the heart (epicardium) or the inside of the heart (endocardium). It is through this catheter that an electrical impulse is delivered to the myocardium by the pulse generator, and the heart is stimulated to contract.

Some patients need a pacemaker to continuously stimulate the heart at a particular rate. This is called a fixed rate pacemaker. Every time you take the person's pulse, it should be regular and within a few beats of the set rate. Notify the RN if the pulse of someone with a fixed rate pacemaker is irregular or varies from the set rate.

Some pacemakers are classified as demand pacemakers, in that they "sense" if the heart is beating on its own and send a stimulus to the heart only if it is not beating at the rate that is set. If the patient's heart rate is faster than what the pacer is set for, the pacer will not send an impulse. Many pacemakers can be set by a physician to work either as fixed rate or demand pacers. Temporary pacemakers are frequently set as demand pacemakers.

When a patient has a temporary pacemaker you should pay close attention to taking the pulse. The pacemaker will be set at a certain rate, often at 75 to 80 pulses/minute. When taking the pulse of a patient who has a pacemaker, you should never get a pulse of less than the set rate by more than 3–5 beats/minute. For example, if the pacer rate is set at 80, the patient should never have a pulse of less than 75 beats/minute. The pulse should be counted for 1 full minute.

The pacemaker is not working properly if the rate is less than the set rate, and the RN should be notified immediately. The patient can have a pulse rate that is faster than the programmed rate but not one that is more than 3–5 beats lower.

Take care to establish a baseline pulse on a patient with a pacemaker. Take the patient's pulse upon waking and at intervals throughout the day, both before and after activity.

Temporary pacers may be inserted in the operating room, in a pacer laboratory, or under emergency situations as part of a CODE. Important care measures when caring for a temporary pacemaker include:

The patient should remain on bedrest for 24 hours after insertion of the pacer to avoid dislodging the electrodes

- Do not adjust any of the dials on the control box. Do not change any settings
- Avoid any pull on the box or wires that may dislodge the pacing electrodes from the heart. Take care when turning, transferring, or ambulating the patient.

Notify the nurse if the connectors from the pacer wires to the electrodes, or any portion of the electrodes, are coming out from under the dressing.

- To decrease the risk of electrical problems. Using sterile technique, wear gloves and reinforce the dressing to cover the wires.
- The RN is usually responsible for changing the pacemaker dressings.
- Keep the box dry. Be careful when bathing the patient.
- Be extremely cautious of electrical safety, make sure all plugs are grounded, and all equipment in the area has been checked out by the clinical engineering department. This includes personal electrical equipment that the patient uses.
- The patient should be encouraged to use battery-operated devices, i.e., shaver, hair dryer.
- The patient should avoid any strong magnetic field as it can cause the pacemaker to

malfunction. These include microwave ovens and magnetic resonance imaging (MRI) equipment.

RESPONSE TO EQUIPMENT ALARMS IN THE INTENSIVE CARE UNIT

ICUs are filled with multiple types of technological equipment. Most equipment has some type of alarm system attached to it to notify the personnel working in those areas that a problem exits. *It is extremely important to recognize each of these alarms and know how to respond to them to ensure that patients receive safe and competent care.*

High/Low Pulse Rate Alarms

Most cardiac monitoring systems have a high-rate alarm and a low-rate alarm. There is usually an audible and visual alarm. Many monitoring systems have different sounds for different level alarms. For instance, high- or low-rate alarms might be an intermittent sound while an alarm that indicates asystole (flat line) might be a continuous sound. When the rate alarm sounds, it means the patient has a pulse rate that is too low or too high, or it is absent. The primary concern when a rate alarm sounds is what is happening to the patient. Always check for a pulse when the alarm sounds. Response should follow these steps:

1. Manually check the pulse. If the patient has a pulse and the rate is above 50 and below 150, reset the alarm if institutional policy permits. Notify the RN.

2. If the pulse rate is below 50 and the patient has no change in level of consciousness, reset the alarm, call the RN, and stay with the patient until the RN arrives. Check the blood pressure while waiting for the RN.

3. If the pulse rate is greater than 150 and the patient has no change in level of consciousness, reset the alarm, call the RN, and stay with the patient until the RN arrives. Check the blood pressure while waiting for the RN.

4. Institute CPR and call for help when the patient has no pulse.

A low rate of 50 or less and a high rate of 150 or more should be reported immediately. It is especially important when accompanied by changes in the patient's level of consciousness, orientation, or blood pressure, or by complaints of dizziness or syncope.

Alarm rate settings should always be documented, and the condition of the patient should be assessed by the RN and noted when alarm parameters are exceeded.

Consult the equipment operations manual for specific information on the monitoring alarms system installed in your areas. The types of alarms can vary, and the operations manual will describe which types your monitoring system has.

Invasive Pressure Alarms

Multiple types of cardiac pressures and intracranial pressures can be monitored on most hard-wire monitoring systems. The most common type of pressure monitored is the systemic blood pressure. It is monitored through an arterial line.

Call the RN if an arterial catheter is dislodged or disconnected, the patient can hemorrhage. All of the intravenous tubing used on arterial lines should have Luer-Lok connectors. If a catheter is pulled out of the artery, direct pressure should be applied to the insertion site for at least 10 minutes and the RN notified immediately.

These lines usually have high- and low-pressure alarms. Remember to check the patient's pulse and level of consciousness in response to an alarm. Reset the alarm only after checking for a pulse. The sounding alarm will bring additional help to the bedside and ensure that you are not alone with the patient.

Use extreme caution when pushing any alarm buttons. Never turn an alarm off. Most monitoring systems have the choice of alarm off, alarm silence, and alarm reset. When you use alarm silence or reset you are quieting the alarm temporarily to allow time to correct the problem that caused the alarm. After a minute or two, the alarm will sound again if the limits are violated. If you turn the alarm off, then no alarm will sound if the limits are violated.

Check and document your patient's cuff blood pressure, pulse, and mental status when alarm limits are exceeded.

Ventilator Alarms

Mechanical ventilators have multiple alarm parameters. They sound for high oxygen percentages, high pressures, low pressures, high and low respiratory rates, and the absence of respirations (apnea). Different alarms call for different actions. Problems can exist with both the ventilator and the patient to cause an alarm situation. An RN or RT will always be close by any patient who is on a ventilator. PCTs may be asked to assist with care and responding to alarms.

The RN or respiratory therapist should always check the patient on the ventilator to decide if the alarms were caused by a machine or patient problem. When ventilator alarms are activated, it could mean the patient is not receiving adequate ventilation.

High-pressure alarms may be caused by excess secretions and require that the patient be suctioned. Moisture trapped in the ventilator circuitry can also cause high-pressure alarms. Tubing should be emptied of trapped water frequently (every 1–2 hours) to avoid this problem. Drain tubing away from the patient's end of the tubing to avoid forcing water toward the patient's airway and predisposing the patient to respiratory infection.

The PCT may be asked to ensure that the patient is being ventilated by using a bag-valve resuscitator apparatus to deliver breaths to the patient while the RN or therapist examines the ventilator for problems. Observe patient for rise and fall of the chest with each ventilation while using the resuscitator bag.

Infusion and Feeding Pump Alarms

Intravenous infusion pumps usually have occlusion alarms, air-in-tubing alarms, and completion alarms.

• Occlusion alarms go off when the IV system is blocked in some way. It may mean that a clot has formed in the IV device in the patient's arm, or the line may be blocked. Take a moment to trace the line from the IV pump to the patient to see if the patient has rolled over and blocked the line or if the line is kinked. Straighten the line and notify the RN.

NEVER open the IV pump and release the line from the pump. Fluid may run wide open into the patient.

• Air in tubing alarms—air in an IV line can be dangerous to a patient because it can act as an embolus and block a blood vessel. The RN will clear the line and identify the cause of the problem.

• Completion alarms signal the end of a bag of fluid. The RN will hang a new IV bag or discontinue the IV.

PCTs are usually not allowed to correct these alarm situations. Notify the RN immediately so that they may correct the alarm situation and restart the infusion. Many intravenous drugs administered by an infusion pump affect the patient's heart action so that an interruption in the infusion could cause serious problems for the patient.

Feeding pumps generally have occlusion and completion alarms. Occlusion alarms occur when the feeding tube becomes plugged. The RN can irrigate the tube with saline or water to flush the formula through the line and restart the feeding. If the completion alarm sounds, close the clamp on the line to stop the feeding and notify the RN so that she/he can flush the line with water or hang more tube feeding.

Record any tube feeding, amount given, and patient tolerance on the diet sheet or vitals record according to institutional policy.

Summary

Multiple types of alarms and interventions will demand your attention in the intensive care setting. In responding to alarms:

1. Know your scope of practice.
2. Know your institutional policies.
3. Observe the patient with RN support.
4. Do not just "treat the equipment."
5. Never turn an alarm off.

If you keep these four points in mind at all times, you will not go wrong.

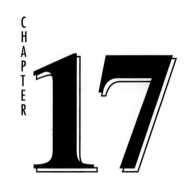
Assisting with Sterile Procedures

KAREN BOLIEK, MS, RN

OUTLINE

Microorganisms

Types

Methods of Transmission

Principles of Asepsis

Personal Grooming

Handwashing
Procedure

Disinfection

Sterilization

Disposable Equipment

Types of Asepsis
Medical Asepsis
Surgical Asepsis

Handling of Sterile Supplies
Opening Sterile Packages
Opening Sterile Trays
Adding Items to a Sterile Field
Sterile Liquids
Applying Sterile Gloves

Implementation of Sterile Technique
Wound Care
Changing Sterile Dressings
Applying Dressings around Drains
Reinforcing a Sterile Dressing
Applying a Wet-to-Dry Dressing

Setting up Intravenous Lines

PREREQUISITE KNOWLEDGE AND SKILLS

- Universal precautions
- Documentation
- Infection process (Chapter 3)
- Communicating with other healthcare providers (Chapter 4)

OBJECTIVES

After you complete this chapter, you will be able to:

- Differentiate between different types of microorganisms.

- Identify how microorganisms are spread.

- Discuss the principles of medical and surgical asepsis.

- List risk factors that may make patients susceptible to infection.
- Explain the ways to control the spread of microorganisms.
- Recall the skills and steps necessary to perform or assist with various sterile procedures.

KEY TERMS

Aerobes Microbes that require oxygen to live

Air Embolism Air bubble in the blood stream that obstructs the flow of blood in a blood vessel

Anaerobes Microbes that live best where there is little or no oxygen

Antibacterial Inhibiting the growth of bacteria

Antibiotic Medication that kills or slows the growth of microorganisms

Antiseptic Agent that slows the growth of microbes but does not kill them

Asepsis Absence of disease-causing microorganisms

Autoclave or Sterilizer Machine that sterilizes equipment

Carrier Person with no symptoms but who can transmit disease

Communicable or Contagious Capable of being spread from one person to another

Contaminate To soil with pathogens

Cross-Infection Infection with a microorganism from another person

Disinfect To destroy most pathogens except spores

Drain Device used to prevent fluid from accumulating in a body cavity or under the skin

Dressing Bandage used to cover and protect a wound

Fomite Object contaminated with germs

Germicide Agent that kills germs

Germ Disease-causing microorganism

Medical Asepsis or Clean Technique Procedure used to prevent spread of germs

Microorganism or Microbe Living thing that can be seen only under a microscope

Nonpathogens Microbes that do not cause disease

Nosocomial Infection Infection acquired in the hospital

Pathogen Any microbe that causes disease

Reinfection Infection more than once with the same microorganism

Sepsis Presence of disease-causing microorganisms

Spores Inactive bacteria with hard shells

Sterile Field Area free of all microorganisms

Sterilization Killing of all microorganisms, including spores

Surgical Asepsis or Sterile Technique Keeping an area totally free of microorganisms

To assist with sterile procedures, it is necessary to understand the principles of aseptic, or sterile, technique. Applying these principles during specific procedures will assure that every precaution is taken to prevent a patient from acquiring an infection. In addition to a discussion of these principles, this chapter will also describe various types of microorganisms, their modes of transmission, and ways to control their spread. Sterile procedures will be explained and illustrated, and the skills required to assist with them will be outlined.

MICROORGANISMS

All around us are tiny living things called *microorganisms*. *Organism* refers to any living thing, and *micro* means very small. Microorganisms are so small, that

although there are millions of them, they can be seen only under a microscope. They live on our skin, hair, clothes, the food we eat, things we touch, and inside our bodies. Microorganisms, also called *microbes*, live and multiply best where there is moisture, a food supply, warmth, and not much light.

TYPES

There are several kinds of microorganisms we are exposed to every day: protozoa, bacteria, fungi (fungus), and viruses. Not all microbes affect our bodies in the same way.

When we use the word *germ* we are usually referring to a type of microorganism called a *pathogen*. Pathogenic microorganisms, or pathogens, are microbes that cause disease. When pathogens invade and multiply in the body, infection occurs, causing damage to the body's tissues. *Staphylococcus aureus* and *Streptococcus* are common pathogens.

Other microorganisms live in our bodies and food and are not harmful; in fact, some microbes are beneficial to humans. These microbes are called *nonpathogenic* because they do not cause disease.

There are cases in which nonpathogenic microorganisms may invade parts of the body where they do not normally live. *Escherichia coli* is a microorganism that lives in and is not harmful to the gastrointestinal system but can cause infection in the urinary system. There are occasions when antibiotics used to treat one infection destroy the microbes that have caused it, but disrupt the balance of nonpathogenic microorganisms that are usually harmless. When nonpathogens increase to levels much greater than normal, they can cause an additional infection in the body.

A final way to differentiate between types of microorganisms is by their need for oxygen. *Aerobic* microorganisms require oxygen to live. *Streptococcus pneumoniae* is an aerobic bacterium that causes pneumonia and flourishes in the respiratory system where there is plenty of oxygen. *Clostridium tetani* is an *anaerobic* microorganism that grows best where there is little oxygen. Tetanus is caused by this microbe and usually develops in deep puncture wounds away from the oxygen-rich surface of the skin.

METHODS OF TRANSMISSION

Many diseases are not caused by pathogens and cannot be transferred from one person to another. However, many diseases are *communicable*, that is, they can be spread by transmission of the microorganisms that cause them. Microorganisms can spread from one person to another in the health care setting in several ways:

- Direct contact transmission occurs by person to person contact. Touching the patient or the patient's blood or body fluids is direct contact. Microbes pass not only from the patient to the health care provider, but also from the health care provider to the patient. Bathing the patient, helping him or her out of bed, and contact with urine and feces are instances when microbes may be directly transferred from one person to another. Direct contact also occurs when droplets of moisture produced by talking, coughing, or sneezing pass between two people less than 3 feet apart.
- Indirect contact occurs by the touching of *contaminated* objects. A contaminated object is one that is soiled with pathogens. Contaminated articles include bedpans, linens, dishes, and pieces of medical equipment that have been used on a patient. *Fomite* is another

word for an article contaminated with infectious microbes.

> Remember, microorganisms are too small to see without a microscope. Articles do not have to look dirty to have microbes living on them.

- Airborne transmission occurs when microbes cling to dust particles or moisture in the air and are inhaled through the mouth or nose.
- Vehicle transmission occurs when microorganisms dwell in food or fluids that are ingested; or drugs, blood products, or fluids administered.
- Vector transmission occurs when an insect such as a fly or tick carries microorganisms from one person to another.

With so many types of microorganisms and ways in which they can spread, it is easy to see how patients in the health care setting are at risk of being exposed to pathogens. Normally we have several lines of defense against infection, such as intact skin, mucous membranes, peristalsis, and the immune system. There are many reasons hospitalized people are susceptible to developing infections:

- People are admitted to the hospital with a variety of different infections that other patients are exposed to. The hospital environment, air, floors, and equipment harbor microorganisms. A number of pathogens are surrounded by a protective shell and survive in a dry state. When air currents move them and they land on a moist surface, such as the mouth, nose, or a surgical wound site, they become active, multiply, and cause infection. Therefore, it is important to remember to keep hospital surfaces as clean as possible and to avoid creating air currents that will circulate microorganisms. Some serious pathogens have developed resistance to antibiotics and are very difficult to destroy. Methicillin-resistant *Staphylococcus aureus* (MRSA) is a microorganism that is resistant to antibiotics.
- Invasive diagnostic and treatment methods such as IVs, Foley catheters, and mechanical ventilators break through barriers that normally protect from pathogens.
- Surgical wounds, burns, and pressure ulcers are ideal sites for the growth of microorganisms. Intact skin provides protection against pathogens. When the skin is broken, it is very easy for harmful microorganisms to enter the body.
- Newborns, debilitated elderly people, and patients compromised by chronic diseases are prone to acquiring infections.
- Certain medications and metabolic disorders depress the body's immune system and decrease its resistance to pathogens.

- Hospitalized patients are in a relatively small space and in close contact with staff, visitors, and other patients who may be *carriers* of disease.
- Patients can be re-infected by the same microorganism more than once. They can also be cross-infected with pathogens from other patients or members of the health care team.

Infections that are acquired in the hospital or health care facility that were not present before admission are called *nosocomial* infections. About 5% of all hospitalized patients develop nosocomial infections. Many of these infections can be prevented.

PRINCIPLES OF ASEPSIS

During the 1800s the death rate in hospitals from infections was very high. Florence Nightingale was one of the first to realize that clean equipment, hands, gowns, and sheets are important to a patient's recovery. Because of her work in infection control, Florence Nightingale has been known as the pioneer of antiseptic principles. Understanding the principles of asepsis can help protect patients, visitors, other staff members, and yourself from harmful microorganisms.

Sepsis is the condition resulting from the presence of pathogenic microorganisms and the poisons they produce in the body. Asepsis means just the opposite—a germ-free condition in which no disease-causing microorganisms are present. Learning how to control the spread of microorganisms is the first step in understanding the principles of aseptic technique.

PERSONAL GROOMING

Good hygiene and attention to personal grooming not only fosters a professional appearance for the PCT, but also helps control the spread of microorganisms. Health care providers should bathe and change their uniforms daily. Hair should be short or worn up, off the collar. Fingernails should be kept short and clean. A wristwatch and simple wedding band are the only pieces of jewelry that should be worn. Germs can live under fingernails, in cracked or chipped fingernail polish, and in rings and other jewelry. Sharp nails and jewelry can scratch the patient, allowing germs to enter through the broken skin.

Cover any cuts or abrasions on your hands with a bandage or gloves. Do not care for patients if you have any uncovered infected lesion on your hands or if you are ill with any communicable disease.

🛑 **STOP** If you are uncertain about contagious conditions you may have, talk with your

supervisor or employee health nurse before reporting to work.

HANDWASHING

The most important procedure in controlling the spread of germs is handwashing. Every member of the health care team must wash his or her hands on arrival to the nursing unit, before and after giving direct patient care, and handling equipment, food, and patient belongings and after using a tissue or the bathroom.

Procedure

1. Before beginning, be sure you have all of the necessary equipment at the sink:

- Soap—Liquid soap is best. Bar soap sits in a pool of water between uses and harbors germs.
- Do not use the patient's soap.
- Paper towels—Cloth towels can harbor germs between washings.
- Warm running water
- Wastepaper basket

2. Wet your hands from 2 inches above your wrists under the running water while keeping your fingertips pointed down.
3. Add plenty of soap and lather well.
4. Rub your hands together in a circular motion, hard enough to create friction to loosen the germs. Thirty seconds is usually long enough to adequately wash your hands unless they are grossly dirty (Fig. 17–1).
5. To clean under your fingernails, rub them across the palm of your opposite hand; if very soiled use an orange stick or nailbrush.
6. Interlock your fingers to clean between them (Fig. 17–1).
7. Keep your hands lower than your elbows all the while

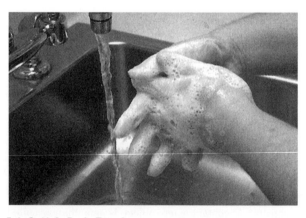

F I G U R E   1 7 – 1

Rub your hands together. Interlock your fingers to clean between them. (From Zakus, S. M: Clinical Procedures for Medical Assistants. 3rd ed. St. Louis, Mosby-Year Book, 1995.)

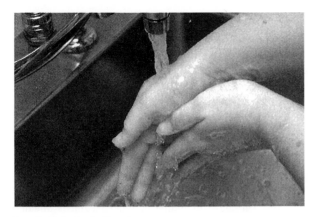

you are washing to keep the soapy water from spreading germs up your arms.

8. Rinse from 2 inches above your wrists to your hands under running water. Rinse with your hands below your elbows with your fingertips pointing down. Be sure to rinse completely. The friction created by rubbing and the soap you use only loosen germs, oils, and dead skin. You remove the loosened matter by rinsing well (Fig. 17–2).

9. Dry your hands thoroughly with paper towels.

10. Turn off the water by using the paper towel to avoid touching the faucet (Fig. 17–3).

11. Throw the paper towel in the wastepaper basket.

🛑 The sink, faucets, and wastepaper basket are considered contaminated. If your hands touch any of them while washing, they are contaminated also and you must start over.

It is impossible to remove all microorganisms from your hands by washing them. Chemicals strong enough to kill all germs would be harmful to the tissue of your skin.

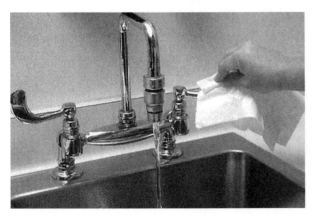

Antibacterial soaps and antiseptics are chemicals safe enough to use on the skin that inhibit the growth and multiplication of microorganisms but do not necessarily kill them.

DISINFECTION

Medical equipment and supplies that are to be reused must first be *disinfected*. Inanimate objects are disinfected by removing, controlling, or destroying as many microorganisms as possible by physical or chemical means. Disinfection does not kill spores. Spores are inactive bacteria that have formed hard shells around themselves. When conditions are right, they become active, multiply, and cause infections. Because of their protective shell, it is very difficult to kill spores.

Chemical *germicides* are used in the health care setting to disinfect contaminated articles. Before placing the article in disinfectant, all gross dirt must be removed with soap and cool water. Articles must be immersed in the disinfectant for varying lengths of time, depending on the type of disinfectant used and the pathogens present.

✔ If you are asked to disinfect equipment, be sure you know the manufacturer's recommendations for the effective use and safe handling of the chemical.

STERILIZATION

Sterilization is the process that destroys all pathogenic and nonpathogenic microorganisms, including spores. Articles may be made sterile by dry heat, steam under pressure, or chemical gas by the use of autoclaves, also called sterilizers. Articles that can tolerate heat are sterilized in pressurized steam autoclaves. Plastics and heat-sensitive equipment are sterilized in gas autoclaves.

DISPOSABLE EQUIPMENT

Many of the supplies used in health care facilities are intended to be used only once, or on one patient alone, and then discarded. The use of disposable equipment is helpful in controlling the numbers of nosocomial infections. Some examples of disposable equipment are plastic bedpans and urinals, thermometer probe covers, hypodermic needles and syringes, and Foley catheters. When contaminated equipment is disposed of properly, pathogens are discarded along with it.

🛑 Do not use disposable equipment more often than intended. You probably do not have the necessary supplies or equipment to clean it properly. Never use disposable equipment for more than one patient.

TYPES OF ASEPSIS

There are two types of asepsis: medical asepsis and surgical asepsis.

Medical Asepsis

Medical asepsis is the practice of procedures and precautions that reduce the number of microorganisms in the environment and inhibit their spread from one person to another. Practicing the principles of medical asepsis is often referred to as using clean technique. Many of the principles of medical asepsis involve things we do every day to promote a clean, healthy environment for our families. We wash our food and refrigerate it to keep it from spoiling. We bathe, wear clean clothes, cover our mouth when we sneeze, and keep our homes clean and free of insects. Because of the many kinds of microorganisms in the health care facility, and the susceptibility of the patients there, extra precautions must be taken to provide a safe environment in the hospital.

Role of the Patient Care Technician in Medical Asepsis

Every member of the health care team, including the patient care technician (PCT), is obligated to practice the techniques of medical asepsis. By recalling the ways in which microorganisms are spread, you can probably think of ways to avoid their growth and transmission. Some of your examples should include the following:

Direct Contact

- Wash your hands before and after giving patient care.

- Use an antiseptic on any cut on your hand and cover with a bandage.

- Use gloves when emptying bedpans and urinals and avoid splashing.

- Wear goggles if there is any danger of body fluids splashing in your eyes.

- Cover your mouth, turn your head, and use a tissue whenever possible when coughing or sneezing and encourage the patient to do the same.

- Do not report to work with any type of communicable condition.

- Wear a mask in the patient's room if he or she has a communicable disease that can be spread by droplets of moisture in the air.

- When using aseptic technique, start cleaning from the cleanest to the least clean area to avoid recontamination.

Patients requiring special isolation precautions such as the wearing of masks should have appropriate signs posted on the outside of their doors. If you have any questions, consult your infection control manual, staff RN, or infection control RN.

Indirect Contact

1. Do not use disposable equipment on more than one patient or on one patient more times than it was intended.
2. Disinfect reusable equipment between uses. Do not use any supplies, including linen, that have touched the floor.
3. Keep a bag taped to the bedrail for disposal of dirty tissues.
4. Do not let dirty linen touch your uniform.
5. Do not share personal items such as razors and combs between patients.
6. Wear gloves when handling contaminated equipment or supplies.
7. Dispose of contaminated supplies in appropriate biohazard containers.
8. Do not store clean and contaminated equipment in the same area. Most hospitals have separate clean and dirty utility rooms.

Airborne

1. To prevent microorganisms from getting into the air, do not shake linen.
2. Damp-dust furniture to keep dust down.
3. Cover your mouth and turn your head when coughing or sneezing.
4. Wear a mask when appropriate.
5. Keep laundry hampers covered.

Vehicle

1. Remove meal trays promptly. If food is to be saved, cover and refrigerate.
2. Assist the patient in washing his or her hands before eating.
3. Wash your hands before handling food.
4. Keep water pitchers covered and water fresh.
5. Do not share food from the patient's tray.

Vector

1. Leave windows closed to keep out insects.
2. Discourage the storing of food in patient rooms to avoid attracting vermin.
3. Do not discard food in patient wastepaper baskets.

Surgical Asepsis

Surgical asepsis is an extension of the practices of medical asepsis used when patients need special protection against microorganisms. Sterile equipment and supplies have undergone a process that destroys all living microorganisms, including spores. Surgical asepsis, also called sterile technique, is the practice of creating a sterile area, or sterile field, and maintaining sterility throughout a procedure.

Maintaining a sterile environment is especially important when caring for patients with wounds. There are many types of wounds in the health care setting. Gunshots, surgical incisions, venipuncture sites, and pressure sores are all examples of wounds. The skin is normally a very effective barrier that protects the body from invasion by microorganisms. When there is a break in the skin due to a wound, microorganisms are given the opportunity to invade the body and cause infections.

Patients with tubes inserted into sterile body cavities for examinations or treatments are also at risk for infection. The bladder is an example of a sterile environment. Foley catheters inserted into the bladder must be sterile.

Principles of Surgical Asepsis and the Role of the Patient Care Technician

 There are many sterile procedures that may only be performed by licensed persons. Carry out only those sterile procedures that are included in your job description and for which you have been adequately trained.

Understanding and following the principles of surgical asepsis will enable you to set up a sterile area and keep it sterile throughout the procedure that you are performing or assisting the RN or physician to perform.

Only sterile items can be used in a sterile field. Sterile items only can touch other sterile items. If an unsterile item touches a sterile one, the sterile item is contaminated and must be replaced.

 If you are not sure whether an item has been contaminated, replace it with a sterile one.

Barriers are used to protect sterile areas from nonsterile ones. It is impossible to sterilize your hands, nose, or mouth. Good handwashing and the use of germicidal soaps can lessen the number of microbes on your hands. Sterile gloves, masks, and gowns protect the sterile field from the microorganisms in and on your body. Sterile drapes protect the sterile field from the unsterile table beneath it. Any time a barrier is permeated, it is considered contaminated.

Any hole in gloves, gowns, masks, or drapes is a source of contamination of the sterile field.

A sterile field must stay dry to remain sterile. Microbes can seep through packages and drapes if they become wet. Moisture-proof drapes prevent transmission of microbes from unsterile to sterile areas. The edges of a sterile package (about 1 inch) are considered contaminated once the package is opened. Keep all sterile supplies well within the borders of the sterile field.

Never reach over a sterile field with unsterile articles. You may drop them onto the sterile field, or microbes from them may fall onto the sterile area. If you are not wearing a sterile gown, microbes from your clothing may also contaminate the field.

Only the top of a table in a sterile field is considered sterile. Only the front of a sterile gown from the waist up to the shoulders is considered sterile. Keep your sterile gloved hands in front of you, above your waist. Open sterile supplies at the time you are going to use them. Supplies left uncovered and unattended may become contaminated.

Remember, microorganisms are too small to see without a microscope. Articles may be contaminated without looking dirty.

Surgical Conscience

Any member of the health care team working where surgical asepsis is necessary must develop a *surgical conscience*. Surgical conscience is based on the golden rule "Do unto others as you would have them do unto you." Any time a patient's safety is at risk because of a break in sterile technique, surgical conscience compels us to acknowledge and correct the situation. It reminds us to accept responsibility for maintaining a sterile field whether we are alone or with others. Health care providers must have the integrity to report accidental contamination committed by themselves or by others in a constructive manner.

HANDLING OF STERILE SUPPLIES

Some supplies you will use come from the manufacturer in sealed, sterile paper or plastic packages. They usually have an expiration date on them indicating how long sterility is guaranteed.

Other supplies are sterilized at the hospital and come in cloth packages sealed with tape. There are indicator strips on sterile packages that change color when the sterilization process is complete. These packages will also have an expiration date.

Before opening any sterile package, be certain that the seal is intact. Make sure no edges of the package have been loosened. Become familiar with the indicator strips so you can recognize properly sterilized supplies. Inspect the package for holes or tears. Any breaks in the protective barrier of the wrapper allow microorganisms to enter, and the package is no longer considered sterile. Do not use any package that is wet or appears to have been wet but has since dried, since it can no longer be considered sterile. Be certain that the expiration date has not passed.

Opening Sterile Packages

Gauze pads, gloves, and culture tubes are examples of sterile equipment that comes in sterile paper packages. These packages are like envelopes that are sealed tightly but have separated edges tabbed for easy opening. Follow these steps when opening any sterile package:

1. Wash your hands.
2. Inspect the package carefully to insure its sterility.
3. Grasp each side of the package at the separated edges and peel it open slowly. Do not tear the wrapper (Fig. 17–4).
4. Be sure you do not touch the inside of the wrapper or the contents of the package. Keep holding onto the edges only.
5. If you are assisting someone else with a procedure, the other person may remove the contents of the package wearing sterile gloves.
6. You may lay the package on a dry table, allowing only the outside of the wrapper to come in contact with unsterile surfaces. The interior of the wrapper is a sterile field.

Opening Sterile Trays

Foley catheter insertion setups, peritoneal dialysis equipment, and IV cutdown supplies come in sterile trays. Some trays are premade by the manufacturer and are double wrapped in plastic and paper. Other trays

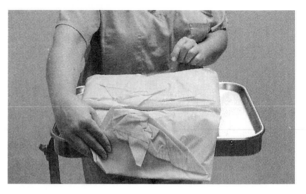

F I G U R E 1 7 – 5

Open the flap farthest from you first. (From Zakus, S. M: Clinical Procedures for Medical Assistants. 3rd ed. St. Louis, Mosby-Year Book, 1995.)

are sterilized in the hospital and come double wrapped in cloth.

The procedure for opening both types of trays is the same:

1. Wash your hands.
2. Inspect the package carefully to ensure its sterility.
3. The edges of the cloth or paper wrapper will be folded neatly on top of the tray. Break the paper seal.
4. Holding on to only the edges, begin unfolding the wrapper by opening the flap farthest from you first. By doing so, you will not reach over the sterile field once it is exposed (Fig. 17–5).
5. Fold back each of the side flaps (Fig. 17–6).
6. Finish by folding open the flap nearest to you (Fig. 17–7).

Adding Items to a Sterile Field

Once a sterile tray has been opened without contamination, you have created a sterile field. Additional sterile items may be added to the field as needed.

1. Follow the steps for opening sterile packages.
2. Hold the package over the sterile field and turn it

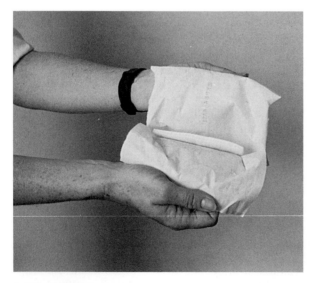

F I G U R E 1 7 – 4

Grasp each side of the wrapper and peel it open. (From Zakus, S. M: Clinical Procedures for Medical Assistants. 3rd ed. St. Louis, Mosby-Year Book, 1995.)

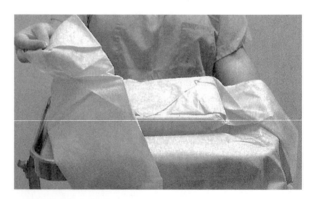

F I G U R E 1 7 – 6

Fold back each side flap. (From Zakus, S. M: Clinical Procedures for Medical Assistants. 3rd ed. St. Louis, Mosby-Year Book, 1995.)

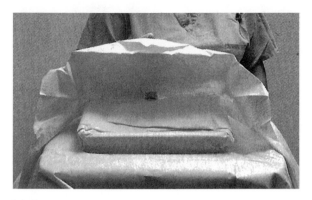

FIGURE 17-7

Fold open the flap nearest you last. (From Zakus, S. M: Clinical Procedures for Medical Assistants. 3rd ed. St. Louis, Mosby-Year Book, 1995.)

upside down, letting the contents fall onto the sterile field (Fig. 17–8).

3. Be careful not to touch the sterile field with the unsterile wrapper.

Sterile Liquids

Sterile liquids are used in cleaning surgical wounds, abrasions, and pressure sores and on special types of dressings. Strict aseptic technique must be followed when opening sterile bottles and pouring sterile liquids.

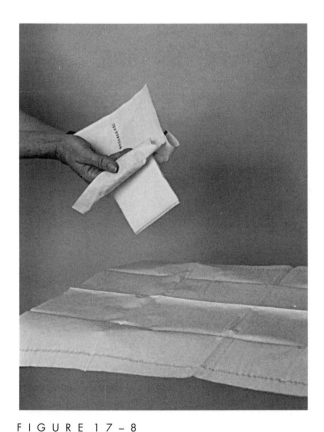

FIGURE 17-8

Let the contents of the package fall onto the sterile field.

1. Wash your hands.

2. Inspect the bottle for sterility. Check the expiration date, safety seal, and for any cracks in the bottle or cap.

3. Remove the cap and place it on the table with the open edge facing up to prevent contamination of the inside.

4. With the label facing up, pour liquid into a sterile container or onto a sterile dressing.

5. Do not touch the edge of the bottle to the container.

6. Use single-dose bottles of liquids when available. If solution remains in the bottle for reuse, replace the cap snugly.

Sterile liquids must be used or discarded within 24 hours after opening. Label the bottle with the patient's name and the date and time it was opened.

Applying Sterile Gloves

As you have learned, it is impossible to destroy all of the microorganisms on your hands. Wearing sterile gloves allows you to touch sterile supplies and open areas on the patient's skin. Careful aseptic technique must be followed to prevent contamination of your gloves while putting them on.

1. Wash your hands.

2. Follow the steps for opening sterile packages by first inspecting for sterility then peeling open the outer wrapper.

3. The gloves will be in an inner wrapper. Touching only the outside of this wrapper, lay them flat on the inside of the opened outer wrapper.

4. Holding on to only the edges, open the inner wrapper from the middle (Fig. 17–9).

5. The gloves will be lying with the palm side up, each with a folded cuff exposing the inside of the glove. This side of the glove will have a thin layer of powder on it to prevent it from sticking to your skin.

6. Pick up a glove by the folded cuff. (When the

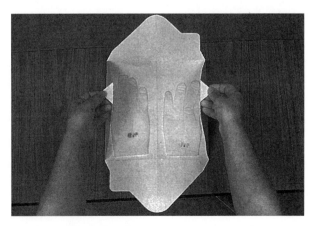

FIGURE 17-9

Open the inner wrapper holding only the edges. (From Taylor, C., et al.: Fundamentals of Nursing: The Art and Science of Nursing Care, 2nd ed. Philadelphia, J.B. Lippincott, 1993.)

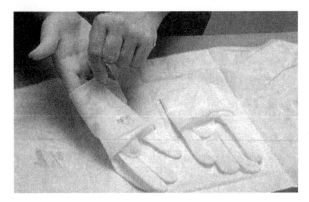

FIGURE 17–10

Hold the glove by the cuff only, and insert the opposite hand. (From Zakus, S. M: Clinical Procedures for Medical Assistants. 3rd ed. St. Louis, Mosby-Year Book, 1995.)

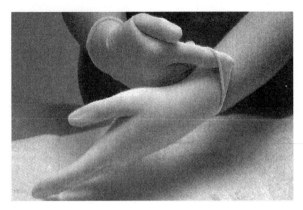

FIGURE 17–12

Pick it up and pull onto your hand. (From Zakus, S. M: Clinical Procedures for Medical Assistants. 3rd ed. St. Louis, Mosby-Year Book, 1995.)

glove is on and the cuff straightened out, this will be the inside of the glove.)

7. Place your opposite hand inside the glove and pull on, still touching only the cuff (Fig. 17–10).

8. Slip your gloved fingers under the cuff of the remaining glove and pick it up, only letting your sterile glove touch the other sterile glove (Fig. 17–11).

9. Place your hand in the glove and pull on (Fig. 17–12).

10. You now may adjust the fingers and cuffs of both, remembering that both gloves are sterile and may touch only each other.

IMPLEMENTATION OF STERILE TECHNIQUE

Once you understand the principles of sterile technique and have practiced with supervision, you will be ready to perform certain procedures and assist with others that require these skills.

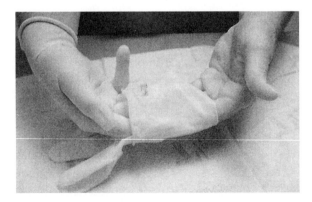

FIGURE 17–11

Slip your gloved fingers under the cuff of the remaining glove. (From Zakus, S. M: Clinical Procedures for Medical Assistants. 3rd ed. St. Louis, Mosby-Year Book, 1995.)

⚖ Remember that there are many procedures that only licensed persons may perform. Do not attempt any procedures for which you have not been adequately trained or which are not in your job description.

Wound Care

Open areas on the patient's skin are a potential source of invasion by pathogens and the development of infections. Strict aseptic technique must be followed to provide the safest environment for your patient.

Changing Sterile Dressings

A dressing is a bandage used to cover and protect a wound. Most dressing changes require a doctor's order, often with specific instructions about what type of dressings to use, how to clean the wound, and how often to change the dressing. Many doctors prefer to change a surgical dressing themselves the first time. Sterile saline is a common cleansing solution used on wounds.

🛑 Check with the RN with whom you are working about the specific details of the dressing change order before beginning the procedure.

The following are the steps performed when changing a sterile dressing:

1. Assemble all of the supplies you will need:
    Sterile dressings as ordered
    Sterile gloves
    Sterile cleansing solution as ordered
    Sterile saline
    Sterile solution container
    Tape
    Clean gloves
    Disposable kit containing scissors and forceps

Moisture-proof pad to protect patient's bed

Mask if patient is at particular risk for infection

Moisture-proof gown if there is danger of soiling your uniform

Plastic bag for contaminated supplies (Most facilities use red plastic bags for contaminated supplies.)

2. Inspect all packages for sterility.

3. Explain the procedure to the patient.

4. Pull the curtain around the patient's bed and/or close the door for privacy.

5. Wash your hands.

6. Put on mask and/or gown if indicated.

7. Lower the rail on the side of the bed you are working on. Raise the bed to a comfortable height for you to work.

8. Put moisture-proof pad on bed.

9. Put plastic trash bag nearby.

10. Cut or tear strips of tape.

11. Open sterile packages and leave on the bedside table.

12. Put on clean gloves. It is not necessary to wear sterile gloves if you do not touch the wound.

13. Remove old dressing. Loosen the edges of the tape and carefully pull toward the wound while gently putting tension on the skin underneath. This will make the tape removal less painful and avoid pulling at the incision site.

Remove the gauze pads one layer at a time.

STOP There may be drains underneath that you cannot see and could easily pull out if you remove the entire dressing at one time.

Drainage from the wound may have dried, causing the gauze pads to stick. Pouring a little sterile saline on the gauze will loosen it and make removal easier and less painful.

Place the soiled dressing in the red plastic trash bag.

14. Remove your gloves and place them in the trash bag.

15. Wash your hands.

16. Pour cleansing solution into sterile container.

17. Put on sterile gloves.

18. Use the sterile forceps from the disposable dressing kit to dip a folded gauze pad into the cleansing solution. Using the forceps will prevent contamination of your sterile gloves. Be sure the cleansing solution drips into the sterile container to avoid contaminating the sterile field with moisture. Always start at the cleanest part of the wound and work toward the dirtiest part. Do not go back over an area you have already cleaned. Use small, circular strokes to clean the wound. Discard soiled gauze pads in the plastic trash bag and use new ones until the entire wound is cleaned.

STOP Do not contaminate the forceps by touching the trash bag with them.

19. Either allow the wound to air dry, or gently pat it dry with sterile gauze.

STOP Do not fan the air to hasten drying. The motion of the air will stir up dust and airborne microorganisms.

Once the area is dry, remove the sterile dressings from the opened package and cover the wound. Common sterile dressings consist of 4 × 4 gauze pads closest to the wound and ABD pads as an outer covering. The amount of wound drainage will determine how many layers of dressings you will need.

20. Remove gloves and discard in red trash bag. Once the wound is covered, you no longer need sterile gloves. In addition, handling tape while wearing gloves is very difficult.

21. While applying gentle pressure, tape the dressing using the least amount of tape necessary to hold it securely in place.

22. Remove all soiled supplies from the patient's room and place in the appropriate contaminated trash area.

23. Wash your hands.

Document the date and time the dressing was changed in the patient's chart. Record any observations you made about the color, consistency, amount, and odor of any drainage and the appearance of the wound and the skin around it. Some hospital policies require that the date, time, and initials of the person changing a dressing be written on the tape in ink.

It is the RN's responsibility to assess the patient's wound. However, you should immediately report bleeding, redness, swelling, pain, drainage, opening of the wound edges, or any sudden change in the wound that you observe.

Applying Dressings around Drains

Various types of drains are inserted into surgical incisions to allow blood and secretions to exit the wound. Preventing the accumulation of fluid under the skin helps the wound heal faster. Hemovacs, Jackson-Pratts, and chest tubes are types of drains you may see. The drain is a pathway into a sterile area of the body, and although the incision may be sutured closed, the drain site is an opening and a potential site of infection. Microorganisms grow best where there is moisture, a food supply, warmth, and not a great deal of light. You can see why a wet surgical dressing is a good place for pathogens to grow.

When you are changing a dressing on a wound with a drain, strict aseptic technique must be followed.

1. Follow the procedure for changing a sterile dressing.
2. Special care must be taken with the drain. Most drains are sutured in place, but careful attention must be paid to avoid pulling out the drain or dislodging it in any way. Using a circular motion, carefully clean around and under the drain, beginning close to the drain and moving out.
3. Because the drain is designed to bring fluids to the surface of the skin, the area around it becomes especially wet. Special gauze pads are placed around the drain to absorb the moisture and protect the surrounding skin.

Premade drain sponges are gauze pads with slits that allow the gauze to be slipped snugly around the drain.

If you do not have premade drain sponges, you can make them by cutting a 2-inch slit in a regular 4 × 4 gauze pad.

STOP Remember to use aseptic technique for all surgical dressing changes. Use the sterile scissors in the disposable kit to cut the slit in the gauze.

Apply several drain sponges at different angles to completely cover the area around the drain (Fig. 17–13).
4. Continue dressing the wound, following the procedure for sterile dressing changes.

Reinforcing a Sterile Dressing

There are occasions when the original surgical dressing is not to be changed. Because of normal drainage, with or without incisional drains, dressings may become saturated with blood or secretions.

As you have learned, protective barriers that have become wet are no longer considered sterile. A wet dressing allows microorganisms from the patient's gown and bed linen to pass through the barrier to the wound beneath it.

Reinforcing the original dressing with dry, sterile supplies helps reestablish a protective barrier against infection.

The following is the procedure for reinforcing a surgical dressing:

1. Assemble all equipment:
   Sterile gloves
   Sterile dressings
   Tape
2. Wash your hands.
3. Explain the procedure to the patient and provide privacy.
4. Inspect the dressing packages for sterility and open them.
5. Put on sterile gloves.
6. Lay the sterile dressing on top of the original one and tape securely in place.
7. Document on the patient's chart the date and time the dressing was reinforced and the color, amount, and consistency of the drainage.

If the reinforced dressing becomes wet with drainage again, the procedure will be repeated.

1. Assemble all equipment:
   Nonsterile gloves
   Sterile gloves

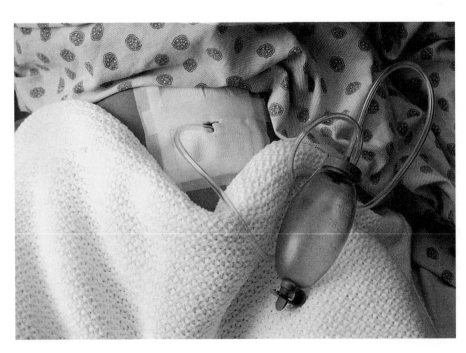

FIGURE 17-13
Sponge around drain.

Sterile dressings

Tape

Red plastic trash bag

2. Wash your hands.

3. Explain procedure to the patient and provide privacy.

4. Put on nonsterile gloves.

5. Gently remove the tape and dressings you added to reinforce the original dressing. Do not disturb or remove any parts of the original surgical dressing.

6. Discard the soiled dressing and your gloves in the red plastic trash bag.

7. Wash your hands.

8. Put on sterile gloves and follow the procedure for reinforcing a surgical dressing.

Be sure to notify the RN each time you reinforce a dressing for him or her to assess whether the amount of drainage is normal or excessive.

Applying a Wet-to-Dry Dressing

Open wounds may be treated with wet-to-dry dressings. As the name suggests, these dressings are put on wet and allowed to dry before removal. As the dry dressing is removed, old dead tissue clings to it and is removed also. Removal of dead tissue helps the wound heal.

Because this type of dressing requires ongoing assessment of tissue healing, it is best for the PCT to assist the RN.

Some surgical wounds and pressure sores are treated with wet-to-dry dressings. Sterile normal saline and Betaine are common solutions used on wet-to-dry dressings.

If the doctor has written the order for a simple wet-to-dry dressing, you will apply it by following these steps:

1. Assemble all equipment:
Sterile gloves
Nonsterile gloves
Sterile gauze dressings
Sterile solution ordered
Tape
Moisture-proof protective pad
Red plastic trash bag
2. Wash your hands.

3. Explain the procedure to the patient and provide privacy. Place the protective pad on the bed.

4. Put on nonsterile gloves.

5. Gently remove old, dried dressing. Take care to avoid tearing new healing tissue.

6. Dispose of soiled dressing and your gloves in plastic trash bag.

7. Wash your hands.

8. Open sterile packages after inspecting for sterility. Pour solution on gauze pads.

9. Put on sterile gloves.

10. Clean the wound, holding moistened gauze pads with sterile forceps. Work from the cleanest area to the least clean. Do not go back over an area you have already cleaned.

11. Dispose of soiled gauze pads in trash bag. Do not contaminate your gloves or forceps by touching the bag.

12. Cover the wound with moistened gauze pads, then apply dry sterile dressings.

13. Remove gloves and discard in trash bag.

14. Tape dressing using the least amount of tape necessary to hold it securely.

15. Remove all contaminated trash from the patient's room.

16. Wash your hands.

Document the application of the wet-to-dry dressing, date and time, solution used, and the condition of the wound and skin around it.

Some orders for wet-to-dry dressings include packing the wound with moistened gauze pads. The PCT may set up the supplies necessary for the procedure and assist with it, but only licensed persons may pack wounds.

SETTING UP INTRAVENOUS LINES

Many patients in health care facilities have IV lines. IV fluids may be administered for a variety of different reasons. Some patients may not be allowed or able to eat or drink. IV solutions provide necessary nourishment such as water, sugar, minerals, protein, and fats. Other patients may receive medications through IV solutions because they cannot take them orally or because the medications work best when given intravenously. Still other patients may need blood or blood products that are also administered through IVs.

Setting up IV lines is a sterile procedure the PCT may be asked to assist with.

This procedure requires you to follow all of the principles of sterile technique you have learned so far. All of the equipment that comes in contact with the patient's blood stream must remain sterile.

In the beginning of this chapter you learned about the different methods of transmission of microorganisms. You know that microbes may be transmitted through direct and indirect contact, through the air, and by vehicle transmission. Administration of IV solutions that have been contaminated is an example of vehicle transmission of microorganisms.

In addition to concerns about sterility, the administration of IV fluids also puts the patient at risk for devel-

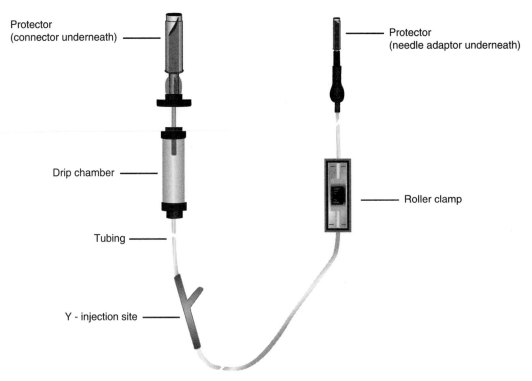

Protector
(connector underneath)

Protector
(needle adaptor underneath)

Drip chamber

Roller clamp

Tubing

Y - injection site

FIGURE 17–14

IV infusion equipment.

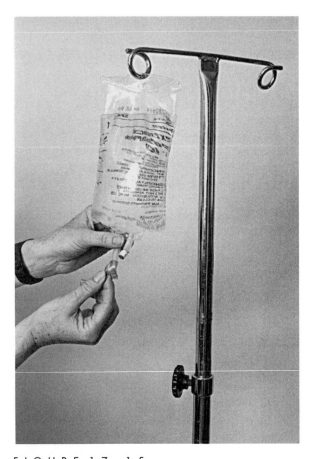

FIGURE 17–15

Remove the protective cap.

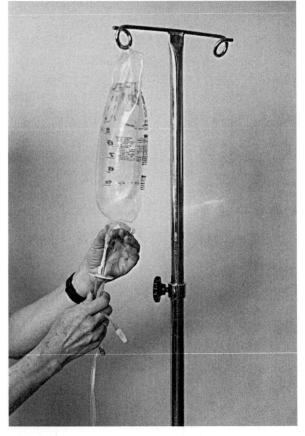

FIGURE 17–16

Spike the bag while maintaining sterility.

oping an *air embolism.* An air embolism is an air bubble in the blood stream that obstructs the flow of blood in a blood vessel. These can be very dangerous, and care must be taken to prevent them. When setting up an IV line you will "prime" the tubing, that is, force all of the air out of it by allowing fluid to run through. There are many types of IV solutions, ways to administer them, and equipment used. In setting up IV lines you will need a bag or bottle of solution, the correct type of administration set, and an IV pole (Fig. 17–14).

⚖ It is the responsibility of the RN to determine the correct IV solution according to the physician's orders, the type of administration set needed, and to actually connect the IV to the patient. State Board guidelines or agency policy may allow PCTs to assist RNs by setting up IV lines.

If you are asked to set up an IV line, you will follow these steps:

1. Assemble all of the supplies you will need:
Bag or bottle of solution as directed; IV administration set; bags require nonvented tubing; bottles, vented tubing
IV pole, standing on rollers, attached to the bed or hanging from the ceiling
2. Wash your hands.
3. Inspect packages for sterility, including checking expiration dates, and open them. IV bags come with clear, heavy outer wrappers. IV bottles do not have outer wrappers. Aside from the areas covered by protective caps, the IV bags, bottles, and administration sets do not have to be kept sterile. You may pick up the contents of these packages without wearing gloves, but be sure the protective caps are in place.
4. IV bags may be wet with condensation when removed from their outer wrappers, but be sure they are not leaking. Check bottles for any cracks. Inspect all solution for cloudiness or particles floating in them.

🛑 Report any concerns about the sterility of IV solutions to the RN before proceeding.

5. If using a bag, hang it on the IV pole. If using a bottle, set it on a table or counter.
6. Close the roller clamp on the IV tubing.
7. Remove the plastic protector from the bottom of the IV bag (Fig. 17–15), or the metal ring, cap, and rubber diaphragm from the top of the IV bottle. As you remove the rubber diaphragm, you will hear air escape from the vacuum inside the bottle.
8. Remove the protective cover from the IV tubing spike and push it firmly into the container using a twisting motion. Do not allow the exposed spike to touch anything except the sterile opening of the bag or bottle (Fig. 17–16).

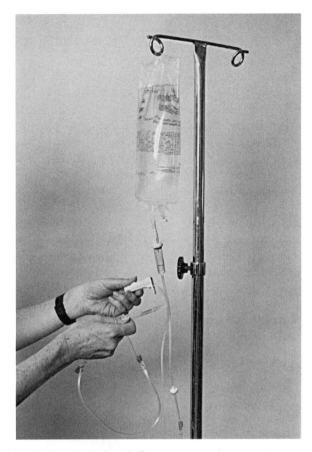

FIGURE 17-17
Run fluid through the tubing to expel all air.

9. Squeeze the drip chamber of the administration set until it is half filled with fluid.
10. Partially open the roller clamp and carefully remove the protective cap at the end of the tubing. Maintain the sterility of the protector; you will need it again once the tubing is primed.
11. Holding the opening over a trash can or basin, let the fluid run through, forcing all air out (Fig. 17–17).
12. Turn the filter upside down and gently tap it to dislodge trapped air bubbles.
13. When all of the air is out of the tubing and filter, close the roller clamp and replace the sterile protective cap.

SUMMARY

Asepsis is everyone's responsibility. Recognition of how organisms are spread is only the first step. Staff must take great care to follow all aspects of medical and surgical asepsis. From handwashing and providing personal care to dressing changes and tube care, PCTs make a difference for patients because the safety of their care can prevent nosocomial infections.

18

Computerization of Health Care

JOYCE BECKER, MS, RN,C

OBJECTIVES

After you complete this chapter, you will be able to:

- List the structures and functions of a computer system.
- Describe how to access patient information using a computer system.
- State how a computer system interacts with the laboratory to obtain results.

- Discuss how a computer system can be used with patient monitoring.
- Identify techniques that increase the successful use of a computer.

KEY TERMS

Computer Virus   A computer virus is a program or set of instructions that was developed by a programmer to experiment with the capabilities of programming. A computer virus usually is set up to automatically copy itself to any diskette used in the system. Viruses "infect" any computer they have access to and interfere with its proper functioning.

Diskettes   Flat circular objects that can store computer data or instructions

Data   Elements of information collected for analysis or calculation

Data Repository   Type of output device that can store data from several different sources

Delete Key   This key moves the cursor back a space; if there is a number or letter in the place it will be erased or taken away

Double Click   Mouse button is pressed and released twice in rapid sequence. This is usually done to open or activate a feature or software

Drag   Clicking on an object, then without lifting a finger or the mouse, moving the object to the desired location

Ergonomics   Science that studies the interaction between people and machines, analyzing workers' body positions and visual fields in relationship to the equipment they are using

Eyestrain   Tenderness or soreness in the eyes that is caused by excessive or improper use of the eyes

Floppy Diskette   A soft plastic flat circular object in a square plastic case that stores data and allows data files from one computer to be transported by the user to a different computer. Floppy diskettes are more easily damaged than hard diskettes.

Function Key   Usually above the numbers on the keyboard, might be a different color; their functions are specific to the various software programs

Hard Copy   Information from a computer that is printed out on paper, often in a report format

Hardware   The physical pieces of the computer system: monitor, keyboard, printer, and the like

Input Devices   Used for moving data from outside the computer system to inside the computer system. Examples include keyboard, mouse, scanner

Keyboard   Data input device that looks like a typewriter with a few extra keys

Logout   Steps or procedures done to exit or leave the computer system

Mouse   Data input device that moves the cursor around the screen, allowing for the selection of different items

Multimedia   Simultaneous use of different media (ways information is communicated), often visual and audio

Numeric Key   Group of numbers that are to the right of the alphabetical keys; "Num Lock" must be selected for these numbers to work. The numbers will be the same regardless of whether you use the ones above the letter or in the number pad

Output Devices   These devices present the computer information or data to the person using the information. These devices include monitors, printers, and speakers

Password   Special code, card, or key that is necessary to use to sign into a computer

Point   Moving the mouse so that the cursor is over or on the command the user wishes to select

Press   Pointing to something and holding the mouse button down. This allows the computer user to see choices, usually hidden on the menu, that are available for selection

Printers   Output devices that prepare a paper copy of the computer data

Shift Key   Produces capital letter or upper case letters; also used in conjunction with numbers on the top of the keyboard that will activate the symbols

Single Click   One pressing and releasing of the mouse button

Soft Copy   Information from a computer that is on a diskette and can be used by other users

Software   Set of step-by-step instructions that directs the computer to perform specific tasks

Space Bar The big key at the bottom of the keyboard that enters a space between words; pressing it once inserts one space; holding it down will insert many spaces

Speakers Output devices that communicate computer information in an audio format

As the world we live in continues to change and expand, the demand for information increases. This explosion of information has caused computers to become part of our daily lives. Society's demand for more information and the ability to perform complex calculations have caused people to rely on computers as part of their daily work. Today, almost every person's work life is touched by computers in some form or another.

Computers are now used for a wide variety of things: accessing our banking accounts with money cards, counting a grocery store's inventory, and reserving a book at the library. Health care is also experiencing the growth of computers. As technology advances it is not unusual for health care providers to be asked to use a computer to assist in caring for patients. The first computers were the size of a room; now computers can be carried in a pocket. Over the years computers have become smaller and faster in their functions.

The way a computer is arranged affects how it functions. In the early days of computers there were mainframes—single, large-capacity computers that received information from terminals. Terminals were essentially a keyboard and monitor without any processing capability. The number of terminals a mainframe could handle was limited, and as technology advanced, this organization became obsolete. In the early 1980s, introduction of personal computers allowed processing of information at the office desk, on a single work station, or at home. As technology continues to advance, networking is used to connect personal computers (PCs) so that software and information can be shared among computers. There are several ways to network computers: cable similar to the kind used with cable television, wire similar to telephone cable, fiber optics similar to long distance telephone lines, and radio transmission or infrared light, which is a wireless method of connecting computers. The benefits of networking computers are sharing information, programs, and equipment, which can increase productivity and access to data and decrease costs of computerization.

For a computer system to operate successfully in an organization, several types of people need to be involved. There are basically two groups involved with the computer system—users and support staff. Users are the actual personnel who will be using the computer system in conjunction with their other job responsibilities. Support staff are personnel with specialized knowledge of how computers work. Their responsibility is to take care of the computers so that they are available for the users.

Depending on the organization, a department of employees may exist or one individual may be responsible for computer support. The department might be called Information Resources or IR. Within the department there might be a title of system administrator or information system personnel. The role of these individuals is to manage the technical side of the computer system. The system administrator is the person who will decide how the computer system is set up and who can answer questions when they arise, fix problems with the system, and plan for growth of the system as computer capabilities increase.

BENEFITS OF USING A COMPUTER

The benefits of using a computer outweigh the time and energy that it takes to learn how to use it. In health care, one of the first benefits is that patient information is more accessible. That means more than one person can look at information at the same time. In a noncomputerized documentation system, if one member of the health care team is using the paper chart, other health care providers must wait before the chart is available. But with a computerized system, one health care provider can read the chart and another could record the intake and output, for example at another computer terminal. People at different locations can also review information; people working in different parts of the hospital or an outpatient clinic can access the information from their desk.

The second benefit of using a computer is that it increases health care providers' ability to communicate. When health care providers need to communicate with one another, they do not have to use the telephone and risk getting a busy signal. The message can be sent by electronic mail, through the computer system, and the people receiving the message can read it at a time that is convenient for them. Computer systems are also used for ordering supplies needed for patient care. Computers are faster and more accurate when calculating information. This can save time and prevent errors that can be harmful to patients.

Another time-saving device for patient care is using bar codes similar to those on groceries for supply items charged to patients. This saves having to write information by hand or peeling off a sticker from a patient charge item and possibly losing it. When bar codes are used, charges for supplies can be automatically entered into the patient's account and inventory can be adjusted, making it possible to keep an accurate record of what supplies are available.

Information on paper requires storage space. Computers can store information on tapes or disks that require less storage space, resulting in fewer files in the medical records room. Using a computer makes it easier to read information. It would not be necessary to "interpret" different people's handwriting, which is difficult and may lead to errors. Computers may also be used in education and training activities for class registration, presenting information, simulations of patient care needs, and maintaining records of class attendance. Computers can display information in graphs, as the patient's weight compared to calorie counts, or amount of food eaten.

One of the most useful benefits of using a computer is the ability to review data and group information to report trends and statistics. For example, by using a computer, health care providers are able to print out a list of patients who are allergic to certain foods or who have fallen within the last week. Benefits of using computers in health care are increasing as technology continues to develop. Soon computers will be as common as other equipment used by health care providers such as thermometers and stethoscopes.

FEARS ABOUT USING COMPUTERS

When learning to use computers remember it takes time to learn new things. It took patient care technicians (PCTs) a while to learn to do the things they do every day now. Remember how long it used to take you to measure blood pressure or count a pulse. It will take some time to learn the computer system, but once learned, things will be quicker and easier. There are people who can help you learn to use the computer. Some people fear that they will be replaced by a computer, but this is not likely. Computers will always require the validation of the caregiver. Some positions may be eliminated, but there will always be people needed to operate the computer systems. Computers cannot run themselves. Another fear is that the computer system can be destroyed. This is also not likely. PCTs, along with other users of the computer systems, will be receiving training and an opportunity to practice using the computer. This is a good time to make mistakes, ask questions, and learn from these errors. Usually during training, no actual patients or situations are used, so this is a good place to practice. Also during regular use on the units, most computer programs have many built-in safeguards and warnings if information is entered in the wrong way. These messages on the screen let the user know what to do next. Various staff will be available to help with the learning of specific computer functions at your setting.

STRUCTURE AND FUNCTION OF A COMPUTER SYSTEM

Computer systems consist of hardware and software. Hardware is the physical part of computer systems. Computer hardware can be divided into several categories: input devices, output devices, and secondary storage devices. Software refers to programs a computer uses to accomplish different tasks.

Input Devices

Keyboard

Input devices are used for moving data from outside the computer system to inside the computer system. The computer system cannot do this by itself, it needs people to put in this information. Major devices used for data entry include a keyboard, a mouse, and a scanner. A keyboard looks like a typewriter but has a few extra keys. Keyboards can be specific to a specific computer system, but several common keys exist (Fig. 18–1).

1. Return or enter: Moves the cursor to the next line or enters the data into the system and then allows you to go on to another feature or item. It can also be an arrow.

2. ESC—the escape key: Allows you to get out of the section you are in; it can undo things, it can back you out one screen at a time.

3. Shift key: Produces capital letters or upper case letters. If you press *Caps lock*, all your letters are capitalized. To get the symbols above the numbers you must press the shift key with the number.

4. Function keys: These are usually above the numbers on the keyboard and can be a different color. They are labeled *F* and a number. During training, these keys will be referred to F10, or F12 keys, and you must press these keys specifically, not an F and a 12. The specific function of these keys varies for each software program.

5. Numeric keys: These are the group of numbers that are usually located to the far right of the alphabetical keys. The *Num lock* must be pressed for these numbers to work. The numbers will be the same regardless of whether you use the ones above the letters or in the number pad. You can use whatever keys your hand is closer to or that you feel more comfortable using.

6. Delete or backspace key: This key moves the cursor back a space. If something (a letter or number) is there it will be erased or taken away.

7. Space bar: The big key at the bottom of the keyboard that inserts a space between words. Pressing it once will insert one space. Holding it down will insert many spaces, until you release the key.

Remember, it takes practice to use any new equipment, a keyboard is no different. It might be helpful to practice typing to learn the key locations. After some practice you will not need to look at the keys as often to enter the information you want.

Mouse

Another common data entry device is the mouse (Fig. 18–2). It is a pointing device that moves the cursor

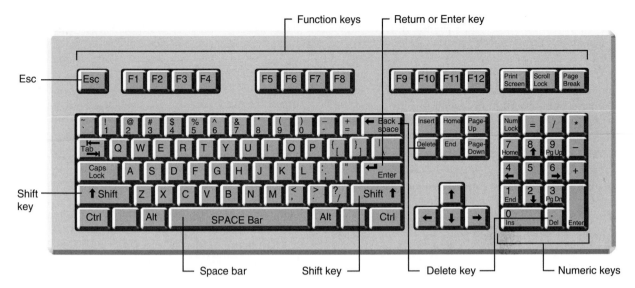

FIGURE 18-1
Keyboard.

around the screen, allowing selection of different things. The cursor is the symbol that marks where the user is on the screen. The cursor can be an arrow, a lighted dash mark, or flashing box. To use a mouse, roll it around on a flat surface; this action moves the cursor around on the screen. It takes lots of practice to use a mouse. A fun way to practice using a mouse is to play computer games such as solitaire. The more you use a mouse, the better your eye–hand coordination will become. There are buttons on top of the mouse that are pressed to activate the command or activity.

1. Single click: One pressing and releasing of the button

2. Double click: The mouse button is pressed and released twice in rapid sequence. This is usually done to open or activate a feature or software. It is not uncommon to click too slowly. With practice one gets faster at clicking. Also the clicking speed can be adjusted to accommodate users clicking at different speeds.

3. Press: Pointing to something and holding the mouse

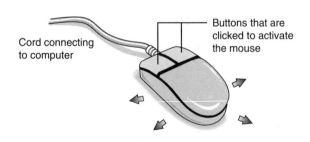

FIGURE 18-2
Mouse.

button down. This allows the computer user to see choices, usually hidden, on the menu that are available for selection.

4. Drag: Clicking on an object and, then without lifting a finger or the mouse, moving the mouse and object to the desired location. This can be practiced by moving cards in solitaire. Dragging is often used for copying files or selecting text.

5. Point: Moving the mouse so that the cursor is over or on the command the user wishes to select.

Other Input Devices

Other devices that can be used for entering data into a computer (Fig. 18–3) are touch screens, scanners, light pens, and voice activation. A touch screen is very simple to use; a finger is used to touch certain areas on the screen to activate features or make choices. The screen responds from the heat or pressure of your finger. Substitutes such as ballpoint pens typically will not work and can be harmful to the computer equipment. A scanner converts patterns into data. Bar codes are commonly scanned to quickly enter data. Entire documents or pictures can also be "scanned" and entered into the computer. Bar codes identify items and can store a large amount of information in a short time. For example, laboratory samples can be scanned along with the patient's bar code to ensure positive identification. Light pens are special devices that are used with special monitors. To use a light pen simply touch the screen with the pen. When using a light pen one can write notes by hand on the screen and the computer can be trained to read the user's handwriting. Light pens can be very expensive and are used only for specialized data entry. Another device for data entry is voice activation. This device

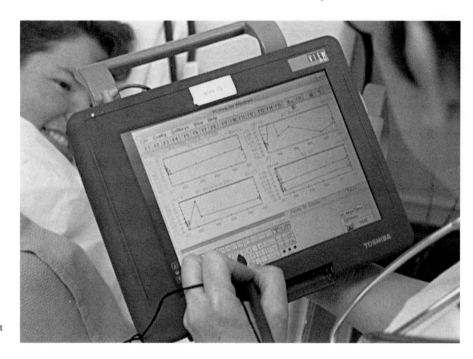

FIGURE 18 – 3
Input device: Touch screen, light pen.

converts speech into a data form that the computer can process. This technology can be used in emergency and operating rooms for recording events when the health care providers' hands are busy working. Initially using a computer required data input from a keyboard, but as technology has advanced, often keyboard skills are no longer necessary to communicate with a computer.

Processing Unit

The part of the computer that really does the work is called the central processing unit, or CPU for short. This is the brain of the system and cannot be seen unless the cover of the computer is removed. The CPU is a collection of chips that are silicon and have electronic elements on them that perform programmed instructions. Chips are small, about the size of a fingernail, but very powerful. Powerful means that the computer can store lots of data and do calculations or functions very fast.

Output Devices

Output devices present the computer information or data to the person using the information in a hard copy (paper) or soft (diskette) copy form. Output devices include monitors, printers, and speakers.

Monitors

Monitors are the display screens that inform users of what is happening with the computer system. It is very important to read the computer screen because there are usually instructions that tell the user what to do next. Monitors vary in size and appearance. Monochrome monitors display only one color, green or amber on black,

while color monitors display from 4 to 1 million colors. Color monitors are more interesting to look at, and colors can be used to highlight certain features. The print on a computer screen can be difficult to see at times. If you have difficulty there are several things you can do that may make the screen easier to see. First, adjust the tilt of the monitor to avoid glare; adjust the brightness and contrast buttons to what is more visible to you. The height of your chair can be adjusted to make it easier to see the screen. If these suggestions do not improve your ability to see, an eye examination may be necessary. Visual problems associated with a computer are often corrected with glasses and some practice time.

Ergonomics

When learning about computer systems it is also important to learn about ergonomics. The word *ergonomics* is from the Greek word *ergo*, which means work, and *nomos*, which means law. Ergonomics is a relatively new science that looks at the interaction between people and machines, analyzing workers' body positions and visual fields in relationship to the equipment they are using. Ergonomics attempts to study and recommend working conditions that will best provide for workers' health, safety, comfort, and productivity.

When using a computer it is important to keep several issues and concepts in mind (Fig. 18–4). The computer screen should be vertical, with the top of the computer screen about eye level and 1 to 2 feet from your eyes. The presence of rotating, tilting, and swiveling mechanisms can allow the PCT to make the necessary adjustment so the computer screen is in proper alignment for them. The computer keyboard has two small flip-down

Do-It-Yourself "Ergonomic Assessment" Checklist

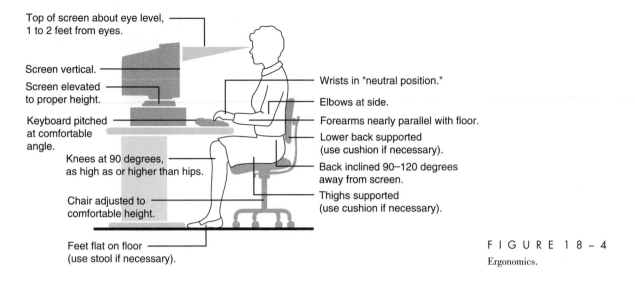

Top of screen about eye level, 1 to 2 feet from eyes.

Screen vertical.

Screen elevated to proper height.

Keyboard pitched at comfortable angle.

Knees at 90 degrees, as high as or higher than hips.

Chair adjusted to comfortable height.

Feet flat on floor (use stool if necessary).

Wrists in "neutral position."

Elbows at side.

Forearms nearly parallel with floor.

Lower back supported (use cushion if necessary).

Back inclined 90–120 degrees away from screen.

Thighs supported (use cushion if necessary).

F I G U R E 1 8 – 4

Ergonomics.

"legs" located at the bottom of the keyboard near the back. When using a keyboard, it should be elevated on its legs to give the user an angled reach for the fingers while the wrist angle should be less than 10 degrees. Wrist pads are available at office supply or computer stores that will elevate and support a person's wrists. When one is properly seated at the computer, forearms should be parallel with the floor and elbows at the body's sides. The chair a PCT is seated in should allow for the lower back and thighs to be supported; knees should be bent at a 90-degree angle or higher than hips. Feet should be flat on the floor; a stool or telephone book can be used to rest feet on if necessary. Following these recommendations will help reduce or prevent the pain and stiffness in the neck, shoulders, and lower back that result from poor posture at the work station. Another helpful hint is to schedule frequent breaks from the computer system. If you are finding that you are making many mistakes and your frustration level is increasing, get up from the computer and do some other aspect of your work and return after a short break. Looking at a computer screen for long periods can cause eyestrain. To decrease the occurrence of eyestrain take a few minutes every 30 to 45 minutes to focus on something off in the distance. This helps the eye use different focusing mechanisms and lets the ones used for close work rest a few minutes.

Printers

Printers are the devices that prepare a paper copy of the data. Basically two types of printers are available—nonimpact and impact. With nonimpact printers, the printing mechanisms do not touch the surface of the paper. These printers are ink jet, thermal, or laser and do not make much noise when printing, which makes them a good choice for patient care areas where extra

noise adds to the stressful environment. With impact printers, the printing mechanism does touch the surface of the paper. These printers are daisy wheel, dot matrix, and plotter printers, which can be noisier but can be a little faster. Regardless of what type of printer is used in your area, it is important to know how to turn it off and on, how to load paper, and how to remedy a paper jam. When reports print that contain patient information, it is crucial that these reports are placed in the patient chart. This allows physicians, ancillary staff, and students to review data. Filing the reports may be a task that the PCT is asked to perform.

Speakers

Audio feedback can be provided to the users from computers through speakers. This provides great technology for training. Users are able to hear a patient's simulated heart beat or instructions of how to do a particular procedure. The computer can give step-by-step instructions. This area of computer application will be expanding rapidly as the numbers of computers equipped for multimedia use increases in the workplace.

Storage Devices

Data that are used by the computer can be stored on hard or floppy drives. Hard drives can also be called fixed drives because they are storage devices that are fixed in a sealed case. This sealed case can be inside the computer or outside the computer in a separate device. Hard drives are the main storage device of the computer. Hard drives store more data and permit faster retrieval than floppy drives. Floppy drives read floppy disks. *Floppy diskette* is an old term that refers to initial 5¼-inch diskettes that were thin and flexible. These diskettes can be easily damaged from heat, radiation, static electricity, and bending. Newer floppy disks are 3½ inches and are thicker, not flexible, and are less susceptible to damage. Floppy disks can store programs or data that can be used for computer systems. Data are usually shared by copying files to a floppy disk and sharing disks. This also serves as a type of input device, as files from one computer can be transferred and worked on in a different computer. Along with files of information, computer viruses can also be shared this way.

Computer Viruses

A computer virus is a program or set of instructions that was developed by a programmer to experiment with the capabilities of programming. A computer virus usually is set up to automatically copy itself to any diskette used in the system. Files copied from a computer infected with a virus to another computer carry the virus with it. Since most computer viruses act by interfering with the way regular computer programs work, much damage could be done in a large work setting or computer network. Most organizations place some restriction on who enters data into each type of computer system. The organization also restricts staff from copying information to their computer from a floppy diskette brought from home or copied from other outside sources. Contact the help desk or system administrator to find out the policy on using diskettes and outside computer bulletin boards.

If you notice someone you do not recognize copying data with a diskette or loading new information into the computer system, ask what he or she is doing. Security may need to be notified.

Symptoms that may indicate that the computer may have a virus include: programs are not operating properly, data are missing, or unusual messages are displaying on the screen. Computer viruses can do a lot of harm to any computer system, resulting in loss of data or inability to use the data that is still there. If you are working on a networked computer these problems can be spread to other users. There are special programs to detect computer viruses, and network system administrators or information system personnel may do routine virus checks. Software programs are also available to check individual computers. Notify the system administrator if the virus checking software indicates that a virus was found on your computer.

Diskettes (Fig. 18–5)

To prevent damage to diskettes and computer data the following safety precautions are recommended:

1. Keep diskettes dry, protected, and away from heat and cold. Transport diskettes in a special carrying case designed for that purpose.

2. Store 5¼-inch diskettes in the paper envelope they came in; be careful not to bend them.

3. When handling 5¼-inch diskettes, touch only the label; do not touch the exposed area, for 3½-inch diskettes do not touch the area under the silver shutter.

4. When putting a diskette into a disk drive, slide the disk gently in with the label side up and toward you.

5. Be careful to store diskettes away from magnets, including electrical appliances, monitors, and phones. Libraries sometimes use magnets for security systems. Have computer disks hand checked.

STOP Label diskettes by using felt-tipped pens. Ballpoint pens can cause permanent indentations on the diskette surface.

FIGURE 18–5
Diskettes.

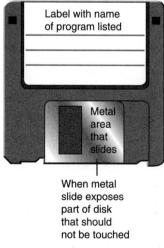

3¹/₂ Diskette

Label with name of program listed

Metal area that slides

When metal slide exposes part of disk that should not be touched

This end goes in the computer

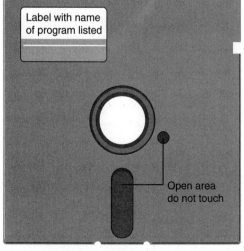

5¹/₄ Diskette

Label with name of program listed

Open area do not touch

This end goes in the computer

Software

Software is the other necessary item for a computer to function. Computer software is a set of step-by-step instructions that directs the computer to perform specific tasks. Computer software provides the instructions to the computer. All computers require software to function. Computer software can be the operating system or the application programs. Operating system software is designed to coordinate the computer hardware components and to supervise all basic operations. Common operating systems are MS–DOS, System (for the MAC), Unix, and Windows (Fig. 18–6). Windows is a graphic operating system used with DOS or MAC that is very easy to learn and use. One advantage of using Windows is that it permits working on one task without closing or completing the other task.

Application software programs are developed to meet specific needs of the user. Common applications in the business world include spreadsheets, word processing, graphics, data base managers, and communication programs such as E-mail. Software in the health care field includes systems to enter orders, document at the bedside, monitor patient vital signs and functions, record medication administration, and inquire about patient information including diagnostic and laboratory test results.

ACCESSING PATIENT INFORMATION

Using Passwords

Because information related to patients is confidential, computer systems often have features that maintain confidentiality.

⚖ Patient information in a computer is confidential; use the information on a "need to know basis, only." Access only the information needed to do your job.

When accessing patient information on a computer system, most times it will be necessary to sign on to the computer using a special key, card, or a password code. Using computer passwords helps to limit computer users to only the information they need, as well as helping to maintain confidentiality. Signing in, using your password, is required before any computer functions can be performed, such as viewing, printing, or entering information. The password is linked to information about the user, such as name, job code, and user limits to computer access. The computer program security usually keeps track of what computer functions the user performed. In most systems no one else should know the password that is assigned to a particular person. Sharing your password is a breach of confidentiality and may be punishable.

 Sharing passwords is not acceptable. Do not share your password with anyone.

Sometimes the system administrator will have access to passwords.

✔ If the password you are trying to use does not work, notify the help desk or the system administrator.

Depending on the requirements of the system, a password can be a combination of numbers and/or letters. Often the user will have control in designing the password. When designing a password, consider making it something unique, using a combination of numbers and letters that would not be readily known by others. A password should be easily remembered by the user, but not so common that others can guess it. Some systems require periodic changing of the password, usually every 6 months. In a computer system the password is the electronic signature of the user. When using a paper system it is not acceptable to have another health caregiver sign his or her name to your work. In a computer system it is not acceptable for someone else to use your password. There are several things that can be done to safeguard a password. First and most important: Never share a password with another health care worker. Also never write down your password where others can find it. Sometimes staff members write their password on a note near the computer terminal or attach the number to their identification tag. Both of these practices should be avoided.

🛑 Computer users should not write their password on the back of their identification tag. Making a list of passwords and placing it near the computer screen is also not acceptable. Both of these practices can allow unauthorized users access to the computer system.

When a password is entered in the computer system, it is displayed on the computer screen as "***," thus eliminating the possibility that the password will be seen by anyone. When you are done using the computer system, it is important to exit the program and log yourself off the computer. If you do not log out, the next user could enter data with your password. You would be responsible for the accuracy of the data even though you did not actually enter the data, because your electronic signature or password would continue to be linked to the data that were entered.

⚖ Always sign out or log off when done using the computer. This prevents other users from entering data that could be attached to your electronic signature.

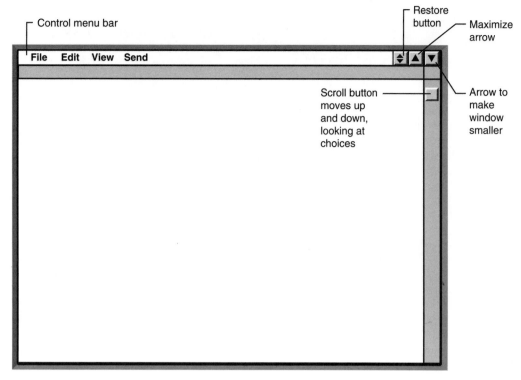

Control menu bar

Restore button

Maximize arrow

| File | Edit | View | Send |

Scroll button moves up and down, looking at choices

Arrow to make window smaller

FIGURE 18 – 6
A window.

TYPES OF HOSPITAL COMPUTER SYSTEMS

Computers entered the health care profession during the 1950's, assisting health care workers in determining patient charges, calculating payrolls, controlling inventory, and analyzing medical statistics. Over the years, technology has advanced and equipment cost has decreased, making computer systems more widely used and available to health care providers.

Patient Admission Process

The patient's admission to a hospital begins with entering data about the patient into a financial or admission system. Information that is stored in this software includes demographic information, insurance details, and names and addresses of emergency contacts. Demographic information includes the patient's birth date, age, sex, employer information if applicable, and status of advanced directives. Once this information is entered into the computer system the patient can be assigned a bed in the system along with the actual bed on the patient care unit. The ability to search this information when looking for the patient and room number can be helpful to visitors who often get lost in the hospital on their way to visit a patient. Once the patient is entered into the computer system, other information can be included, like orders, documentation, and care planning. As the patient's condi-

tion changes and he or she is transferred to various units in the hospital, the patient can also be transferred in the computer system to a new bed with a few keystrokes. Once patient information is in the system it can be shared with users in various locations in the hospital. When the patient is discharged from the hospital, the bed will become vacant, ready for the next patient, but the patient data will be saved and available for access at a later date. These data can be accessed by a permanent chart copy that has been printed or by a data repository that allows access at a later date.

Documentation Systems

Computerization helps in gathering and storing data about each patient. Currently, computers can be used for charting patient information, planning care, monitoring patient functions, and ordering patient supplies. Bedside documentation systems allow documentation wherever patients are (Fig. 18–7). Computerized methods for recording patient information and observations are some of the most available nursing computer applications. There are several different approaches to charting patient information depending on the software and equipment used, but there are some overall similarities.

The patient charting system usually has an electronic library of frequently used words or phrases arranged in subject categories. The health care provider then chooses the phrase that best describes the patient's condition.

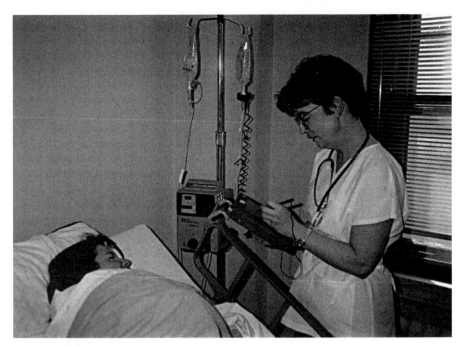

F I G U R E 1 8 – 7
PCT at bedside.

This information is then stored in the computer where it can be viewed later by looking at a review screen. Depending on the software's features, patient's data can be compared and manipulated in the computer. This would allow data to be viewed in a graphical format or make it possible to compare, for example a patient's weight to fluid intake and output. The patient information can be printed out in a flow sheet or report format for filing in the medical record and possibly storage.

There are many advantages of computerizing the documentation of patient care activities. Because reports from a computer are more legible than handwritten notes, they decrease reading time and increase the accuracy of reading. Using a computer also saves time; it is easier and quicker to pick the necessary items to chart from a list of choices. Because information is entered where it happens, there is an increase in accuracy of the entry. Software systems can be designed to prompt the caregivers for information, which can serve as a reminder of what needs to be done for the patient. This prompting also serves as a teaching tool by providing a guide for the necessary entries. Research processes are easier because the computer can search the data using standardized terminology. The computer can verify, for instance, that all diabetic patients have blood glucose monitoring ordered. Health care providers will spend less time writing notes, which will provide more time to care for patients.

 When charting patient information on a computer system it is important to remember to be accurate because other people have immediate access to the information that you are charting.

Chart information as you collect it. Charting as you go fills the medical record with more accurate information because you are not relying on your memory. Recording information when it happens takes less time because you do not have to wait until the end of the shift to record everything and have to reconstruct the situation or remember the information. Charting as it happens also decreases transcription errors and lost data.

When charting on a computerized system it is important to chart on the correct patient; always read the screen for the patient's name and room number to verify you are charting on the correct person. It is also important to understand the meaning of what you are charting and to understand the screens you will be entering data into. When charting information it is important to review information that has been charted; another caregiver may have already charted the information you are charting. It is a good habit to review the patient's previous charting so that you know what is happening with the patient. This review-patient-charting feature can also be used when giving a change-of-shift report. You will receive training on how to use the computer system where you work. It is important to practice and ask questions. You will need to make sure you know how to fix mistakes in data entry and how to handle simple problems with the computer equipment.

Material Systems—Monitoring Supplies

Computer systems can be used to communicate with various departments in the patient care setting. For example, if you need a particular item, such as a bedpan, from the supply department it is possible to send the supply department a message with the computer and either have them send the bedpan to you or have it available for your pick up at a scheduled time. This computerized ordering not only makes it easier to count items on hand, it also can alert the purchasing department when certain items need to be ordered. Reports can be generated to show peak usage times and the most frequently used items. Using electronic messages eliminates the phone call, which also can eliminate having to be put on hold during busy times. Also, the person in the supply department does not have to stop work and answer the phone. Supply departments can code items to be ordered at a specific time and/or frequency.

Patient Monitoring Systems

Coronary care units and pacemaker clinics were the first users of patient monitoring systems. Computers were initially used to monitor patient heart rhythms to notify health care providers of variations from normal standards. Currently there are computer systems available to monitor patient's heart rhythm and rates, temperature, and respiratory rates. Advanced monitoring of pressures from arterial blood, central venous blood, and intracranial space is also available. Computerization of patient monitoring frees the health care providers from the technical role of watching machinery, which allows them to focus on providing care and attention to the patient and family. In the future, PCTs will be using computerized monitoring systems to measure a patient's temperature, blood pressure, pulse, and respiratory rate. Research studies have revealed that the use of computerized cardiac monitoring increases early detection of abnormal heart rhythms, which contributes to a decrease in deaths of coronary care patients. These systems also help compare a patient's earlier condition to what he or she is currently experiencing.

Computerized Laboratory Systems

Computer systems connecting hospital laboratories with patient care units and physician offices are increasingly common. Laboratory systems begin with the physician's order of a specific test; the order is then entered into the system by health care personnel, or it may come from a computerized laboratory system. The PCT may be asked to perform such data entry duties. The next step is obtaining the laboratory specimen, which is also a duty the PCT can do (see Chapter 21). The specimen needs to be labeled and then sent to the laboratory for testing purposes. Once the test is complete the laboratory technician will enter the test results into the computer system where health care personnel can access the results. If the laboratory test is one that can be done at the patient's bedside, after the PCT performs the test the results can be entered into the computer system.

INFORMATION THE LABORATORY PROVIDES TO HEALTH CARE UNIT

- The status of the requested test:
  Ordered but specimen not received
  Specimen received but results not available
  Test completed, results available
- If the results are out of the normal range, results that are either low or high will be marked
- Information on how the specimen needs to be collected, what color tube the blood must be in, or if the sample needs to be refrigerated
- Information on the quantity that needs to be collected for the test to be run

INFORMATION PCTs PROVIDE TO THE LABORATORY

- What laboratory test is needed; what is ordered by the physician
- The laboratory specimen label with patient information
- How the test should be run—stat or routine

It is not usually within the PCT's role to know the significance of specific laboratory values; the PCT should report the results to the RN caring for the specific patient. Most often PCT's responsibilities will be related to obtaining and sending specimens. It will be possible to print laboratory results and file them in the chart; this also might be assigned to a PCT. Some computer laboratory systems have the ability to graph laboratory results over the patient's hospital stay. The personnel who are most interested in this information are usually physicians; the PCT may need to assist the physician with this activity in the computer system.

Maintaining Patient Safety

Computers can assist in keeping the patient safe. Bed-check systems exist in which sensors are placed under a patient's mattress that will alarm when the patient attempts to get out of bed unattended. PCTs will be trained how to put the bed-check equipment in place and troubleshoot any equipment malfunctions. PCTs have valuable information about patient's activity levels and abilities. This information can be used to recommend a specific patient for a bed-check system. If you feel that a patient's safety level can be increased with a bed-check monitor, ask the RN to order one for the patient. Patients still need to be checked on by hospital personnel even if a bed-check system is in use.

It is also possible to computerize the patient call-light system. Depending on the software package, it is possible for a patient to put on the call light and someone from the command station can answer the light and use a beeper to dispatch a caregiver to meet that patient's request. The PCT will be required to know how to answer the patient's light from the command station, know how to dispatch a caregiver to assist the patient, and know how he or she can respond to a page from the command center (see Chapter 19). An advantage of computerizing the call-light system is that patient calls can be logged, average response time can be monitored, and caregivers can respond without visiting the nursing station, which can save a PCT some steps. Also by knowing what the patient needs, the care provider can be more prepared before entering the patient's room. Monitoring patient requests may also be used to determine staffing needs of the unit.

Computers in Education

If you have not experienced using a computer as a teacher, it is probable that you will in the future. Computer-assisted instruction programs (CAI) are educational experiences presented via a computer. A common use of CAI is instruction in cardiopulmonary resuscitation (CPR). To use computerized CPR the PCT would enter his or her identification code and select what aspect of CPR to review or be evaluated on. The computer system then will provide various patient situations and wait for the participant's response. There will be computer sensors that will be connected to the resuscitation manikin that will give the participant feedback; for example, if the compression was too deep or if the breath entered the victim's lungs. The computer program allows the user to practice as much as he or she wants before being tested on the skills of CPR. The advantage of using CAI is that it allows the learner to progress at a pace best suited to him or her, allowing for repetition of information whenever the user needs it. CAI learning can be done at the time most convenient to the learner, not when the instructor is available. CAI is most effective when it is supplemented with personal instruction to assist with computer problems and evaluate learning. Regardless of the computer software or technology, computers should be used to assist health care providers to administer the best possible care for patients. The responsibility of the PCT with CAI is to follow the directions and complete the modules or lessons

that are assigned. If the PCT is having difficulty with the program there is always a staff person assigned as a resource person who can answer questions or troubleshoot the computer if the user is experiencing difficulties. Additional commonly used programs that are available in the CAI format include infection control, safety procedures, body mechanics, and medical terminology. A variety of CAI programs are available as health information for the general public as well as in teaching health care personnel.

TECHNIQUES FOR COMPUTER SUCCESS

Learning to use a computer can be scary. Remember what it took to learn the other duties of the role as a PCT: time, patience, and practice. Using a computer is no different; allow time to grasp the concepts of the computer software system; be patient while learning a system. Remind yourself of what you have learned in the past and that you can learn to use the computer also. Spend time practicing to use the computer—do not give up. The information below can assist in learning the computer system but is not a substitute for the specific computer training received at the place of employment.

HINTS FOR USING COMPUTER SYSTEMS

1. Be accurate in data entry—Information in a computer system is immediately available to other members of the health care team, so it must be accurate. To increase accuracy, it is recommended to read the screen for instruction about the required information that must be entered. Reading the screen is also a good thing to remember if you get confused and forget what to do next. Often the screen will prompt you for the information that is required or spark your memory of what to do next, often in a line of text at the bottom of the screen. When in doubt read the screen.

2. Review information on the computer screen before entering it—Double-check the information that you entered prior to sending it to the system. This is especially true of numbers and patient names. Always check to see if things are spelled correctly if you used narrative notes. The computer software program will sometimes help you maintain accuracy by giving you a message when you enter something that could possibly be out of range, like a blood pressure reading of 376/30. If this is attempted, the system will stop and send you a message asking if you are sure about this entry. Software packages are designed for human beings, and human beings make mistakes. These mistakes can be corrected in the computer system by using editing or modification features

that your computer training personnel will teach and the software will support.

3. Practice, practice, practice—When learning to use a computer system, practice using it in your job every opportunity you can. The sooner you use the training in the patient care setting the more information you will remember.

CONFIDENTIALITY

Patient information is confidential. This does not change when patient information is stored in a computer. The institution that you work for will have policies and procedures related to confidentiality that you will need to follow. It is important that you read these policies and procedures to understand what they mean. If you have questions, consult your manager or supervisor. It may be necessary for PCTs to sign a confidentiality agreement; as with any agreement, make sure you understand what you are signing. Once again, talk with your manager or supervisor if you have questions or do not understand what is in the agreement. Depending on how your computer system is set up, your password may give you access to only certain computer functions. For example, you may be able only to enter data about activities of daily living (ADL) and not information about treatments. The features and information you can access depend on job responsibilities. Information accessed through the computer system should be shared only with other health care providers based on what information they need to do their job. It would be a violation of confidentiality if you share information with another health care worker just because it is interesting. If you are in doubt if you should repeat any particular information, the answer probably is that you should not.

STOP Looking up information on a computer system that is not needed to do the PCT's job is a violation of patient confidentiality.

Computer printouts also need to be properly disposed of because of the patient information the printouts contain. It is necessary for the PCTs to dispose of computer printouts at their facility, where the document will probably be shredded. If you happen to take a paper with patient information on it home with you, either black out the patient's name or tear the report into small pieces before disposing of the report. Patient information is always private.

As a PCT, you should be able to enter data quickly once you have learned the system. Just as some PCTs can make beds in a flash or bathe patients quickly, you will see some PCTs who operate the computer system very quickly. It is not necessary for you to be a computer expert, but you should not be slowed down by the computer system once you have learned how to operate it. You will find that your speed increases with practice and use.

One way to increase your speed with the computer system is to practice as much as possible. If your facility has a training room, visit it often to practice. Computer trainers can provide you with training exercises. If you have questions or problems with the computer system, ask someone in your area to review things with you; your supervisor or manager can also offer assistance. The people who provided the computer training also can answer questions and help you solve problems. Take the initiative to use the computer system as often as possible in your daily work.

Resources to contact if assistance is needed to learn how to use the computer system include educators, trainers, clinical nurse specialists, managers, and the information systems' help-desk staff.

SUMMARY

As a PCT it is very likely that using a computer system will be part of your job responsibilities. It takes time to learn to use computer systems, but the computer can assist in providing patient care in a more accurate and time-efficient manner. Allow time to learn to use the computer by practicing and asking for assistance from trainers. With some practice, the computer will become easy to use and will assist the PCT in providing quality patient care.

Cross-Training Options for the Multiskilled Partner

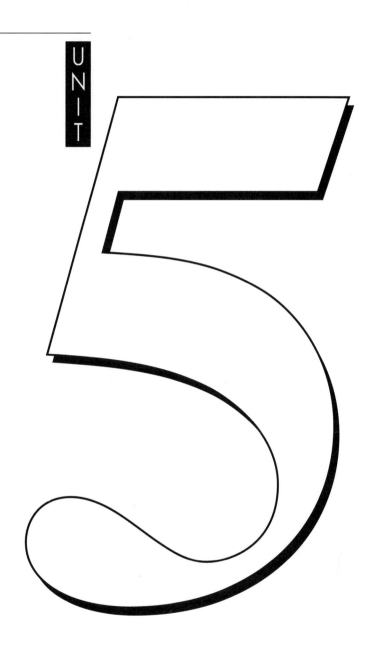

Clerical Skills

SHELLEY UNCAPHER, BS Ed., BS, BA, CHUC
SHERRY SPEER, BA, CHUC

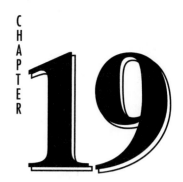

PREREQUISITE KNOWLEDGE AND SKILLS

- Customer service skills
- General hospital policies and procedures
- Hospital departments and their functions
- Computer skills
- Confidentiality

OBJECTIVES

After you complete this chapter, you will be able to:

- Recognize and interpret common medical abbreviations and terminology.

- Utilize common communication devices (pagers, patient call system, telephones).

- Discuss routine phone calls and the appropriate action to take with each.

- Explain common pager guidelines.

- Describe general patient calls and the action to take with each.

- Discuss a typical shift routine.

- Explain the clerical worker's role in handling the patient chart.

- Prepare a patient chart with standard chart forms.

- List supplemental chart forms and describe their use.

- Discuss census transactions and the clerical worker's role in each.

- Identify the four different categories of physicians' orders.

- Describe the order transcription process.

- Classify physicians' orders by department.

KEY TERMS

Acronyms Word formed from the first letter of each word in a series of words

Admission This process is followed when a new patient arrives at the hospital; includes placing patient in a room and creating an in-patient chart

Advance Directives Instructions by patient, given before admission, regarding medical treatment preferences

AMA Against medical advice

Clerical Worker Person who maintains paper flow and nonclinical tasks on patient care unit

Laboratory Values Results of blood tests ordered; many tests have normal limit ranges

Laboratory Work Blood tests ordered by physician to diagnose or monitor a patient's condition

Legal Document Official papers required by established rules and laws

Paging System System used by hospital to deliver messages or announcements to staff

Medical Record Collection of documents that record patient information during hospital stay

Process Series of steps to complete a task

Requisitions Forms used to order tests, treatments, or supplies

Stat To be done immediately

Transcribe To transfer information from physician's orders to various forms used on patient care unit

UNIT ORGANIZATION AND ROUTINE TASKS

In many health care facilities today, clerical responsibilities are being delegated to the patient care technician (PCT). This chapter will cover the major clerical responsibilities needed to facilitate patient care at any institution. Additional tasks may be included by each individual institution to ensure the ongoing, efficient functioning of the patient care unit.

Paging and other types of communication such as answering the telephone and patient call lights and greeting/directing patients and visitors are considered routine tasks for the PCT serving in a clerical role. Other routine tasks include transcribing physicians' orders, completing requisitions, assembling and maintaining patient charts, ordering supplies, and processing patient charges. Other tasks may be incorporated into the role at other facilities.

Clerical components of the PCT's role include much more than answering phones and taking messages. Today's clerical role encompasses many skills that are required of administrative assistants and executive assistants. These skills include organization, accuracy, an understanding of priorities on the patient care unit, and good listening and communication skills.

Organization, the arrangement of tasks into some semblance of order, is the glue that holds everything together. Organization is necessary to keep everything flowing on the unit. The clerical person must be able to keep himself or herself aware of where things are placed and what goes together. A patient's chart does not help anyone if it is

not in order. The same can be said for the general nursing station, which is primarily the clerical person's work space. The PCT serving in a clerical role will be asked many times where items are kept. If these items stay organized and in their place, others will be able to get forms and supplies on their own without directions or assistance. The clerical person's work will not need to be interrupted to fill another person's needs each and every time. This allows both workers to be more efficient.

The clerical component also requires that PCTs organize their time. This will help ensure that work gets done in a manner that will allow the other departments to do their part to care for the patient. If laboratory work is ordered later than the time requested by the laboratory, the results may not be available when the physician is on the unit to see the patient. This will ultimately delay treatment to the patient. Organization will help the PCT handle more tasks and improve the efficiency of the patient care unit. In turn, the organized PCT will be able to cope with the many demands of the role.

Accuracy is another skill needed for the clerical role. The PCT will handle many items throughout a typical shift in which information processing is required. The ability to receive and transmit messages, physicians' orders, and other requests accurately is a minimum expectation. It is better to ask questions or verify information before passing along information than to communicate it incorrectly or incompletely.

Another necessary skill is the ability to set priorities or to arrange tasks (and then complete them) according to their level of importance. The PCT should complete tasks resulting from a crisis or emergency situation first before moving on to items that should be completed within or by a certain time. Many tasks on the patient care unit should be completed as soon as possible. The effective PCT is able to rank those tasks to complete the most important tasks first. An understanding of the priorities on the patient care unit will also help make unit operations better. It is important to learn the priorities of the unit and the expectations of those with whom you work. This alone will help improve the unit operations and alleviate many frustrations among the staff.

Good listening and communication skills are required so that the PCT can handle tasks independently. When the admitting representative needs to place a new admission on the unit, good communication skills will make that admission flow smoothly. Poor communication could lead to hard feelings, difficult or strained working relationships, and at the very worst, a poor perception of the hospital by the patient. What if the patient ends up lying on a cart in the hallway instead of going to his or her room because someone did not communicate that the room had not been cleaned yet? Do you think the patient would be happy about the care? Communication to the admitting area about the dirty room could have expedited the cleaning process and have been passed along to the patient, who would understand the short wait in the lobby. Often, listening to others will help the PCT anticipate their needs and improve situations. It is certainly easier to work with people who tell you what they expect of you, and the job will be much easier if you in turn listen to what the person said and can act appropriately.

Good communication skills also go a long way in streamlining operations. Interpersonal skills as well as intradepartmental and interdepartmental communication are required. All types of communication require common courtesy and adherence to general customer service policies and procedures.

Communications

In any hospital, communication is essential to keeping the patient care unit functioning efficiently. Communication is defined as the sending and receiving of a message. While most communication takes place with the patient by the many technicians, RNs, and physicians involved with the patient's care, additional communication takes place at the central reception area or nursing station on each patient care unit. Because this communication is integral to positive satisfaction among patients, visitors, staff, physicians, and administrators, excellent customer service skills are essential. It is important to remember that often the person in this area is making the first contact with a patient or visitor at your facility. A patient may form a poor first impression in a matter of minutes because of a problem or perceived problem not being handled correctly here. When you are speaking with

others, it is imperative to treat each person with courtesy and respect. Remember the golden rule to always treat others as you want to be treated. Eye contact and appropriate listening skills are essential components of good customer service.

While the nursing station is often a hectic place, it is important to remember that each person/call/request deserves your undivided attention. If the patient/visitor is told help is on the way, help should be sent, even if it means making yourself a note and crossing it off when you accomplish the task or helping the patient yourself. (Refer to Chapter 4 for additional information regarding dealing with difficult people.) In any type of communication, it is necessary that everyone speak the same language. In the medical profession, this language is often one of abbreviations and acronyms. Some of the most common abbreviations found in health care today are found in the appendix at the back of this book.

The abbreviations listed in the Appendix are only a part of those usually used in health care. Additional abbreviations are used for specific diagnoses. A list of diagnoses and their abbreviations is too extensive to include here. Many hospitals also have abbreviations for the different buildings in their facility. During orientation to this new position, the PCT should become familiar with these.

In communicating with the various personnel and departments, it is imperative that the PCT understand the equipment that will be used and proper procedures for handling it. Communications equipment common to most health care facilities includes the telephone (both single-line and multiline styles), pagers/beepers (verbal, digital, long distance), patient call system, and computer system. Below are some general guidelines for operating each piece of equipment. Because each facility uses different systems, new PCTs should refer to any operating manuals at their facility for specific operating instructions.

Phones

The single-line telephone is found in many hospitals and functions primarily like a home telephone. Often these are found in out-of-the-way areas such as physician lounges, staff lounges, and conference rooms. Generally only one person can use this type of phone at a time. The multiline phone has several different phone lines all coming into a central receiver. This phone is often equipped with a hold button and sometimes other specialty buttons as well. It is important that the PCT learn to operate any type of telephone efficiently.

Generally, when incoming calls are being answered, promptness is the key. Calls should be answered within the first 3 rings, but preferably after the first ring. When picking up the phone (to answer the call), state your unit or location, name, and title so the caller knows immediately if the correct location has been reached. Listen attentively to the caller and concentrate on the caller's needs. If the person being called is not immediately available, ask if the caller can hold for a moment while you locate the appropriate person or information needed. If it will take more than a moment to locate the person or information requested, offer to take a message.

A good message includes the caller's name, business or relation to patient, phone number, reason for calling, date, and time. It is also a good idea to write your name or initials on the note so that the person may check with you if questions arise.

If, for some reason, the caller needs to be placed on hold, first ask permission to do so. If the caller agrees to be placed on hold, press the hold button and return the receiver to its appropriate location on the phone. If the phone does not have a hold button, check with the facility's communications department for the best way to place a caller on hold so that the caller does not hear conversations that are not intended for him or her. If someone is placed on hold, remember to check back periodically to let the caller know that he or she has not been forgotten. The institution does not want to give the impression that the caller is on "eternal" hold.

While functioning in the clerical position, the PCT will field many different types of calls and it is important to handle them in the best possible manner. Table 19–1 is a guideline. Most hospitals have policies and procedures that dictate how certain calls should be handled. Consult these for your best response to certain calls.

In all hospitals, good judgment is expected to prevail. If there is ever any question about what your response to a caller should be, *ask.*

Some hospitals have limitations put on their phone systems by the communications department. These limitations help the patient care units by restricting unwanted callers from reaching certain areas without prior permission. Examples of these include allowing incoming calls to come into a patient care area via one outside line or only during certain times of the day, and restricting phones from dialing long distance. Check with your hospital to see what limitations have been placed on the phone system in your area.

Occasionally the PCT may be asked to place an outside call as a representative of the hospital. Plan the call by having all necessary information available before dialing the phone. Identify yourself and state the reason for your call so that the receiver can help or direct your call to someone who can help.

Almost all phones are capable of transferring callers from one number to another number. The process for doing this, however, varies greatly with each phone sys-

TABLE 19–1
Handling Different Types of Calls

REQUEST	ACTION
Patient condition/patient information	Generally the condition that is reported to the information desk and/or newspaper can be given out. Any other information should be handled by the patient's RN.
Offer abnormal laboratory values	If comfortable in reporting them and your hospital allows it, write down the information as neatly as possible and immediately inform the patient's RN. Some hospitals have policies that require the RN to take this information.
Schedule patient test/appointment	Take a complete message and inform the patient's RN. This message may require that the patient's current therapy be altered because of special preparations.
Patient census transaction	Take a complete message and inform the charge RN. This message may require that a follow-up phone call be made to another area such as admitting or another patient care unit.
Physician's order	Locate the patient's RN or charge RN. Verbal orders may be handled only by RNs in most facilities.

tem. This is a very nice feature that, when used correctly, can prevent a lot of frustration for the caller. If used incorrectly, this transfer feature can disconnect the caller or send the call to the wrong destination, either of which increases the caller's frustration level. Be sure to ask how to transfer calls using your hospital's phone system.

Paging Systems

Hospitals may use several different types of paging systems for different tasks. The simplest paging system is the overhead paging mechanism that is activated by the hospital telephone operator. To have someone paged on this system, the PCT will need to know the first and last name of the person to be paged. When this is known, dial the hospital operator (0) and ask to page the requested person. Sometimes the operator will need to be given a complete message such as, "Will the family of John Doe please return to the 8th floor." Usually these types of overhead pages are used for patients, family members, and staff who do not carry a pocket pager. These pages reach the majority of the hospital complex, but are difficult to hear in certain areas like the cafeteria because of the regular activity that occurs there.

Pocket pagers come in all styles and sizes with slightly different methods to activate and send a message. The most common will be discussed here. One type is the long-distance pager usually used by a physician or hospital administrator. This pager can receive messages at a farther distance from the hospital than can other pagers. To activate the pager, dial the pager number just as if calling an outside number. A phone will then ring just as if a phone number had been dialed. When the ringing stops, a series of beeps will sound. At this point, dial the phone number that the person should call followed by the pound (#) sign.

Another type of pager that is commonly used is carried by hospital staff. These pagers can carry either digital or voice messages, depending on the type of pager. A digital pager protects confidentiality and allows the receiver to have a record of the calls. A voice pager gives a one-time voice message. To activate either of the pagers, dial the appropriate four-digit code. Some facilities have an access code that must be entered prior to entering the four-digit code. Most paging systems will prompt the user, either by voice message or tone, when to enter the message.

Paging guidelines that should be followed regardless of the type of pager used include:

- Allow at least 5 minutes for a page to be returned before paging again.
- The charge RN is generally responsible for coordinating calls for the physicians, especially during the off shifts.
- When asked to page someone, remember who requested the page so you can route callers appropriately when they call back.

Do not page physicians to give them laboratory values unless directed to do so. Many times the physician will need to alter the patient's treatments or medications, and the RN is needed for this.

Patient Call System

Every hospital has some type of call system to enable the patient to contact the RN. Some systems are sophisticated and do not require a person (usually the person responsible for the clerical functions) to answer the patient's call. Other systems, like those found in most health care facilities, require a person to answer the patient's call, find out the patient's needs, and "dispatch" the appropriate person to handle the call. All patient rooms have a call button at the bed (either in the bed's handrail or a cord-type button) to alert the nursing staff of the patient's needs. Emergency call buttons are also located in patient bathrooms, public restrooms, and sitz bath areas.

When you are answering a patient call, it is important that the specific operations for the unit are known so that communication can be handled appropriately.

When answering a call, remember to write down the patient's name, room and bed number, and the request. Some facilities also require that this information be written on a special form that is later used for reference and following up on patient requests.

Some newer patient call systems also record the time of call, the time it was answered, and the time that someone went into the room to complete the call automatically.

When you are answering a patient call, it is important to speak clearly into the phone or speaker so the patient can hear and understand. It may not be easy to understand patients since their speaker is often at their side and not close to their head. If you do not understand their request, repeat what you thought you heard and ask for verification. Just as in using the phone system, it is important to remain calm and courteous. Every patient's request is important, and the clerical person's responsibility is to handle each request efficiently, regardless of the nature of the call and the activity going on at the time.

The procedure to handle a patient request depends on the type of request. A request for help with elimination (bathroom, bedpan) or for water, ice, to turn lights on/off, and so on, will usually be handled by the PCT. Some hospitals may ask the clerical worker to handle these types of calls. Check before doing so to make sure this is in accordance with hospital policies and procedures. Requests for medications, IVs, information about tests, orders, and questions about care will generally be directed to the patient's RN.

Some general guidelines when answering patient calls follow:

Notify the patient's RN *immediately* any time a call is received that may signify a change in patient status. These would include calls such as "I'm bleeding," "I'm having trouble breathing," "My roommate needs help," and "I'm having chest pain." Also listen for clues such as crying, vomiting, and screaming to help determine the urgency of the call. Generally a patient call placed from the bathroom would also indicate an urgent call.

1. Write down all requests whether the call needs to be handled by you personally or by someone else.

Interruptions may occur, and it may be necessary to refer to notes about requests that have not been fulfilled.

2. Direct the call to the most appropriate person as often as possible. For instance, do not page the RN to get the patient some water unless the PCT is unavailable and you cannot handle the request personally.

3. Page someone to fulfill the patient's request as soon as possible. To a patient waiting in bed, 5 minutes may seem like an eternity.

4. Remain calm and courteous. "May I help you, Mr. Jones?" would be an appropriate way to answer a patient call.

5. Let the patient complete the request before you disconnect the conversation. The patient may feel unimportant if not given a chance to finish the request. If you are not sure you heard correctly, repeat it and ask for verification.

6. Always acknowledge a patient's request. Tell the patient how the request will be addressed, with a statement such as "I will let your nurse know."

7. Answer each call promptly regardless of the number of times the patient calls. Some patients will call quite frequently. They may be frightened and just want to hear that someone is there with them and they are not alone.

STOP Learn of any special patient needs at the beginning of the shift. Leave a note on the patient case system if a patient is hard of hearing, has a tracheostomy, is deaf, or has other communication deficits.

Computer System

In these days of technology, almost every hospital has some type of computer system on the patient care unit. The system may be used to obtain laboratory results, enter physicians' orders, or update admission/discharge/transfer information. In most facilities, these systems are utilized by the clerical coordinator of the patient care unit as well as other members of the patient care staff. (Please refer to Chapter 18 on computers for additional information.)

Routine Responsibilities

A typical shift routine might include the following responsibilities and expectations:

1. Obtain a thorough report from the previous shift.

2. Complete any pager schedules or changes as required.

3. Call consults or other messages as needed.

4. Continuously update the unit census during the shift by adding new admissions and transfers in, and subtracting any discharges, transfers out, and deaths.

5. Transcribe physicians' orders as quickly as possible by communicating orders to other departments either by computer or requisition, and verbally to the patient's RN.

6. File reports and other forms as they arrive on the unit. Forward reports for patients no longer on the unit to the appropriate unit or Medical Records Department.

7. Prepare charts as needed for patient census transactions such as admissions, discharges, and postoperative patients.

8. Maintain charts with extra blank forms for physicians' orders and progress notes and other forms as needed.

9. Accurately record vital signs and intake and output.

10. Order and stock supplies. Ordering supplies such as chart forms, tape, pencils, and other clerical needs is an important but sometimes forgotten responsibility for the person substituting in the clerical role. Supplies should be inventoried weekly or biweekly and ordered appropriately to be available when needed. Remember that these supplies are as important to patient care as are the clinical supplies such as bandages and thermometers.

THE PATIENT CHART

The patient's medical record is a permanent legal record that belongs to the hospital. It must be treated with care and confidentiality like other legal documents such as birth certificates and marriage licenses. It must be maintained and stored according to the legal policy of the institution.

Because the medical record is the legal record of the patient's hospital stay, it is admissible as evidence in court cases.

A patient's chart serves many purposes, but on a patient care unit it will be used as the primary means of communication between the physician and staff responsible for the care of the patient. The patient's chart can also be used for planning patient care, educational purposes, and research. The patient's chart is a carefully documented record of the patient's diagnosis, plan of care, treatment by the medical staff, and patient condition at discharge from the hospital.

When a patient is discharged, the chart is sent to the medical information management department. This department is responsible for examining the patient chart and verifying that it is appropriate and complete. The chart will then be filed where it can be retrieved if needed. If the patient is readmitted, the medical staff may request that a chart from a previous admission be forwarded to the patient care unit.

Medical/Legal Considerations

Everything that is written in the chart is part of the permanent record. All staff who document in the chart must follow basic rules. Responsibility for the maintenance of the chart while the patient in on the patient care unit is assigned to the clerical worker. Here are a few chart maintenance guidelines:

- Make all entries permanent; always use blue or black ink or a computer printer; never use a pencil.
- The patient's name must appear on every record page.
- Sign every entry that you make with your first initial, last name, and title.
- Record the time and date of all entries—include day, month, year, and time of day (usually military time).
- Abbreviations may be used according to the list of approved abbreviations.
- Never delete material in the record by scratching out, using correction fluid, obliterating with felt tip markers, typing XXXXXs, etc.

If an error is made in charting, draw a single line through the error, and write the word *error* along with your initials and the date. *Do not* cover the error with correction fluid, labels, or other means.

Since the chart is considered a legal document, an acceptable method for correcting errors must be used. If the chart forms are imprinted with an incorrect imprint or label, the form may be destroyed if no notations have been made. If the chart form has notations, the form cannot be destroyed. The correct information may be imprinted in another area near the incorrect imprint: Make a line or an X through the incorrect information, write *error* with your first initial, last name, and title nearby.

Confidentiality

The clerical worker is responsible for managing the verbal and written communication processes on the unit. By the nature of these responsibilities, the PCT has access to a great deal of patient-related information, and all of this information is considered confidential. The PCT and all medical staff are expected to treat patient information in a confidential manner, sharing it only with those who have a need to know. Health care workers are not to reveal information to the patient, family members, visitors, other staff, or their friends. Never discuss any patient information except when necessary for patient care purposes.

Discussion of patient information should be conducted outside of the patient's and visitor's range of hearing. Be aware of others at the desk when discussing patients. Information may be overheard and misunderstood, creating unnecessary worry, anxiety, or even panic for the patient or family member. Never talk about patients in the hallways, elevator, cafeteria, or any other place where there is a danger of being overheard.

Refer all telephone calls and requests for information from the police, the media, legal agencies, or other agencies, to the RN manager or assigned administrator on call. Do not even discuss general patient information. If asked, politely refuse to reveal any information, and then quickly change the subject.

Only authorized persons such as physicians and staff should have access to the chart. Always know the status of the person using the chart. Never give the chart to a relative or friend because of a request to see the chart. The protection of the patient's chart is one of the clerical worker's responsibilities.

Patients have a right to review the information in their medical record, but must request access by signing an authorization form. The clerical worker must follow the policy at the institution to have copies made of a patient's chart.

The Basic Chart

The forms that make up a patient chart are kept in some type of chart holder. This holder may be made of vinyl or metal and can be opened from the top, bottom, or side, depending on the style used at your institution.

The chart forms are usually placed into sections separated by chart dividers kept in the sequence designated by the hospital. The patient's name, room, service, and doctor are identified on labels placed on the chart holders. The charts are kept in slots, numbered by rooms on the unit, of a chart rack when they are not in use. Many types of chart racks are available.

Each chart form must be identified with the patient's information by an imprint. When each patient is admitted, an imprinter card is created in the admitting department. This card may be made of plastic or metal and is used to imprint the patient information onto the chart forms, requisitions, consults, and any other form used by the patient during the hospital stay. Some institutions will print labels on the computer when a patient is admitted and use them to identify the patient's forms and requisitions. If this system is utilized, then an imprinter card would not be necessary.

The patient's name, age, sex, medical record number, address, and attending physician's name are usually included on the imprinter card or label. A manual or electric imprinter is used to transfer the information from the imprinter card to any form requiring the patient's information.

Standard Chart Forms

All chart forms will have the name of the institution printed somewhere on the form and a space for the patient's information. There are common types of *standard chart* forms found in any hospital and used in all patient charts. There are also *supplemental chart* forms that may be added to the patient chart, depending on the care and treatment.

There are several forms that are considered standard:

Face sheet or information form (Fig. 19–1)
Admission agreement or general hospital consent form (Fig. 19–2)
Physician's order forms (Fig. 19–3)
History and physical record
Physician's progress notes (Fig. 19–4)
Laboratory reports
Medication administration records (Fig. 19–5)
Nursing flow sheets and progress notes (See Chapter 15)
Graphic or clinical record (Fig. 19–6)
Discharge summary sheets (Fig. 19–7)
Kardex (Fig. 19–8)

Face Sheet or Information Form

The face sheet or information form is generated when the patient is admitted to the hospital. It contains personal information about the patient, such as name, address, telephone number, medical record number, admission diagnosis, attending physician, next of kin, and insurance information.

Admission Agreement or General Hospital Consent Form

This form is signed by the patient on admission. It authorizes the physicians and staff to provide care during the patient's stay. Sections may also be included for advance directives and release of medical information (to insurance companies for financial reimbursement). Advance directives are legal documents that advise caregivers, including the patient's physician, on the measures that should be taken to keep the patient alive. Every state has different laws that pertain to these directives, and as a result they are handled somewhat differently in every institution. Some institutions may require advance directives to be filed with physician's orders or progress notes so that the physician is constantly reminded of their presence.

Physician's Order Forms

The physician's order form or doctor's order sheet is a very important form used by the physician to record requests for care and treatment procedures for the patient. All orders for the change or cancellation of procedures and treatment must be recorded on the order sheets also. Orders are transcribed to other records and forms to use as guidelines by nursing for patient care. Many institutions will use physician's order forms with duplicate copies. Copies may be sent to the pharmacy or given to patient care staff to eliminate errors in the transcription

process. The original sheet is always kept with the patient's chart.

History and Physical Record

Every patient admitted will have a medical history taken and an initial physical assessment completed by an attending physician, resident, or other designated person. This assessment is recorded on the history and physical record. This report may be handwritten in ink or may be dictated and typed by a medical transcriptionist.

Physician's Progress Notes

The physician's progress note is a form for the doctor to record the patient's progress during a hospital stay. Notes will include observations, impressions, and recommendations of any physician who examines the patient. Most hospitals require notes to be written within a certain time frame. In some institutions, the progress note and doctor's order sheet may be combined on one form.

Laboratory Reports

Laboratory tests are requested by the physician, and the results are recorded on the laboratory report. These reports are most commonly in the form of computer-generated reports. Multiple results may be included in the same report. The frequency that this report is generated will be determined by laboratory staff.

Medication Administration Record

A chart form used for recording all medications given to the patient by the nursing staff is called the medication administration record. Whenever a new order or change in a current medication order is requested by the physician, the nursing staff transcribes the name of the medication, dosage, route, and frequency from the physician's order form to this form. The recording of requested medications is a task included in the order transcription procedure that may be assigned to the clerical worker in many hospitals.

Nursing Progress Notes

The nursing progress notes are provided for the documentation of the RN's observations of the patient, such as the patient's behavior and response to treatments ordered by the physician. In some facilities, all staff caring for the patient may record patient progress on a multidisciplinary progress note.

A *nursing data base, nursing admission record,* or *nursing history form* may be used by the RN as initial assessment of the patient upon admission. The RN or other patient care staff member will compile a short history from the patient or a family member if the patient is unavailable or unable to answer questions. Questions

Text continued on page 342

Name: Last, First, Mi		Maiden Name	Room No.		Adm. No.	Med. Rec. no.		Adv. dir.
Street Address		City	State		Zip		County	
Telephone	Sex	Race	Marital Status		Birthdate		Age	
Social Security #	Religion	Birth Place	Valuables	Info. By		Pa. Int.	Adm. Int.	
Adm. Date	Adm. Time		Prev. Adm. Date			Prev. Disch. Date		
Attending Physician		Address	City	State		Zip	Telephone	
Transferring Facility Name		Address	City	State		Zip	Telephone	
Referring Physician		Address	City	State		Zip	Telephone	
Personal Physician		Address	City	State		Zip	Telephone	
Next of Kin Name			Relationship		Telephone Number			
Street Address		City		State		Zip		

INFORMATION COLLECTED AND STORED IN MEDICAL RECORDS MAINTAINED BY THE UNIVERSITY MEDICAL CENTER IS CONFIDENTIAL. THIS INFORMATION IS THE PROPERTY OF THE PATIENT AND THE MEDICAL CENTER. THE PHYSICAL FORM OF THE INFORMATION (FILES, DATA BASES, MICROFORM, PRINTOUTS, ETC.) IS THE PROPERTY OF THE MEDICAL CENTER.

PATIENT DISPOSITON: ☐ HOME ☐ ICF/SNF ☐ AMA ☐ EXPIRED ☐ AUTOPSY ☐ CORONER ☐ OTHER HOSP.

D/C DATE: SUMMARY DICTATED — DATE INITIALS

DO NOT WRITE IN THIS SPACE — AWAITING SIGNATURE / DATA COMPLETION / RECEIVED / ASSEMBLED / CODING COMPLETE / ANALYZED / PERMANENT FILE

INSURANCE COVERAGE - PRIMARY

Insurance Agency	Agency Code	Telephone	Subscriber Name	Relationship
Street Address		City	State Zip	County
Claim/Case/Policy #	Recipient #	Group #	Plan Code	Void Date
Assignment	Certification Group	Telephone	Authorized By	Days Auth.
Auth./Reference #	Benefits			

INSURANCE COVERAGE - SECONDARY

Insurance Agency	Agency Code	Telephone	Subscriber Name	Relationship
Street Address		City	State Zip	County
Claim/Case/Policy #	Recipient #	Group #	Plan Code	Void Date
Assignment	Certification Group	Telephone	Authorized By	Days Auth.
Auth./Reference #	Benefits			

FIGURE 19-1
Face sheet or information form.

GENERAL CONSENT

CONSENT FOR MEDICAL TREATMENT

Knowing that I am suffering from a condition requiring hospital care, I hereby consent to such hospital care covering all diagnostic procedures and medical treatment by my physician, his assistants or his designees as may be necessary in his judgment. I am aware that the practice of medicine and surgery is not an exact science and I acknowledge that no guarantees have been made as to the results of treatments or examination in the hospital.

CONSENT FOR RELEASE OF MEDICAL INFORMATION

The hospital and physicians providing care to me are authorized to release any medical information necessary to process applications for financial coverage for services rendered during this admission to the third party payors and their agents. The release of information may include diagnoses and treatments, including HIV testing, AIDS, ARC, psychiatric, drug and/or alcohol related diagnoses. Release of information may also include any information requested to determine coverage, medical necessity or other benefits determination. To enable follow-up and continuity of my medical care, The University Medical Center is authorized to release medical records and/or medical information to physicians providing such care. I understand that I may revoke this authorization at any time except to the extent that actions based on this authorization have been taken. This form has been fully explained to me and I certify that I understand its contents.

MEDICARE - MEDICAID - CHAMPUS CERTIFICATION

I hereby authorize The University Medical Center to release information and request payment. I certify that the information given by me in applying for payment under CHAMPUS or Titles XVIII and XIX of the Social Security Act is correct. I authorize release of all records to act on this request. I request that payment of authorized benefits be made on my behalf. I understand that care rendered during this admission is subject to review by the designated Peer Review Organization. I have received information from The University Medical Center (in the Medicare or CHAMPUS Beneficiary Letter) indicating my rights while a Medicare or CHAMPUS hospital patient.

FINANCIAL RESPONSIBILITY

The undersigned, in consideration of hospital services to be rendered by The University Medical Center to the below named patient, does agree to pay The University Medical Center on demand all charges for services and incidentals incurred on behalf of said patient. I authorize direct payment of surgical and medical benefits to the attending physician or to whomever he/she designates. I also authorize direct payment of all other hospital benefits to The University Medical Center. The benefits referred to herein would be payable to me if I did not make this assignment and include Major Medical Insurance. I understand that I am responsible to the hospital and the physicians, respectively, for charges not covered by this agreement. I also understand that some hospital and physician services may not be covered by insurance or other health care coverage and I agree to pay the hospital and physicians, respectively, for services not covered by such plans. **(NOTE: Medicare recipients are only responsible for medicare deductibles, coinsurance, and non-covered items.)**

ACKNOWLEDGEMENT OF ADVANCE DIRECTIVE INFORMATION

State and Federal laws require that I be made aware of my right to make health care decisions for myself including my right to accept or reject medical and/or surgical treatment. In the event I become unable to make informed decisions regarding the administration of life-sustaining treatment, I understand that I now may express my wishes to accept or reject life-sustaining treatment in a written document called an ADVANCE DIRECTIVE.

☐ Yes   ☐ No   I HAVE prepared written ADVANCE DIRECTIVES regarding my health care. ADVANCE DIRECTIVES have been copied and incorporated into the medical record: _____ (Emp. Initial)

☐ Yes   ☐ No   I would like to discuss ADVANCE DIRECTIVES further with the hospital's in-house resources.

ACKNOWLEDGEMENT OF RECEIPT: My signature acknowledges my receipt of written information on ADVANCE DIRECTIVES, my other health care decision making rights, and the hospital's policy and procedure for implementing ADVANCE DIRECTIVES.

RELEASE OF SOCIAL SECURITY NUMBER FOR MEDICAL DEVICE TRACKING

I hereby authorize the release of my Social Security number to the manufacturer of any medical device I receive while a patient at The University Medical Center, in accordance with federal law and regulations. I further understand that my Social Security number may be used by the manufacturer to help locate me if there is a need to contact me with regard to this medical device. I release The University Medical Center from any liability that might result from the release of this information.

PATIENT SIGNATURE (or authorized party)	RELATIONSHIP	DATE	
WITNESS	DATE	Addressograph	
SECOND WITNESS (for verbal consent)	DATE		

GENERAL CONSENT

Admission agreement or general hospital consent form.

USE BALL POINT PEN · PLEASE WRITE FIRMLY

PHYSICIAN'S ORDERS

DATE/TIME	PHYSICIAN'S ORDERS	INDICATE WITH "THIS BRAND ONLY" IF AN EQUIVALENT PER HOSPITAL FORMULARY MAY NOT BE DISPENSED.

FIRST/SECOND Call circle one   Dr _____ @ _____
Physician(s) or Group   Phone or Pager #

FIRST/SECOND Call circle one   Resident _____ @ _____
Service   Pager #

ALLERGIES/REACTION: NKA ☐

① ← DO NOT USE THIS SHEET UNLESS A NUMBER SHOWS

Addressograph

PHYSICIAN'S ORDERS

FIGURE 19–3

Physician's order forms.

HISTORIES, PHYSICALS AND PROGRESS NOTES

Entry on this sheet will include THE ADMISSION, HISTORY AND PHYSICAL EXAMI-
NATION completed by the medical student and housestaff. All progress notes will be
written by, or under, the direct supervision of a physician or dentist licensed under the
laws of the STATE. Entries by medical students must be signed by them and
countersigned by a licensed physician.

Approved format for recording lab results:

WBC $>$ $\dfrac{\text{Hgb}}{\text{Hct}}$ $<$ P/T $\dfrac{\text{Na}}{\text{K}}$ | $\dfrac{\text{Cl}}{CO_2}$ $<$ BUN, Glucose, Creatinine

Hematology   **Chemistry**

ADDRESSOGRAPH

Date 19	Condition of Wound, Drainage, Removal of Stitches, Consultation, Change in Diagnosis, Complications, Condition on discharge, Instructions to Patient, Signed by Recording Physician each time.

PROGRESS NOTES

F I G U R E   1 9 – 4

Physician progress notes.

MEDICATION ADMINISTRATION RECORD				DIAGNOSIS								
SHIFT	Date	Date	Date	Date	Date	Date	Date					
11–7												
7–3								ROOM				
3–11												

NOTE:			Date →									
Drug, Dosage Form		Dose	Route									
Frequency	Administration Times											
Drug, Dosage Form		Dose	Route									
Frequency	Administration Times											
Drug, Dosage Form		Dose	Route									
Frequency	Administration Times											
Drug, Dosage Form		Dose	Route									
Frequency	Administration Times											
Drug, Dosage Form		Dose	Route									
Frequency	Administration Times											
Drug, Dosage Form		Dose	Route									
Frequency	Administration Times											
Drug, Dosage Form		Dose	Route									
Frequency	Administration Times											
Drug, Dosage Form		Dose	Route									
Frequency	Administration Times											
Drug, Dosage Form		Dose	Route									
Frequency	Administration Times											
Drug, Dosage Form		Dose	Route									
Frequency	Administration Times											

☐ NO KNOWN ALLERGIES   ☐ ALLERGIES

Checked by _____   ☐ MEDICATIONS FROM HOME

FIGURE 19–5

Medication administration records.

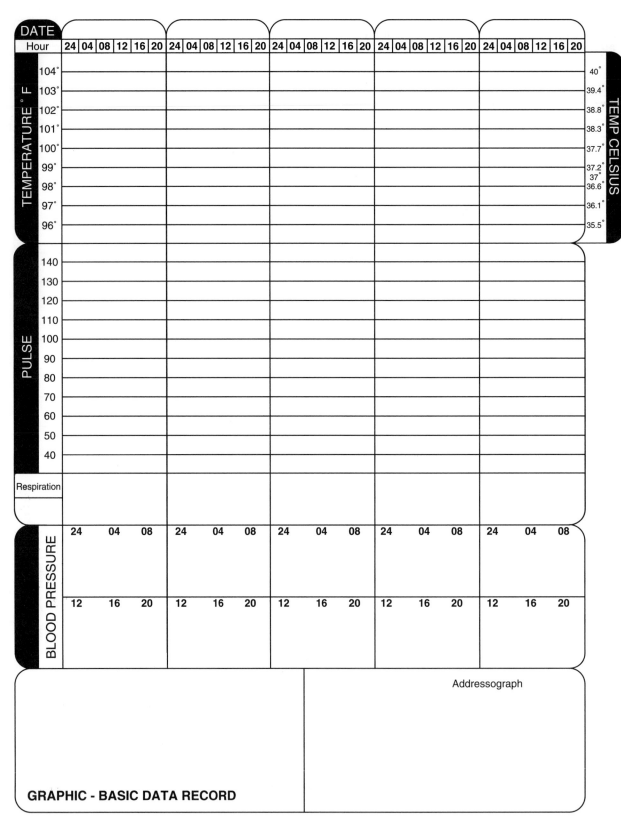

GRAPHIC - BASIC DATA RECORD

F I G U R E 1 9 – 6
Graphic or clinical record.

DISCHARGE ORDER/INSTRUCTIONS

☐ DISCHARGE _____
DATE

DOCTOR SIGNATURE/DATE ————————————
RESIDENT SIGNATURE/DATE ————————————

INSTRUCTION PROVIDED

Activity ☐ No Restrictions   ☐ Restrictions

Medications ☐ None Prescribed   ☐ Prescriptions

Diet ☐ No Restrictions   ☐ Special Diet

Wound Care

Resources ☐ None Required

Special Instructions: Hospital contact no: _____   Physician no: _____

APPOINTMENTS   Physician   Specialty   Phone   Date

I HAVE RECEIVED AND UNDERSTAND THESE DISCHARGE INSTRUCTIONS
SIGNATURE OF PATIENT/FAMILY _____ Date _____
RN _____ Date _____

DISCHARGE ORDER/INSTRUCTIONS   Addressograph

FIGURE 19–7

Discharge summary sheets.

CODE STATUS Date _____	# NURSING KARDEX	**ADDRESSOGRAPH**
CONDITION Date _____ critical ☐ fair ☐ poor ☐ satisfactory ☐		
Admit Date	**Medical Problems/ Surgical Procedure**	

ALLERGIES:

TPR	**DAILY HYGIENE**	**FAMILY INFORMATION**
BP	Complete ☐ Partial ☐	
WEIGHT	Shower ☐ Shampoo ☐	
SPECIAL CHECK		
Urine	Other	
Chemstrip		
Hemastix		
Guaiac	**MOUTH CARE**	**DIET**
Circ		
Neuro	Dentures: Upper ☐ Lower ☐	
		NPO
	SKIN CARE	Reason
		Hold tray on for
ACTIVITY UAL ☐ BR ☐ BRP ☐		Feed ☐ Assist ☐
Ambulation ☐		
	DRESS/GROOM self assist total	
Chair ☐		**TUBE FEEDINGS**
PROSTHESIS/HANDICAP/SENSORY LOSS	**ELIMINATION**	Residual Q_____
	Foley	
POSITIONING		
Turn ☐	Bowel	Calorie Count
	Last BM _____	
TUBES/TUBE CARE		I & O
		FLUID RESTRICTIONS
	MODE OF TRAVEL	_____ cc's per day
	Wheelchair ☐ Cart ☐	Nursing | Dietary | IV
	O₂ ☐ IV Pole ☐	D
		E
	SAFETY PRECAUTIONS	N
	Restraint	
ISOLATION	Security Room ☐	
Type	Side Rails ☐ High Risk Fall ☐	
Date		

F I G U R E   1 9 – 8

Kardex.

DISCHARGE PLANNING

Anticipated DC Date _____
        To_____
Continuity of Care _____
        To_____
    Date Completed_____
Needs: (equipment, home health visits, etc.)

Social Worker _____

DATE	INTRAVENOUS THERAPY

DATE	DAILY LAB WORK	Line Draw ☐	DATE	SPECIMENS	DONE

DATE	ONE-TIME LAB ORDERS	REQ. SENT

DATE	DIAGNOSTIC TEST/APPOINTMENTS	DATE DONE	DATE	PHYSICIAN CONSULTS	DATE CALLED	DATE DONE

DATE	ALLIED PROFESSIONAL CONSULTS	DATE CALLED	DATE DONE

FIGURE 19–8
Continued

include a brief medical and social history, information about the patient's activities of daily living, present illness, and any medications the patient may be taking currently. Discharge plans are usually discussed at this time. The patient's vital signs, height, weight, and any allergies/reactions are recorded.

 It is common practice to record all patient allergies in red ink.

A *nursing flow sheet* is used to record daily nursing care activities.

Graphic or Clinical Record

This form is utilized as a graphic representation of the patient's vital signs in a given period. Vital sign frequency is ordered by the physician. In some institutions, it is the clerical worker's responsibility to record the vital sign information from the flow sheet to the graphic record.

Discharge Summary Sheets

Discharge summary sheets may be used to prepare the patient for discharge. They usually include instructions for the patient to follow after leaving the facility. A nursing discharge summary may document the patient's condition at the time of discharge. A physician's discharge summary will summarize the diagnosis and treatment of the patient while in the facility.

Kardex

The Kardex is the form used to record the procedures, treatments, medications, and tests for the patient. The patient care staff will use this as a reference to create a care plan for each shift. This form is used only as a worksheet and is not considered a legal document. It can be discarded when the patient is discharged. Accuracy in transcribing information from the physician's orders to the Kardex is vital.

Each of these standard forms will be included in the patient's chart in some format. Each institution has a form that provides the same function if it does not have one of the specific forms previously discussed.

Supplemental Chart Forms

In addition to the standard chart forms, supplemental chart forms may be added according to the specific needs of each patient. Some common supplemental forms are reviewed here.

Records of Surgery

Various forms are required to document a surgical procedure on a patient. The forms are used by the sur-

geon, the operating room staff, the anesthesiologist, and the postanesthesia care unit (also known as recovery room) staff. Some forms may be initiated before surgery such as a consent form and a preoperative checklist. Other forms may be added during the surgical procedure such as an operating room record and record of anesthesia. Another form may be added by nursing staff in the postanesthesia care unit. If tissue was removed during the operation, a surgical pathology consult may be initiated. Additional responsibilities for surgery will be discussed later.

Therapy Records

Therapy records will include documentation from several departments, including social work, respiratory therapy, physical therapy, occupational therapy, nutritional therapy, radiation therapy, and others. Often these forms are used in a fashion similar to progress notes and to record treatments and patient response to these treatments. This information may also be documented on a multidisciplinary progress note.

Consultation Forms

In some cases the physician may want to get the opinion of another physician or specialist in a particular area. A consultation form will be initiated and placed on the patient's chart. The area consulted may record any observations or information requested on this form. Often a consultation is dictated, and the results return in a typewritten form.

Special Medication Records

In many facilities, special records are kept when a patient is being given certain types of medications. Two of the most common medications that are recorded on a special record are anticoagulants and insulin. Records of insulin administration are often documented on a diabetic record and include blood and urine tests performed to monitor the effects of insulin.

Consent Forms

In health care facilities today, there are numerous situations that require the patient, or person responsible for the patient (if the patient is not competent for any reason), to grant permission to perform procedures on the patient. Consent forms for surgery and other procedures are legal agreements between the patient and the physician. Always follow the consent procedures at your institution.

Managing the Patient Chart

As the person performing the clerical role on the patient care unit, one of your main responsibilities is maintenance of the patient chart. Responsibilities that may be included:

- Properly identify the chart with the patient's name and location.
- Ensure proper identification of each form in the patient chart.
- Place all chart forms in proper sequence.
- Replace charts in chart rack or designated area.
- Add or replace chart forms and order sheets as needed.
- File chart forms, results, and reports as they are generated and sent to the unit.
- Assist any staff in locating the patient's chart.
- Know the identity and medical relevance of persons accessing the chart.
- Keep a record of the location of a patient's chart when it is removed from the patient care area.
- Check often for physician's orders and transcribe.

CHART PROCEDURES

The Admission Procedure

The admitting office is responsible for notifying a patient care area that a patient is being admitted. The admitting office will relay information regarding the patient, including name, age, physician's name, diagnosis, and medical record number, if the patient has previously been admitted. The clerical worker will communicate with the charge RN to determine what bed the patient may be placed in (the admitting office will need this information) and if the patient being admitted needs any special equipment. The admitting office is responsible for sending a face sheet and consent forms with the patient or to the unit shortly afterward, accompanied by the patient's imprinter card. A patient identification band will also be generated and is often placed on the patient at this time.

✔ Contact the admitting office for missing face sheets, consent forms, or identification bands. These pieces should be with the patient and chart at all times.

A patient's admission is considered *routine or elective* if the date of admission is previously scheduled by the attending physician. A routine admission will usually arrive to the floor escorted by an admitting representative, transporter, or volunteer. Some patients are admitted through the emergency department and their admission is considered an *emergency*. Usually the patient care staff will move the patient to the unit after an RN in the emergency department calls report to an RN on the unit

receiving the patient. Additional emergency department documentation will accompany the patient and be placed on the patient chart with the other forms. No matter how the patient enters the hospital, a new inpatient chart must be initiated to document the hospital stay.

A supply of preassembled standard forms needed for each admission is called an admission packet. The contents of the packet may vary from unit to unit, but will include all standard forms discussed previously as well as additional supplementary forms necessary for the patient's diagnosis and treatment. All the forms must be imprinted with the patient's information and placed in proper order in the patient chart, labeled with the patient's information, for the patient care staff to document the patient's diagnosis, treatments, and progress. This process may seem long and complicated with all the different forms and places to insert the patient's name, but after a little practice, the entire process will take only a few minutes. The clerical worker should try to have as much paperwork as possible prepared before the patient actually arrives to the unit. The goal is to have the patient admission process completed before the RN has completed the admission assessments and documentation.

As soon as the patient arrives to the unit, notify the RN assigned to care for the patient and the physician responsible for the patient's admission. Someone on the patient care team is responsible for greeting the patient and providing orientation to the room. The physician may need to know that the patient is in the assigned room and meet with the patient to make an initial assessment. Doctor's orders for the plan of patient care are usually generated after this step. Occasionally the physician may have assessed the patient's status already, and orders will accompany the patient to the floor with the other admission paperwork.

Other steps of the admission process include creating bed cards and door tags for the patient's room; creating a nursing Kardex for documentation of doctor's orders; completing a census transaction summary; and entering the patient's name on other unit forms such as an inpatient listing, dietary information sheet, charge vouchers; team assignment sheet; nursing service report, and any other form utilized by the patient care unit. It may be helpful to make a list of all the necessary entries and keep them for future reference, because it can be difficult to remember all the steps when asked to cover the desk occasionally.

Steps to follow for the admission procedure:

1. Get the patient information from the admitting office (name, diagnosis, physician, medical records number), and check with the RN for bed availability.

2. Prepare an admission packet, and label the patient's chart.

3. Notify the nurse and physician when the patient arrives to the unit.

4. Imprint standard and any supplemental chart forms, including the face sheet and consent forms, and place in proper order in the patient's chart.

5. Identify the patient on all unit forms. Keep a list for reference.

The Discharge/Expiration Procedure

Patients leave the hospital on the order of a physician, by signing themselves out against medical advice, or if they die. The steps to follow for each procedure are similar, with additional steps for patients leaving against physician's orders and for patients who die.

The routine discharge begins when the physician writes the order for discharge. The order may include directions to arrange for a follow-up visit, prescriptions, and medical discharge instructions to be completed before the patient leaves the unit. The clerical worker may be responsible for contacting the business office to determine if there are any financial issues the patient must address before leaving. The RN must always be notified before the patient leaves the floor. This is done to make sure the RN has made final assessments and given all the information needed to the patient.

After the patient leaves the unit, his or her name must be removed from all the unit forms. The patient chart forms are removed from the chart holder and fastened together into a discharge chart order according to a prearranged procedure. All patient charts will be returned to the medical information management department for processing.

Check to make sure that all the forms are properly identified with the patient's information and properly completed.

If the patient is being transferred to another medical facility, it is also considered a discharge. Additional forms, such as an information summary for the continuity of care (COC), may be completed by the physician, nurse, or clerical worker to be sent with the patient to the new facility. An information summary may also be completed if the patient requires medical assistance in the home setting. A copy of this form will go with the patient, and another copy will be kept in the patient's chart.

On occasion a patient decides not to remain in the hospital even though the physician advises against discharge. This patient is classified as leaving against medical advice (AMA). If this situation arises, steps must be taken to protect the hospital and staff from liability in case of serious medical consequences to the patient. The RN and physician may talk to the patient; if the patient still insists on leaving, the physician will ask the patient to sign a release form. If the patient refuses to sign, this is documented by the staff. Once the release is signed and the patient is aware of the possible consequences of

premature discharge, the clerical responsibilities are the same as for a routine discharge.

When a patient dies, the procedure is the same as the discharge procedure except that additional forms, such as a death certificate, autopsy consent, and release of body, must be initiated. Some facilities require a donation request form for families who wish to donate organs and/or tissue. The physician, nurse, and/or the mortician are responsible for getting signatures, but the clerical worker must be able to identify the forms and prepare them for the staff to use. Once these forms are completed, the steps to follow are the same as the routine discharge procedure.

Steps to follow for the discharge/expiration procedure:

1. Transcribe the discharge order and follow through with any requests such as follow-up appointments.

2. Notify the RN when the patient is ready to leave to ensure that all the necessary discharge information has been completed and given to the patient.

3. Remove chart forms from the chart holder and fasten together. Send the chart to the medical information management department for further processing.

4. Remove the patient's name from unit forms.

5. If the patient is leaving AMA, make sure a release form is signed and the situation is documented.

6. If the patient is transferring to another medical facility, make sure the COC forms have been completed.

7. If the patient has died, make sure the death certificate and other death forms have been completed.

The Transfer Procedure

There are times when it may be necessary to move a patient to another room or unit during a hospital stay. Any of these room changes are classified as a patient transfer. A patient may be transferred in (a patient comes to your unit), or transferred out (a patient leaves your unit), or transferred within (a patient remains on your unit, but moves to another room). There are several circumstances that may result in a transfer:

- The patient may have a change of condition. The patient's condition may become unstable, and an intensive care unit required, or stable, and an intermediate care unit is needed.

- There may be a change in diagnosis. Some units will specialize in more specific skills (chemotherapy, dialysis, labor and delivery, etc.), and the physician may want the patient moved to the specialty area.

- Isolation may be required.

- Special equipment (traction, ventilator, etc.) may be required.

- The patient may need to be closer to the desk for special observation.

- The patient or family requests a private room.

• The patient does not get along with his or her roommate.

Transfer Out

Before a transfer can occur, the physician must write a transfer order. The clerical worker is responsible for contacting the patient's care team and then arranging for a bed by calling the admitting clerk. The admitting office will locate a bed on the new unit. After receiving the new room assignment, the clerical worker should call the receiving unit to confirm the room and to give any other information that the new unit may require.

When the room is available, the RN from the patient's current unit will call report of the patient's condition to the RN on the receiving unit. The patient care staff will be responsible for getting the patient ready and transporting the patient, while the clerical worker is responsible for gathering the patient's chart and other paperwork to send with the patient.

It is possible that a patient may be transferred immediately. This is usually a situation in which the patient needs to be transferred to an intensive care unit after a Code Blue is resolved. The process to transfer out may be the same, but some additional steps must be taken. Special equipment (such as a portable monitor) may need to be ordered while you are trying to organize the paperwork. Often the patient's belongings may not go to the intensive care unit and must be packed, labeled, and either given to the family or sent to a storage location. Steps to follow for the transfer-out procedure:

1. Transcribe orders for transfer and notify patient care team.
2. Notify admitting office to arrange for a room.
3. Call the receiving area to confirm room number and to give any other necessary information.
4. The patient's RN will call the patient's status report to the RN in the receiving area.
5. Prepare the patient's information by gathering the chart and all the miscellaneous forms (Kardexes, medication administration records, and so on).
6. Send the imprinter card with the patient's chart.
7. Remove the patient's name from all unit forms.

Transfer In

Because it is the responsibility of the admitting office to arrange a room for the patient, the admitting clerk will notify the unit that a patient is expected. The clerical worker notifies the charge RN who assigns an RN to care for the patient.

✔ When the transferring unit calls to ask if the receiving area is ready and to give report to the patient's RN, ask if any special supplies or equipment will be needed.

After arriving at the unit the patient care staff will orient the patient to the room and make initial assessments while the clerical worker completes the patient chart and unit forms. It may be necessary to make new identification tags for the patient's room and chart, place Kardexes into the appropriate holders, and imprint any chart forms that may need to be added to the current chart. Any new orders or changes in current orders must be transcribed and documented appropriately.

Steps to follow for the transfer-in procedure:

1. Admitting office notifies unit of expected patient.
2. Sending unit should confirm the readiness of the new room.
3. The RN receiving the patient will take report of the patient's condition from the RN sending the patient.
4. After the patient arrives, change identification tags for the room and chart, place Kardexes, and add any new chart forms as needed.
5. Identify the patient on all unit forms.

The Operative Procedure

A patient may have *elective* or *emergency* surgery. *Elective* surgery will be scheduled in advance, and the patient may be admitted the day of surgery or the day prior to surgery. Admission-day-surgery patients have had preoperative testing in an outpatient area prior to admission and are admitted to an inpatient care unit after surgery and recovery care are completed. Some patients may be admitted prior to surgery to allow time for diagnostic studies and tests before surgery. Any abnormal test results may require further investigation before the patient is taken for surgery. Elective surgery is usually scheduled and performed during the day, but emergency surgery may take place at any time. Because of the nature of emergency operations, all clerical workers must be ready to prepare a patient's chart for surgery at any time.

The clerical worker will identify patients scheduled for surgery on an operating-room schedule. This schedule will list information such as the patient's name, age, medical record number, surgical procedure to be performed, scheduled time, and estimated length of the procedure.

Preparing a patient for surgery requires completion of clinical and clerical tasks. The tasks to be completed are indicated on a preoperative checklist. Clerical tasks to be completed on the preoperative checklist may vary according to the policies of the hospital.

It is vital for the preoperative checklist and any preoperative orders to be completed before the patient leaves the unit for surgery. It is often the policy of a hospital that surgery cannot be performed unless all the required reports, information, and tasks are performed.

The operating room will call the unit before the patient's scheduled time to notify the patient care staff to give any preoperative medications that may have been ordered and to prepare the patient to be transported to the surgical area.

Immediately following surgery, the patient is usually sent to the recovery room or postanesthesia care unit (PACU) until he or she has recovered from the effects of the anesthesia. An RN in PACU will call the patient's RN to give a condition report before transporting the patient back to the unit.

✔ This is a good time to order any equipment or supplies, such as oxygen and/or suction set-up, that the patient may need when returning from surgery.

When the patient arrives on the floor, the patient care staff will assist the patient into bed and perform initial postoperative assessments. The clerical worker is responsible for organizing the operating reports under the appropriate section in the chart and transcribing any postoperative orders as soon as possible. *All* preoperative orders are automatically discontinued unless the physician writes to resume preoperative orders. Often these new orders require a new Kardex and MAR to be initiated.

Steps to follow for operative procedures

Prior to surgery:

1. Identify patients scheduled for surgery.
2. Prepare and complete the preoperative checklist.
3. Notify the appropriate staff when the operating room calls for the patient.

After surgery:

4. Inform the RN when the patient arrives in the recovery area.
5. Organize patient chart forms.
6. Transcribe postoperative orders; initiate Kardexes and medication forms when necessary.

ORDER TRANSCRIPTION

Any medical procedure performed on the patient requires an order by the physician. An order will include things such as medications, diet, activity level, diagnostic tests and procedures, and therapeutic procedures. The written orders are a permanent part of the patient's medical record and are considered legal documents like any other documentation in the chart. After the orders are written, the clerical worker is responsible for transcription of the orders and the RN is responsible for carrying out the orders for patient care. In some institutions the RN is also responsible for reviewing the orders transcribed by the clerical worker for accuracy and signing off on them.

Transcription is the process used to communicate the written order to the area responsible for completing the order. For example, if an order is written for vital signs to be obtained every 4 hours, the clerical worker ensures that the information is communicated to the patient care staff. If an order is written for a chest X-ray, the clerical worker ensures that the requisition is completed and the arrangements are made for the patient to be transported to the radiology department. The transcription of orders is one of the most important responsibilities of the clerical worker.

✔ Accuracy is vital. An inaccurately transcribed order may result in errors in treatment that may have a serious effect on the condition of the patient.

The forms used in order transcription are the physician's order sheet and the Kardex. The physician's order sheet is a form on which the physician writes all the patient's orders, dates them, and signs them in blue or black ink. As stated before, the physician's order sheet becomes part of the patient's permanent legal record.

A Kardex, created from physician's orders for a specific patient, categorizes the orders for easy reference by the patient care staff. Caregivers will refer to the Kardex when creating a care plan for each patient on each shift.

Information that will not change during the patient's stay may be written on the Kardex in ink. This includes the patient's name, age, admission date, and physician. Different colors of ink may be used to highlight specific information, such as writing information about allergies in red ink. Most information is recorded in pencil so it can be erased when an order is cancelled or changed.

Usually, all Kardexes for patients on a unit are kept in a Kardex holder at or near the nursing station. The type of Kardex system used may vary widely from one hospital to another, but the purpose of the form is similar. Like all forms previously discussed, the clerical worker needs to become familiar with the types of forms used in his or her own institution.

The main areas of the Kardex:

Activity: Refers to the type of activity and ambulation the patient will be allowed (UAL, BR, and the like).
Diet: Refers to any nutritional needs of the patient (diet order, tube feeding, fluid restrictions, or food allergies).
Treatments: Refers to a wide variety of procedures that need to be performed by the patient care staff and includes orders for monitor parameters, wound care, and so forth.
Diagnostic tests, consults, and appointments: Refers to diagnostic testing and consultations such as radiology and electrocardiography.
Daily laboratory work: Refers to the laboratory tests to be performed on a routine basis.

The methods in which orders may be presented:

Written: Most orders will be written by the physician on

a physician's order form. Each order must be written completely, following the same rules as any documentation in the chart, as discussed earlier, with the date, time, name, and title included in each entry.
Verbal and telephone: A physician unable to go to the patient care unit to write orders may call the unit and speak with an RN. An RN may then write the order as verbalized by the physician. In some institutions, other registered staff (pharmacist, respiratory therapist, or dietician) may also write orders as requested by the physician. These orders must be written exactly as given by the physician. Verbal and telephone orders may be carried out immediately, but must later be cosigned by the physician who gave the order.
Computer: As technology advances, more and more methods are created to decrease the number of misinterpretations of written and verbal orders from the physician. Some computer systems allow the physician to input orders directly into the computer. A legible printout is created, and orders are immediately sent to the appropriate area by the system. This can be done from the physician's office or by modem from home. Many interpretation errors from handwritten orders can be eliminated with this method.

Main Categories of Orders

Physician's orders can be categorized into four main areas:

Standing Order

Once this order is written, it will remain unchanged until the physician writes another order to specifically change or discontinue the order. Most orders fall into this category.

vital signs q4h
$O_2$2L/NC
CBC qAM

One-Time or Limited Order

The doctor may want a medication or treatment given only once or for a short time. This will be indicated by a qualifying phrase such as "give one tonight and one in the morning." This type of order is automatically discontinued after being completed.

ABG on room air
Theophylline level in AM
Restoril 15 mg PO × 1

Stat Order

This type of order must be completed immediately and is usually written in emergency situations. Because these orders are urgent they must be transcribed first, and the patient care staff must be notified immediately.

Stat CXR
Stat ECG in event of chest pain
Obtain CBC, lytes immediately on arrival to floor

PRN Order

This type of order is carried out according to the needs of the patient and can be either a standing order or a one-time order.

MOM 30 cc PO PRN
If unable to void, may straight cath PRN
Compazine 10 mg IM q6h prn nausea

Transcription Process

Steps to follow in transcribing orders:

1. Identify

The first step is to identify that there is an order to be transcribed. Each hospital will have a method to indicate that an order has been written. The order may be located in the patient's chart or in a separate physician's order book. Some hospitals may use an order sheet with copies that need to be sent to various designated departments (such a medication order copy goes to Pharmacy). All new orders will have a current date and signature and be flagged or placed in the selected area. It is vital to read and interpret physician's orders accurately.

 Never guess at an illegible order.

2. Prioritize

The next step is to determine if the order should be done stat or ASAP. These types of orders must be done first before orders of lower priority are transcribed. The RN will need to be notified whenever there is an indication of high-priority orders.

3. Kardex

After priority is determined, the next step is to document the order on the patient's Kardex. Be sure to write the order exactly as the physician wrote it.

4. Forms / Requisitions / Consults

Many services and equipment require some type of requisition to be completed. Select the appropriate one, imprint it with the patient's information, fill in date and time needed and any other information necessary, and sign your name if required.

STOP It is essential that the correct patient's imprinter card is selected. An incorrect imprint may cause the wrong patient to receive the test. Always double check the name on the requisition with the name on the order to ensure accuracy.

5. Medication Administration Record (MAR)

A medication order will consist of the name of a drug, the dose or amount, the route of administration, and the time to be given. Medication orders may need to be recorded on an MAR if required by your institution. The MAR is a part of the permanent patient record and therefore must be documented in ink. In many hospitals it is the responsibility of the clerical worker to assign the times for the medications to be given according to the policy in that institution. Transcribing medication orders requires extreme accuracy because errors may be detrimental to the patient. Additional training may be required prior to transcribing medications onto the MAR.

6. Communicate

After the order is written on the Kardex and any requisitions and MARs are completed, it may be necessary to verbally communicate some orders. The RN may need to be notified that there is a change in IV, or you may need to call another department to order supplies or schedule a test. The next step in the process is to communicate a written order to the area that requires the information so the order can be completed.

7. Sign-off

When all orders have been communicated either verbally or by requisition, the orders must be signed by the person who recorded them to indicate that the orders were properly transcribed. The date, time, first initial, last name, and title are indicated in red ink to offer proof that the order was noted.

To reduce the chance of error, the same process should be followed each time an order is transcribed. It may help to make small marks or checks on the order sheet to indicate each order as it is completed. This is especially useful when the unit is busy and interruptions occur. If each item is marked after completion, it is easier to return to the items that still need to be completed. Each time a set of orders is completed, ask yourself the following questions:

Is it written on the Kardex?
Are all the necessary forms completed?
Have the medication records been completed?
Has the order been communicated?

Classification of Orders

Orders can be classified or separated into several main categories to assist the caregivers in determining the course of action to take in completing the physician's orders.

Therapeutic Procedures

The transcription of therapeutic procedure orders will require communication of the order to the responsible department by telephone, requisition, or computer. The order will also be transcribed to the Kardex for patient care reference and follow-up. Examples of therapeutic procedures include orders for respiratory or inhalation therapy, physical medicine and rehabilitation, traction, occupational therapy, speech therapy, and pain management.

Diagnostic Procedures

Any orders used to diagnose and/or monitor the patient's condition are considered diagnostic procedures. Radiology tests, such as CXRs and CT, as well as cardiology tests such as electrocardiography, Holter monitoring, stress testing, and others all fall into this category. After completing the appropriate requisition, these orders must be communicated to the patient care staff so that any necessary preparations can be completed before the patient's test. The type of preparation necessary and the extent to which the clerical worker is responsible will vary.

The patient's chart will go with the patient to most procedures. It is the clerical worker's responsibility to have the chart ready to go. This may include adding specific forms, imprinter card, or other specific items.

Dietary Procedures

While a patient is in the health care facility, the physician is responsible for ordering the specific type of diet the patient is to receive. The requested diet is communicated to the dietary department by means of a diet sheet that contains the patient's name, room number, and diet. Other systems may include the use of requisition forms, dietary Kardexes, or the computer.

The clerical worker will notify the dietary department before each meal of any new changes in current diet orders, and of any patients who are transferred, discharged, or expected to be out of the room at mealtime. New diet orders and changes in diet orders must be documented on the patient care Kardex at the time the order is transcribed. Examples of diet orders are *standard* (regular, soft, full liquid, clear liquid), *therapeutic* (low cholesterol, no cardiac stimulants, sodium restrictions, diabetic), and *tube feedings* (Ensure, Sustacal, Osmolite, Jevity). Other diet orders that relate to nutritional needs but are not considered diets are *force fluids* or *fluid restrictions, nutrient calculations* (calorie counts), *NPO,* and *consults for the dietician.* Other dietary-related responsibilities for the clerical worker may be to check and reorder the nourishment supply for the patient care unit or order an extra meal tray for a friend or family member of the patient.

Patient Care Procedures

Patient care procedures (or nursing treatment orders) may originate partly from the physicians and partly from the RN. They include most of the treatment required to manage the patient's condition. This type of order is performed by the patient care staff and rarely involves other departments except for supplies to carry out a procedure. Because of the broad range of patient care activities required, it is difficult to effectively categorize them here. The following are examples of patient care procedure orders: vital signs and weights *(VS q4h, wt qd);* activity *(BR, UAL, OOB);* positioning and body alignment *(elevate HOB, Fowler's position);* observation *(circ check, neuro check);* I&O; dressings *(wound dressing change bid);* elimination and catheterizations *(SS enema, cath prn);* bedside testing *(Accucheck ac and hs);* personal hygiene *(may shampoo hair);* restraints; isolation; drains, tubes, and catheters; transfusions; suction and irrigation; binders; bandages; heat and cold applications; irrigations; comfort and safety measures; skin protection; and anything else a doctor may order for the patient to be carried out by the patient care team.

When transcribing patient care procedure orders the clerical worker's most important responsibility is to communicate the order to the appropriate person. Determining who will perform the task is regulated by the policies and procedures of the health care facility.

Laboratory Procedures

Laboratory tests are vital diagnostic tools for monitoring a patient's condition and for planning prescribed treatment. The physician may order various laboratory tests on blood, sputum, urine, stool, spinal fluid, and other tissues and fluids.

It is the clerical worker's responsibility to interpret abbreviations the physician uses to order laboratory tests. Laboratory requests will be either stat or routine. *Stat* indicates specimens are to be gathered immediately and sent to the laboratory to be run before all other laboratory requests. *Routine* laboratory work refers to tests that may be ordered on a scheduled basis, such as daily, or on a one-time basis, such as an admission battery. Specimens for most routine laboratory work are obtained each morning unless it is ordered for a specific time.

Once a physician's order for a laboratory test has been identified, the clerical worker's main concern is to complete the appropriate requisition form (or appropriately enter the order into the computer) to send to the laboratory with the specimen. With a little practice, most laboratory tests will become familiar. Utilize the laboratory guide from your institution for tests that are unfamiliar.

It is important to be familiar with the laboratory subdivisions in your institution. The size of the institution will determine the number and configuration of the laboratory area. In large institutions there may be many specialized divisions, while in smaller institutions there may be a general division. More specialized requests may be sent to outside laboratories. It would be nearly impossible to identify all possible divisions of the laboratory and tests performed in the divisions, but the following can be used for general guidelines:

Chemistry: Tests the amount of elements (for example—Na, K, Mg, glu, drug levels) in a specimen. May be performed on blood, urine, stool, spinal fluid, and any other body fluid.

Hematology: Tests the amount of cells (for example—CBC, Hgb, ESR) and their quality in a specimen. May be performed on blood, urine, stool, spinal fluid, and any other body fluid. Urinalysis is often performed by this division.

Coagulation (often combined with hematology): Tests the ability of the blood specimen to clot (for example—PT, PTT, bleeding time).

Microbiology (may also be referred to as bacteriology): Tests to identify and measure the amount of disease-causing microscopic organisms present in a specimen such as blood, urine, stool, sputum, vaginal secretions, wound drainage. Other subdivisions within the microbiology division: (1) *Bacteriology* (also known as bacti): Tests specimens by growing them in a culture, identifying the bacteria, and testing for antibiotic sensitivity. This process is called culture and sensitivity, or C&S. (2) *Serology* (or immunology): Tests body fluids for immune bodies present if exposed to disease (for example—HIV, hepatitis, legionella). (3) *Mycology:* Tests specimens to identify fungi. (4) *Parasitology:* Tests specimens for organisms that live off other organisms (for example—O&P).

Cytology (also known as pathology): Studies the cells obtained from body tissues to determine cell type and to detect cancer or a precancerous condition (for example—Pap smear, biopsies).

Blood bank: Responsible for typing and crossmatching of patient blood, obtaining blood for transfusions, storing blood components, and keeping records of blood transfusions and donors. Any order for blood or blood component transfusion automatically indicates that the blood will be typed and crossmatched. Type and crossmatch is the test that determines the patient's blood type and compatibility. Examples of blood bank requests—PRBC, platelets, FFP, direct and indirect Coombs.

Medications and IV Fluids

In many hospitals, transcription of medication orders also falls under the clerical components of the PCT role. In other hospitals, this task is given to a pharmacy technician or nursing personnel who may be more familiar with medications. It is important for anyone caring for the patient to know the different types of medications, dosing instructions, automatic stop orders, and the names of some common medications.

In general, administration of medications can be categorized into four types: routine, stat, one-time, and prn. Routine medications are those that are given at specified intervals throughout the day

Lasix 20 mg po bid

Stat medications are those that should be given immediately

Lasix 20 mg IV stat

One-time medications include any that should be given in preparation for a test or procedure

*Demerol 50 mg IM with atropine 0.4 mg IM
on call to OR*

PRN medications are given only if the patient needs or wants the medication

Dilaudid 1 mg IM q4hr prn pain

The PCT's familiarity with abbreviations will be beneficial when transcribing medication orders. Standard administration times are usually set for each patient care unit or hospital, based on abbreviations such as bid, qd, hs, tid. It is important to know these times if the PCT will be transcribing medication orders onto an MAR or into a computer system.

Even though a patient care unit may have standard administration times, administration of some medications will not fit into a normal schedule. This is determined by the type of medication. For example, *antibiotics* are usually given around the clock unless ordered differently by the physician. Common antibiotics include penicillin, gentamicin, tobramycin, amikacin, bactrim, Cleocin, Keflex, Unasyn and cefaclor. *Anticoagulants* such as Coumadin (warfarin) and heparin are usually scheduled at specific times also. *Hypoglycemic* medications needed by diabetic patients are usually given before meals. Common hypoglycemic medications include regular Insulin, Lente Insulin, NPH Insulin, Tolinase, glipizide, Micronase, Orinase and Diabinese. *Cardiac* and *antihypertensive* medications for patients with heart and blood pressure problems are routinely given around the clock. Common medications in this class include digoxin (Lanoxin), Lopressor, Apresoline, Minipress, Vasotec, atenolol, quinidine, procainamide, verapamil, nitroglycerin, Cardizem, isosorbide dinitrate, and Capoten. *Pulmonary* medications such as theophylline, Slo-bid and terbutaline are also normally given around the clock. *Narcotic* medications to help alleviate a patient's pain include Demerol (meperidine), Dilaudid (hydromorphone), Seconal, morphine, pentobarbital, Percodan, Percocet, codeine, phenobarbital and fentanyl. *Laxatives* help alleviate a patient's constipation. They are usually given on an as-needed basis. Common laxatives include Colace, Dialose, Dulcolax, Metamucil, milk of magnesia, Peri-Colace, and Doxidan. *Sleep* medications help a patient get to sleep. Common sleep-inducing medications include Dalmane, Halcion, Restoril, Seconal, and Placidyl.

Physicians' orders for narcotics automatically expire in 3 days (72 hours). To be given longer than that, the physician must write another order. Anticoagulant medication orders also expire in 3 days. Antibiotic orders expire at different times, depending on their intended use.

Intravenous solutions are also considered medications as they are dispensed from the pharmacy. These include maintenance solutions, "drips," and intravenous piggyback medications. Maintenance solutions include mixtures of dextrose, sodium, and/or chloride concentrations and sometimes some additives such as potassium. These solutions are always ordered with specifics about the solution and a rate:

D5.45 NaCl c̄ 20 mEq KCl at 75 cc/hr

Drips are solutions of a specific medication such as aminophylline, dobutamine, dopamine, insulin, and heparin. These medications are almost always given using an IV pump to regulate the amount of fluid in drops (gtts) per minute. They will be ordered similarly to a maintenance solution.

Heparin 5000 units in 500 cc D5W at 30 gtts/min

Intravenous piggyback (IVPB) medications are ordered with a frequency

Ancef 1 gm IVPB q6 hr

Miscellaneous orders

This is a catchall group for any orders not included in the previous list. A miscellaneous order usually indicates a special task to be performed or some type of limitation to be understood. Examples of miscellaneous orders: consults with other departments or physicians, leave of absence, restraints, requests for medical records or X-rays, DNR, and no release of information orders.

SUMMARY

As health care changes, the roles and responsibilities performed by health care workers will also change. In many parts of the country, the clerical role is being incorporated into the role of the PCT. Success in the clerical aspects of the PCT role will involve additional training specific to the institution and its policies and procedures.

Electrocardiogram

JUANITA McDONOUGH, MN, RN,C, CCRN

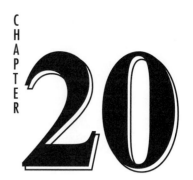

PREREQUISITE KNOWLEDGE AND SKILLS

- Basic anatomy of the chest
- Basic anatomy of the heart

OBJECTIVES

After you complete this chapter, you will be able to:

- State purpose of 12-lead ECG.

- List major structures of the heart.

- Describe the flow of blood through the body.

- Describe the normal electrical pathway of the heart, including the relationship between rhythm strips and electrical activity.

- Demonstrate the correct site location, preparation, and lead placement for a 12-lead ECG using a manikin or student model.

- Obtain a 12-lead ECG using a portable ECG unit and a student model.

- Identify potential causes and interventions when a poor tracing occurs.

- List common emergency clinical situations and describe the role of the patient care technician (PCT) in these situations.

- Recognize common dangerous rhythms that need reporting to the RN.

- Identify methods of preparing children for procedures.

- Discuss special considerations for lead placement when obtaining a 12-lead ECG from a child.

K E Y   T E R M S

Artery   Blood vessel that carries blood away from the heart

Atria   Chambers of the heart that receive blood

Automaticity   Heart's ability to generate and transmit an impulse without stimulation from nervous system

Capillary   Smallest blood vessel. Food and oxygen pass from the capillaries to the cells in exchange for waste products

Diastole   Resting phase of the cardiac cycle during which the heart muscle relaxes and the chambers fill with blood

Electrical Conduction   Process of impulses traveling through the cardiac cells causing the heart muscle to contract and relax, and thus causing heart to beat

Electrocardiogram (ECG)/12-lead ECG   Recording of the electrical impulses of the heart; often referred to as a 12-lead ECG since it provides 12 different recordings, or views, of the heart's electrical activity

Intercostal   Between ribs

Leads   "Pictures" of heart taken from different angles

Systole   Phase in cardiac cycle during which heart contracts, propelling the blood out of the ventricles and into the pulmonary and systemic circulations

Vein   Blood vessel that carries blood toward heart

Ventricles   Chambers of heart that pump blood

Electrocardiograms (ECGs) are recordings of electrical impulses of the heart. The ECG is recorded by applying electrodes to specific locations on the body surface and connecting them to a 12-lead electrocardiograph. Electrocardiograms are often referred to as 12-lead ECGs since they provide 12 different recordings, or "pictures," of the heart's electrical activity. Some institutions interchange the terms ECG and EKG; both terms are acceptable. The ECG records the amount of voltage generated by the heart and the time required for that voltage to travel through heart tissue.* It is one of the tools utilized by the physician to determine conditions of the heart, such as: (1) heart rate and rhythm; (2) evidence of a new or past heart attack; (3) disturbances due to electrolyte imbalance (especially potassium) or cardiac medications; (4) enlarged or thickened chambers of the heart; (5) inflammation of the lining of the heart (endocardium); and (6) effectiveness as a pacemaker.†

STRUCTURES OF THE HEART

A brief review of the structures of the heart is helpful in understanding the heart's electrical activity. A more detailed description of the entire cardiovascular system is in Chapter 7.

The adult heart weighs less than 1 pound, and is about the size of a fist. It lies diagonally in the mediastinum, an area above the diaphragm and between the lungs. A major part of the heart wall is made up of cardiac muscle (Fig. 20–1).

Chambers

The heart has four chambers: the right atrium, left atrium, right ventricle, and left ventricle. The atria are smaller than the ventricles and have thinner walls. The atria *receive blood* and the ventricles *pump blood*. The right atrium receives blood from the head, arms, and trunk of the body. The left atrium receives blood from the lungs. The right ventricle pumps blood to the lungs for oxygenation. The left ventricle, which has the task of pumping blood to all parts of the body, is the heart's most muscular chamber.

Valves

Atrioventricular valves are located between the atria and the ventricles and provide for one-way blood flow. The *tricuspid valve* allows the blood to flow from the right atrium to the right ventricle. The *mitral valve* allows the blood to flow from the left atrium to the left ventricle.

Semilunar valves are located between the ventricles

Electrocardiography: A Better Way. Booklet prepared by Burdick, Inc. Milton, Wisconsin, p. 12.

†*Goldschlagher, N. and Goldman, M.: Principles of Clinical Electrocardiography. East Norwalk, Connecticut, Appleton & Lang, 1989, p.1.*

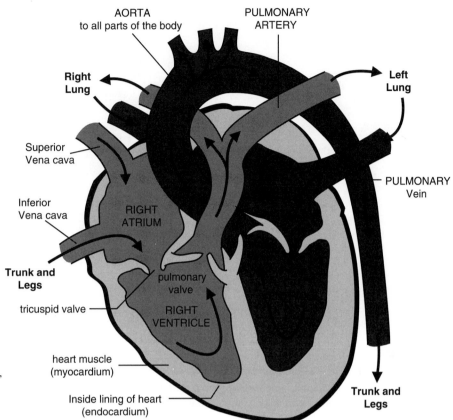

AORTA
to all parts of the body

PULMONARY
ARTERY

**Right
Lung**

**Left
Lung**

Superior
Vena cava

PULMONARY
Vein

Inferior
Vena cava

RIGHT
ATRIUM

**Trunk and
Legs**

pulmonary
valve

tricuspid valve

RIGHT
VENTRICLE

heart muscle
(myocardium)

**Trunk and
Legs**

Inside lining of heart
(endocardium)

FIGURE 20–1

Basic anatomy of the heart: right atrium,
right ventricle, inferior vena cava,
superior vena cava, and pulmonary
artery; left atrium, left ventricle, aorta,
pulmonary vein.

and the pulmonary artery and the aorta. The *pulmonary valve* allows the blood to flow from the right ventricle to the lungs. The *aortic valve* allows the blood to flow from the left ventricle to the systemic blood supply.

Great Vessels

Blood moves in and out of the heart through several large vessels. The right atrium receives venous blood from the systemic circulation through the *superior* and *inferior vena cava.* Blood leaves the right ventricle and enters the pulmonary circulation through the *pulmonary artery.* The pulmonary artery divides into right and left to transport blood from the heart to both the right and left lung. The four *pulmonary veins,* two from the right side of the heart and two from the left side, carry oxygenated blood from the lungs to the left atrium. The aorta delivers blood from the left ventricle to the systemic vessels that supply the body.

Blood Vessels

Arteries are vessels that take the blood *away* from the heart. *Veins* are vessels that *return* blood to the heart. Arteries and veins are connected by a network of tiny vessels called *capillaries.* The capillary walls are very thin, which enables them to provide a rapid exchange of oxygen and waste by-products between the blood and the cells.

CARDIAC CYCLE

Contraction and relaxation of the heart muscle produce a pumping action. Each contraction and the relaxation that follows constitute a cardiac cycle (Fig. 20–2). During relaxation, termed *diastole,* blood fills the ventricles. The contraction that follows, termed *systole,* propels the blood out of the ventricles and into the pulmonary or systemic circulation.

During diastole, systemic blood from the head and arms returns to the right atrium from the *superior vena cava.* Blood from the trunk and legs returns to the right atrium through the *inferior vena cava.* The right atrium fills and distends, pushing open the tricuspid valve. This permits blood to fill the right ventricle. At the same time, blood from the pulmonary circulation is carried via the pulmonary veins to the left atrium. As the left atrium fills, it pushes the mitral valve open, and blood flows into the left ventricle.

During systole, the heart muscle contracts, creating pressure that opens the pulmonary and aortic valves. Blood is ejected into the pulmonary and systemic circulation.

ELECTRICAL ACTIVITY OF THE HEART

Continuous, rhythmic repetition of the cardiac cycle (systole and diastole) depends on the continuous, rhyth-

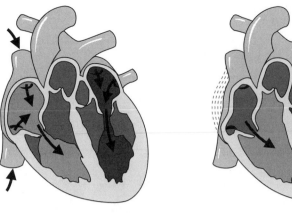

During diastole, the ventricles and atria fill passively

The atria contract, squeezing blood into the ventricles

During systole, the ventricles contract, squeezing blood into the aorta and pulmonary arteries

F I G U R E   2 0 – 2

Diagrams of three hearts with arrows showing flow of blood during the cardiac cycle.

mic transmission of electrical impulses. As the electrical impulse passes from cardiac cell to cell, it stimulates the muscle to contract. After the impulse passes, the muscle relaxes. This process—impulses traveling through the cardiac cells causing the heart muscle to contract and relax and thus causing the heart to beat—is called *electrical conduction.*

The heart has the ability to transmit an impulse without stimulation from the nervous system. This automatic pacemaker—the ability of the heart to generate and transmit its own electrical impulse—is called *automaticity.*

Electrical Pathways

The heart's contraction begins with an impulse generated by specialized cells in the sinoatrial node (SA node) in the right atrium near the superior vena cava (Fig. 20–3). These cells trigger a chain reaction that sends the impulse to the atrioventricular node (AV node). The electrical impulse continues on through the Bundle of His to the right and left bundle branches, and through the Purkinje network. The impulse travels throughout the heart with a wave of muscle contraction following close behind. The voltage created by this impulse can be detected on the skin and recorded by the electrocardiograph.

Combining Electrical and Mechanical Events

Electrical impulses are recorded on the ECG graph paper. The ECG complexes, or tracings, are described with certain letters and combinations of letters, for example, P, QRS, and T. Each impulse causes a mechanical event (atrial or ventricular contraction) that is recorded on the graph paper.

The impulse leaving the SA node causes the atria to contract and is recorded on the graph paper as a *P*

wave (Fig. 20–4). Ventricular contraction, caused by the impulse traveling through the pathways to the Purkinje network, is recorded on the graph paper as the *QRS complex.* The *T wave* represents the heart's resting period, as the cells prepare themselves for another impulse.

INDICATIONS FOR AN ELECTROCARDIOGRAM

The physician will order an ECG to be obtained "routine" or "stat." Routine ECGs are usually obtained in the early morning so that they will be available for the physician during morning patient rounds. Routine ECGs may also be ordered as part of the preparation for a

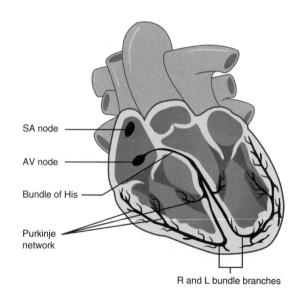

SA node

AV node

Bundle of His

Purkinje network

R and L bundle branches

F I G U R E   2 0 – 3

Normal conduction pathways.

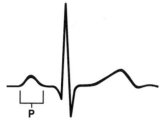

The P wave represents
the impulse that causes
the atria to contract

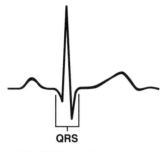

QRS

The QRS complex
represents the impulse
that causes ventricular
contraction

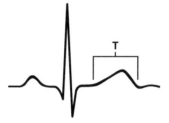

T

The T wave represents
the phases in which the cells
prepare themselves for
another impulse

FIGURE 20–4

Relationship between rhythm strips and electrical activity.

procedure, such as an operation or cardiac catheterization.

 Stat ECGs need to be obtained without delay.

A stat ECG will be ordered anytime the physician needs *immediate* information, as when the patient is experiencing chest pain or changes in his or her cardiac rhythm. Often, stat ECGs are requested during emergency situations. It is important that the patient care technician's (PCT's) speech and actions be calm and competent so that the patient does not become frightened. Be careful not to make statements that might alarm the patient or family members.

EQUIPMENT

Electrocardiograph

The electrocardiograph (Fig. 20–5) is the instrument used to obtain the 12-lead ECG. Today's instruments represent the state of the art in electronics. They are portable and easy to use. A basic understanding of the functions of the instrument is an essential part of your training.

The three basic functions of the electrocardiograph are *input, signal processing,* and *output display.*

INPUT. Sensors in the electrocardiograph serve as receiving antennas for the electrical activity of the heart. Electrodes placed on the patient direct the impulse into the ECG instrument for processing and display.

SIGNAL PROCESSING. Inside the instrument is the solid-state circuitry, which amplifies the signal (impulse) and converts the electrical activity into mechanical action on the display.

OUTPUT DISPLAY. The output is displayed on paper. Older instruments, referred to as *analog ECG machines,* write with heat in the tip of a stylus. The heated stylus reacts with chemically treated paper to produce an ECG tracing. Analog machines require a standardization test before each use. Refer to the equipment manual for specific standardization instructions. It takes only a few seconds and will ensure that the machine is recording correctly.

Newer digital machines utilize thermal array technology, which is achieved by heating dots as the paper moves across the printhead. Digital machines require no manual standardization adjustments, since the machine will automatically adjust itself.

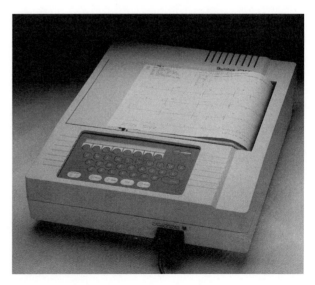

FIGURE 20–5

Electrocardiograph. (Courtesy of Burdick Corporation.)

ECG Electrodes

Electrodes are used on the limbs and the chest to "collect" the electrical impulses and feed them into the ECG instrument. Often the electrodes are referred to as sensors. Both terms are acceptable. Some patients may prefer being connected to a "sensor" rather than an "electrode." Reusable electrodes (Fig. 20–6) require special conduction gel. Disposable electrodes (Fig. 20–7) are an alternative to bulbs and gels; they eliminate the potential for cross-contamination and leave no messy cleanup after removal.

STOP However, disposables must be removed after each use. If left in place, they can scorch the skin in the event that the patient requires defibrillation during CPR. Be aware that mixing disposable electrodes with reusable electrodes can produce an unreliable ECG tracing.

Paper

ECG graph paper is specially marked to assist with measuring the ECG complex and allowing physicians to interpret cardiac voltage. Keep your machine stocked with plenty of paper.

PATIENT PREPARATION

Consult

An order is required to obtain an ECG. Complete the necessary paperwork for the consult. The consult should state why the ECG is being ordered (for example, chest pain, fainting, rhythm problems). A copy of the ECG and the consult must be sent to the electrocardiography department or the physician for interpretation.

Incomplete or inaccurate paperwork will delay the interpretation and processing of the ECG.

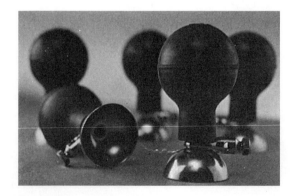

F I G U R E 2 0 – 6
Reusable electrodes.

The consult needs to be completed thoroughly for proper processing. A consult generally includes the patient's name, ID number, primary or requesting physician, consulting department (i.e., Cardiology), procedure requested (i.e., 12-lead ECG), admitting diagnosis, a list of cardiac medications the patient is taking, and pertinent patient information such as a history of chest pain.

Patient Relaxation

The ECG will have better quality tracing if your patient is relaxed and comfortable during the procedure. Smile, try a friendly greeting, explain the procedure, and answer any questions. Assure the patient that the procedure is harmless and painless. Your calm, competent manner will help him or her to relax.

Patient Comfort and Privacy

Have the patient lie on a bed or examining table with arms placed comfortably at his or her side. Use a small pillow to support the head; if the patient is uncomfortable, place an extra pillow beneath the knees for additional comfort. If necessary, have the patient remove any clothing above the waist and uncover the lower legs, but provide privacy by closing the door or drawing the curtain around the bed. Keep the patient covered until it is time for electrode placement.

Recording Position

Many PCTs find it most convenient to work from the patient's left side—where the heart is. Plug the cord into a power source *away* from the patient. Never run the power cord under the patient's bed. This precaution helps prevent electrical interference in your recordings.

Skin Preparation and Patients with Special Considerations

Skin is a poor conductor of electricity. Use of a gel with the reusable electrodes and the gelatin backing on the disposable electrodes help to maximize "pickup" of the impulse from the skin. A few minutes spent preparing the skin will help prevent the need to repeat the procedure because of a poor-quality tracing.

OILY SKIN. Rub the skin with an alcohol pad where the electrode will be placed. Acetone (applied with a 4 × 4 gauze) can also be used to help remove skin oils and lotion, increasing the conductivity of the skin. Dry the skin with a gauze pad. Do not be afraid to rub briskly.

DIAPHORESIS. Diaphoretic, or sweaty, patients need to have the skin prepped first with alcohol and then allowed to dry, both to cool the skin and assist with the evaporative effect. Next, prepare the skin with acetone, again letting it dry thoroughly before placing the electrodes.

HAIRY CHEST. Attempt to separate hairs to allow for electrode placement. If necessary, shave the chest,

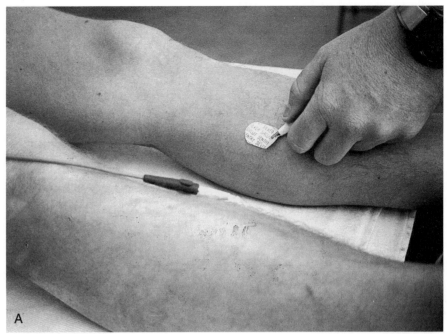

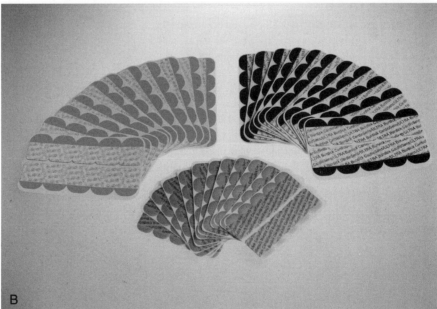

FIGURE 20-7
A and *B*, Disposable electrodes.
(Part B, courtesy of Burdick
Corporation.)

but *only* where the electrode will be placed. Obtain permission from the patient. Assure him that a tiny area is sufficient. Rub the shaved area with an alcohol pad and let the skin dry before placing the electrodes.

TREMORS. If your patient has tremors due to medications or a medical condition (Parkinson's disease, elevated temperature), placement of the arm electrodes onto the shoulders will help decrease the tremor's effect on the quality of the tracing. At times, the clinician will simply attempt to get the best-quality tracing possible then make a notation about the tremors on the consult or ECG tracing.

LARGE-BREASTED WOMEN. Placement of the chest electrodes does not change if a female patient has large breasts. Simply lift the left breast and place the electrodes (V_4 and V_5 will be most affected) in the proper location.

If the patient has a bandage or injury preventing proper lead placement, make a note of this on the consult and tracing. Do your best to place leads as accurately as possible.

LEAD PLACEMENT

Lead placement includes *limb leads,* in which electrodes are placed on the patient's arms and legs, and

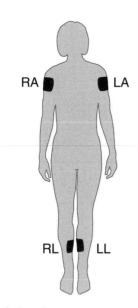

F I G U R E 2 0 – 8

Electrode placement for limb leads.

chest leads, in which electrodes are placed in specific locations on the chest surface. The limb leads are used to record six leads, or pictures, of the heart. Lead 1, lead 2, and lead 3 are called *standard limb leads*. The *augmented limb leads* include aV_R, aV_L, and aV_F. The chest leads include V_1, V_2, V_3, V_4, V_5, and V_6. Together, the limb leads and chest leads total the 12 leads viewed on the standard 12-lead ECG. Remember, precise lead placement is essential. Improper lead placement may produce an inaccurate ECG and one that is not reproducible.

Limb and Augmented Leads

The electrodes are placed on fleshy parts of the limbs—*never* on wrists, ankles, or shins (Fig. 20–8). The

fleshy part minimizes the chance of unwanted muscle artifact, or interference, in your recordings. If the patient has had a limb amputated, place the electrode above the amputated site.

Chest Leads

Knowing the precise placement positions for the 6 chest electrodes is essential (Fig. 20–9). It is necessary, first, to find the correct intercostal positions (intercostal means "between the ribs"). The first intercostal space is between the first and second ribs, *not* between the clavicle and the first rib. (Note: the clavical does not count as a rib.) Placement of the electrodes:

V_1: At the fourth intercostal space at the right margin of the sternum

V_2: At the fourth intercostal space at the left margin of the sternum

V_3: Midway between position V_2 and V_4

V_4: At the fifth intercostal space at the left midclavicular line. In most patients, this will fall directly below the nipple line

V_5: At the level of V_4, but on the left anterior axillary line

V_6: At the position of V_4, but on the midaxillary line (center of the armpit)

CONNECTING THE CABLES

Position the connectors so that the cables point *toward* the patient's feet (Fig. 20–10). Avoid large loops. Make sure the lead cable lies flat against the patient and follows the contour of the body (Fig. 20–11).

Do not forget to make sure that the proper lead wire is

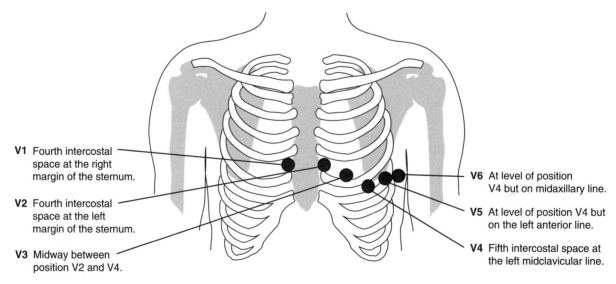

V1 Fourth intercostal space at the right margin of the sternum.

V2 Fourth intercostal space at the left margin of the sternum.

V3 Midway between position V2 and V4.

V6 At level of position V4 but on midaxillary line.

V5 At level of position V4 but on the left anterior line.

V4 Fifth intercostal space at the left midclavicular line.

F I G U R E 2 0 – 9

Placement of chest electrodes.

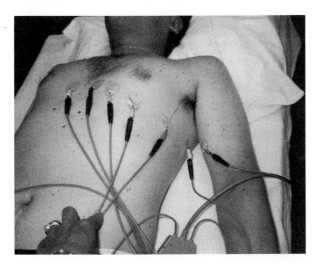

F I G U R E 2 0 – 1 0
V lead placement on chest.

connected to the proper electrode (refer to color code, Fig. 20–12). The lead wires are color-coded and stamped with abbreviations (RA for right arm, and so on).

OBTAINING A TRACING USING THE BURDICK 550 MACHINE (DIGITAL MACHINE)

In general, most electrocardiographs operate with similar instrumentation. The steps utilized with the Burdick

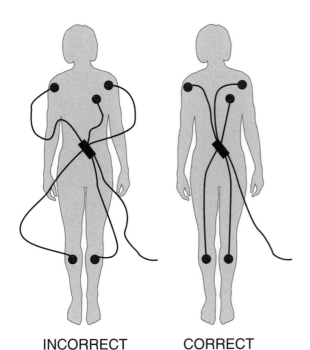

INCORRECT   CORRECT

F I G U R E 2 0 – 1 1
Incorrect and correct cable placement.

STANDARD LIMB LEADS			
LEAD	SENSORS CONNECTED	CODE COLOR	
			BODY
LEAD 1	LA and RA	RL	GREEN
LEAD 2	LL and RA	LL	RED
LEAD 3	LL and LA	RA	WHITE
		LA	BLACK

AUGMENTED LIMB LEADS			
LEAD	SENSORS CONNECTED	CODE COLOR	
			BODY
aV_R	RA and (LA-LL)	RL	GREEN
aV_L	LA and (RA-LL)	LL	RED
aV_F	LL and (RA-LA)	RA	WHITE
		LA	BLACK

CHEST LEADS				
LEAD	SENSORS CONNECTED		CODE COLOR	
			BODY	INERT
V_1	V_1 and (LA-RA-LL)	V_1	BROWN	RED
V_2	V_2 and (LA-RA-LL)	V_2	BROWN	YELLOW
V_3	V_3 and (LA-RA-LL)	V_3	BROWN	GREEN
V_4	V_4 and (LA-RA-LL)	V_4	BROWN	BLUE
V_5	V_5 and (LA-RA-LL)	V_5	BROWN	ORANGE
V_6	V_6 and (LA-RA-LL)	V_6	BROWN	VIOLET

F I G U R E 2 0 – 1 2
Lead arrangement and coding.

550 machine will apply to most digital electrocardiographs.

When the patient is comfortably positioned and the limb leads and chest leads have been properly placed, you are ready to obtain the ECG.

1. Plug in the portable electrocardiograph.
2. Push power button "on."
3. Main menu will appear on screen; press "ACQUIRE ECG."
4. Press EDIT.
5. Enter patient information:
   Last name
   First name
   Patient ID number
   Age
   Sex
   Race
   Location
   Clinician's initials or identification number
6. Press "ACQUIRE ECG."
7. Press "ACQUIRE 12 LEAD."
8. ECG will print out. The machine will automatically print two ECGs.

9. Write on ECG any variations in lead placement or reason for poor-quality tracing (eg, patient tremors).

10. Screen will read "COMPLETION OF SAVE."
   • directory will appear (save only ECG tracings that are to be read by the physician)

11. Turn off machine.

12. Remove electrodes from limbs and chest. If a gel was used, clean sites with gauze or a warm washcloth.

13. Assist patient to a comfortable position and re-place blanket for warmth.

🛑 **STOP** Return bed to low position, have siderails up if ordered, place the patient's call light within reach.

14. Place one copy of the ECG in the patient's chart.

✍ Send the second copy of the ECG with the consult to be read by the physician. Include billing information at this time, if this is your employer's policy.

OBTAINING AN ECG USING AN ANALOG (STYLUS) ELECTROCARDIOGRAPH

Patient preparation and lead placement remain the same regardless of the type of electrocardiograph. The analog machine uses a hot stylus to "draw" a picture of the ECG tracings.

1. Plug in the machine.

2. Turn lead selector switch to STD and adjust stylus to center of graph paper.

3. Move record switch to 25-mm-per-second position and run for a few seconds to adjust centering of stylus. Perform standardization test at this time. Refer to equipment manual for specific standardization instructions.

4. Turn lead selector to leads I, II, III and run 8–12 inches of tracing. Proceed in same manner for leads aV_R, aV_L, aV_F.

5. Turn lead selector switch to V leads and run 4–6 inches of recording of each lead. You may need to readjust the stylus as you proceed through the V leads.

6. Obtain two tracings: one for the patient's chart and one to be sent to the physician for interpretation.

7. Tear off tracing from the machine. Immediately mark it with the patient's name, ID number, age, room number, the day's date and time, and your initials or identification number.

8. Write on ECG any variations in lead placement or reason for poor-quality tracing (eg, patient tremors).

9. Turn off machine.

10. Remove electrodes from limbs and chest. If a gel was used, clean sites with gauze or a warm washcloth.

11. Assist patient to a comfortable position and re-place blanket for warmth.

🛑 **STOP** Return bed to low position, have siderails up if ordered, and place the patient's call light within reach.

12. Place one copy of the ECG in the patient's chart.

✍ Send the second copy of the ECG with the consult to be read by the physician. Include billing information at this time, if this is your employer's policy.

Transmission by Modem

Your institution may have a method of sending ECGs through a phone jack, commonly called modem transmission. A phone line is plugged into the electrocardiograph, and all ECGs are transmitted to a receiving line, generally in the Cardiology Department.

🎓 Refer to the equipment manual for specific modem transmission instructions. Frequency of transmission will depend on your institution's policies.

Troubleshooting

If the ECG recorded only cardiac voltage, the PCT would obtain a flawless ECG tracing every time. Unfortunately, the electrocardiograph records every kind of electrical voltage it can find. As a result, artifact, or interference, from muscle movement, respirations, or electrical voltage in the room can make the tracing difficult to read. Also, improper skin preparation or electrode application can increase skin impedance. High impedance will hamper the ability of the electrode to send the impulse to the electrocardiograph. Refer to Figure 20–13 for a troubleshooting guide.

NO BASELINE TRACING. If the ECG has no baseline tracing, check your machine cable and all connections. Once you have established that all cables and connections are correct, check the machine to ensure that it is set to obtain a tracing.

BASELINE WANDER. If you are convinced your patient is lying still, yet the tracing appears to wander or drift, check for the following problems:

1. Improper electrode application: Electrodes that are applied by straps may be applied too tightly or too loosely. Mixing reusable electrodes with disposable electrodes may cause baseline wander.

2. Improper gel application: Too little gel or the wrong type of gel can also cause baseline wander. Do not use ultrasound gel. Make sure the conduction gel is designed for ECGs. Check disposable electrodes for drying.

	Skin Impedance	Muscle Movement	Electrical Continuity	Electrode
No Base Line			Check all connections Check ECG machine set-up	Check for dry-out; insufficient gel
Base Line Wander	Prep skin Rub briskly with gauze	Stop patient movement	Check ground connection	Dirty electrodes or cables Check for mixed electrodes
Intermittent Signal			Check for loose connections	Check for dry-out Check for loose electrode

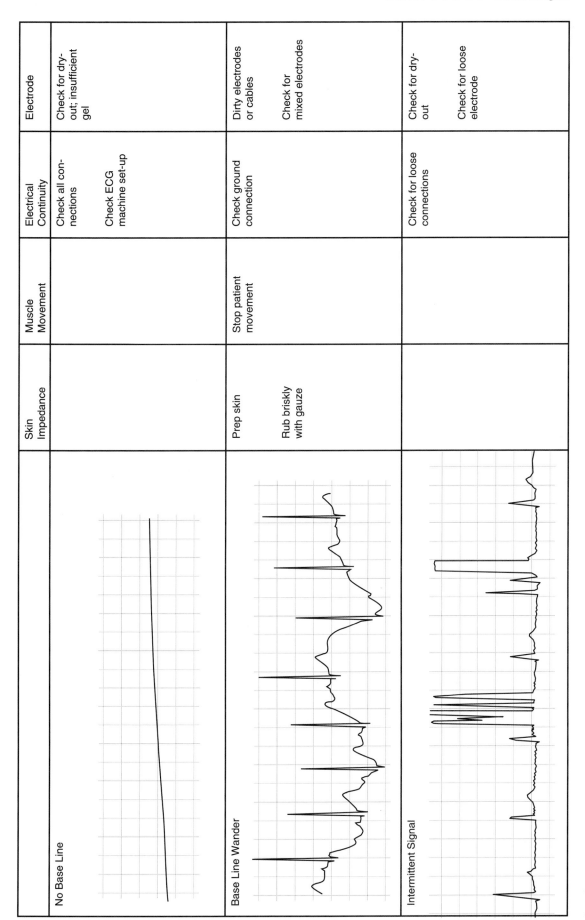

FIGURE 20-13
Troubleshooting guide.

	Skin Impedance	Muscle Movement	Electrical Continuity	Electrode
"60-Cycle" / AC Noise	Prep skin; Rub briskly with gauze	May be caused by uncontrollable muscle tremor; Try relaxation techniques; Check for patient touching metal	Check ground connection; Turn off fluorescent lights and other equipment; Check for cable position; No loops away from a cord	Check for dry-out; insufficient gel; Dirty electrodes or cables
Motion Artifact	Prep skin; Rub briskly with gauze	Stop patient movement; Move limb electrodes; Try relaxation techniques	Turn off fluorescent lights and other equipment; Check for loose connections	Check for dry-out; Check for loose electrode
Low Amplitude	Prep skin; Rub briskly with gauze		Check gain setting	Recheck electrode and cable placement; Check for dry-out

FIGURE 20-13
Continued

3. Poor skin impedance: Reevaluate your skin preparation. Rub area briskly with alcohol pad and let the skin dry before attaching electrodes.

4. Dirty electrodes: Check the reusable electrodes for cleanliness. Gels can cause erosion, which will decrease the electrodes' ability to conduct the impulses. Clean the electrodes and cables after each use.

5. Using reusable and disposable electrodes: Remember that mixing reusable electrodes with disposable electrodes may cause an unstable ECG tracing.

6. Electrical continuity: Check the power cord for a proper ground connection (must have a *3-prong* plug), and check the cable for proper attachment.

AC NOISE. Also known as 60-cycle interference, AC noise is caused by electrical activity. Check for the following:

1. Poor skin impedance: Reevaluate your skin preparation. Rub area briskly with alcohol pad and let the skin dry before attaching electrodes.

2. Electrical continuity: Check the power cord plug for a proper ground connection (must have a *3-prong* plug) and check the cable for proper attachment.

3. Improper gel application: Too little gel on reusable electrodes can cause AC interference. Check disposable electrodes for drying.

4. Electrical interference from other machines and equipment: Check to make sure the electrical cord is plugged into an outlet *away* from the electrocardiograph. If possible, turn off the equipment that is the likely interference source. Be sure to check with the RN before turning off any machines. Often, rotating the patient's bed away from the direction of the probable source of interference is sufficient to obtain a good ECG tracing. Even fluorescent lights can cause AC interference; turn off lights.

5. Looping of cables: Position the connectors so that the cables point *toward* the patient's feet (see Fig. 20–10). Avoid large loops. Make sure the lead cable lies flat against the patient and follows the contour of the body (see Fig. 20–11).

6. Patient position: Check to see that the patient's limbs are not in contact with the bed frame or other metal.

7. Tremors: On rare occasion, a 60-cycle effect can be seen with fine muscle tremors. Be certain the electrodes are placed on fleshy parts of the limbs. Have the patient place hands—palms down—under the buttocks. If this does not decrease the tremors, have the patient shake the limbs and then relax. Ask the patient to breathe deeply. Obtain the best possible tracing and make a notation on the ECG.

INTERMITTENT SIGNAL. Instability of the tracing may cause a signal to "come and go," leaving an intermittent ECG recording. Check for the following:

1. Electrical continuity: Check the power cord for a proper ground connection (must have a *3-prong* plug) and check the cable for proper attachment.

2. Poor connections: Check cables and electrodes for loose connections or improper application. The green, or ground, lead is most often the cable causing interference.

MOTION ARTIFACT. Also known as somatic tremor, motion artifact is caused by muscle movement. Check for the following:

1. Patient anxiety: Perhaps the patient is apprehensive about the procedure or worried about the results of the ECG. Attempt to alleviate any fears or concerns. Utilize distraction techniques such as asking the patient to stare at a spot on the ceiling or to count backward from 100. If possible, postpone the ECG until the patient is less anxious.

2. Involuntary muscle movement: Tremors and uncontrollable muscle jerks may be associated with nervous disorders. Be certain the electrodes are placed on fleshy parts of the limbs. Have the patient place hands—palms down—under the buttocks. If this does not decrease the tremors, have the patient shake the limbs and then relax. Ask the patient to breathe deeply. Obtain the best possible tracing and make a notation on the ECG.

3. Poor connections: Check cables and electrodes for loose connections or improper application. Prep the skin with an alcohol pad.

LOW AMPLITUDE. Low amplitude will cause the tracing to be small and unreliable. Check for the following:

1. Poor connections: Check cables and electrodes for loose connections or improper application. Prep the skin with an alcohol pad.

2. Equipment adjustment: Check the ECG gain settings and adjust for a higher gain.

DANGEROUS RHYTHMS/WHEN TO GET HELP—RIGHT NOW!

The ECG tracing is read and interpreted by the physician, and the PCT's job is to obtain the tracing. You may, however, observe some unusual rhythm or rate changes that will require immediate notification of the RN. Remain calm. Be careful not to make statements that might alarm the patient or family members.

Bradycardia, or excessively slow heart rate, (Fig. 20–14) can make the patient feel lightheaded and weak. If you observe a heart rate less than 60 or if the patient complains of dizziness or sweating, notify the RN immediately.

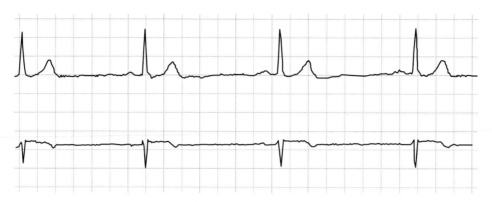

FIGURE 20–14
Bradycardia.

Tachycardia, or excessively fast heart rate, (Fig. 20–15) can also cause the patient to feel lightheaded. If you observe a heart rate greater than 110, notify the RN immediately.

Abnormal rhythm: If the patient's ECG shows beats that are wide and bizarre compared to the other beats (Fig. 20–16), notify the RN. Abnormal beats may be a sign of heart problems.

Chest pain: If the patient complains of chest pain, discomfort, or shortness of breath, notify the RN immediately. Stay with the patient until the RN and physician have evaluated the patient's status. Be prepared to obtain a stat ECG. Remember that your calm, competent manner will help the patient remain calm. Do not say anything that will alarm the patient.

PEDIATRIC ECGs

Preparing a Child for an ECG

Children are less anxious about a procedure when given specific rather than general information. For exam-

ple, "We are going to do a test," may alarm a youngster. Introduce yourself to the child; tell him about the procedure and allow time for questions; use nonthreatening words like stickers or "stickies" rather than electrodes. For example, "Hi, _____ . My name is _____ . I have a special machine that will tell how your heart is working. It won't hurt at all. Just like it doesn't hurt when you have your picture taken with a camera. I am going to put these stickers on your arms, legs, and chest. Now hold very still so the machine can draw the picture." Older children can participate by applying the arm and leg electrodes.

If the child is apprehensive, demonstrate electrode placement using a toy or a parent's arm. Encourage parents to stay in the room. For infants and very young children, have parent gently hold the child in a relaxed manner on his or her lap. By contrast, adolescents may prefer to be alone. Attempt to soothe the infant with a pacifier or a bottle. At times, an ECG for an irritable infant may need to wait until the baby falls asleep.

After you have obtained the ECG, talk about the procedure. Provide support and positive feedback. Stickers, verbal praise, or a trip to the playroom can reward a child for his cooperation. In a pinch, disposable electrodes can be used as "prizes."

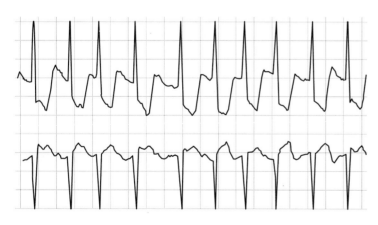

FIGURE 20–15
Tachycardia.

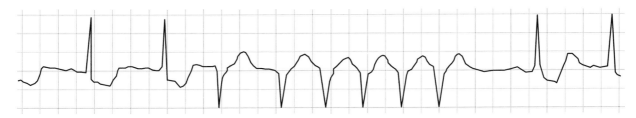

F I G U R E 2 0 – 1 6
Abnormal beats.

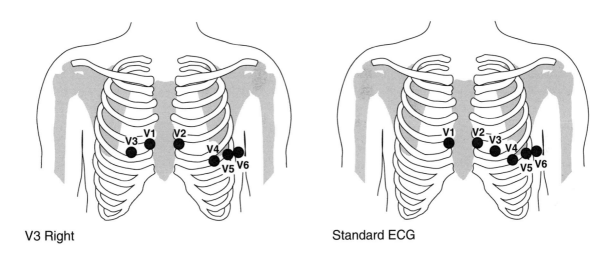

V3 Right   Standard ECG

The placement of the 11 electrodes for a pediatric ECG

Chest Leads: (may need to trim sensors)

V1   4th Intercostal Space, *Immediately to the right of sternum*

V2   4th Intercostal Space, *Immediately to the left of sternum*

V4   5th Intercostal Space in the mid-clavicular line**
          **note: V4 must be placed prior to V3.

V3   Placed between V2 & V4

V3   Right: Placed in exactly the V3 position only on the right side
          of the chest***
          ***note: This is done on pediatric patients from 0-10 years old.

V5   In the anterior axillary line horizontal to V4

V6   In the mid axillary line horizontal to V4

Limb Leads:

RA	Right arm, upper arm	full size sensor
LA	Left arm, upper arm	full size sensor
RL	Right leg	full size sensor
LL	Left leg	full size sensor

Remember: When doing pediatric ECGs, you must do two separate ECGs
with age groups for 0 to 10 years. One is done normal as
in all other age groups and the other is done with the V3
Right.

F I G U R E 2 0 – 1 7
Lead placement in children.

Lead Placement

Disposable electrodes for the chest leads may need to be cut lengthwise if the patient's chest is too small. Trim as little as possible. Limb leads do not need trimming except for use with very small or premature newborns. Obtain an ECG using standard electrode placement and procedure. V_6 must be placed precisely in the midaxillary line, since it offers the best view of the left ventricle. Proper placement is especially important in small children, because even small differences in electrode location can make a difference in the ECG.

For children 10 years and younger, obtain an additional tracing with V_3 placed in exactly the V_3 position but on the *right* side of the chest (Fig. 20–17). The second tracing, with the V_3 sensor on the right side, is called a V_3 *Right*. We obtain a V_3 Right on infants and children for two reasons: (1) The chest gets too crowded with all 6 sensors on the left side. (2) Infants are born with a certain degree of right ventricular enlargement. The V_3 Right position offers a good view of the right ventricle.

✓ If the electrocardiograph has filters, make sure they are turned off when obtaining ECGs on children. Filters are used to decrease artifact, but in children they will distort the QRS complexes and alter the ECG.

SUMMARY

A routine ECG offers 12 leads, or views, of the heart. The PCT utilizes precise lead placement to obtain an accurate, reliable tracing. The more you practice the art and science of electrocardiography, the more efficient you will become and the greater asset you will be to your health care team.

Venipuncture and Point of Care Testing

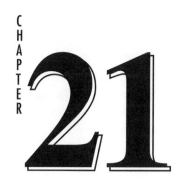

CHAPTER 21

MILDRED PERLIA, MSN, RN

ESTHER JONES, MS, RN

LORETTA PIOMBO BENTON, MS, RN

OUTLINE

General Principles for Venipuncture and Point of Care Testing

Venipuncture
Equipment/Supplies
Identification and Preparation of the Patient
Common Sites
Tourniquet
Cleansing the Site
Labeling
Infection Control
Storage/Processing
Quality Control
Reporting/Documentation Issues
Key Points

Blood Glucose Monitoring
Visual Method of Blood Glucose Monitoring

How Blood Glucose Meters Work
Quality Control
Infection Control
Supplies and Equipment
Patient Preparation
To Obtain a Capillary Blood Specimen
Lancing Devices
Reporting and Documenting Findings
Meter Maintenance
Key Points

Miscellaneous Specimen Testing
Stool Specimens
Test for Fecal Occult Blood
Gastric Specimens
Urine Specimens
Key Points

PREREQUISITE KNOWLEDGE AND SKILLS

- Universal precautions
- Personal protective equipment
- Urine and stool specimen collection
- General documentation principles
- Infection control methods
- Safety measures with hazardous waste
- Patient identification procedures

O B J E C T I V E S

After you complete this chapter, you will be able to:

- Explain how to prevent infections when performing specimen collection and testing procedures.
- Describe the procedure for venipuncture and capillary puncture.
- Identify common venipuncture sites.
- Describe how a blood glucose meter is used.

- Identify factors that affect the accuracy of blood glucose measurement.
- Participate in laboratory practice of selected specimen collection and testing procedures.
- Describe the quality control mechanisms required in specimen collection and testing procedures.
- Discuss competency requirements.

K E Y   T E R M S

Biohazardous Medical Waste   Waste contaminated with potentially infectious materials such as blood

Capillary   The smallest of the blood vessels; the blood vessel accessed in a finger or heel stick

Competency   Demonstration of proficiency for a given procedure

Glucose   Sugar

Infection Control   Measures taken to prevent the spread of infection

Ketones   Metabolic by-products that can be found in urine

Occult   Hidden or unseen

pH   Refers to the alkalinity or acidity of a solution

Quality Control   Measures to assure the accuracy and safety of a procedure and/or equipment

Universal Precautions   Infection control procedures used to prevent contact or potential contact with blood or body fluids

Venipuncture   Puncture of a vein

Venipuncture and point of care testing are procedures performed daily in most hospitals. Especially with the development of glucometers, capillary blood testing has become routine and provides accurate and immediate results. Bedside specimen testing, or point of care testing, refers to any patient test done outside the laboratory. Venipuncture refers to obtaining a blood sample at the bedside for testing that is usually done inside the laboratory. This chapter will examine the procedure for venipuncture and point of care testing procedure of bedside glucose monitoring, testing for fecal occult blood, and the use of reagent strip for urine tests.

GENERAL PRINCIPLES FOR VENIPUNCTURE AND POINT OF CARE TESTING

EQUIPMENT

Mechanical equipment must be tested for accuracy. Supplies must be used according to their date specifications. Chemical solutions or test strips must be stored according to the manufacturer's directions, kept dry and away from heat or freezing temperatures. Some supplies may need to be kept away from light or exposure to air.

ACCURACY

Accuracy is essential as treatment decisions are made on the basis of test results.

QUALITY CONTROL

Quality control measures are described for each procedure. This includes proper patient identification, following universal precautions, using the approved steps for the procedure and equipment.

PERFORMANCE SKILL

Before performing any procedure, you will need to learn how it is done and what will be expected of you. Even if you have already learned this procedure, you may be asked to demonstrate your knowledge. That demonstration of proficiency is called competency. Some procedures call for an annual or more frequent demonstration of competence.

DOCUMENTATION

Your work is documented according to your institution's policies. All procedures must be documented.

REPORTING

Report results to the RN promptly.

INFECTION CONTROL AND UNIVERSAL PRECAUTIONS

Follow infection control measures. This includes hand-washing, using medical aseptic technique (Chapter 17), maintaining cleanliness of materials and equipment, and preventing cross-contamination of supplies. Universal precautions, that is, treating blood and body fluids as if they were infectious, even if you know they are not, should be followed diligently. Personal protective equipment (PPE), usually gloves, masks, shields, and gowns, should be available at all times. Always discard PPE immediately following the procedure. PPE should not be worn outside of the patient's room. Sharps are always discarded in the sharps container.

VENIPUNCTURE

Collection of blood for laboratory testing is one method to provide information on a patient's condition. Results of blood tests can be used to identify a patient's status, confirm a diagnosis, monitor a patient's condition, identify the extent of the patient's disease, and guide treatment decisions. There are several methods used to obtain blood for testing. In this section the focus will be on venipuncture. In venipuncture, a metal needle is inserted into the inner aspect of the vein, at which time blood is withdrawn. The step-by-step procedure, beginning with the gathering of equipment/supplies, will be described.

Equipment/Supplies

Before any blood is drawn, a physician must write an order. The order specifies the name of the test(s) the patient is to have, e.g., fasting blood sugar; when the test is to be done, i.e., in early AM—may specify time, e.g., 6:00 AM; and how often the test is to be done, i.e., daily, times 3 days. Always check to make sure that an order has been written and contains the information you need to perform the blood draw.

 Consult the RN whenever you are unsure or unclear about a blood specimen order.

Once the order has been obtained, the next step is to gather your equipment. Some of the items you choose will depend on the method selected to collect the blood sample. The vacuum tube, butterfly needle/vacuum tube, and needle-syringe are three methods for drawing blood that will be described in this section. The following equipment is needed:

- Black pen
- Tourniquet

- Gloves (latex or vinyl)
- Sterile dry gauze 2 × 2 pads or cotton balls
- Adhesive bandages
- Washcloth/Chux or chemical warm pack
- Blood collection tubes—vacuum tubes
- Plastic hazardous materials bag for delivery (depends on institution's policy)

Vacuum Tube Method

- Vacuum tube holder
- Sterile blood collection needles for vacuum tube holder. These needles are double-ended and are designed specifically for the holder.

Butterfly Needle/Vacuum Tube Method

- Butterfly needle
- Luer-tip vacuum tube needle
- Vacuum tube holder

Needle-Syringe Method

- Sterile syringes
- Sterile needles (usual needle size for an adult, 19–21 gauge; for children, 23–25 gauge)*

The specific laboratory test(s) ordered will guide the selection of the blood collection tubes. The vacuum tubes come in different sizes and are color coded—red, blue, lavender, gray, and so on, to denote whether an additive is present. Different types of additives work in different ways. One additive may extend the life of the cells present in the blood; another may prevent clotting of the blood; whereas another may prevent distortion of the cells in the blood.†

✔ The color-coding of the vacuum tubes for the various laboratory tests may vary by institution; therefore it is necessary to refer to the Laboratory Reference/User's Guide of your agency.

In addition to knowing what color vacuum tube applies to what laboratory test, the sequence in which you collect the tube is crucial when drawing multiple samples. This is to prevent cross-contamination between tubes containing additives and tubes with no additives. Additionally, certain tubes must be mixed immediately after collection to ensure proper mixing of the additive with the blood sample. Mixing is done by gently inverting the tube 5 to 10 times. Never shake the tube. Refer to your institution's policies and procedures for mixing, sequence of tube collection, and amount of sample to be collected.

---

*Perry, A.G., and Potter, P.A.: Clinical Nursing Skills and Techniques. St. Louis, C.V. Mosby, 1994.
†Garza, D., and Becan-McBride, K.: Phlebotomy Handbook, 3rd ed. East Norwalk, Connecticut, Appleton & Lange, 1993.

✔ A common cause for sample rejection by the laboratory is improper collection of a specimen, i.e., wrong tube, incorrect mixing, contamination, and insufficient amount.

The completion of laboratory requisitions and labels will vary from one institution to another. Some institutions will use computer-printed bar-coded labels for the specimens and printout sheets, which eliminates the need to complete requisitions, whereas other institutions use the laboratory requisitions.

The requisition is filled in by hand and has coded labels attached that are affixed to the specimen(s) once collected. Whether they are computer generated or handwritten, the laboratory requires the following information:

- Patient's full name
- Patient's medical record/hospital number
- Patient's room number
- Patient's age and sex
- Physician's full name
- Test(s) requested
- Date and time of specimen collection
- Collector's name or initials

Other information that the laboratory may need to know is the route of collection, ie, venipuncture or capillary stick and how the specimen is to be processed—stat, routine, priority, pre-op, and the like. Each institution will define its processing system, or turn-around times for results, what information must be documented for a specimen to be processed, and what forms are to be used.

📓 When filling out a requisition, print clearly and complete all information required. If working with a computer-generated document, review all information for accuracy.

✔ A common cause for specimen rejection by the laboratory is a specimen submitted without the required patient information.

Identification and Preparation of the Patient

The next step is to identify and prepare the patient for the procedure. Identification of the patient is crucial, as it will eliminate the error of collecting a blood specimen from the wrong patient. The identification is done by checking the patient's hospital band against the laboratory requisition or paperwork. In some instances, in addition to checking the band against the requisition the patient may also need to state his or her name. Each institution

has its own policies on how identification of a patient is to be done. Whatever system is used, all information *must* match.

📣 If there are any discrepancies, however minor, let the RN know. *Do not* proceed until all discrepancies have been clarified and corrected.

Once you have correctly identified the patient, it is good practice to explain what you are about to do. Let the patient know what procedure will be performed, how long it will take, and what he or she may experience. This can help to reduce some of the anxiety the patient may be feeling. It is also good practice to talk to patients during the procedure to prepare them for what they will feel and see. For example, "At this time, Mrs. Smith, I will be inserting the needle into your skin; you may feel a slight pinch."

⚖ A patient asking you for a detailed explanation of why certain laboratory tests are being performed and/or questioning you about his or her disease/condition creates a situation in which you need to get the RN or physician involved.

Discussing the patient's diagnosis, choices of tests, and selection of treatment regimens are not in the PCT's scope of practice.

Positioning the patient for the procedure is important for successful venipuncture and comfort. The preferable positions for venipuncture are supine or semi-Fowler's in bed or sitting in a recliner chair. Some people have a tendency to faint in response to seeing blood or having their blood drawn. These positions prevent injury in case of fainting and also allow for stabilizing the extremity. If a recliner chair is not an option, then having a patient sit in a low chair is preferable.

 Standing is not an option for this procedure.

Prior to selection of a vein, all equipment should be prepared and easily accessible to you. Clear and clean a work area and set out your equipment.

Place equipment easily within your peripheral vision so that you can keep your eyes on the venipuncture site while reaching out for the vacuum tubes. Opening packages and placing items in the order of use will eliminate the need for you to stop or interrupt the procedure.

Always make sure that you have extra equipment with you in case of contamination or defects.

Wash your hands, don gloves, and proceed with vein selection. Glove selection depends on personal preference and skin allergies. If your skin becomes irritated by latex gloves, use vinyl instead. Examination gloves, and not sterile gloves, are appropriate.

Common Sites

Blood can be drawn from various sites such as the arm, hand, foot, heel, and upper chest region (Fig. 21–1).

The arm is always the first site for obtaining a blood specimen. When the arms cannot be accessed or they are unsuitable for the blood draw, the other sites are explored. When working with infants and children, heels and/or fingers are utilized. Heel and finger sticks are capillary punctures and are performed to obtain small amounts of

blood for testing. In the section, Blood Glucose Monitoring, capillary puncture is described in detail.

The subclavian vein, located in the upper chest region, is used for blood draws once a central line has been inserted.

STOP Blood draws from central lines are performed by the RN or physician.

Since the arm is the most frequently used site, the median cubital and cephalic veins are the first choices. These veins tend to be larger, fuller, and close to the skin, and drawing from them tends to be less painful for the patient. Once you have located a vein, feel and trace its path over the arm or hand.

If extremity veins are not easily seen or felt there are a few special techniques that can be performed:

- With a tourniquet in place, have the patient make a fist; gently massage the arm downward toward the hand. (This will increase blood flow into the vein.)

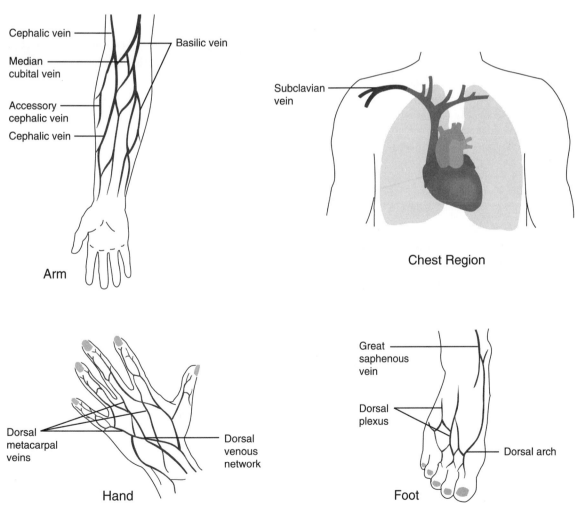

FIGURE 21–1
Sites for venipunctures.

- Tap the veins sharply several times with the index and second finger. (This may cause the vein to dilate. Repeated tapping may cause the vein to spasm and close down and make it more difficult to do the venipuncture.)

- Lower the extremity, ie, the arm, below the level of the heart.

- Apply a warm washcloth and cover with a chux, or apply an activated chemical warm pack, to the site for about 5 minutes. Let the patient know that this will make the blood draw easier for them and you'll be back in 5 minutes.

When selecting a site there are certain areas to avoid:

- IV sites

- Cannula, fistula, vascular graft in the arms of patients who are on dialysis

- Mastectomy (never draw from the side where the mastectomy was performed)

- Excessive scarring

- Stroke—do not use affected arm

- Hematoma

Tourniquet

When applying a tourniquet, it should be placed 4 to 5 inches above the site and must be released after 1 minute; this is done to avoid hemoconcentration of the blood sample and hematoma formation in the tissue. There are several types of tourniquets. The two most commonly used are the flat (latex or vinyl) sponge and the Velcro type. Penrose drains are also commonly used as tourniquets. Each type has its advantages and disadvantages. The type your institution has selected will determine what tourniquet you will become accustomed to using. The tourniquet should be tight enough to hold venous blood in the arm, but not so tight that it stops arterial circulation. Check to make sure there is a radial pulse after a tourniquet is applied to the arm. This assures that you did not apply the tourniquet too tightly and did not block arterial circulation.

Cleansing the Site

After the site has been located, cleanse the area with an alcohol wipe, starting in the center and working out in a circular motion. Allow the alcohol to dry completely before needle insertion. Some locations may require cleansing of the site with betadine.

STOP Never blow on the site. *Avoid* touching the site after cleansing. If it is touched, cleanse it again to avoid contamination.

Procedure

Vacuum Tube Method (Figs. 21–2 to 21–9)

1. Assemble the equipment. With the vacuum holder in one hand, insert the rubber covered end of the double-ended needle into the holder with the other hand. Twist

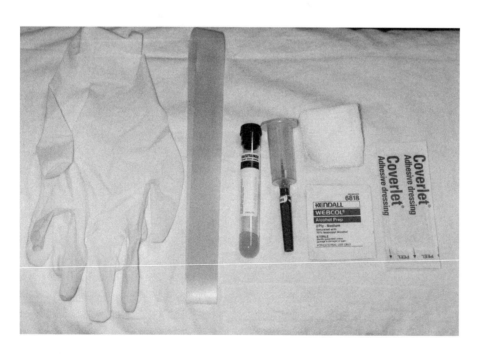

FIGURE 21–2
Equipment for vacuum tube method.

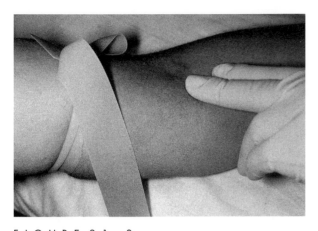

F I G U R E   2 1 - 3
Location on arm vein.

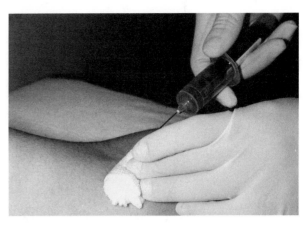

F I G U R E   2 1 - 6
Blood collected, gauze applied, and needle removed.

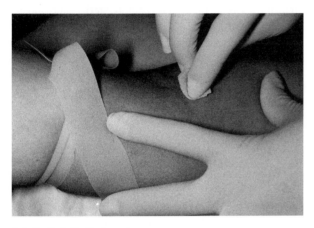

F I G U R E   2 1 - 4
Cleansing site.

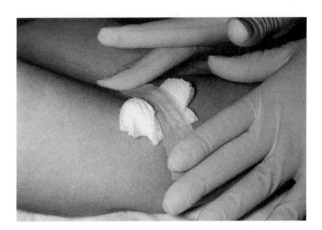

F I G U R E   2 1 - 7
Adhesive bandage applied over gauze.

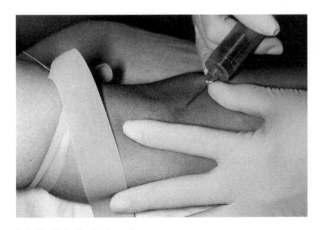

F I G U R E   2 1 - 5
Insertion of needle.

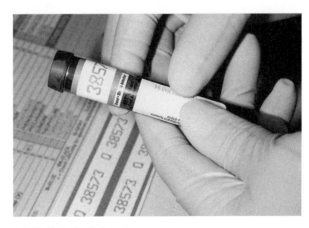

F I G U R E   2 1 - 8
Specimen labeled.

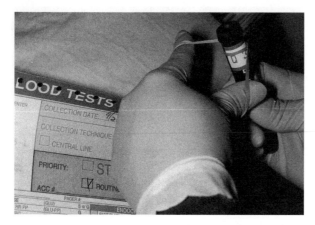

F I G U R E 2 1 – 9
Requisition fastened to the specimen with a rubber band.

the needle in place until it is secure. Arrange vacuum tubes in the order in which they will be filled.

2. Insert the appropriate vacuum tube into the vacuum holder until the rubber stopper touches the rubber covered needle. *Do not* penetrate the rubber stopper with the needle at this time, as the tube will lose its vacuum seal.

3. Carefully remove the needle's cap.

4. Grasp the vacuum holder and vacuum tube in one hand. Position the thumb of your other hand 1 to 2 inches below the puncture site, pull the skin down, and hold firmly in place. This makes it easier to puncture the skin, and hold the vein in place.

5. Line up the needle with the vein, with the needle bevel up. While inserting the needle at a 30–45 degree angle, puncture the skin and enter the wall of the vein. You will feel some resistance and then a "give" as the needle penetrates the vein's wall.

6. Grasp the vacuum holder firmly, bracing your hand

against the patient's arm to stabilize the holder. Push the tube forward, penetrating the rubber stopper with the multi draw needle. Use care to avoid advancing the needle any further.

7. Allow the vacuum tube to fill.

8. The tourniquet should be removed as soon as the last tube to be filled has been placed. Never leave the tourniquet on for more then 1 minute.

9. If there are multiple tubes, hold the vacuum holder with the free hand bracing against the patient's arm to avoid movement of the needle in the vein; with the other hand remove the filled tube gently. Insert the next tube. Repeat steps 6, 7, and 9 as needed. The rubber on the covered needle is self-sealing. When one tube is withdrawn, the rubber seals over the needle and prevents bleeding from occurring during the change of vacuum tubes.

10. When collection is finished, remove the last tube from the vacuum tube, gently apply sterile gauze to the site, and remove needle. Apply pressure to the site immediately after the needle is withdrawn. Putting pressure on the site with the needle still in place causes more pain as well as trauma to the tissues. Ask patient to lift arm and apply pressure while holding the gauze in place. Pressure should be applied for 1 to 2 minutes. Once all bleeding has stopped an adhesive bandage is applied.

These techniques will not only contribute to successful outcomes, but will reduce the chance of a hematoma forming at the site. Removing the tourniquet before the last tube is filled reduces the backflow pressure of venous blood, and less blood will seep into tissues after the needle is removed. Pulling the last tube before removing the needle reduces the chance of any remaining vacuum in the tube drawing blood into the tissues.

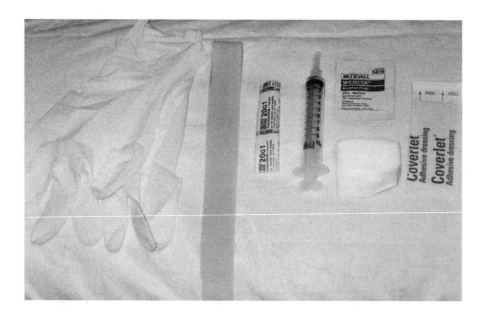

F I G U R E 2 1 – 1 0
Equipment for needle-syringe method (tube for blood is included but not shown).

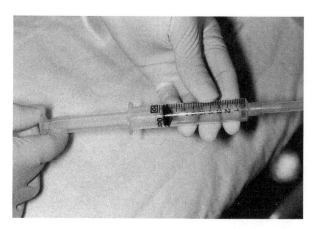

FIGURE 21-11
Needle secured to the syringe.

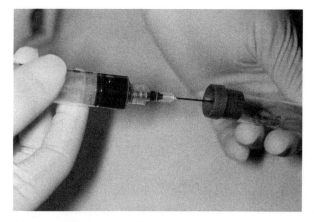

FIGURE 21-13
Needle penetrating rubber stopper of tube.

Needle-Syringe Method (Figs. 21–10 to 21–14)

STOP Great care should be taken when using this method because of the risk of needlestick injury when transferring blood to vacuum tubes.

1. To assemble the sterile needle and syringe, hold syringe in one hand and with the other hand twist needle into Luer tip of syringe. Twist until needle is secured. The size of the syringe you will use depends on the total amount of blood you need to collect. Follow tourniquet application and skin preparation as described earlier.

2. Check the plunger to make sure that it is functioning correctly.

3. Carefully remove the needle's cap.

4. Grasp the syringe with needle attached in one hand. With the other hand position your finger 1 to 2 inches below the puncture site, hold the skin as previously described to stabilize the vein.

5. Line up the needle with the vein, with the needle bevel up. While inserting the needle at a 30–45-degree angle, puncture the skin and enter the wall of the vein.

You will feel some resistance and then a "give" as the needle penetrates the vein's wall.

6. Slowly draw back on the plunger and withdraw the amount needed for the test.

7. Release the tourniquet as soon as blood flow has been established.

8. When collection is finished, apply sterile gauze to the site and remove the needle. Ask patient to lift arm and apply pressure while holding the gauze in place. Pressure should be applied for 1 to 2 minutes. Once all bleeding has stopped an adhesive bandage is applied.

9. Transfer blood into the vacuum tube. There are two ways this can be done. One way is to remove the needle from the syringe and remove the rubber stopper from the tube. Then gently inject the blood into the tube. The second way is to penetrate the rubber stopper with the needle in place and allow the vacuum from the tube to draw the blood out from the syringe. This system tends to be quite risky as the potential for needlestick injuries, blood exposure, or contamination of the sample is great. Refer to your institution's policies regarding the approved transfer procedure.

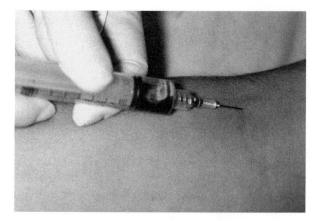

FIGURE 21-12
Needle inserted; syringe plunger gently pulled to fill syringe.

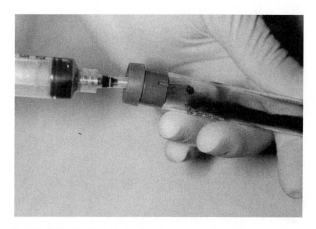

FIGURE 21-14
Transferring blood from syringe to vacuum tube.

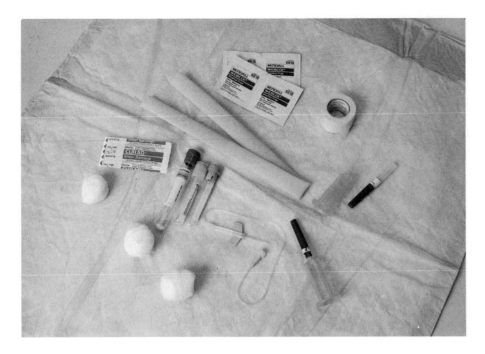

Equipment for butterfly
needle–vacuum tube method.

Butterfly Needle/Vacuum Tube Method (Figs. 21–15 to 21–19)

This method is actually a combination of the other two methods. In this process a standard 21-gauge butterfly needle is used for the venipuncture. A special vacuum tube needle is used. It comes with a Luer tip at one end, to fit into the Luer end of the butterfly needle tubing. The other end has the standard multi draw needle tip. The process is as follows:

1. Assemble equipment. Connect the Luer tip to the end of the butterfly tubing and insert the multidraw tip into the vacuum tube holder. Lay out all tubes in the order in which you are to draw them. Have gauze pad, cotton balls, a 2-inch long piece of tape, and adhesive bandage available. Have an extra venipuncture device available.

2. Apply tourniquet and identify venipuncture site. Although this device is particularly helpful when drawing blood from hand veins, it can be used at any site. Palpate to find a full, compressible vein. Remove tourniquet before cleaning site if it has taken much time to locate the site. Clean site, as previously discussed, with alcohol and let dry.

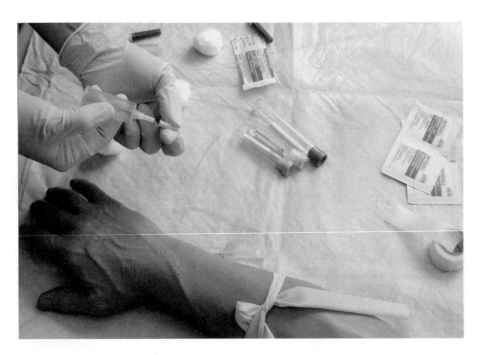

F I G U R E 2 1 – 1 6
Connecting vacuum tube holder to
butterfly tubing.

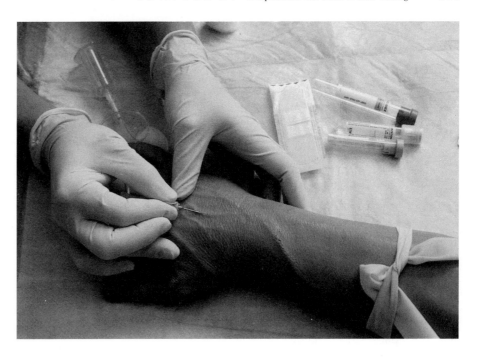

FIGURE 21–17
Insertion of butterfly needle device.

3. Reapply tourniquet. With nondominate hand, pull skin back 1–2 inches below venipuncture site to stabilize the vein. Hold the wings of the butterfly needle, keeping the bevel of the needle up. Insert the needle at a 20–45-degree angle through the skin directly into the vein. An advantage of this system is that blood return will be visible in the tubing if venipuncture has been successful. Flatten the angle of the needle, and insert 1/4 inch. Use a 2-inch piece of tape to temporarily stabilize the needle. *Keep a portion of one hand on the device at all times to maintain device securely in place.*

4. Use other hand to advance first vacuum tube into holder and on to needle. After tube fills, remove and continue to fill remaining tubes. Gently invert each tube 5–7 times to mix additives. One advantage of this system is that there is no danger of advancing the needle into the patient's arm when changing tubes. After the last tube has been inserted, release tourniquet.

5. After last tube has been filled, remove it. Hold patient's arm, loosen the tape holding the device, gently place gauze or cotton ball over site, remove needle, and apply pressure to the site. Pressure should be applied for 1–2 minutes.

Ask patient if there is anything else you can do for

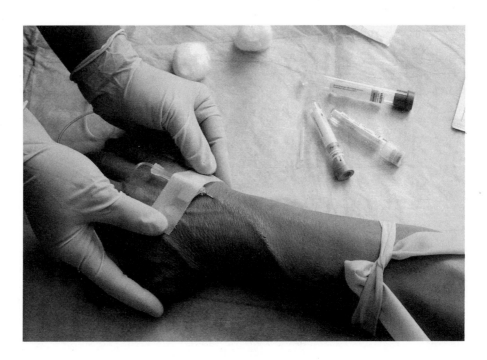

FIGURE 21–18
Stabilizing the device.

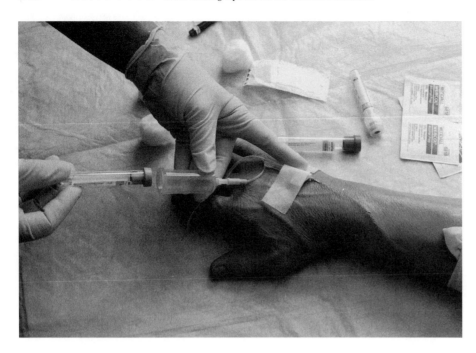

F I G U R E 2 1 – 1 9
Holding the site and inserting
vacuum tube into holder.

him or her before you leave. Place patient in position of comfort, and place call bell within reach.

If there is excessive bleeding, bleeding that persists longer than 5 minutes, notify the RN for assistance. Stay with patient and apply pressure.

Labeling

Labeling of specimens is critical. Labeling should be done at the patient's bedside to decrease the chances of error such as mislabeling. In most institutions, tubes are labeled after collection has been completed and not before. The individual collecting the specimen must be the one who labels the samples. Refer to your institution's policies and procedures regarding correct labeling of specimens. If you have used more than one vacuum tube, take extra care to get the right label on each tube. In some cases more than one test could be run on the same specimen from one tube, and more than one label may be applied to the same tube. Your laboratory may send one computer label per tube and automatically perform all possible tests from each type of tube. Since laboratories use a variety of equipment to perform testing, a variety of procedures are used. It is important to follow your agency policies. Once the specimen is labeled and requisition is completed, the requisition is either fastened to the specimen with a rubberband, or the specimen and requisition are placed in a plastic biohazard bag for delivery to the laboratory.

A common reason for specimen rejection by the laboratory is unlabeled or improperly labeled samples.

Infection Control

Universal precautions/blood and body fluid precautions are strictly followed when performing venipuncture procedures. Latex or vinyl gloves are worn during the procedures. Once the procedure has been completed, the gloves are removed. Wearing gloves outside of the patient's room places others at risk.

Principles of handwashing using medical aseptic technique, discussed previously in Chapter 17, should be used to prevent the spread of germs from staff to patient.

Proper disposal of used equipment is an important infection control measure. Items should be separated into two categories, sharps and nonsharps. These items are then disposed of in the appropriate biohazard medical waste containers.

STOP To prevent needlestick injuries, needles are never recapped. Needles are disposed of directly into the sharps container. If a needlestick injury occurs, report to your supervisor immediately.

Storage/Processing

Once the specimen is labeled, you need to know how the sample is to be preserved during the time from collection to its arrival at the laboratory. Preserving the sample correctly is necessary for testing of the specimen to provide valid results.

Sample preservation relates mainly to the temperature at which the sample should be maintained and the length of time in which the laboratory must receive the specimen. There are three levels of preservation: cold, warm, and room temperature.

• Sample preserved *cold:* The sample is placed on ice or

in cold water or is refrigerated. An example would be arterial blood gases (ABGs), usually drawn by a professional, but the PCT may put the sample in a bag of ice and take it immediately to the laboratory.

- Sample preserved *warm:* Prior to sample collection the tube may be warmed to 98.6°F and/or the sample is placed in warm water.

- Sample preserved at *room temperature:* Sample is collected and sent "as is" to the laboratory with no temperature alteration. This is the usual routine for blood specimens.*

The length of time in which the specimen must be received by the laboratory is also important. The time frames depend upon the testing being done, and these times are defined by the laboratory and the institution. Generally, any specimen should go to the laboratory within an hour.

✔ A common reason for specimen rejection by the laboratory is improper preservation and/or the laboratory receives the specimen late.

There are different ways to get the specimen to the laboratory. A pneumatic tube system may exist in the institution. The tube system provides efficiency by reducing the transportation time while also eliminating the expense of a laboratory transporter physically picking up the specimens at different locations throughout the hospital. The main drawback of this system is the possibility of breakage and contamination due to improper packaging of the sample.

A transport carrier is another means of getting the sample to the laboratory. The transport carrier is a person who makes rounds throughout the hospital at designated times and physically picks up the specimens and delivers them to the laboratory. This allows for transportation of some specimens that cannot be sent by tube. In addition, special pickups can be coordinated with the carrier to address priority situations.

In self-delivery the individual who collects the samples hand-carries them directly to the laboratory. This is often the preferred method for "stat" situations.

Quality Control

- Ensure that all patients are properly identified.
- Make certain that vacuum tubes are not expired.
- Label all specimens at the bedside.
- Check all equipment prior to use.
- A maximum of 2 venipuncture attempts is allowed. (This will be determined by institution policy.)

*Garza, D., and Becan-McBride, K.: Phlebotomy Handbook, 3rd ed. East Norwalk, Connecticut, Appleton & Lange, 1993.

- Wear appropriate personal protective equipment, i.e., gloves.
- Transport items to the laboratory in a timely fashion.
- Ensure preservation of specimen.
- Be sure that all patients are wearing an ID band.

Reporting/Documentation Issues

Report to the RN the following information:

- Success of blood collection, type of test drawn, time specimen(s) collected, and information relating to the delivery of the specimen to the laboratory
- Unsuccessful in blood collection: Number of attempts made, inability to obtain adequate amount, patient refused, or other issues
- Status of puncture site: Site clotted well, continued to bleed for a short period, or excessive bleeding
- How the patient tolerated the procedure

Document the following items:

- Date and time of sample collection
- Site
- Laboratory test(s) performed
- How the specimen was preserved for pickup or delivery to the laboratory
- Time and route of delivery
- How the patient tolerated the procedure

📓 Record information on the requisition, patient chart, and unit laboratory specimen log, as appropriate.

Key Points

- Identify the patient correctly.
- Make sure all paperwork is completed accurately and clearly.
- Label specimen at the patient's bedside to avoid error.
- Maintain good infection control practices.
- Report results of procedure to the RN.
- Be familiar with your institution's policies and procedures relating to laboratory testing and venipuncture.
- Avoid the common causes of specimen rejection by the laboratory.
- Understand the steps used in the three methods of venipuncture (Fig. 21–20).

BLOOD GLUCOSE MONITORING

Fingerstick blood glucose monitoring (FSBG) is a method by which a drop of blood is applied to a reagent

VENIPUNCTURE COMPETENCY CHECKLIST

NAME: _____   UNIT: _____

DATE: _____   EMPLOYEE NUMBER: _____

	PERFORMANCE CRITERIA	COMPETENCY DEMONSTRATED
1.	Obtain physician's order	
2.	Assemble Equipment/Supplies a. Vacuum Tube Method c. Butterfly Needle/Vacuum b. Needle-Syringe Method Tube Method	
3.	Prepare appropriate requisitions/paperwork	
4.	Identify patient and explain procedure	
5.	Set up work environment a. Lighting b. Equipment	
6.	Position patient	
7.	Wash hands and don gloves	
8.	Select extremity - arm	
9.	Techniques for distending veins a. Application of tourniquet b. Patient exercising limb c. Application of warmth	
10.	Selection of appropriate vein site	
11.	Skin preparation	
12.	Perform venipuncture a. Vacuum Tube Method c. Butterfly Needle/Vacuum b. Needle-Syringe Method Tube Method	
13.	Collect specimen in correct order and mix accordingly	
14.	Release of tourniquet done smoothly and quickly	
15.	Inspect site, apply gauze and adhesive tape to site	
16.	Label specimen	
17.	Clean work area a. Safe disposal of sharps and non-sharps b. Safe disposal of medical waste and non-medical waste c. Removing and discarding gloves d. Handwashing	
18.	Preservation of specimen	
19.	Packaging and routing of specimen	
20.	Report results of the procedure to the Registered Nurse	
21.	Documentation	
22.	Quality Control Standards	

Code: S = Satisfactory   U = Unsatisfactory

Validated/Observed by:_____   DATE: _____

F I G U R E 2 1 – 2 0

Veinipuncture competency checklist.

strip, and the results are read visually or by glucometer. In the past, urine was the standard by which glucose levels were measured. However, measuring glucose levels by testing urine has several drawbacks. The results are not quantitative; in other words, an actual numerical glucose level cannot be determined. This method indicates only if extra glucose is being passed in the urine, low glucose levels cannot be identified this way. Checking urine depended on the patient's being able to void. The results were read by strip and thus were dependent on the accuracy of the reader and the urine concentration. FSBGM was revolutionized when blood glucose meters were developed in the mid-1980s. These meters became the standard for blood glucose testing. Early meters were large, bulky, very expensive, and designed for hospital use. The age of technology has produced smaller, less expensive meters for home and hospital use. Today, glucometers are readily available and are the recommended method for testing blood glucose levels.

For patients who have diabetes mellitus, blood glucometers offer a quick, easy, and accurate method to keep track of their blood glucose level. The therapeutic goal of FSBG monitoring is to keep the blood glucose level as near to normal as possible. Blood glucose levels can be measured at home, at work, while traveling, in the hospital, clinic, and laboratory settings.

FSBG monitoring uses capillary blood. Blood glucose monitoring performed in the laboratory is usually done on venous or arterial blood samples. When FSBG monitoring is done in the home, visually or by meter, factors such as cost, age, visual acuity, and the ability to operate the meter are important.

Visual Method of Blood Glucose Monitoring

In this method, the patient applies a drop of blood to a reagent strip and waits the recommended time, then dry- or wet-wipes the blood off the reagent strip. The patient visually reads the color changes on the strips by comparing the strip to the legend on the bottle. There are several drawbacks to this method. Although this method is quick, easy, and less expensive, it is also less accurate and dependent on correct timing and no visual impairment by the person reading the strip.

How Blood Glucose Meters Work

There are many different types of blood glucometers available on today's market. Meters that are small, easy to operate, and accurate are in great demand. Many insurance companies now pay for the purchase of glucometers, and consumer rebates are sizable. Glucometer reagent strips, however, are expensive to purchase, especially for patients on fixed incomes. Many glucometers work by reflecting light; these are called reflectance meters; others use an electrical chemical reaction.

The reflectance meters shine light on the strip when it is inserted; the light is reflected by the strip and picked up by the photoelectric eye, which changes the light to an electric current. The machine will give a digital readout of the blood glucose when the strip has been read. The strip will change colors—light or dark. The color is darker if the strip has more glucose and lighter if it has less glucose.* Reagent strips may be wet-washed, dry-wiped, or not wiped before being inserted into the glucometer. Each type of meter requires particular strips as well as specific treatment of strips after the blood is applied. Wet wash involves rinsing the reagent strip with water once the blood has been in contact with the strip for the prescribed interval. Dry wipe involves wiping the reagent strip with a cottonball after the prescribed contact interval. No-wipe reagent strips allow insertion of the strips directly into the machine without wiping or rinsing. These various methods can cause inaccuracies because of timing factors and too little or too much wiping and blotting. Reagent strips are very sensitive to heat, cold, and moisture—they need to be kept dry and moisture free.

STOP Do not use reagent strips if strips are discolored; they will provide inaccurate test results. Always check the expiration date on reagent strips and control solutions. Do not use if it is beyond the manufacturer's recommended date. Use only the reagent strips recommended for the glucometer you are using.

✓ Mark the date testing materials were opened. Quality control testing solutions should not be used more than 6 months after opening.

Quality Control

FSBG monitoring is a laboratory procedure that is performed outside of the laboratory. Laboratory procedures that are performed outside the laboratory are designated near-patient testing or point of care testing. When nursing or other ancillary personnel perform bedside glucose monitoring, although it is performed outside of the laboratory, it is still under the laboratory's province for quality control. Regulatory and credentialing agencies such as the Joint Commission on Accreditation of Healthcare Organizations (JCAHO), Health Care Financing Administration (HCFA), College of American Pathologists (CAP), and National Committee for Clinical Laboratory Standards (NCCLS) set standards for quality control. These standards specify written policies and procedures on the use and maintenance of glucometers, quality control testing documentation, training programs, documentation of who is qualified to operate the glucometer, and proficiency testing.†

---

*Guthrie, D.W. and Guthrie, R.A.: Nursing Management of Diabetes Mellitus. New York, Springer Publishing Company, 1991.
†Walker EA: Quality assurance for blood glucose monitoring. Nursing Clinics of North America. 28(1):61–69, 1993.

Quality control testing is performed to detect differences in testing that may result because of operator, glucometer, or materials errors. Quality control is designed to monitor differences and to determine when they exceed acceptable limits. Hospitals and regulatory agencies set quality control limits. Many of the newer glucometers have a computerized quality control mechanism. This mechanism provides a written document when quality control checks are done. A user ID code identifies the operator, and repeated testing errors can be tracked to the person who performed the test.

Quality control testing involves using low, normal, and high level solutions. Testing solutions come prepackaged with a specific glucose concentration. The solutions are used in place of blood when performing an example FSBG test. Levels are determined for each glucometer in use on a daily basis. Quality control also consists of meter maintenance and cleaning on a daily basis.

Proficiency testing is a means of external quality control. The laboratory receives specimens from external agencies, and these are tested on internal glucometers. The purpose of proficiency testing is to compare internal test results with external test samples.

We tend to think that someone who has performed FSBG testing for a long time should be an expert. Studies have demonstrated, however, that the skills of the operator/user tend to deteriorate over time. Quality control and the development of competency help to ensure that the operator/user remains proficient in the skills necessary to perform FSBG monitoring. JCAHO requires that personnel who perform FSBG monitoring be assessed at periodic intervals for competency. There is no specified time, but most institutions follow yearly schedules of competency testing. Competency may be assessed by observing technique and performance of quality control or proficiency testing.* Records are maintained to document competency of glucometer users and quality control checks of each glucometer.

FSBG monitoring accuracy can be affected by timing, underwiping or overwiping, insufficient blood sample, defective equipment, defective testing materials, and human error. Good quality control monitoring will ensure proper performance and technique as well as that materials and equipment are functioning properly (Fig. 21–21).

Infection Control

Performing FSBG monitoring involves coming in contact with blood-borne pathogens. The use of handwashing and appropriate personal protective equipment can help prevent the spread of germs and reduce exposure to blood-borne pathogens.

*Belanger, A.C. Point-of-care testing: The JCAHO perspective. Medical Laboratory Observer. 26(6):46–49, 1994.

STOP Hands should be washed before performing FSBG. Both the PCT and patient should wash their hands. The PCT washes the patient's hand or extremity if the patient is unable to do so.

1. Wash hands using medical aseptic technique as discussed in Chapter 3.
2. Blood and body fluid precautions are used to protect the health care worker and patient by preventing the spread of blood-borne pathogens. Use personal protective equipment when performing FSBG monitoring.
3. Dispose of equipment properly. Discard contaminated disposable equipment and sharps using your institution's policy and procedure for biohazardous waste.

STOP Needles and sharps should not be bent or recapped. Sharps should be disposed of in a puncture-resistant container and all contaminated materials disposed of in the biohazardous waste container.

Supplies and Equipment

Assembling supplies and equipment is an important step that enables the user to perform in a efficient and organized manner.

Supplies and Equipment for Performing Blood Glucose Monitoring

Glucometer
Blood glucose reagent strips
Antiseptic wipe/alcohol prep pad
Disposable gloves
Lancet or automated lancet
Cotton ball (optional)
Paper towel
Washcloth and/or soap and water

Supplies and Equipment for Performing Quality Control

Glucometer
Blood glucose reagent strip
Disposable gloves
Quality control solutions

STOP Gloves should be worn when performing blood glucose monitoring as well as quality control testing and meter maintenance because the glucometer is contaminated with blood.

Patient Preparation

Properly preparing the patient for bedside glucose monitoring is an important step. Part of patient prepara-

SAMPLE

GLUCOMETER QUALITY CONTROL CORRECTIVE ACTION LOG

Type of meter _____ Meter Number _____

Date _____ Meter Location _____

Laboratory Review _____

1. Meter operator instructions:
    For quality control ranges that exceed acceptable limits or if meter displays error or failure, record in the record below the date and the code for the corrective action that was taken.

    To determine the appropriate corrective action code, perform desired quality control level (Low, High, Normal).

    1) Make sure control level on meter and control bottle match.
    2) Make sure code number on reagent test strip and meter match.
    3) Check expiration date on reagent strip and control bottle. Discard expired materials.

2. Retest the quality control solution that was out of range. Keep retesting until failed/error is not displayed or if unable to correct, record "F."

DATE	CODE	DATE	CODE

QUALITY CONTROL CORRECTIVE ACTION CODE:

1. When performing quality control testing: Low, High, or Normal.

    a) Failed/error not displayed: Stop here; meter may be used for patient testing.
    b) Failed/error displayed: Record "A" in code box; clean the meter optical system and test area.

2. Retest quality control solution that was out of range.

    a) Fail/error not displayed: Record ("B") for corrective action code.
    b) Fail/error displayed again: Obtain new bottle of quality control solution that was out of range.

3. Retest the quality control solution that was out of range.

    a) If failed/error not displayed: Record "C" in corrective action code. Stop here; meter may be used for patient testing.
    b) Failed/error displayed again: Open new package of test strips.

4. Retest the quality control solution that was out of range.

    a) Failed/error not displayed: Record "D" for Corrective Action Code.
    b) Fail/error displayed: Record "F." Label the meter "Do Not Use" and follow your institution's policy for replacement of the glucometer.

FIGURE 21-21

Glucometer quality control corrective action log.

tion includes explaining the procedure to the patient. Explaining the procedure to the patient helps you to assess the patient's level of knowledge about the procedure as well as to allay anxiety.

1. Identify the appropriate patient by checking the patient's identification bracelet and calling him or her by name.

2. Introduce yourself to the patient and shake hands. This is not only polite, but it allows you to note if the hands feel cold. If the hands feel cold, it is an indication of less blood supply to the hands at the time. If the patient's hands are cold, you will be less likely to have a successful fingerstick. Explain that you will be doing a fingerstick to check blood sugar. The procedure works better if the person's hands are warm, so you will put a warm washcloth on the hand and wrap it in a Chux to increase circulation to the hand. Explain that you will check someone elses blood sugar while the wrap warms the person's hand and be back in 5–10 minutes. This saves the patient a stick and you time.

3. Explain the procedure you are going to perform. Be aware of cultural and age-related differences. Ask if the patient has been performing FSBG testing at home. If so, does he or she have any particular helpful hints?

4. Have the patient wash his or her hands. If the patient is unable to wash the hands, the PCT washes the patient's hands to prevent the spread of microorganisms.

5. Position the patient comfortably in bed or in a chair with a bedside table for support.

Procedure

To Obtain a Capillary Blood Specimen

Capillary blood can be obtained by skin puncture. It is generally quicker and less painful than venipuncture.

1. Wash hands (patient and performer).
2. Apply gloves.
3. Select and prepare puncture site (allow alcohol to dry). If the patient is experienced, ask if there is a site preference.
4. Utilize techniques to increase blood supply. Besides the warm wrap described earlier, other techniques include letting the arm dangle below heart level, gently massaging the arm and then the hand, pushing blood flow toward the fingers.
5. Perform skin puncture using lancet or automated lancing device. Follow the procedure outlined by the manufacturer of the device you are using.
6. Obtain a full hanging drop of blood.

Washing the performer's and patient's hands decreases the number of microorganisms and provides an opportunity to determine the skin integrity. The sides of fingers,

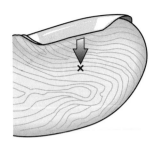

FIGURE 21-22
Fingerstick site.

toes, and heels are the most commonly used puncture sites (Figs. 21–22 and 21–23). Earlobes are also used. These areas are chosen because they have more capillary circulation and fewer nerve endings, and thus tend to feel less pain. The second and third finger are most commonly chosen. Feet should never be used with a diabetic patient, and with any adult, only with permission of the physician or RN. Heel sites are primarily used with infants and neonates. Rotate sites and do not use areas that are swollen or in which the skin is broken. Cleanse the skin with antiseptic and allow it to dry completely before puncturing the skin.

STOP If the alcohol is not allowed to dry, it mixes with the blood and can cause variance in test results as well as sting the patient's finger. Alcohol is a drying agent; do not overuse it.

Lancing Devices

Lancing devices can be hand held or automated. The automated device controls the depth of the puncture more than the hand-held devices. Lancets may be completely or partially disposable. The trend today is toward a totally disposable device. If the device is partially disposable

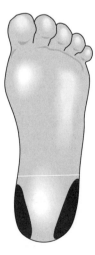

FIGURE 21-23
Heelstick site.

and portions of it come in contact with the patient's blood, make sure that the platform is changed after each use. There have been instances of HBV transmission when disposable lancet platforms were not changed after each patient use. Utilize gravity and milking motions of the extremity to get a good blood return before puncturing the skin. Milking the extremity after the skin has been punctured can cause dilution of the blood glucose and may result in a lower glucose reading. Position the lancet against the skin with moderate, firm pressure. Set timer on glucometer, if appropriate, immediately after the blood drop has been obtained.

🛑 Dispose of a lancet immediately after use.

🛑 Do not press lancet against the skin too tightly, as this might create a deeper puncture. Gently squeeze the finger pad until you get a full hanging drop of blood to apply on the reagent strip. Do not smear the blood.
The instant the drop of blood touches the reagent strip, it starts the chemical reaction.

Allow the blood to remain on the reagent strip the required length of time, and dry or no-wipe before inserting it into the glucometer. Read the results visually, or a digital reading will appear on the glucometer screen when the test results are complete.

Apply light pressure with clean gauze until the puncture site bleeding stops. If the patient is taking medication to thin the blood (anticoagulants), hold the site longer. Automated lancets work well because they allow for more control of the depth of the puncture site. Avoid bony sites. Washing the site with warm water or wrapping it in a warm cloth promotes vasodilation and increases blood flow to the area. This may also increase bleeding after the puncture. Discard sharps in a puncture-resistant container. Discard reagent test strip in biohazard waste. Remove gloves and wash hands.

Reporting and Documenting Findings

📝 Reporting and documenting glucometer results both verbally and written are an important aspect in completing glucometer testing.

Most institutions have critical values. Critical values refer to the lowest and highest level for glucose readings. If the glucose reading falls lower or higher than your institution's set critical value, repeat the test and follow your institution's policies for documenting and reporting.

✏️ If the values are above or below normal, or quite different for the particular patient, or if you observe any differences in the patient's

condition, alert the RN so she can assess the condition of the patient and initiate appropriate treatment. You need to know your institution's critical values for glucometer testing.

📝 The results of your glucometer reading will be recorded on the patients diabetic record (Fig. 21–24).

Meter Maintenance

Regulatory agencies require glucometers to be cleaned at least once a day.

📝 Document daily cleaning according to your institution's policy and procedures.

Most glucometers are cleaned with water and mild detergent or alcohol swabs, as needed.

🛑 Wear appropriate PPE equipment when cleaning meters.

🛑 Alcohol should not be used to clean some glucometers because it can damage the internal components. Alcohol should not be used over clear plastic view screens as it "clouds" the screen over time.

Most machines are battery operated and have varying signals to indicate when the batteries need changing. Follow the manufacturer's recommendation for battery changes. If a meter malfunctions and you are unable to clear it by troubleshooting, follow your institution's policy for malfunctioning meters. See Figure 21–25 for a sample glucometer competency checklist.

The development of the glucometer has revolutionized blood-glucose monitoring. The newest technology is the development of a noninvasive device that will be able to read blood glucose levels by means of infrared monitoring. The extremity is inserted into the device, and readings are based on the absorption of different light frequencies. The impact this development will have for patients, who will no longer need to puncture their skin 3–4 times a day, will be significant.

Key Points

• Remember the therapeutic goal of blood glucose monitoring is to keep the blood glucose level as near to normal as possible.

• Ensure quality of testing materials by always checking expiration dates on reagent strips and control solutions.

• Practice blood and body fluid precautions.

		Insulin				Urine	Cap. Glucose	Serum Glucose		SAMPLE DIABETES RECORD	
Year											
Date	Time	Type	Dose	Route	Site	Ketones	Gluco-meter	Lab. Value		Comments	Initial

Initial	Signature & Title	Initial	Signature & Title	Initial	Signature & Title

F I G U R E 2 1 – 2 4

Sample diabetic record.

GLUCOMETER CLINICAL COMPETENCY

NAME:_____ UNIT:_____

DATE: _____ EMPLOYEE NUMBER:_____

PERFORMANCE CRITERIA	COMPETENCY DEMONSTRATED
1. Performer washes hands and patient's extremity using medical aseptic technique.	
2. Correctly assembles the equipment required for a blood glucose check.	
3. Correctly demonstrates calibration of the glucometer.	
4. Correctly matches the code number on display in the machine with the code number on the reagent strips.	
5. Correctly demonstrates quality control of the glucometer using the low, normal, and high glucose control solutions.	
6. Correctly verbalizes the sequence of steps involved in performing a blood glucose check.	
7. Correctly performs capillary puncture.	
8. Correctly disposes of sharps and biohazard materials.	
9. Correctly states the procedure for cleaning the glucometer.	
10. Correctly demonstrates the removal and replacement of the battery.	
11. Correctly documents the daily maintenance of glucometer.	
12. Correctly documents and reports test results.	

CODE: S = Satisfactory   U = Unsatisfactory

Validated by:_____ **RN   DATE:**_____

FIGURE 21-25

Glucometer clinical competency checklist.

- Quality control testing and meter maintenance should be performed daily according to your institution's policies.
- Know your institution's critical values for glucose levels.
- Document glucometer results and report abnormal results to the RN.

MISCELLANEOUS SPECIMEN TESTING

In this section, tests and specimen collection of stool and urine are described. Elimination of waste products from the body is a natural process. Waste products, called stool, feces, or excrement, are passed through the rectum. This process may also be referred to as a *bowel movement* or *defecation*. Elimination schedules vary from individual to individual so that "normal" may mean a daily bowel movement, but equally "normal" may be every few days for others. Stools are described by color, consistency, odor, amount, and shape.

Stool Specimens

Some stool specimens are sent to the laboratory for diagnostic testing.

1. Supplies
   - Bedpan or commode
   - Laboratory requisition or label
   - Wooden applicators
   - Specimen container
   - Gloves

2. Patient preparation
   - Verify the order.
   - Identify the patient.
   - Explain the procedure.
   - Instruct the patient to notify you when he or she is able to have a bowel movement.
   - Instruct the patient not to void in the stool specimen.
   - Instruct the patient not to put toilet tissue in the stool specimen.
   - Provide privacy.

3. Infection control/Universal precautions
   - Wash your hands, using medical aseptic technique, before and after the procedure. Document the test results on the patient's record.
   - Always wear latex or vinyl gloves when handling stool specimens.
   - Keep the outside of the specimen container clean and free from contamination from the specimen.

4. Quality control
   - The specimen may need to be refrigerated or taken to the laboratory immediately, depending on the type of test ordered. Using the 3-bottle collec-

tion system stabilizes the stool with various additives. In this case, the specimen can be maintained at room temperature. It should be taken to the laboratory within an hour. The patient should void prior to collection of the stool specimen.
- The specimen should be collected in a clean bedpan or specipan collector used in the commode.

Procedure

1. Wash hands and put on gloves.
2. Transfer the specimen into a specimen container using wooden applicators; 1–2 tablespoons of stool is sufficient. Often a prepared set of 3 containers is used, each with its own fixative or reagent inside. Fill all 3 containers with stool to the fill line indicated. Make sure lids are on tightly.
3. Label the specimen with the patient's name, date, and time of collection.
4. Place the specimen container in a clean, impervious plastic bag for delivery to the laboratory or place in designated area for laboratory pickup. Attach requisition form.
5. Document on the patient's record the time the specimen was collected and sent to the laboratory.
6. The bedpan should be cleaned and the applicators wrapped in a paper towel and discarded. Follow your institution's policy and procedure for medical waste.

Consult the requisition slip, laboratory guide, or the RN about method of storage of the specimen or if immediate delivery to the laboratory is required.

Test for Fecal Occult Blood

Stool specimens may also be tested for occult blood at the bedside or point of care. Occult blood, or blood that is not visible in the specimen, may be identified by performing a simple test on the specimen. A cardboard slide with guaiac paper and a developer composed of hydrogen peroxide and alcohol are used. Collect the specimen as described above.

1. Supplies
   - Slide
   - Wooden applicator
   - Developing solution

- Bedpan or specimen container
- Gloves

2. Patient preparation
   - Verify order.
   - Identify the patient.
   - Explain the procedure.
   - Instruct the patient to notify you when he or she is able to have a bowel movement.
   - Instruct the patient not to void in the stool specimen.
   - Provide privacy.

3. Infection control/Universal precautions
   - Wash your hands using medical aseptic technique before and after the procedure.
   - Always wear latex or vinyl gloves when handling stool specimens.

4. Quality control
   - Check the expiration date on the slide and developer.
   - Slides and developers should not be exposed to extreme temperatures. Store at 59–86°F.
   - Protect developer from light and keep tightly capped.
   - Use caution with the developer to prevent contact with eyes or skin.
   - Specimen should be collected in a clean bedpan or specimen container.

5. Testing
   - Open front flap of slide.
   - Using the applicator, apply a thin smear of the stool specimen to one of the boxes on the slide.
   - Using a clean area on the applicator, obtain a second sample from another part of the specimen and apply a thin smear to the other box on the slide. Close the slide.
   - Open flap on the back of the slide. Apply 2 drops of the developer over each box on the slide containing the smear.
   - Read results in 30–60 seconds, depending on the manufacturer's directions. Any trace of blue on either box indicates a positive result or that occult blood may be present.
   - After the results have been read, the reliability of the slide should be demonstrated. The reliability of the slide and developer is tested by applying a drop of developing solution on the mid-lower section of the slide on the performance control area. Correct performance of the slide and developer is indicated by the appearance of blue in 10–30 seconds. See manufacturer's directions for exact time.
   - Make patient comfortable and dispose of equipment following your institution's policy for medical waste.

- Wash hands.
- Record bowel movement on I&O record. Record results of guaiac testing. Report test results to the RN.

A more simplified testing procedure is available also. This involves placing a small amount of stool on special occult-blood–testing paper, turning the paper over, and placing 2 drops of reagent solution on the paper in back of the stool. If a blue ring forms, the test is positive and must be documented and reported. The test you use will be dependent upon the materials used at your agency (Fig. 21–26).

Gastric Specimens

The same type of testing for occult blood is performed on stomach contents. The sample may be from nasogastric tube drainage or vomitus. A sample of the drainage, which looks red or brown or black, is placed on the occult-blood–testing cards or paper as indicated in stool testing. The procedure is the same.

 If the patient has eaten red meat within 3 days of the test, the test may give a false positive.

Urine Specimens

Fluid wastes passed through the urethra are called urine. This process may be referred to as *voiding, urination,* or *micturition.* It is often necessary to measure urinary output and to describe the color of the urine. Urine specimens may be sent to the laboratory for diagnostic testing. Sometimes, clean-voided midstream specimens are required.

Clean-Voided Midstream Urine Specimens

Following is the procedure for dependent patients:

1. Supplies
   - Bedpan or urinal
   - Laboratory requisition or label
   - Clean/sterile urine specimen container
   - Cotton balls, gauze, or towelettes and antiseptic solution (These may also come prepared in a disposable kit.)
   - Gloves

2. Patient preparation
   - Verify the order.
   - Identify the patient.
   - Explain procedure.
   - Instruct patient to notify you when able to void.
   - Provide privacy.

3. Infection control/Universal precautions
   - Wash your hands using medical aseptic technique before and after the procedure.

```
┌─────────────────────────────────────────────────────────────────────┐
│           TEST FOR FECAL OCCULT BLOOD COMPETENCY CHECKLIST            │
│                                                                       │
│   NAME:_____      UNIT:_____   │
│                                                                       │
│   DATE: _____      EMPLOYEE  NUMBER: _____   │
└─────────────────────────────────────────────────────────────────────┘
```

PERFORMANCE CRITERIA	COMPETENCY DEMONSTRATED
1. Collect supplies Slide Wooden applicator Developing solution Bed pan or specimen container Gloves	
2. Identify patient and explain procedure for specimen collection	
3. Wash hands and use gloves	
4. Check expiration date of slide	
5. Apply specimen to slide	
6. Use developing solution on specimen and quality indicator and read results correctly	
7. Document results	
8. Dispose of supplies/equipment using medical waste requirements	

CODE: S = Satisfactory   U = Unsatisfactory

Validated by:_____   **RN   DATE:** _____

FIGURE 21–26

Test for fecal occult blood competency checklist.

- Use latex or vinyl gloves during the procedure and when handling urine specimens.
- Keep outside of container clean and free from contamination from the specimen. Apply lid to the container tightly.

4. Quality control
   - Urine specimens are usually refrigerated while waiting for laboratory pickup, or taken to the laboratory immediately, depending on the type of test ordered.

Procedure

1. Female patients
   - Place patient on bedpan.

- If patient has a discharge, wash the perineal area with soap and water.
- Separate folds of the labia.
- Clean with cotton balls, gauze squares, or towelette moistened with the antiseptic solution. Discard wipe after each cleansing swipe to prevent cross-contamination of the area.
- Wipe each fold of the labia, alongside of the meatus.
- Wipe meatus.
- Always use a downward direction.

2. Male patients
   - Retract foreskin on the penis if patient is not circumcised.
   - Using the cotton balls, gauze, or towelettes moistened with the antiseptic solution, cleanse the area around the meatus and then the meatus, using

a circular motion. Discard each cotton ball after each wipe.

3. All patients
    *   Instruct patient to begin voiding (bedpan or urinal).
    *   After patient has voided about 30 ml and when the stream has gained force, collect urine in the clean/ sterile specimen container.
    *   Close the container. Avoid touching the inside of the container. Apply lid tightly.
    *   Label the specimen with the patient's name, date, and time of collection.
    *   Send to the laboratory with the requisition identifying this as a clean-voided midstream urine specimen.
    *   Place the specimen container in a clean, plastic biohazard bag and attach requisition. Place for delivery to the laboratory or refrigerate prior to laboratory pickup.
    *   Document on the patient's record the time the specimen was collected and sent to the laboratory.
    *   Clean and store or dispose of equipment. Follow your institution's policy and procedure for medical waste.

4. Independent patients
    *   Instruct the patient how to obtain own specimen.
    *   Include information about how to handle the specimen container.
    *   Patient should wash hands before and after procedure.
    *   Follow above steps to give patient sufficient information.
    *   Document on the patient's record as above.

 Consult RN to determine patient's ability to perform procedure independently.

Catheter Specimens

Sterile urine specimens may be collected via a straight catheter or from a Foley catheter. The RN usually is responsible for collecting these specimens.

A specimen for culture and sensitivity gathered in a culture tube requires only 10 ml of urine.

Routine Urinalysis

Routine urine specimens may be ordered that do not require the sterile technique of a midstream specimen. To collect a routine urine specimen, approximately 30 ml of voided urine is poured into the collection container

designated by the agency. The specimen is labeled and handled the same as other specimens.

24-Hour Urine Collection

Often physicians will order urine to be collected over a 24-hour period. This is not a sterile procedure. A general routine for a 24-hour urine collection involves:

1. Inform the patient of the test. Instruct the patient, if he or she is able to be up to void, to always void into the specimen pan provided in the commode and to save all urine. The patient should not have a bowel movement in the pan with the urine.

2. Post signs at the door to the patient's bathroom to save all urine. Empty all urinals and bedpans into the collection bottles.

3. Prepare the collection bottles. Some tests require use of a stabilizing agent to keep the urine from changing until the test is done. Two common agents are boric acid tablets (2 per 2-liter bottle) and an HCl solution. If used, these are to be added to the bottles prior to collection. Call your agency laboratory to learn if preservatives are to be used. If preservatives are not used, all urine must be kept refrigerated or on ice throughout the 24-hour collection period.

4. Fill a washbasin with ice and place next to the commode. Keep urine collection container packed in ice during entire collection period. Change ice as needed.

5. Use container designated by agency. Label with patient information. Identify as bottle #1, and identify start date and time. Usual start time is 7 AM, and urine is collected through 7 AM the next day. The first voided specimen in the morning of the first day is discarded. That urine has been collecting in the bladder prior to the start of the 24-hour period. Save *all* urine after that.

6. If a new bottle is needed, label it with patient information, and as bottle #2.

7. The next morning, or end of the 24-hour period, *do save* the first void in the AM, since that urine has been collecting during the time identified.

8. Send all bottles to the laboratory with the requisition fastened to one of them with a rubberband. Mark on the requisition the number of bottles sent, and the start and end date and time. Document this information also on the patient chart and on the unit specimen log.

Urine Testing Using Reagent Strips (Fig. 21–27)

Urine may be tested at the bedside or point of care by using reagent strips. In this way, one can quickly test the urine for variety of contents, including pH levels and presence of ketones or blood. While tests for glucose can also be done using reagent strips, this method has, for the most part, been replaced with the more accurate

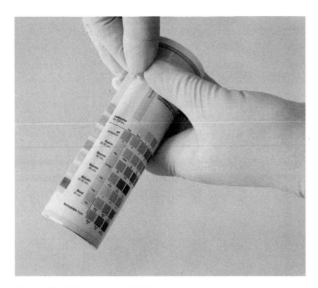

FIGURE 21-27
Reagent strip testing.

procedure of blood glucose testing described in the section Blood Glucose Monitoring. A reagent strip is a firm plastic strip with pads of substances that will produce a chemical reaction. Reagent strips may have multiple pads for a variety of tests or may have only one pad. When using reagent strips, always follow the manufacturer's directions and pay particular attention to the time frame for reading the results.

1. Supplies
   • Bedpan, urinal, or specimen container
   • Appropriate reagent strip
   • Gloves

2. Patient preparation
   • Verify test order and type of test to be performed (ketones, blood, pH)
   • Identify the patient.
   • Explain the procedure to the patient.
   • Instruct the patient to notify you when able to void.
   • Provide privacy.

3. Infection control/Universal precautions
   • Wash your hands using medical aseptic technique before and after the procedure.
   • Always wear latex or vinyl gloves when handling urine specimens.

4. Quality control
   • Urine specimen should be fresh and tested within 1 hour of collection. Usually the first voided specimen in the morning should not be tested since it has been collecting all night. This may make the readings less accurate.
   • Check the expiration date on the reagent strip container.

• Reagent strips should not be exposed to extreme temperatures. Store at room temperature no greater than 85°F. Do not freeze.
• Protect reagent strips from light and keep container tightly capped.
• Do not remove small packets of desiccants (granules that absorb moisture) placed in bottle in order to keep the reagent strips dry.
• Hold the reagent strip on the top edge; do not touch the portion with the reagent pads.
• Reading the results at the specified time is critical.
• Keep the reagent strips in their original bottle.
• The laboratory may test a reagent strip against a known specimen each time a new bottle is opened to confirm the reliability of the strips.

Procedures

1. Wash hands and put on gloves.
2. Collect fresh urine specimen in a clean, dry container.
3. Remove reagent strip from bottle and immediately replace bottle cover securely.
4. Immerse reagent strip in urine completely but briefly.
5. Remove immediately tapping strip or sliding across edge of container to remove excess urine.
6. Hold strip in a horizontal position to prevent dripping of urine onto your hands and also to prevent mixing of reagents.
7. Compare reagents to color code on bottle at time specified for individual reagents.
8. Strip should be held close to the color chart but not touching it, to avoid soiling of the chart and bottle.
9. Clean equipment and discard reagent strip. Follow your institution's policy and procedure for medical waste.
10. Wash hands.
11. Document the test results on the patient's record. Report results to the RN (Fig. 21–28).

Key Points

• Always use universal precautions when working with stool or urine specimens.
• Keep outside of specimen containers free from contami-

URINE TESTING USING REAGENT STRIPS COMPETENCY CHECKLIST

NAME:_____   UNIT:_____

DATE: _____   EMPLOYEE NUMBER: _____

PERFORMANCE CRITERIA	COMPETENCY DEMONSTRATED
1. Collect supplies Bed pan or specimen container Reagent strips Gloves	
2. Identify patient/explain procedure for specimen collection	
3. Wash hands and don gloves	
4. Check expiration date of reagent strip	
5. Dip strip and read results correctly	
6. Document results	
7. Dispose of supplies/equipment using medical waste requirements	

CODE: S = Satisfactory   U = Unsatisfactory

Validated by:_____ **RN   DATE:** _____

FIGURE 21–28
Urine testing reagent strip competency checklist.

nation with the specimen. Secure lids tightly before placing in biohazard bag and sending to laboratory.

• Record the date and time a specimen is collected.

• Store specimens properly.

• Check expiration dates of testing supplies.

• Document test results and report results to the RN.

APPENDIX 1

Tri-Council for Nursing Statement on Assistive Personnel to the Registered Nurse

Nursing is an essential component of health care, and the consumer of health care needs to be assured of the availability, accessibility, and quality of nursing care. It is in the spirit of this responsibility that this statement related to the use of assistive personnel has been developed. Historically, unlicensed personnel have assisted registered nurses in the delivery of patient care. However, in recent years, with economic demands driving the delivery system, there have been increasing concerns about the role of assistive personnel. It is extremely important to use assistants in a manner that assures appropriate delegation or assignment of nursing functions and adequate direction and supervision of individuals to whom nursing activities are delegated.

Patient care is delivered today by a staff mix of Registered Nurses (RN), Licensed Practical/Vocational Nurses (LPN), and unlicensed personnel in assistive roles. The term "assistive personnel" is used to recognize the trained/unlicensed health care worker who is employed with the continuum of acute hospital care to home health, ambulatory and long term care. Two categories of assistive personnel are generally recognized: the patient care assistant to whom the RN delegates or assigns aspects of nursing care and who functions under the supervision of the Registered Nurse, and the unit assistant who supports the nursing care system through a variety of non-nursing activities.

Many clinical settings are revising the staff mix needed for the delivery of patient care because of changing patient needs, the economics of reimbursement, and demand driven shortages of nursing personnel. A variety of manpower models are being explored and refined as the industry strives to balance quality and cost issues. The ultimate aim is to reallocate nursing and non-nursing activities to enable the registered nurse to focus on the patient. Specific models are best crafted at the point of delivery of care.

The nursing profession is accountable for the quality of the service it provides to the consumer. This includes the responsibility for developing nursing policies and procedures and setting the standards of practice for the nursing care of populations being served. It is further incumbent on the nursing profession to define the appropriate educational preparation and role of any group providing services within the scope of nursing practice. The State Board of Nursing is responsible for the legal regulation of nursing practice for the RN and LPN and should be responsible for the regulation of any other category of personnel who assists in the provision of direct nursing care. Professional and statutory provisions require that when the RN delegates and assigns direct nursing care activities to LPNs and assistive personnel, appropriate reporting relations are established and the RN supervises all personnel to whom these activities have been delegated. In all situations, registered nurses and licensed practical nurses are responsible and accountable for their respective individual nursing activities. These relationships should be made explicit in workplace policies.

(Registered Professional Nurses and Unlicensed Assistive Personnel, Appendix, p. 45. American Nurses Association, Washington, DC, 1994.)

American Association of Colleges of Nursing
One DuPont Circle, Suite 530
Washington, DC 20036
202–466–6930
FAX 202–785–8320

American Nurses Association, Inc.
600 Maryland Avenue, SW
Suite 100 West
Washington, DC 20024-2571
202–651–7000
FAX 202–651–7001

American Organization of Nurse Executives
840 North Lake Shore Drive
Chicago, Illinois 60611
312–280–5213
FAX 312–280–5995

National League for Nursing
350 Hudson Street
New York, New York 10014
212–989–9393
FAX 212–898–3710

APPENDIX 2 _____

Common Abbreviations Used in Health Care

Hospital Services

Cardio, CVL, CV	Cardiovascular
D/S	Dental surgery
Derm	Dermatology
Endo	Endocrinology
EENT	Eye, ear, nose, throat
Fam Med, FM	Family medicine
Gen Med, GM	General medicine
GU	Genitourinary
Gyn	Gynecology
Heme	Hematology
Inf Dis, ID	Infectious disease
Neuro, Neu	Neurology
N/S	Neurosurgery
OB	Obstetrics
Onc	Oncology
Opath, Eye	Ophthalmology
Ortho, O/S	Orthopedics, orthopedic surgery
Peds	Pediatrics
P/S	Plastic surgery
Psych	Psychiatry
PVS	Peripheral vascular surgery
Ren	Renal
Surg	Surgery
T/S	Thoracic surgery

Related to Census

Adm	Admission
AMA	Against medical advice
D/C	Discharge
DOS	Day of surgery patient
Exp	Expiration
I/P	Inpatient
LOA	Leave of absence
Obv	Observation patient
O/P	Outpatient
POD	Postoperative day
T	Transfer

Related to Hospital Employees

CHUC	Certified health unit coordinator (also known as Administrative associate with patient-focused care)

CNA	Certified nursing assistant
DO	Doctor of Osteopathy
HA	Hospital aide
HO	House officer (Resident, Intern)
LPN	Licensed practical nurse
MD	Doctor of Medicine
MSW	Master of Social Work; Medical Social Worker
PCA	Patient care assistant or associate
PCT	Patient care technician
RD	Registered dietician
RN	Registered Nurse
RPh	Registered Pharmacist
RPT	Registered Physical Therapist
RRT	Registered Respiratory Therapist
SNA	Student nursing assistant

Related to Hospital Departments

ASU	Ambulatory surgery unit
BICU	Burn intensive care unit
CCU/CICU	Coronary care unit/Coronary intensive care unit
CSS	Central sterile supply
ED, ER	Emergency department/Emergency room
ICU	Intensive care unit
L&D	Labor and delivery
MICU	Medical intensive care unit
MR	Medical records
NICU	Neonatal intensive care unit
OR	Operating room
OT	Occupational therapy
PACU	Postanesthesia care unit
PAS	Patient access services (registration)
PICU	Pediatric intensive care unit
PT	Physical therapy
RT	Respiratory therapy
SICU	Surgical intensive care unit
SPD	Supply processing and distribution

Related to Laboratory Tests

ABG	Arterial blood gas
bili	Bilirubin
BS	Blood sugar (also known as glucose)
BUN	Blood urea nitrogen
Ca	Calcium
CBC	Complete blood count
CCU	Clean catch urine
C/S, C&S	Culture and sensitivity
Chem 6	Chemistry battery (Na, K, Cl, CO_2, bun, creat)

chol	Cholesterol
Cl	Chloride
CO_2	Carbon dioxide
creat, cr	Creatinine
CSF	Cerebral spinal fluid
diff	Differential
ESR, Sed Rate	Erythrocyte sedimentation rate
ETOH	Alcohol (ethanol)
FBS	Fasting blood sugar
Fe	Iron
FFP	Fresh frozen plasma
Fib	Fibrinogen
glu	Glucose
hgb	Hemoglobin
hct	Hematocrit
H/H	Hemoglobin and hematocrit
K	Potassium
lytes, electrolytes	Chemistry battery (Na, K, Cl, CO_2)
Mg	Magnesium
Na	Sodium
O & P	Ova and parasite
Plt	Platelet
PRBC	Packed red blood cells
PT	Prothrombin time
PTT	Partial thromboplastin time
RBC	Red blood cell
T&C	Type and cross
T&S	Type and screen
TIBC	Total iron binding capacity
TP	Total protein
WBC	White blood count
U/A, UA	Urinalysis

Related to Time

ā	Before
ac	Before meals
am	Before noon
ASAP	As soon as possible
ATC	Around the clock
bid	Twice daily
c̄	With
D,d	Day
H,h,hr	Hour
hs	Hour of sleep (bedtime)
min	Minute
p̄	After
pc	After meals
pm	Afternoon
q	Every
qd	Every day
qh	Every hour
q_h	Every (number of) hours
qhs	Every bedtime
qid	Four times a day
qod	Every other day

s̄	Without
stat	At once, now
tid	Three times a day
x	Times
x̄	Except
wa	While awake
wk	Week

Related to Activity

ad lib	As desired
as tol	As tolerated
BR	Bedrest
BRP	Bathroom privileges
BSC	Bedside commode
ch	Chair
crt	Cart
HOB	Head of bed
NWB	No weightbearing
OOB	Out of bed
ROM	Range of motion
UAL	Up ad lib

Related to Temperature, Pulse, Blood Pressure, and Respiration

ap	Apical pulse
ax	Axillary
BP	Blood pressure (S = systolic, D = diastolic)
HR	Heart rate
irr	Irregular
NC	Nasal cannula
R, r	Rectal
T, temp	Temperature
TPR	Temperature, pulse, respiration
VS	Vital signs (temperature, pulse, blood pressure, respiration)

Related to History and Physical

c/o	Complains of
COC	Continuity of care
DNR	Do not resuscitate
dx	Diagnosis
F/U	Follow-up
H/O	History of
H&P	History and physical
hx	History
NKA	No known allergies
NKDA	No known drug allergies
R/O	Rule out
R/T	Related to
S/P	Status post

Related to Orders

MAR	Medication administration record
NO	Nursing order
TO	Telephone order
VO	Verbal order

Related to Tests/Procedures

AAS	Acute abdominal series
BaE	Barium enema
bx	Biopsy
CAT scan	Computerized axial tomography
CPR	Cardiopulmonary resuscitation
CS	Chemstick, Chemstrip
CT	Computed tomography
CVP	Central venous pressure
CXR	Chest X-ray
ECG/EKG	Electrocardiogram
EEG	Electroencephalogram
EGD	Esophagogastroduodenoscopy
I&O, I/O	Intake and output
KUB	Kidney, ureter, bladder
LWS	Low wall suction
MRI	Magnetic resonance imaging
NG	Nasogastric
PCXR	Portable chest X-ray
PFT	Pulmonary function test
post op	Postoperative
pre op	Preoperative
SBFT	Small bowel follow-through
SS	Soap suds (enema)
UGI	Upper gastrointestinal
UO	Urinary output

Related to Dietary

AAT	Advance as tolerated
ADA	American Diabetic Association
cal	Calorie
cal ct	Calorie count
Cl Liq	Clear liquid
FR	Full restriction
FS	Full Strength
NPO	Nothing by mouth
reg	Regular
TF	Tube feeding

Related to Quantities, Measurements, and Medications

AAOC	Antacid of choice
ASA	Aspirin
Fr	French (catheter gauge)
g, gm	Gram
gr	Grain
gtt	Drop
HW, hep well	Heparin well
IM	Intramuscular
IV	Intravenous
IVP	Intravenous push
IVPB	Intravenous piggyback
KCI	Potassium chloride
KVO	Keep vein open
L	Liter
LOC	Laxative of choice
LR	Lactated Ringer's
mcg	Microgram
mEq	Millequivalent
mg	Milligram
ml	Milliliter
NaCl	Sodium chloride
NS	Normal saline
PCA	Patient-controlled analgesia
PCN	Penicillin
PO	By mouth
PR	By rectum
Rx	Prescription
SL	Sublingual
SQ	Subcutaneous
supp	Suppository
TKO	To keep open
TPN	Total parenteral nutrition
u	Unit

Symbols

$>$	Greater than
$<$	Less than
#	Number, gauge, or pound
♂	Male
♀	Female
√	Check
°	Hour, degree
↑	Increase, raise, elevate
↓	Decrease, lower
△	Change

Page numbers in *italics* refer to illustrations; those ending in the letter t refer to charts.